# Scaling Biodiversity

We know that there are millions to tens of millions of plant and animal species, but we do not know enough to be able to describe the patterns and processes that characterize the distribution of species in space, time, and taxonomic groups. Given that in practical terms it is impossible to understand the intricacies of the relationships between all the organisms and the dynamics of populations and communities in all spatial and temporal scales, other approaches must be used. Scaling rules offer one possible framework, and this book offers a synthesis of the ways in which scaling theory can be applied to the analysis of biodiversity. *Scaling Biodiversity* presents new views on quantitative patterns of the biological diversity on Earth and the processes responsible for them. Written by a team of leading experts in ecology who present their most recent and innovative views, this book will provide readers with the state of the art in current ecology and biodiversity science.

DAVID STORCH is a researcher and university teacher at Charles University in Prague and former international Fellow of the Santa Fe Institute. He teaches courses on animal ecology, macroecology and community ecology.

PABLO A. MARQUET is a Professor at the Pontificia Universidad Católica de Chile, and a researcher at the Center for Advanced Studies in Ecology and Biodiversity and Instituto de Ecología y Biodiversidad, and former international Fellow of the Santa Fe Institute.

JAMES H. BROWN is a Distinguished Professor in the Department of Biology at the University of New Mexico.

**Ecological Reviews**

*Ecological Reviews* will publish books at the cutting edge of modern ecology, providing a forum for volumes that discuss topics that are focal points of current activity and likely long-term importance to the progress of the field. The series will be an invaluable source of ideas and inspiration for ecologists at all levels from graduate students to more-established researchers and professionals. The series will be developed jointly by the British Ecological Society and Cambridge University Press and will encompass the Society's Symposia as appropriate.

*Biotic Interactions in the Tropics: Their Role in the Maintenance of Species Diversity*
Edited by David F. R. P. Burslem, Michelle A. Pinard and Sue E. Hartley

*Biological Diversity and Function in Soils*
Edited by Richard Bardgett, Michael Usher and David Hopkins

*Island Colonization* by Ian Thornton
Edited by Tim New

# Scaling Biodiversity

Edited by

**DAVID STORCH**
*Charles University, Prague, and the Santa Fe Institute*

**PABLO A. MARQUET**
*Pontificia Universidad Católica de Chile, Santiago, and Center for Advanced Studies in Ecology and Biodiversity and Instituto de Ecología y Biodiversidad, the Santa Fe Institute*

**JAMES H. BROWN**
*University of New Mexico, Albuquerque, and the Santa Fe Institute*

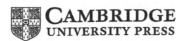
CAMBRIDGE
UNIVERSITY PRESS

CAMBRIDGE UNIVERSITY PRESS
Cambridge, New York, Melbourne, Madrid, Cape Town, Singapore, São Paulo, Delhi

Cambridge University Press
The Edinburgh Building, Cambridge CB2 8RU, UK

Published in the United States of America by Cambridge University Press, New York

www.cambridge.org
Information on this title: www.cambridge.org/9780521699372

First published 2007

*A catalogue record for this publication is available from the British Library*

ISBN 978-0-521-87602-5 hardback
ISBN 978-0-521-69937-2 paperback

Additional resources for this publication at www.cambridge.org/9780521699372

Transferred to digital printing 2009

# Contents

The color plates are situated between pp. 366 and 367*
*These plates are available for download in colour from
www.cambridge.org/9780521699372

# Contributors

SEBASTIAN R. ABADES
Center for Advanced Studies in Ecology
and Biodiversity (CASEB) and
Departamento de Ecología, Pontificia
Universidad Católica de Chile, Casilla
114-D, Santiago, Chile

ANDREW P. ALLEN
National Center for Ecological Analysis
and Synthesis, 735 State St., Suite 300,
Santa Barbara, CA 93101, USA

BRENDAN J. M. BOHANNAN
Center for Ecology and Evolutionary
Biology, University of Oregon, Eugene,
Oregon, OR 97403–5289, USA

LUÍS BORDA-DE-ÁGUA
Department of Plant Biology, University
of Georgia, Athens, GA 30602, USA

JAMES H. BROWN
Department of Biology, University of
New Mexico, Albuquerque, NM 87131,
USA, and The Santa Fe Institute,
1399 Hyde Park Road, Santa Fe,
NM 87501, USA

JÉRÔME CHAVE
Laboratoire Evolution et Diversité
Biologique, UMR5174 CNRS – Université

Paul Sabatier, 118 route de Narbonne,
31062 Toulouse, France

GUILLEM CHUST
Laboratoire Evolution et Diversité
Biologique, UMR5174 CNRS – Université
Paul Sabatier, 118 route de Narbonne,
31062 Toulouse, France

ANDREW CLARKE
Biological Sciences, British Antarctic
Survey, NERC, High Cross, Madingley Road,
Cambridge CB3 0ET, UK

RICK CONDIT
Center for Tropical Forest Science,
Smithsonian Tropical Research Institute,
Unit 0948, APO AA, 34002–0948, USA

DAVID J. CURRIE
Ottawa-Carleton Institute for Biology,
University of Ottawa, Box 450, Station A,
Ottawa, Ontario, Canada K1N 6N5

ANTHONY F. G. DIXON
School of Biological Sciences, University
of East Anglia, Norwich NR4 7TJ, UK

KARL L. EVANS
Biodiversity and Macroecology Group,
Department of Animal and Plant Sciences,

University of Sheffield, Sheffield S10
2TN, UK

KEVIN J. GASTON
Biodiversity and Macroecology Group,
Department of Animal and Plant Sciences,
University of Sheffield, Sheffield S10
2TN, UK

MURRAY GELL-MANN
The Santa Fe Institute, 1399 Hyde Park
Road, Santa Fe, NM 87501, USA

JAMIE F. GILLOOLY
Department of Zoology, University of
Florida, Gainesville, FL 32611, USA

JESSICA GREEN
School of Natural Sciences, University of
California, P.O. Box 2039, Merced, CA
95344, USA

JOHN HARTE
Energy and Resources Group and
Ecosystem Sciences Division, College of
Natural Resources, University of California,
Berkeley, CA 94720, USA

STEPHEN HARTLEY
School of Biological Sciences, Victoria
University of Wellington, P.O.B. 600,
Wellington, New Zealand

FANGLIANG HE
Department of Renewable Resources,
University of Alberta, Edmonton, Alberta,
Canada T6G 2E1

TOMÁŠ HERBEN
Department of Botany, Faculty of Science,
Charles University, Benátská 2, CZ-128 01
Praha 2, Czech Republic, and Institute of
Botany, Academy of Sciences of the Czech
Republic, CZ-252 43 Průhonice, Czech
Republic

STEPHEN P. HUBBELL
Department of Plant Biology, University of
Georgia, Athens, GA 30602, USA, and
Smithsonian Tropical Research Institute,
Unit 0948, APO AA 34002–0948, USA

TIMOTHY H. KEITT
Section of Integrative Biology, University of
Texas at Austin, Austin, TX 78712, USA

PAVEL KINDLMANN
Institute of Systems Biology and Ecology,
Academy of Sciences of the Czech Republic,
and Faculty of Biological Sciences,
University of South Bohemia, Branigovska
31, 370 05, Czech Republic, and Agrocampus
Rennes, UMR INRA/ENSA-R Bi03P, 65 rue
de Saint-Brieuc, 35042 Rennes Cedex,
France

WILLIAM E. KUNIN
Earth and Biosphere Institute, School of
Biology, University of Leeds,
Leeds LS2 9JT, UK

FABIO A. LABRA
Center for Advanced Studies in Ecology and
Biodiversity (CASEB) and Instituto de
Ecología y Biodiversidad (IEB) and Departa-
mento de Ecología, Pontificia Universidad
Católica de Chile, Casilla 114-D,
Santiago, Chile

JACK J. LENNON
The Macaulay Institute, Craigiebuckler,
Aberdeeen AB15 8QH, UK

PABLO A. MARQUET
Center for Advanced Studies in Ecology and
Biodiversity (CASEB) and Departamento de
Ecología Pontificia Universidad Católica de
Chile, Casilla 114-D, Santiago, Chile, and
Instituto de Ecología y Biodiversidad (IEB),
Facultad de Ciencias, Universidad de Chile,
Casilla 653, Santiago, Chile, and The Santa
Fe Institute, 1399 Hyde Park Road, Santa Fe,
NM 87501, USA

GÉZA MESZÉNA
Department of Biological Physics, Loránd
Eötvös University, Pázmány Péter stny. 1/C,
H-1117, Budapest, Hungary

BEÁTA OBORNY
Department of Plant Taxonomy and
Ecology, Loránd Eötvös University, Pázmány
Péter stny. 1/C, H-1117, Budapest, Hungary

MICHAEL W. PALMER
Botany Department, Oklahoma State
University, Stillwater, OK 74078, USA

IVA SCHÖDELBAUEROVÁ
Institute of Systems Biology and Ecology,
Academy of Sciences of the Czech Republic
and Faculty of Biological Sciences,
University of South Bohemia, Branigovska
31, 370 05, Czech Republic

ARNOŠT L. ŠIZLING
Center for Theoretical Study, Charles
University, Jilská 1, 110 00-CZ Praha 1,
Czech Republic

DAVID STORCH
Center for Theoretical Study, Charles
University, Jilská 1, 110 00-CZ Praha 1,
Czech Republic, and Department of
Ecology, Faculty of Science, Charles
University, Viničná 2, 128 44-CZ Praha 2,
Czech Republic, and The Santa Fe Institute,
1399 Hyde Park Road, Santa Fe, NM 87501,
USA

GYÖRGY SZABÓ
Research Institute for Technical Physics
and Materials Science, P.O. Box 49, H-1525,
Budapest, Hungary

CHRISTOPHE THÉBAUD
Laboratoire Evolution et Diversité
Biologique, UMR5174 CNRS – Université
Paul Sabatier, 118 route de Narbonne, 31062
Toulouse, France

GEOFFREY B. WEST
The Santa Fe Institute, 1399 Hyde Park
Road, Santa Fe, NM 87501, USA

ETHAN P. WHITE
Department of Biology, Utah State
University, Logan, UT 84322, USA, and
Department of Ecology and Evolutionary
Biology, University of Arizona, Tucson, AZ
85721, USA, and Department of Biology,
University of New Mexico, Albuquerque,
NM 87131, USA

# Foreword

ROBERT M. MAY

*(Lord May of Oxford)*

*University of Oxford*

One of the appealing things about physics is the existence of invariance principles and conservation laws, which provide the basis for powerful simplicities
and generalizations (if the laws of physics are the same at all times and places
then, for example, momentum is conserved). Extending this, if we are presented
with a set of equations describing how a physical system behaves – the
Navier–Stokes equations describing fluid flow, for instance – then we can
immediately set about recasting them in terms of appropriately dimensionless
variables (coordinates of space and time rescaled against the system's characteristic lengths and time) and dimensionless combinations of other parameters
(the Reynold's Number, which is essentially the ratio between inertial and
viscous forces, for example). Such scaling laws then allow us to construct a
small model of a racing yacht, or Formula I car, or airplane, and test its fluid
dynamical behavior in an appropriately constructed testing tank or wind tun-
nel. On the back of an envelope, we can explain why the V-shaped waves break
away from the bow of a ship in deep water at an angle of $\theta = 19.5°$ ($\tan \theta = 1/2\sqrt{2}$),
independent of the ship's speed, a result first established by Kelvin in 1887.

A particularly notable example of the use of dimensional arguments was
given in the 1950s by G. I. Taylor, the leading fluid dynamicist involved in the
Manhattan Project at Los Alamos (an appropriate example in the context of this
book, perhaps, given the geographical proximity to Santa Fe). In an atomic
explosion, there is an essentially instantaneous release of a large amount of
energy, $E$, from what is effectively a point source. The subsequent spherical
shock wave propagates into the surrounding air, of density $\rho$, with the pressure
behind the early-stage wave front being vastly larger than the air pressure. It
follows that the only physical factors determining the radius of the spherical
shock wave front, $R$, are $E$, $\rho$, and the elapsed time, $t$. In terms of the basic scaling
dimensions of mass, length and time (M, L, T), these three independent variables
have dimensions $[E] = ML^2T^{-2}$, $[\rho] = ML^{-3}$, $[t] = T$; $R$ has dimensions $[R] = L$. To get
the scaling relation between $R$ (dimension L) and $t$ (dimension T), we eliminate
M among $[E]$, $[\rho]$ and $[t]$ to get $L^5 \sim T^2$. This implies $R \sim t^{2/5}$ or a straight line with
slope 1 when $\ln R$ is plotted against $(2/5) \ln t$. Taylor used the data from a series of

high-speed photographs of the fireball expanding over the test site in Nevada to verify this result, and then further used the $y$-axis intercept of this line to estimate $E \sim 10^{21}$ erg. He published this simple and elegant analysis in 1950, causing a furore among the military bureaucracy; although the film was not classified, the energy release figure was Top Secret (for a more detailed account, see Barenblatt, 1996).

These ideas have made their way into several areas of biology, mainly at the level of the physiology and behavior of individual organisms. D'Arcy Thompson's *On Growth and Form in Biology* (see particularly Bonner's 1961 abridged addition, with commentary) is one notable early example. Further developments and applications are surveyed by Berg (1983), Vogel (1988) and others. The first sentence in Berg's book begins "Biology in wet and dynamic". His book elaborates this theme, brilliantly drawing out the distinction between those organisms whose physical dimensions in relation to the medium through which they move are such that inertial forces dominate (e.g. airplanes, or us walking down the street) and those where the medium's viscosity dominates (e.g. bacteria propelled by rotating flagella). Here the scaling questions involve the above-mentioned dimensionless Reynold's Number, $\mathrm{Re} \sim \rho v L / \mu$, where $\rho$, $v$ and $\mu$ are the density, relative velocity, and viscosity of the fluid, and $L$ is the "characteristic length" (diameter of pipe or channel for internal flows; maximum length of a solid object – submarine or bacterium – moving with relative velocity $v$ against the fluid). More broadly, it is fascinating to see how scaling laws can illuminate biological issues as varied as how prairie dogs ventilate their burrows, how tiny worms withstand high pressures, or why a mouse walks away when it falls down a mineshaft but we break and horses go splat.

Going beyond Berg's "Wet and dynamic", I particularly like the application of these ideas first made in 1680 by Giovanni Alfonso Borelli, and later independently presented by John Maynard Smith (1968), to show that, to a good approximation, the characteristic height to which an animal can jump (i.e. lift its center of gravity) is common to all, fleas to horses (around one meter). This result, sometimes called Borelli's Law, is derived as follows. The energy needed to lift an animal of mass $m$ (which scales as $L^3$, where L is the animal's characteristic length scale) to a height $h$ is $mgh$, where $g$ is the acceleration due to gravity. This energy is provided by the animal's downward force on the ground, $F$, multiplied by the distance through which the force moves (the leg extension giving the uplift, which is of the order of L). The force $F$ is limited by the mechanical strength of the limb, which scales as $L^2$. Hence we have $h = FL / mg \sim L^2 \times L / L^3$. That is, $h$ is, to a rough approximation, independent of the animal's characteristic size. Obviously there are fluctuations around this characteristic height, set by particular adaptations to the animal's life history, but even so the rule holds remarkably well across the animal kingdom. This and other examples are to be found in Maynard Smith's wonderful little book on *Mathematical Ideas in Biology* (1968), whose cover is a schematic diagram illustrating the above calculation for a jumping mouse; the Russian edition has replaced this schematic diagram with a socialist-realist mouse!

The dynamics of the spread of an infectious disease within a host population also can, in simple limiting circumstances, be illuminated by dimensional analysis and scaling laws. Suppose we have an infection which is transmitted directly by contact between susceptibles (S) and infected/infectious (I) individuals, in a homogeneously mixed population. Individuals recover (R) from the infected/infectious phase after a characteristic interval D, thereafter being immune. If a few infected individuals are put into a wholly susceptible population, the resulting equations for this so-called SIR system can be put in dimensionless form, and the shape of the consequent epidemic curve is seen to have a form that depends only on the single dimensionless parameter, $R_0$, which measures the average number of secondary infections produced by an infected/infectious individual in the initial stages, when essentially everyone is susceptible. The total number ever infected as the epidemic sweeps through the population, $I$, is given by $I = 1 - \exp(-R_0 I)$; the fraction of the population who are infected/infectious at the peak of the epidemic is simply $y_M = 1 - (1 + \ln R_0)/R_0$ (Anderson & May, 1991, ch. 6). This dimensionless quantity $R_0$ is called the basic reproductive number, and it can among other things be used to assess the proportion of the population we need to vaccinate in order to protect against a possible epidemic (i.e. to drive the population's effective basic reproductive number below unity); this fraction is $1 - 1/R_0$. Although the shape of the epidemic curve depends only on $R_0$ in this simple limiting case, the timescale over which an epidemic unfolds – possibly eventually extinguishing itself, or possibly oscillating to settle at a state of endemic infection – involves other parameters (such as D and the rate at which new susceptibles enter the population by birth or migration). Interestingly, ecologists have long recognized the importance of what they call a population's "basic reproductive rate", $R_0$. When Roy Anderson and I first emphasized the central role played by $R_0$ in epidemiological theory, we underlined the basic relationship with ecologists by using their conventional terminology – "reproductive rate" – even though we recognized that $R_0$ was dimensionless, not having the dimension of 1/(time) which "rate" would strictly imply. Later epidemiological workers, incensed by such terminological inexactitude, have prevailed in establishing "basic reproductive number" as approved usage; ecological texts, however, remain unrepentant in their time-honored use of "reproductive rate".

More generally, of course, computationally sophisticated studies aimed at better understanding of HIV/AIDS, foot and mouth disease, SARS, avian H5N1 flu, and much else deal with heterogeneities in individual behavior and transmissibility, in guiding public health policy. The basic understanding provided by scaling relations, however, remains important (Keeling *et al.*, 2003; Keeling, 2005).

Efforts to apply such scaling considerations to observed patterns of biological diversity are, in general, more recent. The present volume, very much in the spirit of the Santa Fe Institute, outlines work on several different levels, beginning with the relation between spatial scale and numbers of species. Later chapters in this rich offering widen the scope to scaling relations involving taxonomic groupings, species–energy relations, latitudinal gradients in species numbers, and more. Some of the work closely parallels the physics-like scaling rules sketched above, while other chapters take a broader view of "power laws" and possible mechanisms causing them.

In my opinion, the complex and contingent workings of evolutionary processes, playing out in an ecological theater which itself undergoes environmental change, mean that we cannot generally expect to find the crisp scaling laws of physics in assemblies of species. But we can sometimes hope to come close, and – at very least – this book shows the quest itself is interesting and informative.

## References

Anderson, R. M. & May, R. M. (1991). *Infectious Diseases of Humans: Dynamics and Control.* Oxford: Oxford University Press.

Barenblatt, G. I. (1996). *Scaling, Self-Similarity, and Intermediate Asymptotics.* Cambridge Texts in Applied Mathematics 14. Cambridge: Cambridge University Press.

Berg, N. C. (1983). *Random Walks in Biology.* Princeton: Princeton University Press.

Bonner, J. T. (ed.) (1961). Abridged edition of D'Arcy Thompson's *On Growth and Form.* Cambridge: Cambridge University Press.

Keeling, M. J. (2005). Models of foot and mouth disease. *Proceedings of the Royal Society of London, Series B,* **272,** 1195–1202.

Keeling, M. J., Woolhouse, M. E. J., May, R. M., Davies, G. & Grenfell, B. T. (2003). Modelling vaccination strategies against foot-and-mouth disease. *Nature,* **412,** 136–142.

Maynard Smith, J. (1968). *Mathematical Ideas in Biology.* Cambridge: Cambridge University Press.

Vogel, S. (1988). *Life's Devices: The Physical World of Animal and Plants.* Princeton: Princeton University Press.

# Preface

This unusual book had an unusual origin. It resulted from a symposium entitled "Scaling Biodiversity" that took place in Prague, Czech Republic, on 19–22 October 2004. The goal of the symposium was to bring together a diverse group of scientists who are applying ideas, approaches, and methods of scaling to address major conceptual questions about biodiversity.

The symposium was cosponsored by the Santa Fe Institute and Center for Theoretical Study, Charles University in Prague and co-organized by David Storch of Charles University, Pablo Marquet of the Catholic University in Chile, James Brown of the University of New Mexico, and Geoffrey West of the Santa Fe Institute. This sponsorship and organizing committee says much about the origin and operation of the workshop, the identity of the invited contributors, and the contents of this book. All of the co-organizers and many of the participants have strong relationships with the Santa Fe Institute (SFI). Much of the funding for the symposium, the activities of the co-organizers that led up to it, and the preparation of this book came from the SFI International Programs. Founded in 1984, the Institute is an interdisciplinary research center in Santa Fe, New Mexico. It is widely regarded as the birthplace and leading center of modern "complexity science". It is a special place that attracts mathematicians and physicists, biologists and ecologists, economists and anthropologists, who are dedicated to working on big, challenging questions in the natural and social sciences. There is a heady atmosphere of intense interaction and collegial collaboration at the Institute, and it results in a special kind of SFI-style science.

The symposium and the resulting book are representative of this kind of science. The participating scientists represent a blend of card-carrying ecologists and interlopers from other disciplines, established scientists and new, young investigators, theoreticians and empiricists. Several of the participants have been affiliated with SFI. Geoffrey West and Murray Gell-Mann are members of the Resident Faculty, James Brown is a member of the External Faculty, David Storch, Pablo Marquet, and Beáta Oborny have been International Fellows, and Timothy Keitt, James Gillooly, Andrew Allen, John Harte, Andrew Clarke, Jessica Green, and Ethan White have all participated in Institute workshops or other activities. That said, however, the other participants in the symposium and authors of this book are fresh faces.

This book and the symposium that gave rise to it represent an initial effort to bring the perspective of scaling to address the challenging topic of biodiversity. Concepts of scaling relations, along with theoretical approaches and analytical methods for studying them, are well represented across the physical, biological, and social sciences. Classic examples of so-called "scaling laws" include the Maxwell–Boltzmann distribution of kinetic energies of gas molecules, the size distribution of heavenly bodies in physics, the three-fourths power scaling of metabolism with body mass, the relationship between body size and longevity, the Gutenberg–Richter distribution of earthquake magnitudes, the Horton–Strahler hierarchy of stream and river orders, the Zipf distribution of word frequencies in languages, and the Pareto distribution of incomes among households. Classic examples in the scaling of biodiversity include species–area and species–time relationships, trophic pyramids, and distributions of abundance, range size, and body size among species.

Indeed, over the last two centuries, and accelerating rapidly in recent years, major empirical patterns of biodiversity have become increasingly well documented: across landscapes and geographic space, ecological and evolutionary time, and organisms of different body sizes, functional groups and trophic levels, and phylogenetic lineages and taxonomic groups. Many of these patterns represent scaling relations with respect to space, time, body size, environmental temperature and productivity, and other variables. Still missing, however, is a theory of biodiversity that can provide a unified, synthetic explanation for these relationships. Indeed, there is no general consensus explanation for the quintessential pattern, the decrease in number of species and many other measures of biological diversity from the tropics toward the poles.

Neither the symposium nor the book reaches definitive conclusions. The contributions do, however, present a special perspective on the state of the science. They focus on scaling as a way to characterize empirical relationships and explore theoretical concepts across the many dimensions and enormous spectrum of biodiversity. They highlight some of the progress that has recently been made, and some of the promising lines of investigation that are currently being pursued. In particular, they showcase the contributions and promise of some of the more theoretical and quantitative approaches to biodiversity. The contributors are interested not only in documenting the patterns of biodiversity with increasing accuracy and detail, but also in understanding the ecological and evolutionary processes that generate and maintain these patterns. Perhaps most importantly, the symposium presentations and book chapters collectively articulate an optimistic vision of biodiversity research. Half a century ago, the eminent ecologist G. E. Hutchinson asked, "Why are there so many species of animals?" Twenty-first century science can see into the farthest reaches of the universe and rapidly sequence the genome of any organism. Hopefully it will soon be able to explain why there are so many species of organisms, and more in tropical rain forests and coral reefs than in arctic tundra and the abyssal plain.

James H. Brown
Geoffrey B. West
Murray Gell-Mann

# CHAPTER ONE

# Introduction: scaling biodiversity – what is the problem?

DAVID STORCH
*Charles University, Prague, The Santa Fe Institute*
PABLO A. MARQUET
*Pontificia Universidad Católica de Chile, CASEB, IEB, The Santa Fe Institute*
JAMES H. BROWN
*University of New Mexico, The Santa Fe Institute*

Biological diversity is the most fascinating phenomenon on the Earth. Biologists, amazed by the splendid variety of life, spent several centuries collecting, describing, and classifying living things. We are still engaged in this endeavor. Some groups, such as birds, mammals, molluscs, and vascular plants, have received most of the attention, while others, such as mites, nematodes, fungi, and prokaryotes, remain very poorly known. Moreover, we are still only beginning to understand in depth the processes that generate and maintain the global biodiversity. Part of our ignorance comes from the complexity of observed biodiversity patterns and of the processes that have produced them. These range from evolutionary events that occurred millions of years ago to contemporary interactions between individual organisms and their environments, from biogeographic processes that play out on the scale of continents and oceans to local interactions that can occur on miniscule spatial scales. Part is simply due to the fact that the diversity of life is determined by a multitude of processes which are unique for each taxon and each environment: each kind of organism has unique features of structure and function, which are due to evolutionary constraints and which affect its strategies for survival and reproduction, each type of habitat has its unique abiotic conditions and biotic composition and its own dynamics, and each land mass and body of water has its own geological, climatic, and organic history. Searching for universal laws might seem to be a hopeless task.

There are, however, general, perhaps universal, patterns of biodiversity, suggesting that they might be due to equally general underlying processes. Biological diversity increases with the area sampled, decreases from the equator towards the poles, and is generally high in hot and humid places. Species richness tends to increase with total abundances of individuals and is promoted by the turnover in species composition of local communities, which, in turn, is affected by habitat heterogeneity and spatial aggregation of individuals. Also, although, or perhaps because, biodiversity is scale dependent, species richness of local ecological communities is always related to the richness of the larger surrounding biogeographic regions. Many potential explanations, some of them mutually exclusive, some not, have been advanced to explain these patterns (see e.g. Gaston & Blackburn, 2000, and Blackburn & Gaston, 2003, for reviews). Discerning between competing explanations requires careful formulation and quantitative testing of formal models relating pattern to processes (Storch & Gaston, 2004).

The study of biodiversity is therefore a sophisticated quantitative modern science. Similarly as in other branches of science, it is necessary to discover and quantify those properties of systems that remain relatively invariant and stable regardless of the system-specific details and intricacies, and to develop formal models that capture the general features of system structure and behavior (Maurer, 1999). Such an approach has been very successful in disciplines such as statistical physics and cosmology, and is best exemplified by the theory and methodology of scaling. Scaling, in its broadest sense, is the effort to discover and explain how some state variable or dynamic parameter changes with some other variable.

Scaling in ecology is perhaps best developed in the context of spatial scaling, i.e. changes in observed patterns with the spatial scale of observation. Ecologists have long been aware that different patterns are apparent and different processes are operating on different spatial scales (e.g. Rahbek & Graves, 2001; Whittaker, Willis & Field, 2001; Rahbek, 2005). Only recently, however, have ecologists and biogeographers been able to reveal *quantitative* rules that describe how the patterns change across scales. This is an important first step toward a true scaling theory that would use models based on first principles to accurately predict such empirical scaling phenomena. Recent progress toward such quantitative treatment of biodiversity based on principles of scaling is the topic of this book.

The chapters in this volume are the written versions of talks presented at a workshop "Scaling Biodiversity", which was held in Prague, Czech Republic, on 19–22 October 2004. The workshop was cosponsored by the Santa Fe Institute and the Center for Theoretical Study, Charles University in Prague. It brought together an eclectic mix of scientists interested in biodiversity and scaling theory. These ranged from empirically oriented ecologists and biogeographers to mathematical biologists and theoretical physicists, and from graduate students and postdocs to eminent senior scientists. The lively interchange of data and ideas by individuals with very different backgrounds, approaches, and methodologies made for a memorable conference. Most participants agreed that the conference substantially broadened their own limited perspectives on biodiversity. It highlighted the many contributions that scaling approaches are now making to the emerging understanding of biodiversity patterns and processes.

The title of this volume thus refers to quantitative approaches to the patterns of biodiversity and the processes that generate them. We start, in the first part, with spatial scaling of species richness and its relationship to the spatial distribution and abundance of individual species. The second part considers other quantitative patterns, such as phylogenetic diversity and species spatial turnover. The third part tackles the role of energy availability, which appears to be a major driver of spatial biodiversity patterns, including the well-known latitudinal biodiversity gradient. The final part is devoted to more synthetic views on processes responsible for scaling phenomena and future perspectives on biodiversity scaling.

## Part I. Spatial scaling of species richness and distribution

The notion that species richness depends on scale of observation is old, dating at least to the beginning of the twentieth century (Arrhenius, 1921; Gleason, 1922). The fact that the number of species on average increases with the area over which the species are counted is obvious, but the exact form of the species–area relationship is not. Empirical species–area relationships can take many forms depending on the spatial scale of study, taxon, environmental and geographical setting, and role of ecological and evolutionary processes (Rosenzweig, 1995). Nevertheless, there are also regularities. The species–area relationship tends to be triphasic – increasing rapidly at small spatial scales, then more slowly and approximately as a power law at intermediate scales, and then increasing rapidly again at the largest spatial scales. The overall shape of the species–area relationship is driven by the interplay between sampling effects, spatial population processes, and species turnover in response to habitat heterogeneity (Storch, Šizling & Gaston, 2003). Whereas the effects of sampling and spatial population processes have been studied comprehensively, and their influences on species–area relationships have been analyzed (e.g. Hanski & Gyllenberg, 1997; Hubbell, 2001), the effects of species-specific requirements in relation to spatially varying habitat structure have been largely neglected. Mike Palmer (Chapter 2) shows that the structure of habitat mosaics – i.e. along a gradient from fine-grained to coarse-grained – predictably affects the shape of the species–area relationship. Moreover, differences among landscapes in how habitat grain changes with spatial scale give testable predictions of how species richness scales with area.

Proximately, the shape of the species–area relationship is given by the spatial structure of the distribution of individual species: if all species had homogeneous distribution and occurred everywhere, species richness would not increase with area, and the more clumped the distributions of the species, the steeper the slope of the species–area relationship (He & Legendre, 2002). Spatial distributions of individuals are almost never random (i.e. Poisson-like) nor simply clumped in large clumps without any internal structure, but rather they tend to be aggregated on all scales of resolution. This has led to the notion that species spatial distribution is fractal – i.e. self-similar – with quantitatively similar patterns of aggregation occurring on every spatial scale (Kunin, 1998), and that fractal species distributions are responsible for observed power-law species–area relationships (Harte, Kinzig & Green, 1999; Šizling & Storch, 2004).

But is spatial distribution of most species really fractal? And how do deviations from fractality affect the increase of species richness with increasing area? Fangliang He and Rick Condit (Chapter 3) show that although the increase of species relative occupancy with spatial scale can be often well approximated by a power law, indicating fractality in spatial distribution, a slightly different model fits even better. This suggests that better tools for analyzing and predicting spatial distribution of individuals, and consequent scaling of species richness, are needed. Jack Lennon and his colleagues (Chapter 4) used an original analytical technique to reveal fractality in the large-scale distributions of South African birds, finding that whereas spatial distributions of some species cannot be distinguished from true fractals, those of other species – especially the more abundant ones – deviate significantly from fractality, revealing less aggregated distributions at fine scales. Together, these two chapters question the generality and usefulness of strictly fractal approaches to species distributions and consequently to biodiversity scaling patterns.

By contrast, fractal patterns represent at least very good first approximations of the geometry of species spatial distributions; the distributions are definitely much closer to fractal than homogeneous or random. Are there biological reasons why the structure of species distribution should be self-similar? Arnošt Šizling and David Storch (Chapter 5) show that a distribution which is effectively indistinguishable from fractal can emerge by random multilevel aggregation driven by a hierarchical distribution of habitat patches, randomly nested within more broadly defined habitat types. This simple null model predicts well not only the observed scale-dependence of species occupancy patterns, but also the observed shapes of species–area relationships, and even the distribution of species abundances. The HEAP model of John Harte (Chapter 6) is similar in many of its tenets and makes similar predictions. This model also assumes random spatial aggregation of individuals on multiple scales, although the aggregation process is based on purely statistical principles rather than defined biological mechanisms (see Harte et al., 2005). However, Harte's chapter shows how the HEAP model can be interpreted in terms of random population growth–extinction processes, and can provide invaluable insights into how the spatial scaling of species abundance, distribution, and diversity are all related to each other.

## Part II.   Alternative measures of biodiversity: taxonomy, phylogeny, and turnover

The number of species co-occurring within an area is only one aspect of bio-logical diversity. Different patterns can be revealed by measuring phylogenetic relationships or similarity and dissimilarity in taxonomic composition between communities. Careful consideration of such alternative measures is especially valuable whenever the concept of species or the definition of taxonomic units seems to be vague or unclear. This is especially true in the case of the hotly discussed issue of microbial biodiversity patterns. Some authors (e.g. Fenchel & Finlay, 2004) claim that macroecological patterns in prokaryotes and unicellular eukaryotes are very different from those typically observed in large, multicel-lular plants and animals. They suggest that microbes are distributed relatively homogeneously across the Earth's surface. The idea is that microbes have phenomenal capacities for dispersal so they eventually colonize and occur everywhere that suitable conditions occur. The result is that similar environ-ments have similar microbial species composition, regardless of their current spatial separation and evolutionary histories. However, as shown by Jessica Green and Brendan Bohannan (Chapter 7), this may be an artifact due to taxonomic resolution. New molecular genetic tools are revealing that a single morphologically recognizable microbial "species" can contain diverse geneti-cally distinct populations, comparable in some cases to much higher taxonomic categories (genera, families, and even orders) of multicellular organisms. Therefore, as new tools reveal the full extent of diversity patterns in microbes, it will be important to incorporate genetic patterns and phylogenetic thinking to elucidate the processes underlying these patterns. In a similar vein, Jérôme Chave and his colleagues (Chapter 8) provide an example of how much addi-tional information can be obtained by incorporating phylogenetic information into a quantitative study of forest biodiversity. Indeed, two hectares of forest with the same number of species can have very different diversity levels in terms of phylogenetic disparity between individuals. This means that the his-tory of speciation and extinction, lineage diversification processes, and biogeo-graphic events can leave important signatures in contemporary biodiversity.

Not only local species richness, but also species composition of communities change over space, especially in local ecological or larger-scale geographic gradients of environmental change. Spatial turnover of species contributes substantially to macroecological biodiversity patterns, because different regions can have very different levels of turnover between local communities. A major problem is how to measure turnover, which may depend on absolute levels of species richness as well as the spatial scale (grain size) of measurement

(Koleff, Gaston & Lennon, 2003). Tim Keitt (Chapter 9) proposes an efficient way of how to measure turnover simultaneously on a continuous range of spatial scales, showing how it depends on both scale and spatial location.

Since turnover in species composition between two sites depends on distance, habitat differences, and dispersal abilities of the organisms, it might seem that only few if any generalizations would be possible. However, Kevin Gaston and colleagues (Chapter 10) show that although various measures of turnover capture different features of the phenomenon, there are still some regularities. Similarity in species composition almost always decreases with distance and, when properly measured, it increases with local species richness and mean species occupancy. Such regularities by themselves cannot distinguish the roles of habitat heterogeneity and limited dispersal in generating turnover in species composition between distant sites; both niche-assembled and dispersal-assembled species assemblages produce the same patterns. Nevertheless, observed regularities reveal the close connection between spatial patterns of species turnover and scaling patterns of species occupancy, abundance, and diversity.

## Part III.  Scaling of biological diversity with energy and the latitudinal biodiversity gradient

Diversity is not equally distributed across the Earth surface; some places are much richer than others. The most notable pattern is the latitudinal gradient of diversity, i.e. the decrease in species richness from the tropics towards the poles (Gaston, 2000; Willig, Kaufman & Stevens, 2003). Andrew Clarke (Chapter 11) suggests that this pattern probably has several causes, ranging from contemporary climate to historical climatic and geological events. Moreover, the pattern is not absolutely universal. Some taxa are actually more diverse at high latitudes and altitudes. Pavel Kindlmann and colleagues (Chapter 12) supply evidence to suggest that these reverse gradients may be caused by negative relationships between the diversity of these exceptional organisms and of the more typical organisms that generate the "normal" gradients prevalent in most other taxa. Regardless of the possible multiple causality of the latitudinal gradient and some deviations from the common trend, however, there is a very strong and general relationship between biological diversity and climate (Hawkins *et al.*, 2003). David Currie (Chapter 13) shows that terrestrial animal and plant diversity scales with key variables of temperature and humidity in essentially the same way throughout the world, so he infers that local ecological conditions constrain diversity so strongly that regional historical effects are relatively unimportant.

Temperature and moisture together largely control productivity, and therefore the quantity of resources available to a given taxon (but see Currie *et al.*, 2004). In addition, however, temperature, through its effect on metabolic rate, could affect species richness through other mechanisms, such as rates of speciation, extinction, and ecological interaction (Allen, Brown & Gillooly, 2002; Brown et al., 2004). Although Currie claims that species richness does not scale with temperature as predicted by metabolic theory, testing the theory is not straightforward. Andrew Allen and coauthors (Chapter 14) show that the deeper development and understanding of metabolic theory leads to slightly different predictions: namely the effect of temperature can be assessed only by comparing communities that contain approximately similar numbers of individuals and are not limited by water availability. This implies that species richness may be affected by the effect of temperature both on productivity through its influence on resource availability and on rates of ecological and evolutionary processes through its influence on metabolic rate. The current version of "metabolic theory" suggests how metabolic rate affects rates of both evolutionary and ecological processes, so its predictions about biodiversity are necessarily quite complex. As far as we know, however, it is the only theory providing quantitative predictions of scaling of species richness with environmental variables.

By contrast, some quantitative patterns relating species richness and energy availability can be derived from the knowledge of scaling of species richness with space. High environmental productivity leading to high species richness is often associated with higher probability of occurrence of individual species and consequently higher species occupancies (Bonn, Storch & Gaston, 2004). This in turn leads to lower species turnover and shallower slopes of the species–area relationships in more productive areas and slower increase of richness with productivity within larger areas (Storch et al., 2005). As shown by David Storch, Arnošt Šizling and Kevin Gaston (Chapter 15), the assumption that the probability of species occurrence scales with both area and productivity is appropriate for realistically predicting both species–area and species–energy relationships, as well as of the interaction between them.

## Part IV.   Processes, perspectives, and syntheses

Many scaling rules mentioned above are based on quite simple geometric considerations and assumptions of static environmental constraints. However, all the patterns are in fact consequences of complex dynamical spatiotemporal processes, and these processes themselves reveal scaling laws. Species richness, for instance, increases predictably not only with spatial scale, but also with temporal window of observation (Preston, 1960), as discussed by Ethan White in his overview of this pattern (Chapter 16). Similarly as in the case of the interaction between the species–energy and species–area relationships, there is a negative interaction between species–area and species–time relationships: species richness increases more slowly with time in large areas. Does such apparent regularity in observed spatiotemporal patterns indicate some universal processes underlying them? What are the relevant processes?

A hotly debated approach assumes that most essential processes can be modeled by treating all species as ecologically equivalent, with the result that community structure is then determined largely by stochastic events of birth, death, and local dispersal (Hubbell, 2001). Luís Borda-de-Água, Stephen Hubbell and Fangliang He (Chapter 17) used the so-called multifractal approach to show that models which assume such neutral dynamics and use realistic dispersal kernels predict scaling patterns of diversity and distribution very similar to those observed in tropical forests. Tomáš Herben (Chapter 18) applies the neutral approach to successfully predict patterns in species invasions, including relationships between richness of native and alien species, and higher susceptibility of islands than mainlands to invasion. These "neutral" models that generate diversity by assuming that all coexisting species share some very general features contrast markedly with traditional "niche models" that generate diversity based explicitly on differences among coexisting species.

Interesting patterns can also emerge when considering just one population of a species not interacting with other species, but constrained by local density dependence, dispersal, and/or habitat patchiness. William Kunin (Chapter 19) demonstrates how spatial structure of populations affects processes (namely local population extinction) that in turn affect population persistence and spatial structure. Beáta Oborny and colleagues (Chapter 20) show how local density dependence and dispersal limitation can lead to a "universal" spatio-temporal scaling behavior, which is independent of the many system-specific details. Indeed, population dynamics in space and time can lead to such phenomena as "critical states" and "scale invariance", which crucially affect population persistence, and which have been observed in complex physical systems. Pablo Marquet and colleagues (Chapter 21) develop similar themes, discussing the extent to which observed population abundances and their fluctuations reveal signs of universal scaling behaviors. As seen in several chapters, many population and community patterns can be approximated by power laws (see also Keitt & Stanley, 1998; Keitt et al., 2002), again suggesting that some universal principles generate uniformity that lurks behind the observed variability.

## Concluding remarks

We believe that this book captures the current diversity of the science of biodiversity. There is excitement and ferment, a heady variety of conceptual approaches, analytical techniques, and mathematical models. The chapters show how much progress has been made in just the last few years. Indeed, the depth of thinking, the number of environmental and historical factors being considered, and the sophistication of mathematical models and statistical analyses have all increased enormously. Many but by no means all chapters and their authors optimistically suggest that there are some general law-like patterns and processes underlying all of the many intricate details: the differences among taxa, environments, and historically and geographically isolated regions.

It is also clear, however, that any such general laws remain elusive. Many of the patterns may seem universal if analyzed in the "right" way, but the neutral and/or more deterministic ecological and evolutionary processes that have generated those patterns remain poorly understood. The chapters in this book amply illustrate the unfinished state of the science. Collectively, the chapters highlight the divergent approaches, contradictory assumptions, predictions, and interpretations, and still unanswered questions. Models that make very different assumptions are able to generate predictions that are very similar to each other and to observed empirical patterns. Alternative hypotheses, which may not necessarily be mutually exclusive, can be difficult to distinguish. There is obviously much unfinished business.

Nevertheless, it is equally obvious that progress is being made and the perspective of scaling is playing a major role. This perspective – the analysis of data and the development of models to understand how biodiversity varies across space, time, environmental conditions, and historical contingencies – has much more to contribute. We hope that some readers will be challenged to address the unresolved issues. And if they do so, we hope that they will find the information in this book to be useful, especially the emphasis on building and evaluating models that explore relationships between the patterns and processes, among the multiple variables and mechanisms, and across the disparate scales of space and time that characterize the enormous diversity of life on Earth.

Neither the workshop nor this book would have been possible without the help of many people. We thank the Santa Fe Institute (SFI) and the Center for Theoretical Study, Charles University (namely its research program MSM0021620845), for their generous support for the workshop and the preparation of this book. We are especially grateful to Barbora Svatá for substantial help in organizing the workshop as well as technical assistance in the days before final manuscript submission. We thank the authors for their effort to write and rewrite chapters so as to improve the overall quality and integration of the book, for their patience and cooperation. We are particularly grateful to Cambridge University Press, and namely Alan Crowden, Clare Georgy and Dominic Lewis, for their assistance with the production of this volume.

## References

Allen, A. P., Brown, J. H. & Gillooly, J. F. (2002). Global biodiversity, biochemical kinetics, and the energetic-equivalence rule. *Science*, **297**, 1545–1548.

Arrhenius, O. (1921). Species and area. *Journal of Ecology*, **9**, 95–99.

Blackburn, T. M. & Gaston, K. J. (eds.) (2003). *Macroecology: Concepts and Consequences*. Oxford: British Ecological Society and Blackwell Science.

Bonn, A., Storch, D. & Gaston, K. J. (2004). Structure of the species–energy relationship. *Proceedings of the Royal Society of London, Series B*, **271**, 1685–1691.

Brown, J. H., Gillooly, J. F., Allen, A. P., Savage, V. M. & West, G. B. (2004). Toward a metabolic theory of ecology. *Ecology*, **85**, 1771–1789.

Currie, D. J., Mittelbach, G. G., Cornell, H. V., *et al.* (2004). Predictions and tests of climate-based hypotheses of broad-scale variation in taxonomic richness. *Ecology Letters*, **7**, 1121–1134.

Fenchel, T. & Finlay, B. J. (2004). The ubiquity of small species: patterns of local and global diversity. *Bioscience*, **54**, 777–784.

Gaston, K. J. (2000). Global patterns in biodiversity. *Nature*, **405**, 220–227.

Gaston, K. J. & Blackburn, T. M. (2000). *Pattern and Process in Macroecology*. Oxford: Blackwell Science.

Gleason, H. A. (1922). On the relation between species and area. *Ecology*, **3**, 158–162.

Hanski, I. & Gyllenberg, M. (1997). Uniting two general patterns in the distribution of species. *Science*, **275**, 397–400.

Harte, J., Kinzig, A. & Green, J. (1999). Self-similarity in the distribution and abundance of species. *Science*, **284**, 334–336.

Harte, J., Conlisk, E., Ostling, A., Green, J. L. & Smith, A. B. (2005). A theory of spatial structure in ecological communities at multiple spatial scales. *Ecological Monographs*, **75**, 179–197.

Hawkins, B. A., Field, R., Cornell, H. V., *et al.* (2003). Energy, water, and broad-scale geographic patterns of species richness. *Ecology*, **84**, 3105–3117.

He, F. L. & Legendre, P. (2002). Species diversity patterns derived from species-area models. *Ecology*, **85**, 1185–1198.

Hubbell, S. P. (2001). *The Unified Theory of Biodiversity and Biogeography*. Princeton: Princeton University Press.

Keitt, T. H. & Stanley, H. E. (1998). Dynamics of North American breeding bird populations. *Nature*, **393**, 257–260.

Keitt, T. H., Amaral, L. A. N., Buldryev, S. V. & Stanley, H. E. (2002). Scaling in the growth of geographically subdivided populations: invariant patterns from a continent-wide biological survey. *Philosophical Transactions of the Royal Society of London, Series B*, **357**, 627–633.

Koleff, P., Gaston K. J. & Lennon, J. J. (2003). Measuring beta diversity for presence-absence data. *Journal of Animal Ecology*, **72**, 367–382.

Kunin, W. E. (1998). Extrapolating species abundances across spatial scales. *Science*, **281**, 1513–1515.

Maurer, B. A. (1999). *Untangling Ecological Complexity? The Macroscopic Perspective*. Chicago: University of Chicago Press.

Preston, F. W. (1960). Time and space and the variation of species. *Ecology*, **29**, 254–283.

Rahbek, C. (2005). The role of spatial scale and the perception of large-scale species-richness patterns. *Ecology Letters*, **8**, 224–239.

Rahbek, C. & Graves, G. R. (2001). Multiscale assessment of patterns of avian species richness. *Proceedings of the National Academy of Sciences of the United States of America*, **98**, 4534–4539.

Rosenzweig, M. L. (1995). *Species Diversity in Space and Time*. Cambridge: Cambridge University Press.

Šizling, A. L. & Storch, D. (2004). Power-law species-area relationships and self-similar species distributions within finite areas. *Ecology Letters*, **7**, 60–68.

Storch, D. & Gaston, K. J. (2004). Untangling ecological complexity on different scales of space and time. *Basic and Applied Ecology*, **5**, 389–400.

Storch, D., Šizling, A. L. & Gaston, K. J. (2003). Geometry of the species-area relationship in central European birds: testing the mechanism. *Journal of Animal Ecology*, **72**, 509–519.

Storch, D., Evans, K. L. & Gaston, K. J. (2005). The species-area-energy relationship. *Ecology Letters*, **8**, 487–492.

Whittaker, R. J., Willis, K. J. & Field, R. (2001). Scale and species richness: towards a general, hierarchical theory of species diversity. *Journal of Biogeography*, **28**, 453–470.

Willig, M. R., Kaufman, D. M. & Stevens, R. D. (2003). Latitudinal gradients of biodiversity: patterns, process, scale, and synthesis. *Annual Review of Ecology and Systematics*, **34**, 273–309.

PART I

# Spatial scaling of species richness and distribution

# CHAPTER TWO

# Species–area curves and the geometry of nature

MICHAEL W. PALMER

*Oklahoma State University*

## Introduction

It is widely appreciated that species distributions and biodiversity can be strongly related to environmental factors. Likewise, it is recognized that increasing environmental heterogeneity with area is one of the determinants of species–area relationships. However, few theoretical treatments of species–area relationships specifically address *how* biodiversity's increase with scale should be related to the geometry of the environment. I hypothesize that this geometry is the underlying reason for the triphasic species–area curve.

## Gradient analysis

One of the oldest, strongest and least contentious generalizations in ecology is that the spatial distribution of species is due, at least in part, to variation in the environment. In particular, the abundance of a species tends to be a unimodal function of important environmental variables (Whittaker, 1975; ter Braak, 1987; Austin & Gaywood, 1994). Such functions are termed species response curves, and graphs of the response curves for all species in a region combined or *coenoclines* (Fig. 2.1) are in almost all ecological textbooks (for example, Begon, Harper & Townsend, 1996; Ricklefs, 2001) and have played important roles in the development of ecological theory (Whittaker, 1972; Shmida & Ellner, 1984; Tilman, 1988). The study of how species respond to gradients in the environment is known as gradient analysis (Whittaker, 1967; Austin, 1987; ter Braak & Prentice, 1988).

The unimodal species response curve is a simple manifestation of a species having an optimum set of environmental conditions. As conditions deviate from the optimum, the species will occur in less abundance. Classic competition theory (for example, Giller, 1984) and its derivatives (for example, Tilman, 1988) dictates that interspecific competition may decrease the breadth of the species response curve – that is, the "realized niche" is less than the "fundamental niche". However, the utility of gradient analysis and the validity of unimodal response curves do not depend on the role or strength of interspecific interactions.

*Scaling Biodiversity*, ed. David Storch, Pablo A. Marquet and James H. Brown. Published by Cambridge University Press. © Cambridge University Press 2007.

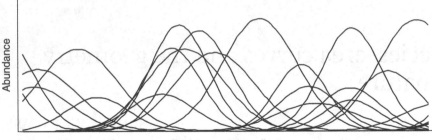

**Figure 2.1** A hypothetical coenocline, consisting of the species response curves of all the species in a community. Although the curves illustrated here are mostly smooth and unimodal (one-peaked), the principles described here will hold with a modest amount of multimodality and noise in abundance.

An obvious consequence of the relationship between species and the environment is the *environmental heterogeneity hypothesis*: you expect to find more species in regions which are spatially variable in the environment (Palmer, 1992, 1994; Rosenzweig, 1995; Kerr & Packer, 1997; Burnett *et al.*, 1998; Fraser, 1998; Cowling & Lombard, 2002; Ewers *et al.*, 2005). This simple hypothesis has been verified in a number of systems (Kerr & Packer, 1997; Burnett *et al.*, 1998). Most environmental variables exhibit distance decay (Journel & Huijbregts, 1978; Burrough, 1981; Palmer, 1990; Bell *et al.*, 1993), meaning that heterogeneity in the environment increases as a function of spatial scale. Therefore, the species–area relationship should be largely determined by environmental heterogeneity (Williamson, 1988; Whittaker, 1998).

### The geometry of heterogeneity and the species–area relationship

One of the biggest challenges in linking gradient analysis to the study of species–area relationships is that we have no comprehensive theory governing the geometry of environmental variation. Some environmental gradients vary smoothly and linearly: for example, the zonation of vegetation on a lakeshore (Nilsson & Wilson, 1991; Grace & Wetzel, 1998). Other gradients may be more spatially unpredictable, such as the distribution of light patches in an old-growth forest with numerous treefall gaps (Poulson & Platt, 1989; Hubbell *et al.*, 1999). Still other gradients, such as soil nutrients (Palmer, 1990) may have an intermediate degree of spatial predictability.

Furthermore, the geometry of environmental heterogeneity can change as a function of scale. While the edge of a lake has a well-defined slope, the distributions of lakes within a county may be not as easy to describe with a few parameters. On a yet broader scale, the frequency of lakes in a continent may be a predictable function of climate. Thus, the component of the species–area curve that is caused by environmental heterogeneity is likely to behave differently at different scales.

## The fractal geometry of the landscape and species richness

Fortunately, the science of Fractal Geometry (Mandelbrot, 1983) allows us to quantify and model the geometry of environmental heterogeneity (Burrough, 1983; Milne, 1992). This is most clearly illustrated by taking a line transect through a landscape (Fig. 2.2). The value of an environmental variable (or "regionalized variable" in the sense of geostatistics) as a function of a linear transect is topologically a line (a 1-dimensional object) embedded within a 2-dimensional space (defined by one spatial axis and one environmental axis). In this case, the environment's fractal dimension ($D$) ranges from 1 to 2. If the environment behaves as a smooth function of position along a transect, the function is very close to a line, and therefore has a $D$ close to 1. If the environment is spatially unpredictable, the graph of environment as a function of position practically fills the plane. As a plane is a 2-dimensional object, $D$ is close to 2. Most environmental variables will have an intermediate degree of predictability, and hence the fractal (or fractional) dimension will be somewhere between 1 and 2.

If we consider a 2-dimensional landscape (not just a line transect through it), a regionalized variable will be topologically 2-dimensional, but embedded in a 3-dimensional space. Its fractal dimension will therefore vary between 2 and 3. This is analogous to a smooth piece of paper being essentially a 2-dimensional object, but a highly crinkled piece of paper will be close to 3-dimensional. If the regionalized variable under consideration is elevation, then all dimensions are spatial.

There is an ample literature providing formal definitions of fractals, fractality, multifractals, self-similarity, self-affinity, and related concepts. Such precise concepts are important for simulations and theoretical treatments of fractals (see Šizling & Storch; Lennon et al.; Borda-de-Água et al.; and He & Condit, this volume). However, the use of fractal dimensions to get an empirical handle on the geometry of nature does not depend on such precise definitions. Most theoretical treatments of fractals involve a self-referent function (Feder, 1988): that is, a mechanism that generates self-similarity. It may be impossible to identify such functions in a complex natural setting; indeed they may not exist. But this is not an impediment for the use of fractal language to describe irregularity in nature.

The accumulation of new environments, and hence new species, as a function of area will differ depending on the fractal dimension. For example, one does not need to traverse a great distance to encounter numerous habitats in a high $D$

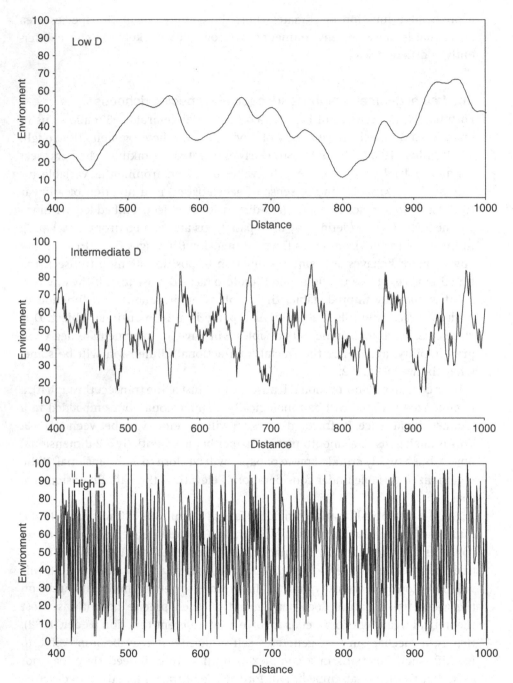

**Figure 2.2** Three hypothetical examples of environmental heterogeneity along transects, ranging from smoothly varying (low fractal dimension) to white noise (high fractal dimension).

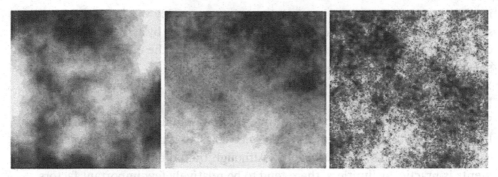

**Figure 2.3** Simulated landscapes of 256 × 256 cells, in which the value of an environmental gradient varies from 0 to 100, as indicated by darkness. From left to right, the landscapes have fractal dimensions of 2.1, 2.5, and 2.9 and were constructed with the midpoint displacement algorithm (Saupe, 1988).

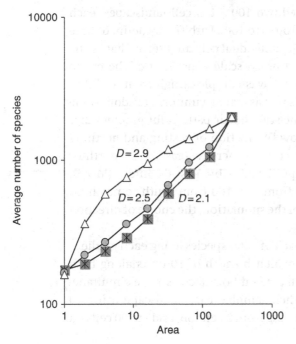

**Figure 2.4** Species–area curves (each point is the average of 10 simulated square quadrats) for landscapes differing in fractal dimension (Fig. 2.3). The environment of each landscape varied between 0 and 100, and each of 2000 species occurred in the landscape wherever the environment was suitable. Each species had a habitat breadth of 10 units, and the midpoint of each species' range was randomly chosen between −5 and 105. The midpoints can fall outside the range of the environment, much as the species optimum may fall outside the environmental conditions in real landscapes (see Fig. 2.1).

environment, in contrast to a low $D$ environment (Fig. 2.2). I illustrate this further by simulating 2-dimensional landscapes (Fig. 2.3). The landscape with the highest $D$ initially accumulates species at the fastest rate, as most environments are sampled at the finest scales (Fig. 2.4). Note that landscape geometry influences not only the location (that is, left to right and up to down position) but also the shape of the species–area relationship.

It is worth noting that the fractal dimension is only one descriptor of environmental texture. Landscapes (real or simulated) with the same $D$ can be generated in different ways. For example, one can generate smoothly varying low-$D$ land-scapes by averaging out random variation (as in Fig. 2.2) or by assigning linear or curvilinear functions of space (as in Fig. 2.3). However, the effects of such on species richness patterns are not likely to be dramatic.

## Multiple gradients

Species composition responds to multiple environmental factors, not just one. Indeed, modern gradient analysis can be viewed as an act of *dimension reduction* (Gauch, 1982; Lepš & Šmilauer, 2003). Although the potential number of gra-dients is practically limitless, there tend to be relatively few important factors determining species composition (Gauch, 1982; Whittaker, 1975). The existence of even two or three factors greatly complicates the relationship between heterogeneity and scale. For example, different variables may have different underlying fractal dimensions.

To illustrate this principle, I simulated two $100 \times 100$ cell landscapes, each with two important gradients (ranging from 0 to 100). I arbitrarily defined three spatial scales: a fine scale consisting of the individual cell, an intermediate scale consisting of a $10 \times 10$ cell block, and a broad scale consisting of the entire landscape. For both landscapes, gradient 1 was complex (high $D$) at an inter-mediate scale: each block of $10 \times 10$ cells was assigned a uniform random value between 0 and 100. Landscape A had fine-scale linear pattern for gradient 2: it varied between 0 and 100 as a linear (low $D$) function of easting and northing within each $10 \times 10$ cell block. The direction of increase (east, west, north or south) was randomly chosen. Landscape B had a broad-scale linear (low $D$) pattern for the gradient 2: it increased from 0 to 100 from south to north (as there is no net directionality to the rest of the simulation, the choice of direction is inconsequential).

I randomly located the midpoints of each of 1500 species along each gradient in each landscape. Each species had a habitat breadth of 10 units along both gradients. A species would only occur in a cell if both factors were simultane-ously within the appropriate range. I then sampled each landscape using 10 replicates of each of 11 spatial scales, ranging from 2 cells on a side to 90 cells on a side, and counted the species in each.

Figure 2.5 illustrates that landscapes A and B have dramatically different species–area curves. Each curve has an inflection. Landscape A has a steep initial slope associated with the fine-scale, low-$D$ gradient. Once several of the $10 \times 10$ cell blocks have been encountered, most of the environmental variation has been sampled, and the curve levels off. In contrast, landscape B has a low initial slope within the blocks, because neither gradient varies appreciably at that scale. The slope does not decrease at broad scales because of the broad-scale, low-$D$ gradient. In other words, an increase in grain (above the scale of the block) invariably leads to sampling new environments.

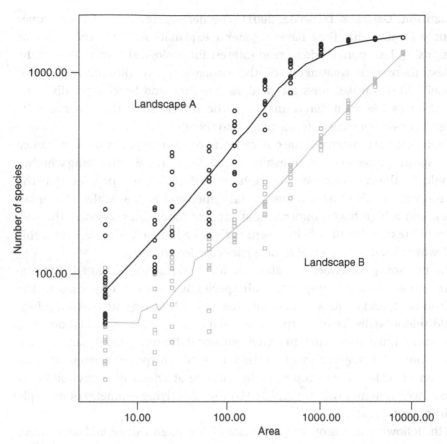

**Figure 2.5** Species–area curves for two hypothetical landscapes, as described in the text. Both landscapes have one gradient with a high $D$ at an intermediate scale. Landscape A has a secondary gradient that has a high fractal dimension at a broad scale, and a low fractal dimension at the fine scale. Landscape B has a secondary gradient with a low fractal dimension on a broad scale. Curves are LOWESS fits.

At intermediate spatial scales, the two species–area curves are parallel. This is undoubtedly due to the fact that gradient 1 is identical between the two landscapes.

I have shown two simple but arbitrary configurations for a two-gradient system. The bewildering variety of *possible* combinations of variables, scales, and geometries might doom any synthetic theory of species–area curves in heterogeneous landscapes (that is, all real landscapes). However, I will argue below that there may be general principles underlying the geometry of the environment, and these could lead to a fuller understanding of the species–area relationship.

### The Environmental Texture Model of the triphasic species–area curve

When viewed over many orders of magnitude of grain, species-area curves tend to be triphasic: they are steep at fine and broad scales and shallow at intermediate scales (Shmida & Wilson, 1985; Rosenzweig, 1995; Hubbell, 2001;

Williamson, Gaston & Lonsdale, 2001). The near-universality of such curves strongly implies that they have a general explanation. Thus, the triphasic relationship has spurred widespread interest for ecological theory. Two of the boldest theoretical treatments of the triphasic curve (Rosenzweig, 1995; Hubbell, 2001) invoke fine-scale random sampling and broad-scale dispersal limitation as the main determinants of the relationship; they do not fully integrate environmental heterogeneity into theory.

Given that the geometry of the environment has a great potential to influence the shape of species–area relationships (Figs. 2.3–2.5), it is worth asking whether it could be the root cause of the triphasic pattern. Here, I propose that the environment tends to have a low fractal dimension at fine scales and broad scales, and a high fractal dimension at intermediate scales. Because the geometry or "texture" of the environment varies as a function of scale, I term this the *Environmental Texture Model of the triphasic species–area curve*.

The previously described simulations, for convenience, assumed that gradients were all equally important, all species had similar responses to the environment, and there was no qualitative noise. Violating such assumptions would undoubtedly have effects on the shapes of species–area relationships. However, I must stress that the Environmental Texture Model has no such assumption: it merely stresses that the rate at which species accumulate as a function of scale will be influenced by the rate at which new environments appear, which in turn will be regulated by the underlying geometry of multiple environmental gradients.

In the following discussion, the definitions of fine, intermediate, and broad scales are admittedly arbitrary. As discussed later, these scales are likely to vary between regions. However, to frame the discussion, I consider "fine" scales to typically be less than a hectare, and "broad" scales to be greater than a million hectares.

## Low *D* at fine scales

At fine scales, spatial variation in the environment is often dominated by topography (Wondzell, Cornelius & Cunningham, 1990; Norton, 1994; Umbanhowar, 1995; Clark, Palmer & Clark, 1999; He, LaFrankie & Song, 2002). Gravity, along with flaking of rock and other erosional processes, tends to decrease roughness or fine-scale complexity in the environment. Indeed, we often take the topographic smoothness of the landscape for granted – the rough, irregular, or complex elements of landscapes are often considered points of special beauty or interest, and occupy a relatively tiny portion of the landscape.

Gravity also tends to even out the water table on a fine scale – so hydrological influences on species composition (Wassen & Barendregt, 1992; Zunzunegui, Diaz Barradas & Garcia Novo, 1998) also tend to have low fractal dimensions.

Variation in soils can influence fine-scale distribution of plant species (Cox & Larson, 1993; Oliveira-Filho *et al.*, 1994; Tuomisto *et al.*, 2002). Substantial fine-scale variation can exist in soils, and have a high fractal dimension (Palmer, 1990). However, rhizospheres are able to integrate over such fine-scale variation (Schmid & Bazzaz, 1987; Evans & Whitney, 1992; Wijesinghe & Hutchings, 1997). Similarly, the mass effect (Shmida & Ellner, 1984; Auerbach & Shmida, 1987; Palmer, 1992; Bengtsson, Fagerström & Rydin, 1994; Onipchenko & Pokarzhevskaya, 1994) or "vicinism" (van der Maarel, 1995; Zonneveld, 1995) will tend to make the *effective* environmental heterogeneity smoother than the *actual* environmental heterogeneity. Not being rooted, most animals will also be able to average out fine-scale variation in the environment.

**High $D$ at intermediate scales**

Imagine a soil map or a vegetation map for a state, province, or small country. More often than not, the soil types or vegetation types (admittedly arbitrary categories) exist as small, often complexly shaped patches scattered throughout the landscape. Perhaps as a root cause of this, topography at such scales often has a high fractal dimension. As scale is increased, the topographic variation that is smooth on the scale of a hill or a valley gives way to the complex (high $D$) variation of multiple hills and valleys.

It is worth noting that as $D$ approaches 3, the landscape can be considered *homogeneous* (*sensu* Palmer, 1988; and Šizling & Storch, 2004). Homogeneity does not refer to within-landscape variation, but rather the fact that the landscape remains similar upon subdivision. It is unlikely that there are scales at which any landscape is truly homogeneous, but it is quite likely that most landscapes exhibit more homogeneity at some scales than at other scales.

It might seem inappropriate to mention anthropogenic patterns in a discussion of triphasic curves. However, there are few large regions untouched by human activities. Given that humans have a profound effect on the geometry of the environment, it would be folly to ignore anthropogenic patterns. It is often said that humans tend to homogenize the landscape. This may be true at the scale of individual fields or other pieces of managed land. When we consider a small number of adjacent pieces of managed land, we have a low $D$: there are predictable, uncomplicated spatial trends. However, at the scale of multiple management units (for example, agricultural fields, forest stands) anthropogenic effects may be "patchy" and hence have indeed a high $D$.

**Low $D$ at broad scales**

The spherical shape of the Earth causes differential heating of its surface. This simple fact, along with the Earth's rotation and tilt, is responsible for smoothly varying patterns of climate (for example, temperature, rainfall). The fact that air and water are fluids, and therefore are well mixed relative to solids, causes fine-scale and intermediate-scale spatial variation (that is, "weather") to be relatively short-lived or smooth. The relationship between climate and species composition is strong

(Retuerto & Carballeira, 1991; Hallgren, Palmer & Milberg, 1999; Qian *et al.*, 2003; Currie, this volume), and has been appreciated for a long time (von Humboldt & Bonpland, 1807). Because climatic variation has a low *D*, increasing the grain will always increase environmental heterogeneity at broad scales.

## Exceptions

The argument that *D* is likely to vary with scale as described above is likely to be less than convincing. There are numerous obvious exceptions. For example, karst topography (a highly dissected geomorphology caused by the dissolution of limestone) illustrates high *D* at fine scales. Similarly, there are counterexamples to "high *D* at intermediate scales". Coastal plain regions may have a broad, smooth spatial gradient related to sedimentation history and groundwater hydrology. Mountains can cause high-*D* spatial variation in climate at relatively fine scales due to adiabatic processes and the rain shadow effect.

The existence of such exceptions gives us the ability to test the Environmental Texture Model. For example, we might expect a coastal plain to lack a well-defined triphasic curve, as increasing area at an intermediate scale will accumulate new environments at a rapid rate. Even if the basic model (low *D*–high *D*–low *D*) is correct, we should expect the shape of the triphasic to vary among regions. The first inflection point for a region with short inter-ridge distances, for example, should be to the left of that for a region with long inter-ridge distances.

## The case of mountainous regions

Mountains represent a particularly interesting but complex challenge to the Environmental Texture Model (Fig. 2.6). The effects of gravity are the same as in nonmountainous regions. Thus, mountains should have low *D* at fine scales (though for various reasons, especially in regions with active orogenesis,

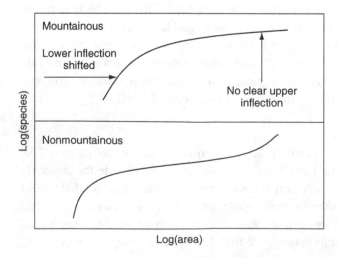

**Figure 2.6** Hypothetical species–area curves for mountainous and nonmountainous regions, as discussed in the text.

I expect fine-scale $D$ to be slightly larger than in nonmountainous regions). However, by definition, mountains are tall. Given the effects of gravity, they will also tend to be broad (with exceptions of some mesas). Therefore, the scale at which low $D$ gives way to high $D$ will be greater in mountainous regions. A high $D$ occurs when multiple mountains or ranges are sampled; adding yet another mountain does not add much to environmental heterogeneity (unless bedrock or other characteristics differ). On a broad scale, we are unlikely to see an upward inflection. This is because the broad-scale (low $D$) climatic gradients are masked by the finer-scale orogenic climatic effects. In other words, a wide range of climates have already been sampled.

## Richness of North American vascular floras in mountainous regions

In order to investigate the potential effect of mountainous regions on species–area relationships, I utilized data from the Floras of North America Project (http://botany.okstate.edu/floras; Palmer, Wade & Neal, 1995; Withers *et al.*, 1998; Palmer *et al.*, 2002; Palmer 2005), which is an attempt to collect all vascular floras (plant species lists) written within North America north of Mexico. To date, my colleagues and I have gathered approximately 8000 references. While about 3000 of these contain valid data (Fig. 2.7), we have only extracted useful information

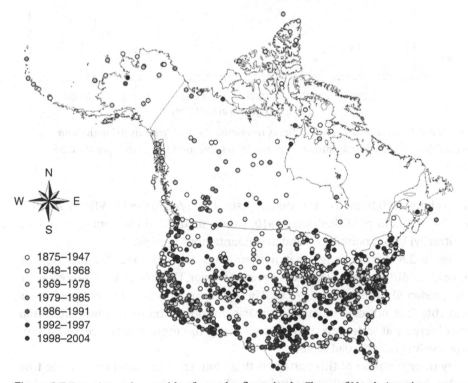

**Figure 2.7** Locations of centroids of vascular floras in the Floras of North America Project, with markers indicating year of study.

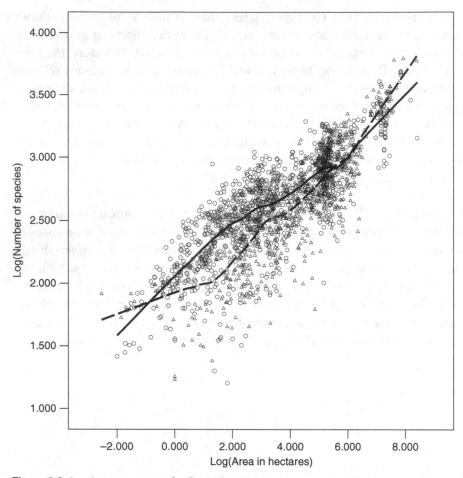

**Figure 2.8** Species–area curves for floras from mountainous regions (triangles and dashed line) and nonmountainous regions (circles and solid line). Lines are LOWESS curves.

from about 2200 floras. For this study, I restrict analysis to the 1815 floras south of 49° latitude and published after 1910. I then subdivided the continent (rather arbitrarily) into mountainous and nonmountainous regions.

Figure 2.8 demonstrates that mountainous and nonmountainous regions have quite different species–area curves. However, the difference is quite unlike the predicted difference (Fig. 2.6). The curve for nonmountainous regions is arguably (but not convincingly) triphasic. In mountainous regions, the initial slow increase at scales less than 10 ha gives way to a more rapid increase without any leveling off at broad scales.

My interpretation of this pattern is that alpine systems are fairly rich at fine scales, because of small individual size. This is coupled with a sampling bias, because botanists studying mountainous regions are more interested in the higher elevations (thus the lowlands will not be sampled with small floras). However, at scales of one to thousands of hectares, there is a steep increase due to the low $D$ nature of the elevation gradient. The mountain curve lies below the other curve at most scales, because of the altitudinal diversity gradient (Odland & Birks, 1999; Grytnes & Vetaas, 2002). The curve remains steep beyond the scale of individual mountains, either because different ranges are truly environmentally different, or because mountainous landscapes are likely to contain high numbers of local endemics. At broad scales, the number of species in mountainous regions surpasses that of nonmountainous regions because of enhanced environmental heterogeneity.

I cannot predict whether the rank speculation of the previous paragraph, or even the empirical patterns themselves, will stand up to more careful evaluation. The data have tremendous scatter that are caused by both methodological and biological factors. Furthermore, floristic data are known to have biases (Palmer, 1995; Palmer et al., 2002). A set of many carefully chosen, nested species–area curves over many orders of magnitude of scale are likely to be of more value than the shotgun approach of Fig. 2.8. Nevertheless, it is clear that the geometry of the environment, perhaps interacting with phylogeny and patterns of long-distance dispersal, plays a critical role in determining the shape of species–area relationships.

## Conclusions

The theory that the geometry of the environment can strongly affect species–area relationships is a rather simple and perhaps obvious one. In fact, geometric explanations have been articulated before:

"In most cases, increasing the area from 1 ha to 10 ha will add very few new species. At this scale, at least for vertebrates, habitats tend to be similar and easily reached by dispersing individuals. By contrast, increasing the area from one-tenth of the continent to the entire North American continent will result in the addition of many new species" (Brown, 1995).

"The pattern of environmental variation is to some extent fractal. This fact, and the variation in the fractal dimension, may, in time, lead to a deeper understanding of the causes of the variability of species–area curves" (Williamson, 1988).

Williamson (1988) recognizes that the slope of the species–area relationship may be directly related to the fractal dimension or "reddened spectrum" of the environment. The Environmental Texture Model can thus be considered an extension of Williamson's thinking to multiple scales and multiple gradients.

It is possible that the reason why geometric explanations have been largely ignored is because they are not very glamorous - or because their parameters are hard to assess. In particular, we need to discover which environmental variables are important, and at which scales. Another downside of a strong geometric signature is that it may obscure other interesting, and more biological, phenomena (such as the "correlation length" of Hubbell, 2001; or the "interprovincial" curve of Rosenzweig, 1995). Indeed, the Environmental Texture Model practically ignores biology (beyond the assumption that species distributions are influenced by the environment); explanations lie in the realm of geomorphology, geology, and climatology.

The Environmental Texture Model complements studies of species of varying spatial distributions (such as Šizling & Storch, 2004; Šizling & Storch, this volume). The species–area relationship is a simple property of the geometry of species distributions *and their covariances*. The environment plays a strong, but not exclusive, role in structuring species distributions. Patterns of interspecific covariance may help distinguish between the environment and other factors influencing the species–area relationship (Wagner, 2003).

It is perhaps most useful to consider the geometric theory to be a null model. It is when biodiversity patterns are *not* simple reflections of the underlying environmental template that we are likely to uncover macroecological phenomena. There needs to be more detailed study of this environmental template, and more focus needs to be directed to nonbiological disciplines such as geomorphology. Distinguishing between the Environmental Texture Model and alternative models (such as those involving sampling effects and dispersal limitation) will prove exceptionally challenging. Or in the words of Williamson 1988, "the techniques needed are appreciably more difficult; the results should be correspondingly more interesting".

## Acknowledgments

I thank David Storch, Ethan White, Jason Fridley, Peter White, and Daniel McGlinn for commenting on the manuscript. I also thank all the participants of the "Scaling Biodiversity" workshop for stimulating discussions.

## References

Auerbach, M. & Shmida, A. (1987). Spatial scale and the determinants of plant species richness. *Trends in Ecology and Evolution*, **2**, 238–242.

Austin, M. P. (1987). Models for the analysis of species' response to environmental gradients. *Vegetatio*, **69**, 35–45.

Austin, M. P. & Gaywood, M. J. (1994). Current problems of environmental gradients and species response curves in relation to continuum theory. *Journal of Vegetation Science*, **5**, 473–482.

Begon, M., Harper, J. L. & Townsend, C. R. (1996). *Ecology*. Oxford: Blackwell Science.

Bell, G., Lechowicz, M. J., Appenzeller, A., et al. (1993). The spatial structure of the physical environment. *Oecologia*, **96**, 114–121.

Bengtsson, J., Fagerström, T. & Rydin, H. (1994). Competition and coexistence in plant communities. *Trends in Ecology and Evolution*, **9**, 246–250.

Brown, J. H. (1995). *Macroecology*. Chicago: University of Chicago Press.

Burnett, M. R., August, P. V., Brown, J. H., Jr. & Killingbeck, K. T. (1998). The influence of geomorphological heterogeneity on biodiversity. I. A patch-scale perspective. *Conservation Biology*, **12**, 363–370.

Burrough, P. A. (1981). Fractal dimensions of landscapes and other environmental data. *Nature*, **294**, 240–242.

Burrough, P. A. (1983). Multiscale sources of spatial variation in soil. I. Application of fractal concepts to nested levels of soil variations. *Journal of Soil Science*, **34**, 577–597.

Clark, D. B., Palmer, M. W. & Clark, D. A. (1999). Edaphic factors and the landscape-scale distributions of tropical rain forest trees. *Ecology*, **80**, 2662–2675.

Cowling, R. M. & Lombard, A. T. (2002). Heterogeneity, speciation/extinction history and climate, explaining regional plant diversity patterns in the Cape Floristic Region. *Diversity and Distributions*, **8**, 163–179.

Cox, J. E. & Larson, D. W. (1993). Spatial heterogeneity of vegetation and environmental factors on talus slopes of the Niagara Escarpment. *Canadian Journal of Botany*, **71**, 323–332.

Evans, J. P. & Whitney, S. (1992). Clonal integration across a salt gradient by a nonhalophyte, *Hydrocotyle bonariensis* (Apiaceae). *American Journal of Botany*, **79**, 1344–1347.

Ewers, R. M., Didham, R. K., Wratten, S. D. D. & Tylianakis, J. M. (2005). Remotely sensed landscape heterogeneity as a rapid tool for assessing local biodiversity value in a highly modified New Zealand landscape. *Biodiversity and Conservation*, **14**, 1469–1485.

Feder, J. (1988). *Fractals*. New York: Plenum Press.

Fraser, R. H. (1998). Vertebrate species richness at the mesoscale: relative roles of energy and heterogeneity. *Global Ecology and Biogeography Letters*, **7**, 215–220.

Gauch, H. G., Jr. (1982). *Multivariate Analysis and Community Structure*. Cambridge: Cambridge University Press.

Giller, P. S. (1984). *Community Structure and the Niche*. London: Chapman and Hall.

Grace, J. B. & Wetzel, R. G. (1998). Long-term dynamics of *Typha* populations. *Aquatic Botany*, **61**, 137–146.

Grytnes, J. A. & Vetaas, O. R. (2002). Species richness and altitude: a comparison between null models and interpolated plant species richness along the Himalayan altitudinal gradient, Nepal. *American Naturalist*, **159**, 294–304.

Hallgren, E., Palmer, M. W. & Milberg, P. (1999). Data diving with cross validation: an investigation of broad-scale gradients in Swedish weed communities. *Journal of Ecology*, **87**, 1037–1051.

He, F., LaFrankie, J. V. & Song, B. (2002). Scale dependence of tree abundance and richness in a tropical rain forest, Malaysia. *Landscape Ecology*, **17**, 559–568.

Hubbell, S. P. (2001). *The Unified Neutral Theory of Biodiversity and Biogeography*. Princeton: Princeton University Press.

Hubbell, S. P., Foster, R. B., O'Brien, S. T. *et al.* (1999). Light gap disturbances, recruitment limitation, and tree diversity in a neotropical forest. *Science*, **283**, 554–557.

Journel, A. G. & Huijbregts, C. (1978). *Mining Geostatistics*. London: Academic Press.

Kerr, J. T. & Packer, L. (1997). Habitat heterogeneity as a determinant of mammal species richness in high-energy regions. *Nature*, **385**, 252–254.

Lepš, J. & Šmilauer, P. (2003). *Multivariate Analysis of Ecological Data using Canoco*. Cambridge: Cambridge University Press.

Mandelbrot, B. B. (1983). *The Fractal Geometry of Nature*. San Francisco: Freeman.

Milne, B. T. (1992). Spatial aggregation and neutral models in fractal landscapes. *American Naturalist*, **139**, 32–57.

Nilsson, C. & Wilson, S. D. (1991). Convergence in plant community structure along disparate gradients: are lakeshores inverted mountainsides? *American Naturalist*, **137**, 774–790.

Norton, D. A. (1994). Relationships between pteridophytes and topography in a lowland

South Westland podocarp forest. *New Zealand Journal of Botany*, **32**, 401–408.

Odland, A. & Birks, H. J. B. (1999). The altitudinal gradient of vascular plant richness in Aurland, western Norway. *Oikos*, **22**, 548–566.

Oliveira-Filho, A. T., Vilela, E., Carvalho, D. A. & Gavilanes, M. L. (1994). Effects of soils and topography on the distribution of tree species in a tropical riverine forest in south-eastern Brazil. *Journal of Tropical Ecology*, **10**, 483–508.

Onipchenko, V. G. & Pokarzhevskaya, G. A. (1994). "Mass-effect" in alpine communities of the northwestern Caucasus. *Veröfflichung Geobotanischen Institutes ETH, Stiftung Rübel, Zürich*, **115**, 61–68.

Palmer, M. W. (1988). Fractal Geometry: a tool for describing spatial patterns of plant communities. *Vegetatio*, **75**, 91–102.

Palmer, M. W. (1990). Spatial scale and patterns of species-environment relationships in hardwood forests of the North Carolina piedmont. *Coenoses*, **5**, 79–87.

Palmer, M. W. (1992). The coexistence of species in fractal landscapes. *American Naturalist*, **139**, 375–397.

Palmer, M. W. (1994). Variation in species richness: towards a unification of hypotheses. *Folia Geobotanica et Phytotaxonomica*, **29**, 511–530.

Palmer, M. W. (1995). How should one count species? *Natural Areas Journal*, **15**, 124–135.

Palmer, M. W. (2005). Temporal trends of exotic species richness in North American floras: an overview. *Écoscience*, **12**, 336–390.

Palmer, M. W., Wade, G. L. & Neal, P. R. (1995). Standards for the writing of floras. *BioScience*, **45**, 339–345.

Palmer, M. W., Earls, P., Hoagland, B. W., White, P. S. & Wohlgemuth, T. M. (2002). Quantitative tools for perfecting species lists. *Environmetrics*, **13**, 121–137.

Poulson, T. L. & Platt, W. J. (1989). Gap light regimes influence canopy tree diversity. *Ecology*, **70**, 553–555.

Qian, H., Song, J. S., Krestov, P., *et al.* (2003). Large-scale phytogeographical patterns in East Asia in relation to latitudinal and climatic gradients. *Journal of Biogeography*, **30**, 129–141.

Retuerto, R. & Carballeira, A. (1991). Defining phytoclimatic units in Galicia, Spain, by means of multivariate methods. *Journal of Vegetation Science*, **2**, 699–710.

Ricklefs, R. E. (2001). *The Economy of Nature*, 3rd edn. New York: W.H. Freeman.

Rosenzweig, M. L. (1995). *Species Diversity in Space and Time*. Cambridge: Cambridge University Press.

Saupe, D. (1988). Algorithms for random fractals. In *The Science of Fractal Images*, ed. H. O. Petigen & D. Saupe, pp. 71–113. New York: Springer-Verlag.

Schmid, B. & Bazzaz, F. A. (1987). Clonal integration and population structure in perennials: effects of severing rhizome connections. *Ecology*, **68**, 2016–2022.

Shmida, A. & Ellner, S. (1984). Coexistence of plant species with similar niches. *Vegetatio*, **58**, 29–55.

Shmida, A. & Wilson, M. V. (1985). Biological determinants of species diversity. *Journal of Biogeography*, **12**, 1–21.

Šizling, A. L. & Storch, D. (2004). Power-law species-area relationships and self-similar species distributions within finite areas. *Ecology Letters*, **7**, 60–68.

ter Braak, C. J. F. (1987). *Unimodal Models to Relate Species to Environment*. Wageningen: Agricultural Mathematics Group.

ter Braak, C. J. F. & Prentice, I. C. (1988). A theory of gradient analysis. *Advances in Ecological Research*, **18**, 271–313.

Tilman, D. (1988). *Plant Strategies and the Dynamics and Structure of Plant Communities*. Princeton, NJ: Princeton University Press.

Tuomisto, H., Ruokolainen, K., Poulsen, A. D., *et al.* (2002). Distribution and diversity of pteridophytes and Melastomataceae along edaphic gradients in Yasuni National Park, Ecuadorian Amazonia. *Biotropica*, **34**, 516–533.

Umbanhowar Jr., C. E. (1995). Revegetation of earthen mounds along a topographic-productivity gradient in a northern mixed prairie. *Journal of Vegetation Science*, **6**, 637–646.

van der Maarel, E. (1995). Vicinism and mass effect in a historical perspective. *Journal of Vegetation Science*, **6**, 445–446.

von Humboldt, A. V. & Bonpland, A. (1807). *Essai sur la Geographie des Plantes*. Paris: Librarie Lebrault Schoell.

Wagner, H. H. (2003). Spatial covariance in plant communities: integrating ordination, geo-statistics and variance testing. *Ecology*, **84**, 1045–1057.

Wassen, M. J. & Barendregt, A. (1992). Topographic position and water chemistry of fens in a Dutch river plain. *Journal of Vegetation Science*, **3**, 447–456.

Whittaker, R. H. (1967). Gradient analysis of vegetation. *Biological Reviews*, **42**, 207–264.

Whittaker, R. H. (1972). Evolution and measure-ment of species diversity. *Taxon*, **21**, 213–251.

Whittaker, R. H. (1975). *Communities and Ecosystems*, 2nd edn. New York: Macmillan.

Whittaker, R. J. (1998). *Island Biogeography: Ecology, Evolution, and Conservation*. Oxford: Oxford University Press.

Wijesinghe, D. K. & Hutchings, M. J. (1997). The effects of spatial scale of environmental heterogeneity on the growth of a clonal plant: an experimental study with *Glechoma hederacea*. *Journal of Ecology*, **85**, 17–28.

Williamson, M. (1988). Relationship of species number to area, distance and other variables. In *Analytical Biogeography*, ed. A. A. Myers & P. S. Giller, pp. 91–115. New York: Chapman and Hall.

Williamson, M., Gaston, K. J. & Lonsdale, W. M. (2001). The species-area relationship does not have an asymptote! *Journal of Biogeography*, **28**, 827–830.

Withers, M. A., Palmer, M. W., Wade, G. L., White, P. S. & Neal, P. R. (1998). Changing patterns in the number of species in North American floras. In *Perspectives on the Land-Use History of North America: A Context for Understanding our Changing Environment*, ed. T. D. Sisk, pp. 23–32. USGS, Biological Resources Division, BSR/BDR-(1998-0003).

Wondzell, S. M., Cornelius, J. M. & Cunningham, G. L. (1990). Vegetation patterns, microtopography, and soils on a Chihuahuan desert playa. *Journal of Vegetation Science*, **1**, 403–410.

Zonneveld, I. S. (1995). Vicinism and mass effect. *Journal of Vegetation Science*, **6**, 441–444.

Zunzunegui, M., Diaz Barradas, M. C. & Garcia Novo, F. (1998). Vegetation fluctuation in mediterranean dune ponds in relation to rainfall variation and water extraction. *Journal of Vegetation Science*, **1**, 151–160.

# CHAPTER THREE

# The distribution of species: occupancy, scale, and rarity

FANGLIANG HE
*University of Alberta*
RICK CONDIT
*Smithsonian Tropical Research Institute*

## Introduction

Species occupancy is typically measured as the number of cells occupied by the species in a study area. Because it is easy to document and interpret and it correlates with species abundance, occupancy is widely used for measuring species rarity and for assessing extinction risk on which conservation decisions are made (Gaston, 1994; Fagan *et al.*, 2002; Hartley & Kunin, 2003; Wilson *et al.*, 2004). Ecologists and conservation practitioners, however, have long realized that occupancy often fails to capture significant spatial features of distribution. It is possible that two species having the same occupancy can exhibit very different patterns (Fig. 3.1). Most species in nature are discretely distributed due to the patchiness of landscapes, or due to intrinsic reproductive or dispersal behavior of the species. An outstanding problem concerning species distribution in space is how to describe the patchiness of a species and to measure the effect of changing spatial scale (cell size) on the patchiness for the purpose of predicting distribution at fine scales from coarse scales.

There are two primary approaches to addressing this question. The first one is to use existing measures and methods to describe patchiness and scale effect. Many fragmentation indices in landscape ecology can be used for this purpose (Turner, Gardner & O'Neill, 2001; Wu *et al.*, 2003). These include edge length (perimeter), the number of patches, perimeter/area ratio and many other indices to capture the spatial features of species distribution. An interesting development on this front is the percolation models for edge length and the number of patches proposed by He and Hubbell (2003). These models unify edge length, the number of patches, spatial scale and abundance and show that the edge length and number of patches of a distribution can accurately be predicted by the abundance of the species and the degree of fragmentation. These models are useful for analyzing and comparing species distributions.

*Scaling Biodiversity*, ed. David Storch, Pablo A. Marquet and James H. Brown. Published by Cambridge University Press. © Cambridge University Press 2007.

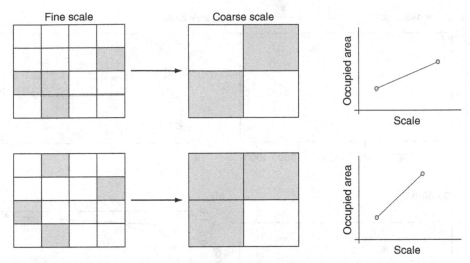

**Figure 3.1** Two species of the same occupancy but different distributions, leading to the difference in the occupancy in the coarse-scale maps and the slope of the occupancy–area relationship. Note the coarse-scale maps are produced by combining four adjacent cells on the fine-scale maps. If all the four fine-scale cells are empty, the coarse-scale cell is designated empty, otherwise occupied.

The second approach is to search for scale invariant properties of species distributions. This includes investigating fractal distribution of species (Kunin, 1998; Kunin, Hartley & Lennon, 2000; Hartley *et al.*, 2004) and employing the negative binomial distribution to quantify and estimate species abundances from coarse-scale distribution maps (He & Gaston, 2000; He, Gaston & Wu, 2002). The fractal method has been shown to be effective in quantifying distribution fragmentation and useful for assessing extinction risk of species, particularly of rare species (Fagan *et al.*, 2002; Wilson *et al.*, 2004). However, these methods meet with limited success in measuring species distributions and estimating abundance, particularly for relatively abundant species (Warren, McGeoch & Chown, 2003; Witte & Torfs, 2003; Tosh, Reyers & Jaarsveld, 2004). More often, the negative binomial method underestimates abundances while the fractal method overestimates (He & Gaston, 2000; Kunin *et al.*, 2000; Warren *et al.*, 2003; Witte & Torfs, 2003; Tosh *et al.*, 2004). Thus, the question about how we may predict distributions across multiple spatial scales remains largely unsolved. The capability to infer distributions across scales is essential for predicting distribution at fine scales from coarse scales, for determining the conservation status of species, and for making management plans and reserve design (Hartley & Kunin, 2003).

The primary objective of this study is to examine the scaling of several common occupancy–area models and thus identify models that may be independent of scale. Scale in this study is referred to as the cell size at which a

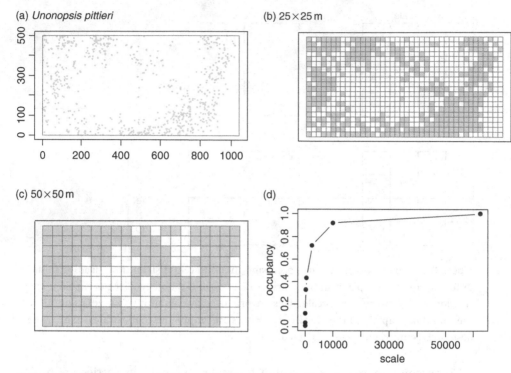

**Figure 3.2** (a) Distribution of 718 stems of *Unonopsis pittieri* in a 50 ha (1000 × 500 m) plot on Barro Colorado Island, Panama. Panels (b) and (c) are the occurrence maps at two mapping scales, and (d) plots the occupancy–area curve, i.e. the relationship between the proportion of occupied area of each map and scale (cell size).

distribution is gridded, and occupancy the proportion of grid cells in which a species is found (Fig. 3.1). First, we introduce several occupancy–area models, and show that a general model unifies them all. We evaluate the scaling properties for three of the models, the power-law model, the Nachman model, and the logistic model, using simulated and empirical data. We then use the three models to estimate occupancy at a fine scale from occupancy at coarse scales, and we compare the slope of occupancy versus area between rare and common species. We conclude with a discussion of the use of the three occupancy–area models for describing species distribution and for conservation practice.

## Occupancy–area models

Plotting species occupancy against spatial scale yields a monotonically increasing curve whose slope is steep at first but gradually becomes flat as scale increases (Fig. 3.2d). Some of the common occupancy–area models are given below. In the following $p$ is occupancy (the proportion of occupied area), $a$ is scale (or cell size), and $c$, $z$ and $k$ are parameters. While $c$ and $z$ must be positive $k$ can be any real number.

the power-law model (Kunin, 1998):  $p = ca^z$,

the Poisson model (Wright, 1991):  $p = 1 - e^{-a}$,

the negative binomial model (He & Gaston, 2000):  $p = 1 - \left(1 + \dfrac{a}{k}\right)^{-k}$,

the Nachman model (Nachman, 1981):  $p = 1 - e^{-ca^z}$,

the logistic model (Hanski & Gyllenberg, 1997; Leitner & Rosenzweig, 1997):

$$p = \frac{ca^z}{1 + ca^z}.$$

These models were originally developed for different purposes by different authors in the form of occupancy–abundance models. In those occupancy–abundance models, the occupancy $p$ is of the same interpretation as in the above occupancy–area models. The only difference is that the scale $a$ is replaced by mean density $\mu$ in occupancy–abundance models (see He *et al.*, 2002, for a detailed description of occupancy–abundance models). Although the derivation of the above occupancy–area models is largely empirical, the replacement of $\mu$ by $a$ is justified because abundance and area are widely found to have a simple linear relationship (Preston, 1962). For instance, the Poisson occupancy–abundance model, written as $p = 1 - e^{-\mu}$, was first developed to describe the relationship between occupancy and abundance (Wright, 1991), the Nachman model was initially used for predicting agricultural pest density from incidence data (Nachman, 1981), and the logistic model was for modeling the species–area relationship (Hanski & Gyllenberg, 1997). These models are now commonly used to describe occupancy–abundance relationships (Gaston, 1994; He *et al.*, 2002; Holt, Gaston & He, 2002). Replacing abundance $\mu$ in occupancy–abundance models by scale $a$, we obtain the occupancy–area curves listed in the above.

Interestingly, the five models can all be written with one general form (He *et al.*, 2002):

$$p = 1 - \left(1 + \frac{ca^z}{k}\right)^{-k},$$

(a)  when $c = z = 1$, the general model becomes the negative binomial model;

(b)  when $k = -1$, it is the power-law model;

(c)  when $k = 1$, it is the logistic model;

(d)  when $k \to \pm\infty$, it is the Nachman model;

(e)  when $k \to \pm\infty$ and $c = z = 1$, it is the Poisson model.

The application of the power-law model to describing species distribution is first proposed by Gaston (1994) and Kunin (1998) and has since become widely used. Beyond this power-law model, however, little is known about the scale-invariant property of other models. In the following, we examine this property for the Nachman and the logistic models together with the power-law model because they have similar linear forms, as given below.

the power-law model: $\log(p) = \log(c) + z\log(a)$,                                    (3.1)

the Nachman model: $\log[-\log(1 - p)] = \log(c) + z\log(a)$,                          (3.2)

the logistic model: $\log\left(\dfrac{p}{1-p}\right) = \log(c) + z\log(a)$.            (3.3)

These three models have the same right-hand terms but differ in their left-hand term. Although the slopes of the three models are not equal, they do change in the same direction, i.e. for a given occupancy if $z$ value is high for the power model, the $z$ values for the Nachman and the logistic models are also high. For a given occupancy at a fine scale small slopes indicate more aggregated distribution, while large slopes suggest more scattered distribution, as illustrated by Fig. 3.1.

## Testing the models

Three sets of data were used to test the performance of models 3.1–3.3: simulated fractal distributions, the local distributions of 301 tree populations in a 50 ha stem-mapped plot from Panama, and the regional distributions of 407 rare plant species of the United Kingdom.

### Random and fractal simulations

Neutral landscape models (Gardner *et al.*, 1987) were used to generate species distributions in an area of size $= 256 \times 256$ cells. The probability of being occupied or empty of each cell was determined by $p$. The neutral distribution models used here include simple random maps and fractal maps. In the simple random maps occupied/empty state of a cell is independent of any other cells, while in the fractal maps occupancy of a cell is spatially correlated with its neighboring cells. The fractal distributions were generated using the random midpoint displacement algorithm (Saupe, 1988). Spatial correlation of a map (i.e. the variance between locations separated by distance $x$) approximately equals $x^{2H}$. Varying $H$ from 0 to 1 corresponds to varying the distribution from extremely scattered to highly aggregated (With, Gardner & Turner, 1997; Turner *et al.*, 2001).

   To illustrate scale effect on distribution, we used a random (lattice) map and a fractal (lattice) map with $H = 0.1$ and calculated occupancy using a pixel size of 1, 2, 4, 8, ..., up to 256 (Fig. 3.3). The relationship between occupancy and scale is shown in Fig. 3.3 for each of the models. Although the power-law occupancy–area curve is linear at small scales, there is apparent curvature when a map approaches saturation (Fig. 3.3a). This curvature has traditionally been explained by the process of space filling near saturation due to finite study area. This concave-down curvature suggests that coarse-scale maps are not useful for estimating occupancy at fine scales. The departure from linearity will overestimate occupancy when extrapolating to smaller scales. The approximate linearity of the

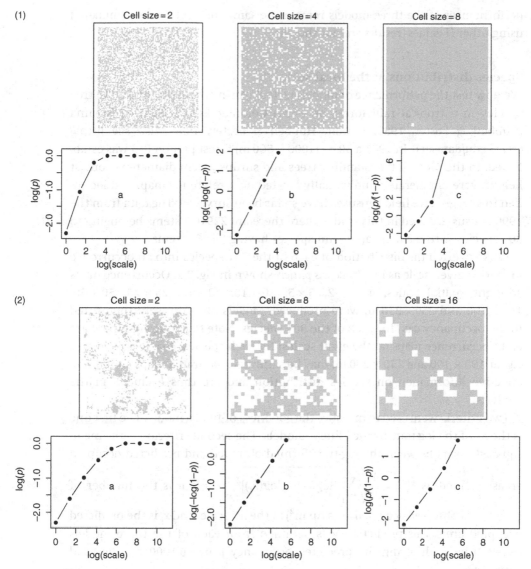

**Figure 3.3** Two simulated distributions at extent $256 \times 256$ cells and their occupancy–area curves. (1) First row shows the simple random maps at three scales: cell size $= 2 \times 2$, $4 \times 4$ and $8 \times 8$. Coarse-scale maps are aggregated from fine-scale maps. The second row shows occupancy–area curves corresponding to the power-law model (a), the Nachman model (b), and the logistic model (c). (2) The fractal distribution simulated with $H = 0.1$ and its three corresponding occupancy–area curves.

Nachman model (Fig. 3.3b) suggests it is a better model for describing the scale dependence, and the linearity seems to hold reasonably well even at near saturation of distribution. The logistic model (Fig. 3.3c) shows concave-up, meaning it will underestimate occupancy if used to extrapolate to smaller scales. The relative performances of the three models remain the same for fractal maps simulated using other $H$ values (results are not shown).

## Species distributions at the local scale

We now test the performance of models (3.1–3.3) using real distributions of tree species in a tropical rain forest on Barro Colorado Island (BCI) of Panama (Hubbell & Foster, 1983; Condit, Hubbell & Foster, 1996; also see http:// ctfs.si.edu/datasets). In 1981 a 50 ha (1000 × 500 m) forest plot on BCI was established. In the plot, all free-standing trees and shrubs ≥1 cm diameter at breast height were enumerated, individually located on a reference map, and identified to species. Five field censuses have so far been surveyed. The data from the 1990 census are used in this study where there are 229 048 stems belonging to 301 species with the most abundant species having 36 060 stems.

We converted the distribution of each of the 301 species into an occurrence map for a given scale as for *Unonopsis pittieri* shown in Fig. 3.2. Occurrence maps at eight spatial scales, $a = 2 \times 2$, $5 \times 5$, $10 \times 10$, $20 \times 20$, $25 \times 25$, $50 \times 50$, $100 \times 100$ and $250 \times 250$ m, were produced. Models (3.1–3.3) were then fitted to the occupancy data for each of the 301 species. Note that although there are eight occurrence maps (at the eight scales) for each species, coarse-scale maps, e.g. at $100 \times 100$ and $250 \times 250$ m, may be saturated. Saturated maps contain no effective information on species distribution and are thus excluded in the analysis.

Two criteria were used to measure the goodness-of-fit of a model. The first one is the $R^2$ of the log-transformed linear models. The second criterion is the mean squared errors between the log-transformed observed and predicted occupied areas, defined as $MSE = \dfrac{1}{n}\sqrt{\sum_{i=1}^{n}[\log(x_i) - \log(\hat{x}_i)]^2}$, where $n$ is the number of scales, $x_i$ is observed occupied area (in m$^2$) at the $i$th scale, and $\hat{x}_i$ is the predicted occupied area. This prediction was obtained from each of the three models (3.1–3.3) by multiplying the predicted occupancy $\hat{p}$ by 500 000 m$^2$ (the total study area).

Distributions of three species and their occupancy–area curves are shown in Fig. 3.4. The Nachman model describes well the scale dependence of species distribution and is clearly superior to the power and logistic models. The shapes of the curves in Fig. 3.4 precisely reflect those simulated in Fig. 3.3: concave-down for the power-law model, more or less linear for the Nachman model, but concave-up for the logistic model. It is worth noting that this general finding also applies to all the BCI species except those rare species with abundance <50. The three models work approximately equally well to those rare species.

To provide an overall judgment on how well the three models fit the BCI data, the histograms of the $R^2$ and $MSE$ for the log-log linear models (3.1–3.3) are

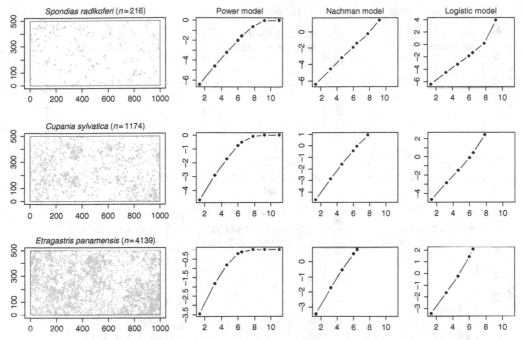

**Figure 3.4** Distributions of three BCI species and their occupancy–area curves. The shape of the power model is typically concave-up, while the logistic model concave-down. The Nachman model seems to be approximately linear. The x-axis of the occupancy–area curves is log(scale), the y-axis is log($p$) for the power model (second column), log[−log(1 − $p$)] for the Nachman model (third column), and log[$p$/(1 −$p$)] for the logistic model (fourth column). Here $p$ is occupancy,

plotted in Fig. 3.5. It is clear that the Nachman model has the largest overall $R^2$ and lowest MSE. The second best model is the logistic model and the power-law model is least satisfactory.

## Species distributions at the regional scale

The performance of models (3.1–3.3) was also tested and compared using 407 rare plant species from the UK (Kunin, 1998; Hartley et al., 2004). Each species was mapped at seven scales with cell size = $1 \times 1$, $2 \times 2$, $5 \times 5$, $10 \times 10$, $20 \times 20$, $50 \times 50$ and $100 \times 100$ km. The occupancy–area curves for three of the species are shown in Fig. 3.6; most of the curves show a slight concave-down shape, which differs from the simulations (Fig. 3.3) and the local-scale BCI data (Fig. 3.4). Previous studies have shown that these UK plant species could be adequately modeled by the power model (Kunin, 1998; Hartley et al., 2004). Our results in Fig. 3.7 support this conclusion. As judged by $R^2$ and the MSE, all the three models describe the occupancy–area curves sufficiently well. There is no definite superior model although the Nachman seems to perform slightly better than the other two models. The indistinguishable results are probably due to the fact that the UK plants are rare species.

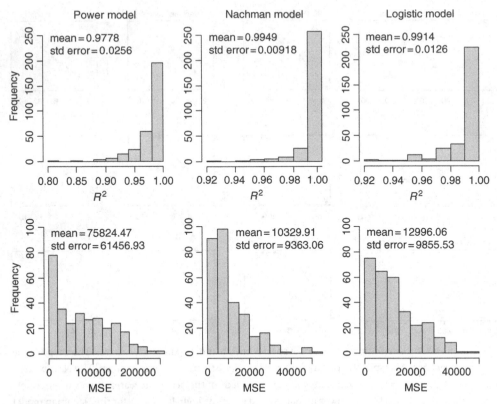

**Figure 3.5** Histograms of $R^2$ and $MSE$ (mean squared errors) indicating the goodness-of-fit of the three models (3.1–3.3) fitting to each of the 301 species distributions. High $R^2$ or low $MSE$ suggests a good fit of a model.

## Estimating occupancy at fine scales from the occupancy at coarse scales

We now turn to use models (3.1–3.3) to estimate occupancy at fine scales from the occupancy at coarse scales for both the BCI and UK data. Two predictions are made here. The first prediction uses the two maps at the coarsest unsaturated scales to predict occupancy at a very fine scale. For most BCI species, this means to use maps at $50 \times 50$ and $100 \times 100$ m to predict occupancy at $2 \times 2$ m. For highly abundant species (>3000 trees) the coarsest unsaturated maps are at $25 \times 25$ and $50 \times 50$ m. For the UK rare species, the coarsest unsaturated maps are $50 \times 50$ and $100 \times 100$ km. They were used to estimate occupancy at $1 \times 1$ km. We also repeated the estimation but used the three (instead of two) coarsest maps to estimate occupancy at $2 \times 2$ m in the case of the BCI species and occupancy at $1 \times 1$ km in the case of the UK species.

The power-law model predicts occupancy well for rare BCI species at $2 \times 2$ m (Fig. 3.8), but overestimates for abundant species because of the curvature in the

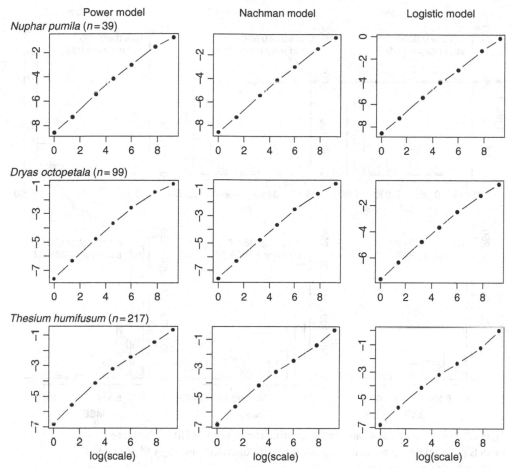

**Figure 3.6.** Occupancy–area curves for three plant species from the UK. The number of occupied cells of the base map (i.e. the map at the finest scale of 1 × 1 km) is 39, 99 and 217 for *Nuphar pumila*, *Dryas octopetala* and *Thesium humifusum*, respectively. The first column is the power model, the *y*-axis is log(*p*). The second column is the Nachman model with *y*-axis log[−log(1 − *p*)]. The third column is the logistic model with *y*-axis log[*p*/(1 − *p*)].

occupancy–area curves (Figs. 3.3 and 3.4). In contrast, the logistic model underestimates due to the opposite curvature (Figs. 3.3 and 3.4). The Nachman model lies in the middle between the power and logistic models and is superior to both, although there is some degree of overestimation. Estimation is much improved by using three maps (Fig. 3.8, bottom row) although this does not change the relative performance of the three models. This result suggests that we should aggregate as many maps as possible (up to saturation) from an observed distribution in order to accurately scale down occupancy at fine scales. Every map up to saturation helps increase accuracy. The Nachman model has the smallest deviation from the observed occupancy (Table 3.1).

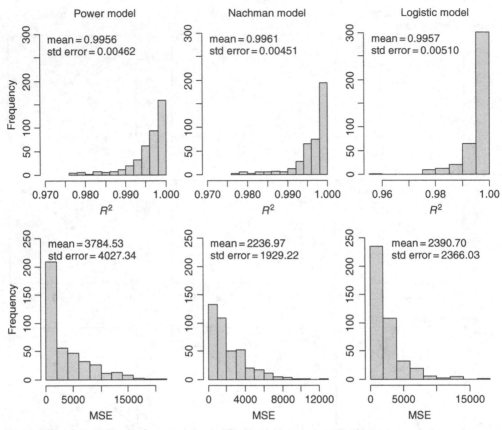

**Figure 3.7** Histograms of $R^2$ and *MSE* indicating the goodness-of-fit of the three models (3.1–3.3) fitting to each of the 407 UK plant distributions. High $R^2$ or low *MSE* means a good fit of a model.

Although a similar result is also observed from the UK data, the difference in the estimation accuracy among the three models is much smaller (Table 3.1, Fig. 3.9). None of the models satisfactorily estimates the occupancy at $1 \times 1$ km from the two coarsest maps, although their performance is substantially improved by using three coarsest maps (Fig. 3.9). Overall, the power model still relatively overestimates the occupancy compared with the Nachman model, while the logistic model underestimates it.

## Comparing the slope between rare and common species
If there is a difference in distribution between rare and common species, the difference should be manifest in the slope of an occupancy–area curve. In other words, the $z$ values of the three models (3.1–3.3) should be correlated with abundance. This correlation is inevitable for abundant species that cover more than 25% of the study area (25% because four fine cells are combined into one coarse cell when scaling up distribution). However, in BCI the most abundant

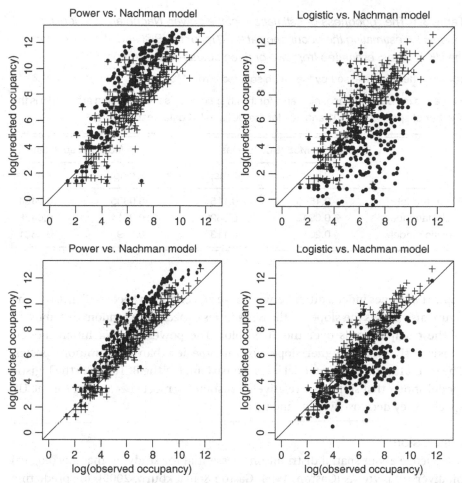

**Figure 3.8** Log-log plot for the estimated occupied area versus the observed area at $2 \times 2$ m scale for the 301 BCI species. The first row is the estimation made from the two coarsest unsaturated maps. The second row is the estimation made from the three coarsest unsaturated maps. Each point represents a species. The crosses are the occupied area estimated from the Nachman model, the filled dots are either from the power model or from the logistic model. If the estimation is accurate, all the points should lie on the diagonal line.

species *Ampea appendiculata* only has 22.89% occupancy at scale $2 \times 2$ m. All the UK plants are rare species, their occupancies are much smaller. Therefore, the slope of an occupancy–area curve for the BCI and UK species should, to a degree, reflect the difference in distribution between rare and common species.

Because abundances for the UK species are unknown, to be consistent we use the occupancy at the finest scale as a proxy for abundance in both data. This means the occupancy at $2 \times 2$ m for the BCI species and occupancy at $1 \times 1$ km for the UK species. The relationships between $z$ and abundance of the species

**Table 3.1** *The "goodness-of-estimation" of the power, Nachman, and logistic models for estimating the occupancy at 2 × 2 m for the BCI and at 1 × 1 km for the UK species, estimated from two or three coarse-scaled maps*

The goodness is assessed by the mean squared errors $MSE = \frac{1}{n}\sqrt{\sum(\log(x_i) - \log(\hat{x}_i))^2}$, where $x_i$ is the observed occupied area for the $i$th species, $\hat{x}_i$ is the estimated area and $n$ is the number of species ($n = 301$ and 407 for the BCI and UK data, respectively).

|  | MSE (BCI species) | | MSE (UK species) | |
|---|---|---|---|---|
|  | 2 maps | 3 maps | 2 maps | 3 maps |
| Power model | 0.1588 | 0.115 | 0.0835 | 0.0484 |
| Nachman model | 0.0942 | 0.0629 | 0.0814 | 0.0438 |
| Logistic model | 0.201 | 0.113 | 0.109 | 0.0501 |

show that slopes indeed differ between rare and common species (Fig. 3.10). The figure also shows the slopes of the BCI species expected by random distribution of the occupied cells over the 50 ha plot. The power and Nachman models consistently predict higher slopes for rare species than for common species. The result for the logistic model is less consistent. For the BCI species the logistic model shows that slopes are relatively constant for most species, but for the UK species they decrease with abundance.

## Discussion

Knowledge about spatial distribution is essential for studying macroecological biodiversity patterns (Gaston, 1994; Gaston & Blackburn, 2000), for predicting the distribution of species in areas where observations are not available (Heikkinen & Högmander, 1994; MacKenzie *et al.*, 2002; Raxworthy *et al.*, 2003), for understanding environmental determination of species distribution (Currie, 1991; Lennon, Greenwoord & Turner, 2000; He, Zhou & Zhu, 2003; Hurlbert & Haskell, 2003), for assessing the effect of landscape fragmentation and climate change on extinction (Thomas *et al.*, 2004; Fagan *et al.*, 2005), and for planning biological conservation priority (Myers *et al.*, 2000). However, the scale dependence of spatial distributions is sometimes considered as a statistical and ecological nuisance that prevents the prediction of species distribution across scales, thus hampering our ability to determine species' conservation status across scales.

Our study has enforced this adverse impression and found that the description of species distributions remains elusive and few species are scale independent in distribution. There exists no universal, genuinely scale-independent model applicable to all species across scales, although the Nachman model is

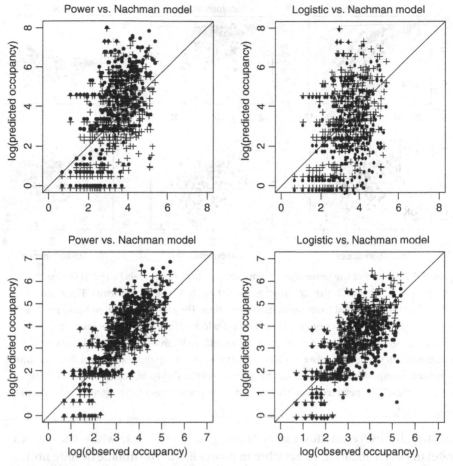

**Figure 3.9** Log-log plot for the estimated occupied area versus the observed area at 1 × 1 km scale for the 407 UK species. The first row is the estimation made from the two coarsest unsaturated maps. The second row is the estimation made from the three coarsest unsaturated maps. Each point represents a species. The crosses are the occupied area estimated from the Nachman model, the filled dots are either from the power model or from the logistic model. If the estimation is perfect, all the points should lie on the diagonal line.

most robust to scaling effect among the three models we tested. From the practical point of view, the Nachman model is superior in two aspects. First, it consistently shows a linear relationship between occupancy and scale up to a certain level for almost all of the species from both the local BCI trees and the regional UK rare plants. Simulation results shown in Fig. 3.3 also reveal the linearity of the Nachman model even at near map saturation (compare the two nearly perfect lines in Fig. 3.3b against the evident curvature in Fig. 3.3a and 3.3c). Second, the Nachman model is apparently the best model for estimating occupancy at fine scales from data of coarse scales. The power-law model

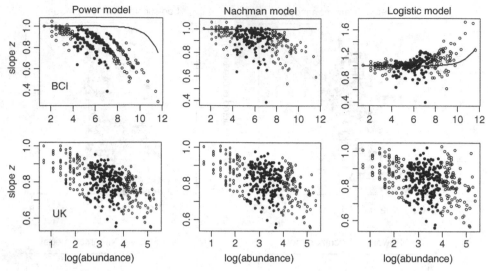

**Figure 3.10** Slope $z$ of the power-law, Nachman and logistic models (3.1–3.3) versus occupancy at $2 \times 2$ m (BCI, the first row) and $1 \times 1$ km (UK, the second row). The curves for BCI are the slope expected from random distribution. They were calculated by: (i) randomly allocating the same number of occupied cells at scale $2 \times 2$ m for each species over the study area, (ii) aggregating up by combining four fine cells to form one coarse scale cell, and (iii) fitting each occupancy–area model to the two scale occupancy–area data. Because only the overall occupancy is known to us the same expected slope cannot be calculated for the UK species. The open circles on the two sides are the species of the 1st and 3rd quantiles of abundance.

substantially overestimates the occupancy at fine scales, while the logistic model underestimates it. The Nachman model lies in the middle despite noticeable overestimation (Figs. 3.8 and 3.9). It is important to note that estimation is significantly improved if occupancy is estimated from three or more maps (see the bottom panels in Figs. 3.8 and 3.9) or if the maps on which the estimation is based are relatively fine-scaled.

An interesting result of this study is that slopes of the three models (3.1–3.3) consistently decrease with abundance except the logistic model for abundant BCI species (Fig. 3.10). Three implications of this result are in order. First, it suggests that there are differences in spatial distribution between rare and common species. Rare species show a tendency of scattered distribution, while common species tend to be more aggregated. Second, the fact that rare species have significantly larger slopes than the common species as predicted by the power-law and Nachman models suggests that rare species fill up space more quickly than common species when scaling up. As a consequence, determination of species rarity based on occupancy at coarse scales can be substantially biased because species of the same occupancy at the coarse scale may have very different occupancies at the fine scale (i.e. the scaling down in Fig. 3.1), conforming to the result of Hartley and Kunin (2003). Third, the dependence of the slope on abundance implies that the slope of a scaling model alone is not sufficient to describe spatial distribution. A good index of spatial pattern ought to be independent of the abundance of species; it has been a methodological challenge to develop such a measure in ecology, and scaling models are no exception.

Whether a species is considered fractal is debatable, depending on how fractal is defined and measured for an empirical distribution which is always of finite size (Cutler, 1993). An important point is that an adequate fitting of the power-law model does not necessarily imply fractal in distribution. Our study is not designed to test the self-similarity properties of species distribution but to investigate the utility of the three occupancy–area models in describing distribution. However, our results show that many species do have similar occupancy–area shapes as those produced from fractal simulations as shown in Fig. 3.3. The breakdown in linearity near map saturation is inevitably caused by space filling due to finite study area. This saturated region is routinely suggested to be excluded from the calculation of fractal dimensions (Halley et al., 2004) although such practice is not the best interest to many applications. From the practical point of view, it is also important to model the curvature as it is an inherent component of the data (Šizling & Storch, 2004).

In summary, we have studied scale-invariant property of species distribution for three occupancy–area models. The findings of the study should shed a light on our understanding of species distribution and provide potentially useful tools for determining the rarity of species for the purpose of conservation. The main results of the study include:

1. No occupancy model is universally superior in describing occupancy data. Among the three models intensively tested in this study, the Nachman model appears to be most robust to scaling effect. It is superior to the power-law and the logistic models in describing species distribution and for predicting occupancy across scales.
2. All empirically observed distributions share a similar occupancy–area shape that increases linearly at small scales but saturates at coarse scales due to space filling. Empirical occupancy–area curves have similar shapes as those simulated from fractal distributions. However, this similarity should not be interpreted as an implication of fractality because the occupancy–area models alone are not appropriate for measuring self-similarity.
3. An important application of occupancy–area models is to estimate species abundance from occupancy. The accuracy is substantially improved if three (or more) rather than two scale maps are used to estimate occupancy at any fine scale. In other words, every coarse-scale map up to saturation is useful for scaling down occupancy at fine scales. The Nachman model which is most robust to scaling effect is a best model for estimating abundance.

4. Distributions are different between rare and common species. The slopes of the log-log occupancy curves are significantly higher for rare than for common species, suggesting that rare species fill up space more rapidly than common species when scaling up. Therefore, determination of species rarity based on occupancy at coarse scales can be substantially biased. If rarity of a species has to be determined and coarse-scale maps are the only data available, the Nachman model must be used to calculate the occupancy at finer scales.

5. The difference among the power, the Nachman and the logistic models for the UK plants seems not to be as evident as for the BCI data. This perhaps reflects the fact that all the UK plants are rare species. Therefore, further testing and comparison of the three models using regional distribution data for both rare and common species are still needed in order to ensure the superiority of the Nachman model at the regional scale.

## Acknowledgments

We are grateful to Jack Lennon and David Storch and many colleagues at the "Scaling Biodiversity" workshop for their very constructive comments, which greatly improved this chapter. We particularly thank Bill Kunin for providing the distribution data of the UK rare plants. This work is supported by the Alberta Ingenuity Fund and the Natural Science and Engineering Research Council of Canada.

## References

Condit, R., Hubbell, S. P. & Foster, R. B. (1996). Changes in tree species abundance in a Neotropical forest: impact of climate change. *Journal of Tropical Ecology*, **12**, 231–256.

Currie, D. J. (1991). Energy and large scale patterns of animal and plant species richness. *American Naturalist*, **137**, 27–49.

Cutler, C. D. (1993). A review of the theory and estimation of fractal dimension. In *Nonlinear Time Series and Chaos*. Vol. I: *Dimension Estimation and Models*, ed. H. Tong, pp. 1–107. Singapore: World Scientific.

Fagan, W. F., Unmack, P. J., Burgess, C. & Minckley, W. L. (2002). Rarity, fragmentation, and extinction risk in desert fishes. *Ecology*, **83**, 3250–3256.

Fagan, W. F., Aumann, C., Kennedy, C. M. & Unmack, P. J. (2005). Rarity, fragmentation, and the scale dependence of extinction risk in desert fishes. *Ecology*, **86**, 34–41.

Gardner, R. H., Milne, B. T., Turner, M. G. & O'Neill, R. V. (1987). Neutral models for the analysis of broad-scale landscape patterns. *Landscape Ecology*, **1**, 19–28.

Gaston, K. J. (1994). *Rarity*. London: Chapman and Hall.

Gaston, K. J. & Blackburn, T. M. (2000). *Patterns and Process in Macroecology*. Oxford: Blackwell Science.

Halley, J. M., Hartley, S., Kallimanis, A. S., Kunin, W. E., Lennon, J. J. & Sgardelis, S. P. (2004). Uses and abuses of fractal methodology in ecology. *Ecology Letters*, **7**, 254–271.

Hanski, I. & Gyllenberg, M. (1997). Uniting two general patterns in the distribution of species. *Science*, **275**, 397–400.

Hartley, S. & Kunin, W. E. (2003). Scale dependency of rarity, extinction risk, and conservation priority. *Conservation Biology*, **17**, 1559–1570.

Hartley, S., Kunin, W. E., Lennon, J. L. & Pocock, M. J. (2004). Coherence and discontinuity in the scaling of species' distribution patterns. *Proceedings of the Royal Society of London, Series B*, **271**, 81–88.

He, F. & Gaston, K. J. (2000). Estimating species abundance from occurrence. *American Naturalist*, **156**, 553–559.

He, F. L. & Hubbell, S. P. (2003). Percolation theory for the distribution and abundance of species. *Physical Review Letters*, **91**, Art. No. 198103.

He, F., Gaston, K. J. & Wu, J. (2002). On species occupancy-abundance models. *Écoscience*, **9**, 119–126.

He, F., Zhou, J. & Zhu H. T. (2003). Autologistic regression model for the distribution of vegetation. *Journal of Agricultural, Biological, and Environmental Statistics*, **8**, 205–222.

Heikkinen, J. & Högmander, H. (1994). Fully Bayesian approach to image restoration with an application in biogeography. *Applied Statistics*, **43**, 569–582.

Holt, A. R., Gaston, K. J. & He, F. (2002). Occupancy-abundance relationships and spatial distribution: a review. *Basic and Applied Ecology*, **3**, 1–13.

Hubbell, S. P. & Foster, R. B. (1983). Diversity of canopy trees in a neotropical forest and implications for conservation. In *Tropical Rain Forest: Ecology and Management*, ed. S. L. Sutton, T. C. Whitmore & A. C. Chadwick, pp. 25–41. Oxford: Blackwell Scientific Publications.

Hurlbert, A. H. & Haskell, J. P. (2003). The effect of energy and seasonality on avian species richness and community composition. *American Naturalist*, **161**, 83–97.

Kunin, W. E. (1998). Extrapolating species abundance across spatial scales. *Science*, **281**, 1513–1515.

Kunin, W. E., Hartley, S. & Lennon, J. J. (2000). Scaling down: on the challenge of estimating abundance from occurrence patterns. *American Naturalist*, **156**, 560–566.

Leitner, W. A. & Rosenzweig, M. L. (1997). Nested species-area curves and stochastic sampling: a new theory. *Oikos*, **79**, 503–512.

Lennon, J. J., Greenwoord, J. J. D. & Turner, J. R. G. (2000). Bird diversity and environmental gradients in Britain: a test of the species–energy hypothesis. *Journal of Animal Ecology*, **69**, 581–598.

MacKenzie, D. I., Nichols, J. D., Lachman, G. B., Droege, S., Royle, J. A. & Langtimm, C. A. (2002). Estimating site occupancy rates when detection probabilities are less than one. *Ecology*, **83**, 2248–2255.

Myers, N., Mittermeier, R. A., Mittermeier, C. G., da Fonseca, G. A. B. & Kent, J. (2000). Biodiversity hotspots for conservation priorities. *Nature*, **403**, 853–858.

Nachman, G. (1981). A mathematical model of the functional relationship between density and spatial distribution of a population. *Journal of Animal Ecology*, **50**, 453–460.

Preston, F. W. (1962). The canonical distribution of commonness and rarity: Part I. *Ecology*, **43**, 185–215.

Raxworthy, C. J., Martinez-Meyer, E., Horning, N. *et al.* (2003). Predicting distributions of known and unknown reptile species in Madagascar. *Nature*, **426**, 837–841.

Saupe, D. (1988). Algorithms for random fractals. In *The Science of Fractal Images*, ed. H. O. Peitgen & D. Saupe, pp. 71–113. New York: Springer-Verlag.

Šizling, A. I. & Storch, D. (2004). Power-law species-area relationships and self-similar species distributions within finite areas. *Ecology Letters*, **7**, 60–68.

Thomas, C. D., Cameron, A., Green, R. E. *et al.* (2004). Extinction risk from climate change. *Nature*, **427**, 145–148.

Tosh, C. A., Reyers, B. & Jaarsveld, A. S. (2004). Estimating the abundances of large herbivores in the Kruger National Park using presence-absence data. *Animal Conservation*, **7**, 55–61.

Turner, M. G., Gardner, R. H. & O'Neill, R. V. (2001). *Landscape Ecology in Theory and Practice*. New York: Springer-Verlag.

Warren, M., McGeoch, M. A. & Chown, S. L. (2003). Predicting abundance from occupancy: a test for an aggregated assemblage. *Journal of Animal Ecology*, **72**, 468–477.

Wilson, R. J., Thomas, C. D., Fox, R., Roy, D. B. & Kunin, W. E. (2004). Spatial patterns in species distributions reveal biodiversity change. *Nature*, **432**, 393–396.

With, K. A., Gardner, R. H. & Turner, M. G. (1997). Landscape connectivity and population distributions in heterogeneous environments. *Oikos*, **78**, 151–169.

Witte, J. P. M. & Torfs, P. J. J. F. (2003). Scale dependency and fractal dimension of rarity. *Ecography*, **26**, 60–68.

Wright, D. H. (1991). Correlations between incidence and abundance are expected by chance. *Journal of Biogeography*, **18**, 463–466.

Wu, J., Shen, W.-J., Sun, W.-Z. & Tueller, P. T. (2003). Empirical patterns of the effects of changing scale on landscape metrics. *Landscape Ecology*, **17**, 761–782.

# CHAPTER FOUR

# Species distribution patterns, diversity scaling and testing for fractals in southern African birds

JACK J. LENNON
*The Macaulay Institute, Aberdeen*
WILLIAM E. KUNIN
*University of Leeds*
STEPHEN HARTLEY
*Victoria University of Wellington*
KEVIN J. GASTON
*University of Sheffield*

## Introduction

Describing and ultimately understanding species distribution and biodiversity patterns is undoubtedly one of the major goals in ecology (Gaston, 2000). Spatial scale is an extremely important issue here, and the topic is deservedly now getting more attention than hitherto (for example, Lomolino, 2000; Whittaker, Willis & Field, 2001). There is considerable interest in applying fractal and related cross-scale analytical methods to species distribution patterns, with a view to describing these patterns parsimoniously, connecting cross-scale species incidence with emergent properties such as the species–area relationship (Harte & Kinzig, 1997; Harte, Kinzig & Green, 1999; Plotkin *et al.*, 2000; Harte, Blackburn & Ostling, 2001; Šizling & Storch, 2004; Kunin & Lennon, 2005), predicting abundance at fine scales from coarse scale information (Kunin, 1998; He & Gaston, 2000; Kunin, Hartley & Lennon, 2000; Gaston, 2003), identifying scaling regions and breakpoints (see Hartley *et al.*, 2004) and detecting scale invariance in populations (Keitt *et al.*, 2002). Although the roots of these cross-scale ideas lie partly in more familiar ecological pattern-analysis methods (for a good summary see Dale, 1998; Fortin & Dale, 2005), they offer exciting new ways of describing and thinking about species distribution patterns that may, ultimately, lead to a much better understanding of the ecological processes involved in their generation.

Despite this large and growing body of work, on the whole surprisingly little is known about the scaling properties of species distribution patterns. Most of the present chapter is concerned with two straightforward and rather fundamental questions about them: (a) do coarse-scale properties of species

*Scaling Biodiversity*, ed. David Storch, Pablo A. Marquet and James H. Brown. Published by Cambridge University Press. © Cambridge University Press 2007.

distribution patterns differ from fine-scale properties and, if so, (b) are there consistent trends in the nature of these differences for most species? In other words, is there a general rule governing how spatial patterns in species distributions (aggregated or random, continuous or patchy) change as one moves between coarser and finer scales of resolution? Does the degree of aggregation in such distribution patterns stay roughly constant for most species across scales, or are there general trends? If there are such trends, do species tend to have sparser, more "random" distributions when mapped at fine scales rather than coarse scales, or alternatively, is the opposite the case, with more clumped or aggregated distributions at fine scales? Do such trends, if evident, suggest that distribution patterns arise from a hierarchical sequence of spatial processes, each with a characteristic scale or range of scales of influence, or do these trends act gradually over a wide range of scales?

To begin to approach these questions, we clearly need some baseline to compare with observed patterns. Is there a single, useful null model for species distribution patterns that would do? A brief digression into commonly used ways of modeling spatial structure may be helpful here (see Dale, 1998; and Fortin & Dale, 2005, for more detail). Perhaps the most familiar spatial pattern is what ecologists usually mean by a "random" pattern, and what statisticians describe as a realization of a homogeneous Poisson process, producing "complete spatial randomness" (CSR; Cressie, 1991). For use as a null model, we reject CSR on the grounds that not only are species distributions conspicuously *not* examples of CSR, virtually *every* spatial pattern in nature, biotic or abiotic, is positively spatially autocorrelated (aggregated). Therefore, we need to consider aggregation. In ecology, this has for the most part meant using variance-mean ratios, $k$ of the negative binomial (Pielou, 1977), mean-variance power laws (Taylor, 1961), and the semivariogram/autocorrelation/spectral decomposition group of methods (Fortin & Dale, 2005). For our purposes, all have shortcomings in terms of arbitrariness and interpretability. For example, $k$ is generally dependent on abundance (Taylor, Woiwod & Perry, 1979) and is sensitive to spatial scale, Taylor's power law (Taylor, 1961) is an empirical description of pattern with parameters that are difficult to interpret, and semivariogram analysis ("universal kriging"; see Cressie, 1991) is primarily concerned with making accurate local predictions rather than detecting general scaling properties. There is ample scope for confusing an inherent scale dependency in methods with a true scale dependency in real distribution patterns. We emphasize that these methods have their own strengths and particular applications, but in order to develop a framework for describing spatial scaling properties of distribution patterns we need to focus on spatial scale directly.

We argue that the most useful null model for species distributions is the fractal paradigm (Mandelbrot, 1983; Hastings & Sugihara, 1993; Falconer, 2003;

Halley *et al.*, 2004), which has been so productive in many areas of science. By definition, a stochastic fractal pattern appears statistically identical at any mapping resolution; a "closer look" at a smaller piece of the pattern on magnification reveals this to be statistically indistinguishable from the whole. At any scale of mapping it is as disordered (in terms of aggregation/ randomness) as at any other scale. This property makes fractals arguably the simplest multiscale distributional model, and thus a natural choice for a null scaling model against which actual distributions might be compared. Yet the use of fractals as a null model for scaling has faced a serious problem in the past: there is no published method (to our knowledge) available to measure the degree to which an observed spatial pattern departs from such uniform scaling behavior. Just as conventional spatial statistics measure departure from CSR (that is: nonrandom levels of aggregation or overdispersion) at a single scale, we need to develop statistical techniques to measure departure from constant scaling (that is: systematic shifts towards more or less aggregated distributions across scales). This chapter will help to fill that gap. By mapping real species patterns at a series of spatial scales, we can make comparisons with the scaling properties of a true fractal pattern. This allows us to quantify and characterize deviations from the fractal null model at particular scales. For example, we can detect whether a real species distribution is more random (less aggregated) at fine than coarse scales, or vice versa. In order to do this, we need to introduce some novel cross-scale modeling and analytical methods.

Our goals in this chapter are roughly fivefold. First, we argue that fractal spatial structure is a useful conceptual and practical null model for species distributions. Second, we introduce a new cross-scale model that allows a range of scaling properties to be described, and systematic departure from fractal scaling to be quantified. Third, we fit this cross-scale model to bird distribution patterns using novel maximum likelihood methods, allowing us to take an individual species distribution pattern and test statistically for differences between its coarse- and fine-scale spatial structure. Fourth, we see how differences found between scaling structure at the species level translate into differences in the distribution and scaling of community (species richness, for example) patterns. Finally, we discuss whether our results can tell us anything about the existence and properties of hierarchical spatial processes involved in determining both species distribution and diversity patterns.

## Methods

First, we describe and comment on the fractal approach, then using it as a conceptual base we develop a more general cross-scale model and finally we apply both models to species distribution patterns of southern African birds.

## The fractal model

The fractal model defines a simple power-law relationship between species incidence and mapping scale (high resolution = fine scale): the total area of occupied quadrats is a (usually fractional) power of the quadrat size used to map a species distribution (Hastings & Sugihara, 1993; Kunin, 1998). As the study area is subdivided using smaller and smaller quadrats, the total area occupied shrinks (but the number of occupied quadrats grows) such that

$$p(s) = p_0 s^{D-2},\tag{4.1}$$

where $D$ is the box-counting fractal dimension, and $p$ is the proportion of quadrats occupied at scale $s$ (quadrat area $= s^2$). The coarsest scale is defined as $s = 1$, a single quadrat covering the entire study area. The parameter $p_0$ is expected to be unity for a stochastic fractal, but typically an empirical fit allows $p_0$ to vary (Hastings & Sugihara, 1993). Currently there is some debate as to the meaning of $p_0$. Originally, Mandelbrot (1983) suggested that this single number summarized the *lacunarity* of a pattern (roughly speaking, the size distribution of "holes" within it), but more recently lacunarity has been described as a function of scale, and not as a single number (Plotnik *et al.*, 1996; Halley *et al.*, 2004).

To draw out the meaning of what is implied by Eq. (4.1), another way of looking at the fractal model is to consider the probability that a particular subquadrat within an occupied larger quadrat is also occupied. In a stochastic fractal pattern, this probability is a fixed value, independent of scale. In other words, if we divide an occupied quadrat into a fixed number $q$ subquadrats, we expect to find a fixed fraction $f$ of them occupied. If we then choose one of these occupied subquadrats and divide it into $q$ sub-subquadrats, then again there will be the same expected fraction $f$ of these occupied (Fig. 4.1a). The box-counting $D$ expected in terms of these parameters (see Falconer, 2003) is

$$D = 2\left(1 + \frac{\log f}{\log q}\right).\tag{4.2}$$

It is clear from this definition, and from the general concept of statistical self-similarity, that for a particular fractal object an occupied quadrat of any size possesses the same amount of disorder in the pattern of occupied subquadrats contained within it: the extent to which the pattern within is random (in the homogeneous-Poisson sense) or aggregated (in the sense of positive spatial autocorrelation) is independent of scale.

There is obviously a connection between $p$ and $D$: if both $p$ and mapping scale are known, then $D$ is determined by Eq. (4.1) (*if* the species truly has a fractal distribution). Since $p$ determines coverage (percentage area occupied), knowing the coverage at a particular resolution means that $D$ is also known. This makes $D$ a less useful way of characterizing different kinds of species distributions, since $D$ has to be relatively large (close to 2) for geographically common species with

COARSE SCALE ⟶ FINE SCALE

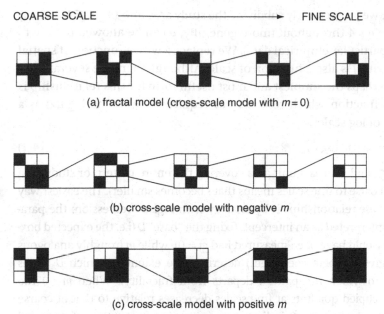

(a) fractal model (cross-scale model with $m = 0$)

(b) cross-scale model with negative $m$

(c) cross-scale model with positive $m$

**Figure 4.1** Spatial scaling behavior of species distribution patterns. The incidence of occupied quadrats (dark shading) at different scales, the proportion of occupied subquadrats on subdivision of occupied quadrats, may or may not show trends across spatial scales. (a) A random fractal distribution: subdivision of every occupied quadrat reveals the same proportion of occupied subquadrats, on average. (b) The cross-scale model (Eqs. 4.2–4.5): a negative value of the $m$ parameter indicates that the proportion of occupied subquadrats within occupied quadrats diminishes at finer scales. (c) The cross-scale model with positive $m$: an increasing proportion of subquadrats within occupied quadrats are occupied at finer scales.

high percentage cover, and small (close to 0) for rare species. This redundancy between $D$ and $p$ disappears if we allow $p_0$ to take values other than unity (see Lennon, Kunin & Hartley, 2002; Šizling & Storch, 2004).

**The cross-scale model**

In order to understand and quantify deviations from the fractal null model, we now relax the assumption of a constant $f$. The proportion of subquadrats occupied within an occupied quadrat can now be permitted to change with scale, as shown in Fig. 4.1(b) and (c). We therefore need a function to describe how $f$ changes with scale. Obviously, it is required that $f$ can grow or diminish at finer scales, but it is also desirable that the function returns a value of $f$ bounded between 0 and 1. Let us rewrite Eq. (4.2) such that

$$f = q^{-\lambda}, \tag{4.3}$$

where $\lambda = 1 - D/2$ in a fractal: a smaller $\lambda$ indicates a larger $D$, and $\lambda$ ranges from zero when $D = 2$, to one when $D = 0$ (see Eq. 4.2). As mentioned above, $q$ is the subdivision factor from one scale to the next. For example, in the case we consider below, we progressively subdivide the study area into $\{4, 16, 64, 256 \dots\}$ quadrats, hence $q = 4$ throughout (more generally, $q$ can be allowed to vary to accommodate particular empirical data). We replace $\lambda$ with a function of spatial scale, meaning that $f$ is also a function of scale. Although there are several ways of doing this, perhaps the simplest and most useful form for this relationship is to use the *logit* function which restricts $f$ as required. We define logit($\lambda$) as a linear function of log scale:

$$\log(\lambda/(1 - \lambda)) = \alpha + m \log s, \tag{4.4}$$

where scale $s \leq 1$, and $s = 1$ is a unit area covering the entire pattern or study area (changing from coarse to fine scales means that $s$ becomes smaller). The easiest way to understand these relationships is by analogy with logistic regression: the parameter $\alpha$ can be interpreted as an intercept, fixing the "base" $D$ (i.e. the expected box-counting $D$ that would have been measured had $m = 0$), while $m$ (roughly analogous to a logistic regression beta coefficient) describes the extent to which $D$ varies (i.e. the degree to which the pattern departs from fractality). When $m < 0$ the proportion of occupied quadrats at fine scales decreases relative to that at coarse scales (Fig. 4.1b), whereas $m > 0$ indicates an increasing proportion of occupied quadrats at fine scales relative to that at coarse scales (Fig. 4.1c). Where $m = 0$ the pattern is fractal ($f$ constant across scales), with a $D$ fixed by the fitted constant $\alpha$ (Fig. 4.1a). A reduced proportional occupancy at fine scales produces less aggregated, more disordered distribution patterns at fine scales compared with coarse scales. Conversely, an increase in relative occupancy at fine scales is indicative of patterns with greater aggregation and reduced randomness relative to coarse scales.

So far, we have developed a way of allowing the proportion of subquadrats occupied at each scale to vary, but have not described explicitly how many quadrats in total are occupied at each scale, in a manner analogous to Eq. (4.1). From Fig. 4.1 it is obvious that the proportion of quadrats occupied at the $j$th scale is the product of the proportion of occupied subquadrats at each subdivision (irrespective of whether a pattern is fractal or not):

$$p(s_j) = \prod_i^j f_i, \tag{4.5}$$

where $s$ is the $j$th scale and the product is across all $f$'s and scales down to scale $s_j$. For example, if at the coarsest scale 50% of subquadrats are occupied ($f = 0.5$), and at the next finer scale 40% of the subcells in these occupied quadrats are also occupied ($f = 0.4$), and similarly at the next finer scale 30% of the sub-subcells are occupied, the proportion of space occupied in the entire pattern after three iterations is $0.5 \times 0.4 \times 0.3$, so $p(s_3) = 0.06$. Equation (4.5) is the general form of the cross-scale model, which in our application incorporates Eqs. (4.3) and (4.4) to model the $f$'s, whereas in the strict fractal model all $f$'s are identical, fixed by $D$ and the subdivision factor $q$ (Eq. 4.2). The type of species incidence–scale

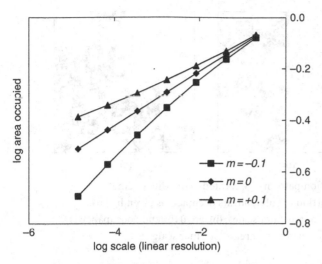

**Figure 4.2** Species incidence (scale–area curves) for a random fractal spatial pattern compared with that under the cross-scale model (Eqs. 4.2–4.5). On log-log axes, a random fractal distribution (equivalent to the cross-scale model with $m = 0$) gives a linear relationship between the total area of occupied quadrats and scale. The cross-scale model with negative $m$ produces downward curvature, representing a reduced area occupied at fine scales relative to coarse scales; a positive $m$ produces an upward curvature relative to the fractal relationship, representing an increased area occupied at fine scales.

relationships and deviations from fractality produced by this logistic cross-scale model are illustrated in Fig. 4.2.

## Synthetic realizations of the cross-scale model

Spatial patterns make it much easier to grasp these scaling relationships (Keitt, 2000). Figure 4.3 shows artificial species distribution patterns with increasing, constant or decreasing occupancy at finer scales, generated using the procedure illustrated in Fig. 4.1 (see Falconer, 2003). This particular scheme produces (for ecological patterns, at least) obvious geometrical artifacts in the form of rough linear boundaries. This is unimportant for our purposes since the shapes used to generate such patterns can take many forms (see Mandelbrot, 1977, 1983); the main feature to be emphasized here is the overall scatter and aggregation of occupied and unoccupied quadrats.

## Model fitting: testing for fractal and cross-scale relationships

No formal statistical test exists to help decide whether or not a pattern is fractal, as far as we are aware. Typically $D$ is estimated by least-squares regression on log-log axes, but the assumptions of regression are violated (conspicuously, the requirements of the independence of data points and constant variance), hence the usual regression statistics are not appropriate for testing the null model of a fractal distribution. This is clearly a shortcoming if we wish to say with any confidence that two fractal patterns have different $D$s, or whether a pattern can reasonably be considered to be fractal at all. In the signal-processing literature (a good example is Balghonaim & Keller, 1998), fractal processes are beginning

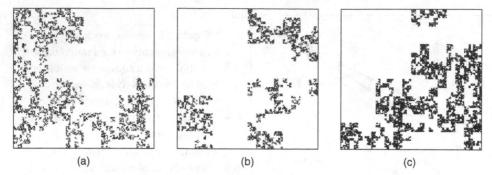

(a)                              (b)                              (c)

**Figure 4.3** Artificial cross-scale distribution patterns, generated using the scheme illustrated in Fig. 4.1, where $f$, the proportion of subquadrats occupied, is given by Eqs. (4.2–4.4): (a) negative $m$, occupancy decreases at finer scales, (b) $m = 0$ (fractal), occupancy is constant at all scales, and (c) positive $m$, occupancy increases at finer scales.

to be approached using more credible statistical methods such as maximum likelihood estimation. Here we develop simple likelihood methods for binary spatial patterns, such as typical presence/absence species distribution data. Relative to linear regression, these methods make better use of the information present within the spatial pattern while incorporating a more realistic error process. They can be used to estimate a single box-counting $D$ (fixed across all scales) or for fitting the parameters of our cross-scale model while providing a statistical test for deviations from fractality.

**Maximum likelihood estimation**

We introduce a maximum-likelihood (ML) estimation method for fitting the cross-scale model; this method allows testing the significance of the $m$ parameter. Since this parameter represents departure from fractality, testing the null hypothesis $H_0$: $m = 0$ also tests the hypothesis that a pattern is fractal, where the expected value of $m$ is zero. The method uses subcell occupancy probability to derived overall likelihoods: see Box 4.1.

Thus, presented with a series of box counts performed at different scales, we could find the ML estimate for $D$ by fitting a constant $f$ using Eq. (4.5) and applying Eq. (4.2) (or simply estimating the mean subcell occupancy directly). But when using the more general cross-scale model we wish to fit a more complex relationship, in which $f$ can vary with scale. In practice, we do this in the same way as described in Box 4.1 for the constant $f$ assumption, but replace $f$ with Eq. (4.4). To test the significance of our ML estimate of $m$, we first fit the model as above, maximizing the likelihood $\theta$ (Eq. 4.6) with respect to both $\alpha$ and $m$ simultaneously. In this likelihood equation, the observed data appear as the number of occupied quadrats at two successive spatial scales, $n_i$ and $n_{i+1}$. We then fit the model again, but this time force $m = 0$ and maximize the likelihood by adjusting $\alpha$ only. Theory tells us that twice the difference between the

---

**Box 4.1    Maximum likelihood estimation using subcell occupancy**

Here is an example using the simplest case where subcell occupancy probability $f$ is a fixed value. Consider dividing a distribution pattern into four quadrats (i.e. $q = 4$). Our initial estimate of the fraction occupied $f$ is the observed proportion of quadrats occupied; say we observe three out of four, so we estimate $f$ at $3/4$. We treat the number of these quadrats occupied (1,2,3,4) as the outcome of three independent Bernoulli trials, plus the single quadrat that must be occupied if the distribution pattern is not empty of individuals. Each of the occupied quadrats is then further divided into four subquadrats; since we have three of these, there may be up to 12 occupied subquadrats in total. Suppose we actually find seven of these occupied; we would then have another estimate of $f$ as $7/12$, and again we can consider this number of occupied quadrats to be the outcome of 9 trials (the three necessarily occupied subquadrats are excluded). Note that the number of trials in the second stage is contingent on the outcome of the first stage. Our best estimate of $f$ would therefore seem to be between $3/4$ and $7/12$, but how do we find it? One way is to make a rough guess at $f$: let us try $f = 0.7$. We can then calculate, using the binomial distribution, the probability of finding two out of three quadrats occupied given three trials each with a probability of success of 0.7 (it is three rather than four trials because at least one subquadrat within an occupied quadrat is always occupied). Call this probability $\pi_1$. Similarly, we can calculate the probability of observing $7/12$ quadrats occupied at the next stage, again given the same trial probability of 0.7. Call this probability $\pi_2$. The overall probability of getting first $3/4$ and second $7/12$ quadrats occupied is $\pi_1\pi_2$. Call this overall probability P. Now imagine varying our initial guess at $f$ from 0.7, and observing how P changes. The ML estimate of $f$ (in this example, 0.625) is that which maximizes P. For the case of a constant $f$, the ML $f$ value is, of course, given simply by the total number of successes divided by the total number of trials (i.e. $0.625 = 10/16$), but this compound probability approach becomes useful in the more interesting case where $f$ varies with scale (numerical maximization is used).

---

log-likelihoods for the two models (first minus second) has a $\chi^2$ distribution with one degree of freedom (Eliason, 1993): significance indicates the probability with which the null hypothesis ($H_0$: $m = 0$, the pattern is fractal) should be rejected. The likelihood, $\theta$, is given by

$$\theta = \prod_{i=1}^{nscales-1} \frac{(qn_i - n_i)!}{(n_{i+1} - n_i)!(qn_i - n_{i+1})!} f_i^{n_{i+1}} (1 - f_i)^{qn_i - n_{i+1}}, \tag{4.6}$$

where $f_i$ is given by Eqs. (4.3) and (4.4).

We make the assumption that the number of occupied subquadrats follows a binomial distribution. As in all statistical analyses, introducing some model for the stochastic nature of the pattern is an unavoidable necessity: clearly, if we did not, hypothesis testing would not be possible, and nothing more could be said. While a binomial model is parsimonious, and an important first step, it should be borne in mind that there are other sampling distributions which may potentially better describe the frequency distribution of the number of occupied subquadrats, while still giving the same expected (mean) number occupied. For example, the number of subquadrats occupied could follow a negative binomial distribution, with the same expected number of subquadrats occupied as before, but with a greater variance: on subdividing occupied quadrats, some quadrats tend to have more occupied subquadrats compared with the binomial distribution, and some tend to have fewer. This scenario still leads to a fractal spatial distribution (if the expected number of occupied subquadrats is a constant), but the appearance of the pattern would change depending on the variance or aggregation parameter of the generating distribution. The change in appearance associated with increasing variation between subsections of the whole is closely related to modern concepts of lacunarity (Plotnick *et al.*, 1996; Halley *et al.*, 2004).

If the generating process was one that increased the variance (between replicates or between scales) then this would have to be incorporated into the ML method, and significance values would change. Any development along these lines would have to take into account $f$ changing with scale and the simultaneous change in the frequency distribution of occupied quadrats at that scale.

## A comparison with the saturation model
The "saturation" model of Šizling and Storch (2004) proposes that species distributions can be described in fractal terms, but the range over which fractal behavior occurs is limited – at some (coarse) scale space suddenly becomes saturated with occupied quadrats. In other words, in moving from coarse to fine scales, the subdivision occupancy probability switches from 1 to a constant value less than 1 (Fig. 4.4; see also Lennon *et al.*, 2002). As before, we made a comparison of the saturation model with our cross-scale model by comparing the log-likelihoods for the cross-scale model with that of the fractal model, but this time we restricted the observed data used in the latter to only those occupancy counts indicating a lack of saturation – where subdividing occupied quadrats into four smaller quadrats did not produce four times as many occupied subquadrats. By truncating the data in this way, we have essentially added another parameter to the one-parameter fractal model – i.e. one describing the scale at which saturation occurs. If the saturation model is a better fit, we expect the difference in log-likelihood of the cross-scale model minus the saturation model to be negative, and approximately >2 to justify considering it a better model (Burnham & Anderson, 1998).

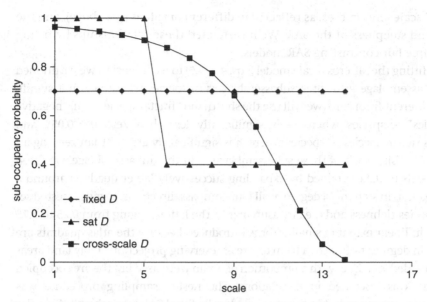

**Figure 4.4** Three different relationships between the probability of occupancy of subcells and scale. For a fractal this probability is constant, for our cross-scale model it changes sigmoidally with (log) scale (negative $m$ example shown), and for the saturation model it switches from less than one to exactly one at a particular critical scale. Scale goes from coarse to fine, left to right.

## Species distribution data

We used spatial distribution data for bird species (excluding marine and vagrant species) in 1858 quadrats (measuring ¼ degree latitude by ¼ degree longitude) covering South Africa and Lesotho (Harrison *et al.*, 1997a,b). Some species had distribution patterns that made them unsuitable for analysis: these were typically species with relatively few records clustered near the coast, which introduces serious difficulties when calculating distributions at coarser spatial scales due to the encroachment of sea into these coarser maps, thus leading to unequal areas of land between different scales of analysis. This affected only five species, leaving a total of 646 for analysis.

## Species–area relationships

Species–area relationships (SARs) emerge from the distributions and abundances of individual species. Potentially an important driver of the SAR is the scaling behavior of these component individual species. Is it possible to predict straightforwardly the scaling behavior of the SAR given only information on the scaling behavior of individual species distributions? By comparing SAR generated using groups of species that have contrasting scaling behavior, we should be able to test this notion directly using the southern African bird distribution data. By "scaling behavior" we mean, principally, both the shape of individual species' scale–area curves, as reflected in different $m$ values (see above), and the shape and steepness of the SAR. We investigated these relationships by fitting five simple but contrasting SAR models.

After fitting the ML cross-scale model (Eqs. 4.3–4.6) to each species, we partitioned the full assemblage into three subassemblages: (i) species where $m$ is not significantly different from zero (we will use the shorthand "fractal species"), (ii) "negative $m$ species" – species where $m$ is significantly less than zero ($P < 0.05$), and (iii) "positive $m$ species" – species where $m$ is significantly greater than zero, again at $P < 0.05$. Using each of these subassemblages and the full assemblage, we fitted SAR models to data obtained by expanding successively larger quadrats around a focal quadrat, in steps of ¼ degree in all four compass directions, to give a nested set of 15 species richness and area measurements, the latter ranging from 0.25 to 7.75 degrees in linear extent (a small error is introduced because the atlas quadrats are defined in degrees rather than from an area-preserving projection). Only land areas were recorded; quadrats with a proportion of ocean were used but the area occupied by ocean was discarded in calculations. The nested sampling procedure was repeated for every quadrat in turn to give a locally fitted SAR for each one. A similar scheme was implemented in Lennon *et al.* (2001). We also generated species richness maps and maps of the slope parameters of the SARs for all three subassemblages and the full assemblage. The two dominant SAR functions were fitted to these data: the power law (Arhennius, 1921) and the logarithmic model (Gleason, 1922). We also fitted the much less commonly used exponential (log(Richness) $= a + b$ Area), and linear (Richness $= a + b$ Area) models (Connor & McCoy, 1979). These four models account for the possible combinations of logarithmically transformed and untransformed axes in richness–area plots. Finally, prompted by the theoretical expectation of a SAR produced by fractal species, namely an upwardly curved relationship on log-log axes (Lennon *et al.*, 2002), we added a fifth model with a doubly logarithmically transformed species richness axis; this implies a relationship of the form Richness $= \exp(c \, \text{Area}^z)$.

Because the three-way partition of the full assemblage described above generates both an unequal number of species in each group, and raises the possibility of different frequency distributions of species range sizes between groups (range size measured as the numbers of quadrats occupied) and because these factors potentially affect the SAR, we defined two additional subsets of species standardized for both species number and the frequency distribution of range sizes. Using the smallest (in terms of numbers of species) of the three partitions, we chose the same number of species from each of the other two partitions, at the same time choosing species with matching occupancy in terms of numbers of ¼ degree quadrats occupied (the finest scale) to make the frequency distributions of occupancy as similar as possible.

If the scaling of individual species drives the SAR, we predict that the fractal assemblage will have an exponential-power-law relationship, based on theory

(Lennon et al., 2002). We expect the full assemblage to follow a power law simply because this is the commonest form of SAR (Connor & McCoy, 1979; Drakare, Lennon & Hillebrand, 2006). The negative-$m$ species should form a subassemblage that produces, relative to the SAR produced by the full assemblage, a SAR that increases more quickly at fine scales but more slowly at coarse scales. This is expected because species with negative $m$ parameters are relatively more sparsely distributed at finer spatial scales when compared with coarser scales, suggesting relatively high beta diversity and so larger $z$ at these finer scales, but as we move to coarser scales the increase in relative evenness of distribution should outweigh this by decreasing both beta diversity and $z$. Of the five models of SAR, we expect the logarithmic model to fit this negative-$m$ assemblage best because the component species have the property of filling space more quickly at first but more slowly later, relative to a power law. By following the same reasoning, we expect the positive-$m$ species to do the opposite, i.e. show shallow slopes on log-log axes for small areas but accelerate at larger areas. This implies a SAR of the exponential-power-law form. We expect none of the assemblages to follow the linear or exponential relationships.

We also predict that positive-$m$ species richness patterns should show more localized hot-spot peaks, because as one moves to finer spatial scales, the proportion of space occupied within occupied quadrats increases, and so relatively dense localized occupancy should generate more localized richness peaks. Conversely, negative-$m$ species should generate patterns of richness that are more even, with again the fractal species being intermediate. This rests on the assumption that all three subassemblages have the same degree of association between species. We see no way to predict in advance the strength of the correlations of the richness patterns between the different subassemblages.

## Results

The majority of species have negative $m$ parameters. Out of the total of 646 species, 504 (78%) have negative $m$ parameters. Of these 504 species, 332 (51% of all species) are significantly different from zero ($P < 0.05$, two-tailed). Of the remaining 142 (22% of all) species with nominally positive $m$ parameters, only 28 (c. 4% of all species) were significantly different from zero. Species indistinguishable from fractal numbered 286 (44% of total). This means that most, but not an overwhelming majority, of southern African bird species distributions are not fractal, tending to be more scattered and having lower relative occupancy when viewed at high resolution (or equivalently, relatively more clumped and contiguous at low resolutions) relative to that expected by the fractal null model. The frequency distribution of $m$ across species, and hence the departure from fractality, is unimodal with a peak just below $m = 0$ and a long tail of negative values (Fig. 4.5).

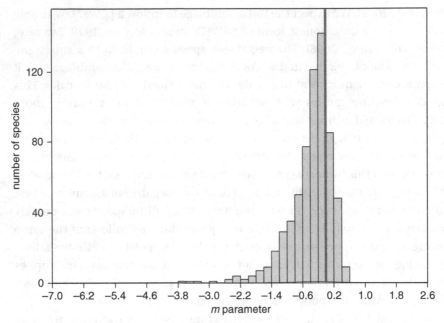

**Figure 4.5** Frequency distribution of $m$ parameters across all species. The $m = 0$ point is marked with a vertical line (median $= -0.270$, lower quartile $= -0.624$, upper quartile $= -0.043$).

We found no evidence that the saturated model is a better description than the cross-scale model: of the 188 species that showed saturation, only 15 gave a negative log-likelihood difference (improved model fit) and only one had a log-likelihood difference less than $-2$, suggesting that the saturation model fits the southern African data rather poorly.

There is a strong relationship between species fine-scale occupancies and their scaling properties (Fig. 4.6). Species that occupy more space (at the finest scale) tend to have more negative $m$ values, and so are more sparse at fine scales compared with coarse scales. This is not explicable simply in terms of rarer species having less information in their distribution patterns, because many relatively rare species show significant differences from fractality, in both directions (both negative and positive $m$). In other words, this trend is not simply a result of low statistical power when considering rare species – for many such species there is sufficient information to reject the null hypothesis that species distributions are fractal.

Partitioning species using the $m$ parameter reveals different spatial distributions of species richness (Fig. 4.7). Our prediction that the positive $m$ assemblage should produce more localized diversity hot-spot peaks than negative $m$ species is in broad agreement with the data. The fractal and the positive $m$ subassemblages have similar patterns of richness ($r = 0.95$,

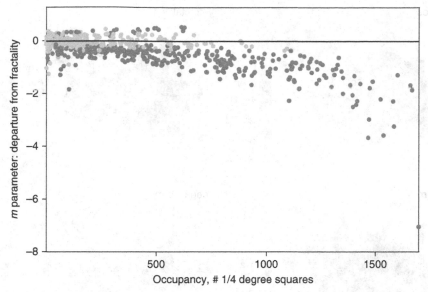

**Figure 4.6** The curvilinear relationship between the $m$ parameter and the commoness/ rarity of species (measured at the finest scale as the number of 0.25° × 0.25° (latitude × longitude) grid cells occupied). Species that tend to have large negative $m$ parameters, and so deviate the most from fractality, are also the commonest. These common species never have a positive $m$, while the rarer species can show a range of behaviors from negative through zero to positive. Dark circles species with $m$ parameters significantly ($P < 0.05$) different from zero; light circles, $P > 0.05$.

$ess = 5.47$, $P = 0.036$; where $ess$ = effective sample size calculated using Clifford, Richardson & Hemon's (1989) procedure). Both show patterns of richness with a more easterly distribution of hot spots when compared with the full assemblage. In contrast, the negative-$m$ subassemblage shows a more westerly distribution and a relatively more even spread of diversity, but is still weakly correlated with the fractal species richness pattern ($r = 0.55$, $ess = 12.2$, $P = 0.025$). This more westerly distribution is probably necessary in that many of these negative-$m$ species are widespread at the finest scale. The positive-$m$ and the negative-$m$ richness patterns are similarly weakly correlated ($r = 0.49$, $ess = 10.7$, $P = 0.07$), but this time the association is not significant. Our expected difference in hot-spot/cold-spot patterning is based on simple (if not simplistic) arguments about individual species scaling. However, the differences in inter-correlation strength between the positive-$m$ subassemblage and the other two subassemblage richness patterns suggest that such individual scaling properties of species can translate into contrasting geographical patterns of richness.

The SAR model parameters fitted to the full assemblage and the three sub-assemblages are given in Table 4.1 and the data plotted in Fig. 4.8. The full assemblage conforms to the power-law relationship (judged by the $R^2$ of OLS

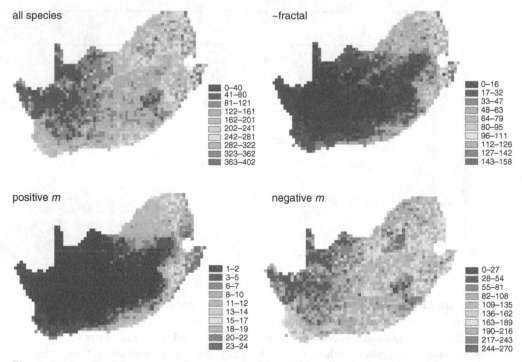

**all species**

- 0–40
- 41–80
- 81–121
- 122–161
- 162–201
- 202–241
- 242–281
- 282–322
- 323–362
- 363–402

**~fractal**

- 0–16
- 17–32
- 33–47
- 48–63
- 64–79
- 80–95
- 96–111
- 112–126
- 127–142
- 143–158

**positive *m***

- 1–2
- 3–5
- 6–7
- 8–10
- 11–12
- 13–14
- 15–17
- 18–19
- 20–22
- 23–24

**negative *m***

- 0–27
- 28–54
- 55–81
- 82–108
- 109–135
- 136–162
- 163–189
- 190–216
- 217–243
- 244–270

**Figure 4.7** Species richness maps for southern African birds. (For color version see Plate 1.)

linear regression). As predicted, the fractal assemblage is fitted best by the exponential-power-law model. In contrast to our prediction, the power-law model is the best fit for the positive-*m* assemblage, but we predicted the behavior of the negative-*m* assemblage correctly in following the logarithmic relationship best. This latter assemblage has the most variation explained by area – more than twice that of the positive-*m* species. However, these assemblages differ in size (numbers of species) and in the frequency distribution of species' ranges (Fig. 4.6). When we standardize all three assemblages by shrinking the number of species in the two more speciose assemblages down to that of the smallest assemblage, the results change to be more uniform across assemblages in terms of SAR slopes (Table 4.1).

The spatial distribution patterns of *z* of the power law mirror those of species richness in each case, but are reversed (Fig. 4.9). Low SAR slopes occur around richness hot spots and high slopes around richness cold spots, in agreement with the findings of Lennon *et al.* (2002), and Storch, Evans and Gaston (2005). Perhaps because of this close relationship with spatial gradients in species richness, there is considerable variation in the slope of the SAR throughout southern Africa. The power law is also a consistently better fit than the semilog model in areas of low species richness, across all subassemblages (in contrast with the findings of Lennon *et al.*, 2002, for British birds).

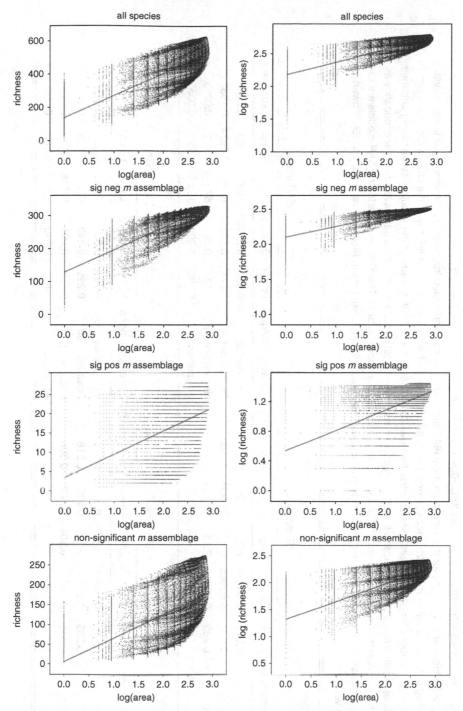

**Figure 4.8** Fitting species–area relationship to southern African bird distribution data. Species richness and area values were obtained by expanding a series of quadrats around each focal quadrat, generating a series of up to 15 richness–area pairs for every focal quadrat (from 0.25 to 6.75 degree quadrats, linear extent). We show only two of the five fitted SAR models here: the log-log power law (right column), and logarithmic model (left column). The large amount of scatter arises from the spatial variation in species richness; see Table 4.1 for fitted parameters.

**Table 4.1** *Species–area relationship models, regression slopes and* $R^2$ *values*

Right side of table: SAR slopes and $R^2$ values for the full assemblage (646 species) and when partitioned into three subassemblages using individual species spatial scaling behavior: positive-$m$ full (28 species), negative-$m$ full (332) and ~fractal full (286). The left half of the table shows a similar partition, but controls for numbers of species in each assemblage (all have 28 species in the subset, the size of the smallest assemblage) and their occupancy at the finest scale. The 28 species chosen from the negative-$m$ and the ~fractal subsets were selected to have as similar occupancy as possible to the positive-$m$ assemblage. The highest $R^2$ value within an assemblage is shown in bold. The abbreviations for the SAR models are as follows. Power, log(richness) vs. log(Area); Exp, log(Area); Log, Richness vs. log(Area); Linear, Richness vs. Area; and Exp(Power), log(log(Richness)) vs. Area.

(a) Regression slopes

| Standardized assemblages | SAR model | | | | | Full assemblages | SAR model | | | | |
|---|---|---|---|---|---|---|---|---|---|---|---|
| | Power | Exp | Log | Linear | Exp(Power) | | Power | Exp | Log | Linear | Exp(Power) |
| ~Fractal subset | 0.271 | 0.00328 | 6.79 | 0.0955 | 0.113 | ~Fractal full | 0.332 | 0.00409 | 59.6 | 0.868 | 0.0858 |
| Positive-$m$ subset | 0.274 | 0.00365 | 6.16 | 0.0934 | 0.035 | Positive-$m$ full | 0.274 | 0.00365 | 6.16 | 0.0934 | 0.1087 |
| Negative-$m$ subset | 0.265 | 0.00265 | 7.15 | 0.0844 | 0.107 | Negative-$m$ full | 0.151 | 0.00151 | 67.7 | 0.761 | 0.0293 |
| | | | | | | All species | 0.196 | 0.00221 | 133 | 1.72 | 0.0355 |

(b) Regression $R^2$

| Standardized assemblages | SAR model | | | | | Full assemblages | SAR model | | | | |
|---|---|---|---|---|---|---|---|---|---|---|---|
| | Power | Exp | Log | Linear | Exp(Power) | | Power | Exp | Log | Linear | Exp(Power) |
| ~Fractal subset | **0.379** | 0.262 | 0.347 | 0.312 | 0.329 | ~Fractal full | 0.496 | 0.333 | 0.355 | 0.333 | **0.507** |
| Positive-$m$ subset | **0.299** | 0.242 | 0.288 | 0.278 | 0.216 | Positive-$m$ full | **0.299** | 0.242 | 0.288 | 0.278 | 0.216 |
| Negative-$m$ subset | 0.585 | 0.266 | **0.602** | 0.371 | 0.506 | Negative-$m$ full | 0.659 | 0.291 | **0.725** | 0.405 | 0.627 |
| | | | | | | All species | **0.606** | 0.340 | 0.548 | 0.403 | 0.598 |

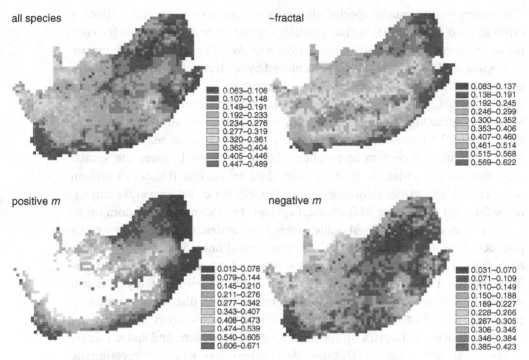

**Figure 4.9** Spatial variation in $z$ of the power-law species–area relationship for southern African birds. The blank (white) areas for the positive-$m$ assemblage occur where there are insufficient data to fit a SAR. (For color version see Plate 2.)

## Discussion

We posed two main questions: (i) are species' coarse-scale distribution patterns different from their fine-scale distribution patterns? (ii) if so, are there consistent trends in how they differ? For the data we have examined, the answer to both questions is a qualified yes: rather more than half the species examined here do not have self-similar distributions, and a large majority of all species differed from self-similarity in the same direction, in simple terms, by being relatively less aggregated at fine than at coarse scales. Most distributions are like Fig. 4.3(a) (negative $m$), a smaller number are indistinguishable from fractal (Fig. 4.3b), and a small minority resemble Fig. 4.3(c). Having said this, a substantial proportion of southern African bird species distributions are statistically indistinguishable from stochastic fractal patterns. While it is likely that the fractal null model was not rejected for some very rare species simply because of lack of information, this issue of statistical power cannot explain the generality of our results – indeed, it can be seen from Fig. 4.6 that the null model is rejected for many rare species. These results strengthen our argument that fractals may serve as a useful null model for species distributions across spatial scales: a baseline against which observed patterns may be judged. Clearly, this is of considerable interest in view of the many other natural phenomena showing fractal properties.

In trying to understand species distributions the issue of recorder effort is often glossed over. It is likely that spatially varying recorder effort partly determines observed species distributions. However, as is the case in many macroecological studies, exactly what role is played by recorder effort in our analyses is unclear. Recorder effort is not spatially random for many reasons, one of which is that human population centers are not uniformly distributed. Moreover, some high richness areas attract more effort because they are more attractive to the human visitor. In fact, it is possible to locate major roads and human population centers in southern Africa quite easily from the spatial distribution of recorder effort for the bird data we analyze (Fig. 5 in Harrison *et al.*, 1997a). The spatial structure of sampling effort can have several contrasting effects on the scaling of individual species. For example, if random omissions are made at the finest scale, such false absences tend to favor the production of negative-*m* distributions from fractal ones. Similarly, if random omissions are made at the coarser scales, this tends to convert fractal patterns into positive-*m* distributions. However, even if effort varies spatially, it is still possible for it to have a limited impact on recorded distribution patterns, providing the effort is not excessively deficient in some areas. If this is the case, it will leave an imprint on species distribution patterns and consequently on their scaling behavior and this should be remembered when interpreting the results presented above.

Why should commoner species tend not to be fractal (or positive *m*)? There is nothing to prevent a species being both common *and* fractal – it can have a fractal dimension close to $D = 2$ and so occupy most (or even all) of the available space. This strongly suggests that the scaling of some important environmental processes common to most or all species sets a limit of some kind, beyond which additional space is occupied in a more random manner (less aggregated at a fixed scale) than expected from a fractal process. Here, we found a preponderance of species with negative-*m* parameters (i.e. decreasing occupancy at finer scales). The same trend was also observed in an analysis of the distribution patterns of rare British plants at scales from 50 km down to 2 km linear resolution (Hartley *et al.*, 2004). However, that study also observed increasing occupancy (i.e. positive *m*) when changing spatial scale from 0.5 km all the way down to 1 m linear resolution. This suggests that in order to capture empirical patterns across a really wide range of scales (six orders of magnitude) we may need to use models that can incorporate systematic peaks or troughs in proportional occupancy as scale changes. The cross-scale model is easily modified to do this: all that is needed is the addition of a quadratic term to Eq. (4.4) in the form of $g(\log s)^2$ where the additional parameter $g$ is fitted using ML in the same way as *m*. In concert with developing more sophisticated models of scaling behavior, further empirical data collected from a wide range of scales, and ideally from a variety of different taxa, are highly desirable.

As far as the relationship between species distribution pattern scaling and diversity scaling is concerned, it has been argued that fractal species distribution patterns do not produce the power law SAR (Lennon et al., 2002; but see Green, Harte & Ostling, 2003; and Šizling & Storch, 2004) – this is certainly true as a mathematical result when dealing with *truly* fractal species, i.e. where individual species occupancy–area relationships follow power laws across all observed scales. Practically, however, the power law SAR may be relatively robust when a mixture of fractal, nonfractal, and quasi-fractal (fractal across a limited range of scales – see Lennon et al., 2002) species are present. This is supported by the approximate linearity of the plots in Fig. 4.8, despite the large proportion of species distribution patterns indistinguishable from fractal (see also Šizling & Storch, 2004). The other side of this coin is that this very robustness makes SAR a blunt tool for understanding spatial variation. If assemblages with markedly different scaling behavior usually result in roughly linear SARs on log-log axes, then clearly the utility of the latter in differentiating between the former may be somewhat limited.

This view is supported by our only partial success in predicting the shape of the three assemblages' SARs from the scaling behavior of individual species. While we correctly predicted that the fractal assemblage should follow an exponential power law, and the negative-$m$ assemblage should fit the logarithmic relationship best, the positive-$m$ species do not behave as expected. Moreover, once these assemblages are standardized to the same number of species and range size frequency distributions, things change. Instead of following the theoretically expected exponential power law, the subset of fractal species follows a power law. The subset of negative-$m$ species continues to fit a logarithmic relationship as before (the positive-$m$ assemblage also does not change because it is the reference assemblage). And while all three subsets do not follow the same SAR, the differences are not great – the power law fits two out of the three subsets best, with the logarithmic marginally better in the third. Why does the fractal subset not behave as expected? One reason could be that although individually these species are statistically indistinguishable from fractal, nonetheless the cumulative effect of small but systematic deviations from fractality across many species may pull the SAR away from the form expected for truly fractal species. Another reason is that the exponential-power-law model is a rough first approximation to the shape of SAR expected from fractal species. It is notable that, despite the very different scaling behaviors of the individual species in these three assemblages, the slopes of the relationships are virtually identical (Table 4.1). Although the assemblage sizes are the same, thus fixing the number of species at an area of the size of southern Africa, and the average richness at the finest scale is also fixed by our standardization of range sizes, this is not sufficient to constrain SAR slopes to be identical across assemblages for two reasons. First, the largest scale used for SAR was only 7.75 degrees, and so there is considerable scope for variation in species richness between assemblages at the coarsest scale. Second, 15 richness versus area points were used, so larger areas do not necessarily dominate the smaller. This suggests, at least as a working hypothesis, that the scaling behavior of individual species may be of secondary importance for slopes of SAR; instead, the frequency distribution of species range sizes may dominate. However, this is not entirely satisfactory when it is remembered that the frequency distribution of range sizes in an assemblage is itself scale dependent, and that the nature of this scale dependency can vary between different assemblages of species (as we have shown here). There is no well-defined canonical range-size distribution but rather a series across spatial scales (Gaston, 2003). So, the notion that SAR slopes can be predicted from species ranges alone is not without difficulties. Clearly, more work needs to be done in this respect, by disentangling species scaling, range sizes and commonness/rarity properties and their contributions to SAR, both empirically and theoretically.

The considerable spatial variation in $z$ and the conspicuous sensitivity of $z$ to species richness gradients (Figs. 4.7 and 4.9; see also Lennon *et al.*, 2001; Koleff, Gaston & Lennon, 2003; and Storch *et al.*, 2005) means that some doubt must be cast on the application of a single value of $z$ throughout a region. When a larger range of scales is considered, focusing on the power-law SAR generates even more difficulty in the form of "triphasic" relationships (examples include Crawley & Harral, 2001; Hubbell, 2001). While the SAR must remain as part of the spatial ecologist's toolbox, a potentially much more powerful approach is to make use of the growing body of knowledge regarding species turnover and beta diversity analysis (see Gaston *et al.*; and Keitt, this volume). This may be particularly important given the current application of SARs in the prediction of global species extinction risk (Thomas *et al.*, 2004).

The three basic types of cross-scale behavior we identify can arise in a number of ways in terms of hierarchical spatial processes (O'Neill *et al.*, 1992; see also Šizling & Storch, this volume). In Fig. 4.10 we show how overlaying a series of "input" patterns (such as environmental constraints) can generate "output" patterns (that is, species distribution patterns) having both fractal and negative-*m* scaling properties (see also Milne, 1997). Here it is envisaged that the output results from a logical "AND" operation performed between input patterns of successively finer grain size, such that species presence at a particular location requires all of the inputs to be "present" or "suitable". In Fig. 4.10(a), the three input patterns all have the same proportion of suitable environment; the output pattern produced is fractal. In Fig. 4.10(b), negative-*m* scaling is produced by the finer scales having less of the suitable environment, while in Fig. 4.10(c) the same negative-*m* scaling is produced by an increase in the number of different environmental factors needed at finer scales. Reversing these trends in Fig. 4.10(b) and Fig. 4.10(c) to run from fine to coarse scales

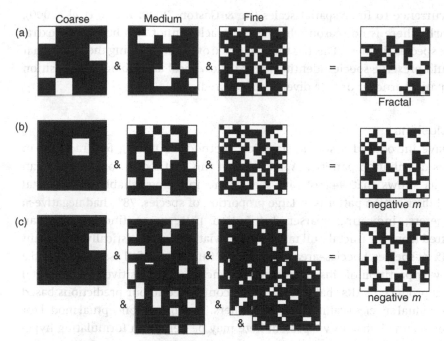

**Figure 4.10** A conceptual model for generating scaling behavior in species distribution patterns. Black squares indicate "suitable" environment (left-hand side) or the "presence" of a species (right-hand side). See text for details.

results in positive-*m* species. Note that these autocorrelated output patterns are produced even when the individual input patterns have no autocorrelation – no internal structure beyond CSR randomness – and indeed even introducing autocorrelation into the inputs will make no difference to the expected scaling of the output pattern. The same cannot be said for correlation *between* input patterns – in this case, positive correlation will tend to favor production of positive-*m* species, while negative correlation will generate negative-*m* species. Going beyond these simple abstractions, it is tempting to hypothesize that energetic and climatic patterns occupy the role of the coarse-grained input, while topographic variation is more important at medium scales nested within the climate envelope, and at fine scales more specific habitat requirements of species, such as soil types or the presence of suitable prey species, are more important (see Rahbek & Graves, 2001; Pearson, Dawson & Liu, 2004). The realized species distribution pattern would then depend both on the proportional coverage and on the number of suitable environments at each scale.

The cross-scale model introduced here, in addition to testing for fractality in species distribution patterns, may prove useful in the prediction of species range sizes and diversity at finer spatial scales than are represented by the available data; the consistent trends observed in the scaling behavior of an individual species can usefully be exploited by using it to extrapolate probability of occurrence to finer spatial scales (He & Gaston, 2000; Kunin *et al.*, 2000); similarly, there is no reason why this approach cannot also be used to extrapolate species richness. This has the advantage over simply using the SAR in that it would preserve species identity, and so allow local assemblage composition and spatial turnover or beta diversity to be predicted.

## Conclusions

We have introduced a simple statistical method for testing for fractality in species distribution patterns. Application of this method to southern African avifauna shows that 44% of bird species are indistinguishable from fractal spatial distribution patterns. A large proportion of species, 78%, had negative-$m$ parameters, indicating sparser distribution patterns at finer scales than expected from the fractal null model; this deviation was statistically significant for 51% of species. Species–area relationships fitted to the full assemblage and a three-way partition of this assemblage into negative-$m$, positive-$m$, and fractal species produced SARs that in some cases conformed to our predictions based on individual species scaling, but not in others. The simple conceptual model for species scaling behavior we present here may be helpful in formulating hypotheses explaining the relationship between the scaling of species distribution patterns and environmental factors.

## Acknowledgments

We are grateful to L. Underhill and the Avian Demography Unit, University of Capetown, for providing access to the data, and the numerous volunteers who contributed to its collection. We thank David Storch, Pablo Marquet, James Brown and Geoffrey West for inviting us to a very productive and successful workshop, and they and the other participants for many stimulating discussions. This chapter was much improved by the challenging and insightful comments from David Storch, Tim Keitt and one anonymous referee.

## References

Arhennius, O. (1921). Species and area. *Journal of Ecology*, **9**, 95–99.

Balghonaim, A. S. & Keller, J. M. (1998). A maximum likelihood estimate for two-variable fractal surface. *IEEE Transactions on Image Processing*, **7**, 1746–1753.

Burnham, K. P. & Anderson, D. R. (1998). *Model Selection and Inference: a Practical Information-theoretic Approach*. New York: Springer-Verlag.

Clifford, P., Richardson, S. & Hemon, D. (1989). Assessing the significance of the correlation between two spatial processes. *Biometrics*, **45**, 123–134.

Connor, E. F. & McCoy, E. D. (1979). The statistics and biology of the species-area relationship. *American Naturalist*, **113**, 791–833.

Crawley, M. J. & Harral, J. E. (2001). Scale dependence in plant biodiversity. *Science*, **291**, 864–868.

Cressie, N. (1991). *Statistics for Spatial Data*. New York: Wiley.

Dale, M. R. T. (1998). *Spatial Pattern Analysis in Plant Ecology*. Cambridge: Cambridge University Press.

Drakare, S., Lennon, J. J. & Hillebrand, H. (2006). The imprint of the geographical, evolutionary and ecological context on species-area relationships. *Ecology Letters*, 9, 215–227.

Eliason, S. R. (1993). *Maximum Likelihood Estimation: Logic and Practice*. Sage University Paper series on Quantative Applications in the Social Sciences, 07–096. Newbury Park, CA: Sage University Press.

Falconer, K. (2003). *Fractal Geometry*. New York: Wiley.

Fortin, M.-J. & Dale, M. R. T. (2005). *Spatial Analysis: a Guide for Ecologists*. Cambridge: Cambridge University Press.

Gaston, K. J. (2000). Global patterns in biodiversity. *Nature*, 405, 220–227.

Gaston, K. J. (2003). *The Structure and Dynamics of Geographic Ranges*. Oxford: Oxford University Press.

Gleason, H. A. (1922). On the relation between species and area. *Ecology*, 3, 158–162.

Green, J. L., Harte, J. & Ostling, A. (2003). Species richness, endemism and abundance patterns: tests of two fractal models in a serpentine grassland. *Ecology Letters*, 6, 919–928.

Halley, J. M., Hartley, S., Kallimanis, S. A., Kunin, W. E., Lennon, J. J. & Sgardelis, S. P. (2004). Uses and abuses of Fractals in Ecology. *Ecology Letters*, 7, 254–271.

Harrison, J. A. *et al.* (1997a). *The Atlas of Southern African Birds*. Vol. 1: *Non-Passerine*. Johannesburg: BirdLife South Africa.

Harrison, J. A. *et al.* (1997b). *The Atlas of Southern African birds*. Vol. 2: *Passerines*. Johannesburg: BirdLife South Africa.

Harte, J. & Kinzig, A. P. (1997). On the implications of species-area relationships for endemism, spatial turnover, and food web patterns. *Oikos*, 80, 417–427.

Harte, J., Kinzig, A. & Green, J. (1999). Self-similarity in the distribution and abundance of species. *Science*, 284, 334–336.

Harte, J., Blackburn, T. M. & Ostling, A. (2001). Self similarity and the relationship between abundance and range size. *American Naturalist*, 157, 374–386.

Hartley, S., Kunin, W. E., Lennon, J. J. & Pocock, M. J. O. (2004). Coherence and discontinuity in the scaling of species distribution patterns. *Proceedings of the Royal Society London, Series B*, 271, 81–88.

Hastings, H. M. & Sugihara, G. (1993). *Fractals: a User's Guide for the Natural Sciences*. Oxford: Oxford University Press.

He, F. L. & Gaston, K. J. (2000). Estimating species abundance from occurrence. *American Naturalist*, 156, 553–559.

Hubbell, S. P. (2001). *The Unified Neutral Theory of Biodiversity and Biogeography*. Princeton: Princeton University Press.

Keitt, T. H. (2000). Spectral representation of neutral landscapes. *Landscape Ecology*, 15, 479–494.

Keitt, T. H., Amaral, L. A. N., Buldyrev, S. V. & Stanley, H. E. (2002). Scaling in the growth of geographically subdivided populations: invariant patterns from a continent-wide biological survey. *Philosophical Transactions of the Royal Society London, Series B*, 357, 627–633.

Koleff, P., Gaston, K. J. & Lennon, J. J. (2003). Measuring beta diversity for presence-absence data. *Journal of Animal Ecology*, 72, 367–382.

Kunin, W. E. (1998). Extrapolating species abundance across spatial scales. *Science*, 281, 1513–1515.

Kunin, W. E. & Lennon, J. J. (2005). Spatial scale and species diversity: building species-area curves from species incidence. In *Biodiversity in Drylands*, ed. M. Shachak *et al.*, pp. 89–108. Oxford: Oxford University Press.

Kunin, W. E., Hartley, S. & Lennon, J. J. (2000). Scaling down: on the challenge of estimating abundance from occurrence patterns. *American Naturalist*, **156**, 560–566.

Lennon, J. J., Koleff, P., Greenwood, J. J. D. & Gaston, K. J. (2001). The geographical structure of British bird distributions: diversity, spatial turnover and scale. *Journal of Animal Ecology*, **70**, 966–979.

Lennon, J. J., Kunin, W. E. & Hartley, S. (2002). Fractal species distributions do not produce power-law species-area relationships. *Oikos*, **97**, 378–386.

Lomolino, M. V. (2000). Ecology's most general, yet protean pattern: the species-area relationship. *Journal of Biogeography*, **27**, 17–26.

Mandelbrot, B. B. (1977). *Fractals, Form, Chance and Dimension*. San Francisco: Freeman.

Mandelbrot, B. B. (1983). *The Fractal Geometry of Nature*. New York: Freeman.

Milne, B. T. (1997). Application of fractal geometry in wildlife biology. In *Wildlife and Landscape Ecology: Effects of Pattern and Scale*, ed. J. A. Bissonette, pp. 32–69. New York: Springer-Verlag.

O'Neill, R. V., DeAngelis, D. I., Waide, J. B. & Allen, T. F. H. (1992). *A Hierarchical Concept of Ecosystems*. Princeton: Princeton University Press.

Pearson, R. G., Dawson, T. P. & Liu, C. (2004). Modelling species distributions in Britain: a hierarchical integration of climate and land-cover data. *Ecography*, **27**, 285–298.

Pielou, E. C. (1977). *Mathematical Ecology*, 2nd edn. New York: Wiley & Sons.

Plotkin, J. B., Potts, M. D., Leslie, N., Manokaran, N., LaFrankie, J. & Ashton, P. S. (2000).

Species-area curves, spatial aggregation, and habitat specialization in tropical forests. *Journal of Theoretical Biology*, **207**, 81–99.

Plotnick, R. E., Gardner, R. H., Hargrove, W. W., Prestegaard, K. & Perlmutter, M. (1996). Lacunarity analysis: a general technique for the analysis of spatial patterns. *Physical Review, E*, **53**, 5461–5468.

Rahbek, C. & Graves, G. R. (2001). Multiscale assessment of patterns of avian species richness. *Proceedings of the National Academy of Sciences of the United States of America*, **98**, 4534–4539.

Šizling, A. L. & Storch, D. (2004). Power-law species–area relationships and self-similar species distributions within finite areas. *Ecology Letters*, **7**, 60–68.

Storch, D., Evans, K. L. & Gaston, K. J. (2005). The species-area-energy relationship. *Ecology Letters*, **8**, 487–492.

Taylor, L. R. (1961). Aggregation, variance and the mean. *Nature*, **189**, 732–735.

Taylor, L. R., Woiwod, I. P. & Perry, J. N. (1979). The negative binomial as an ecological model and the density-dependence of $k$. *Journal of Animal Ecology*, **48**, 289–304.

Thomas, C. D., Cameron, A., Green, R. E. *et al.* (2004). Extinction risk from climate change. *Nature*, **427**, 145–148.

Whittaker, R. J., Willis, K. J. & Field, R. (2001). Scale and species richness: towards a general, hierarchical theory of species diversity. *Journal of Biogeography*, **28**, 453–470.

# CHAPTER FIVE

# Geometry of species distributions: random clustering and scale invariance

ARNOŠT L. ŠIZLING
*Charles University, Prague*
DAVID STORCH
*Charles University, Prague, and The Santa Fe Institute*

## Introduction

Spatial biodiversity patterns are tightly related to the patterns of spatial distribution of individual species. It has been recognized that the spatial distribution of individuals is never random nor homogeneous within some well-defined clusters but is aggregated on many spatial scales: individuals form clusters which themselves are aggregated into larger clusters and so on. The most useful way to capture these patterns is with fractal geometry, which treats such patterns as self-similar sets (Kunin, 1998; Halley et al., 2004). Indeed, it has been shown that species spatial distribution is often close to fractal (Virkkala, 1993; Condit et al., 2000; Ulrich & Buszko, 2003) and that the assumption of fractality of species spatial distribution is appropriate for deriving multispecies macroecological patterns, namely the species–area relationship (Harte, Kinzig & Green, 1999; Šizling & Storch, 2004). By contrast, species sometimes reveal distributions that deviate from strict fractality (Hartley et al., 2004; He & Condit, this volume; Lennon et al., this volume). More importantly, although there are several ways in which fractal distributions could emerge (Halley et al., 2004), there is no strong biological reason why species spatial distribution should be exactly fractal, i.e. it is unclear which biological processes should produce fractal distribution.

Here we show that species spatial distributions which are very close to fractal can emerge from random processes leading to aggregation on several spatial scales. These processes have relatively straightforward biological interpretation and the spatial patterns they produce are in many parameters effectively undistinguishable from classical fractals. Moreover, when we compose together many spatial distributions resulting from these simple processes, we obtain relatively realistic species–area relationships, as well as a frequency distribution of occupied areas which is close to the observed distribution of species abundances. We thus propose a null model of the geometry of species distribution which is biologically reliable, realistic, and more general than is the fractal distribution.

*Scaling Biodiversity*, ed. David Storch, Pablo A. Marquet and James H. Brown. Published by Cambridge University Press. © Cambridge University Press 2007.

## Self-similarity and hierarchical aggregation

There is a wide range of possible types of spatially aggregated distributions, and for our purpose it is useful to distinguish self-similarity from fractality. Self-similarity is often taken as synonymous to fractality, but as we will show, fractal distribution can in fact be treated as a rather specific type of self-similar distribution. A geometric object is self-similar, according to Hastings and Sugihara (1993), "if it can be written as a union of rescaled copies of itself". The problem is the exact nature of the rescaling. Imagine that we have a broad-scale spatial pattern which is patchy on this broad scale of resolution (in ecology these patches can represent, for example, patches of suitable macrohabitat). A self-similar structure emerges by replacing these patches with patterns *similar* to the original patchy pattern. The resulting structures can be very different, depending on the exact meaning of *similarity*, as we will show. Anyway, it is useful to see the emergence of self-similarity as a hierarchical, top-down process, where we obtain the whole structure by a downscaling performed in discrete steps. If we apply an unlimited number of these steps, we would obtain a real, mathematically self-similar set – but in the real world we always have a limited number of these replacements. In the following text we will be dealing only with self-similar structures emerging from a finite number of steps, and will call these steps the *levels of aggregation*. Self-similarity is, in this view, a property that links two subsequent levels of aggregation to one another.

This hierarchical approach to self-similar structures has clear advantages. Most importantly, structures which originate by this process are interpretable in terms of biological processes acting within each level of aggregation. We can imagine, for instance, that the largest patches (i.e. within the zero level of aggregation) correspond to broadly defined macrohabitats characterized by particular climate or elevation. The next level of aggregation can represent habitat patches characterized by particular vegetation, and subsequent levels can be formed for instance by patches of resources. The observed spatial distribution of a species then can form the next level of aggregation, as not all available habitat patches can be occupied, and patterns of occupancy within available habitat patches are given by spatial population (and/or metapopulation) dynamics. The pattern aggregated on many scales of resolution can therefore reflect the nested nature of habitat hierarchy, and also the hierarchical nature of spatial population processes. This hierarchical nature alone obviously does not ensure any regularity concerning the similarity of patterns observed at various levels of aggregation (i.e. self-similarity) or even fractality, but we will show that simple statistical assumptions concerning the nature of these hierarchical processes can lead to surprising regularities.

Note that this hierarchical approach to some extent reconciles two very different approaches to the multiscale nature of ecological systems. One of these approaches, the hierarchical concept of ecosystems (Allen & Starr, 1982) takes seriously the fact that ecological processes differ in different spatial and temporal scales, and treats ecological systems as hierarchical, where each scale has its own rules of behavior. By contrast, the scaling approach consists of looking for patterns which are actually independent of scale, i.e. for scale invariance. We will show that some types of scale invariance can emerge even if we assume different processes acting on each scale – simply because these processes, albeit different, can have something in common, even if it is something whose nature is purely statistical.

## Fractals

Fractals are self-similar structures where the "similarity" is defined in a particular way; classically through particular geometrical projections leading to various structures called "self-similar sets (sensu stricto)", "self-affine sets" and "random fractals". Similarity is there defined as the proportional lessening of the original pattern in the case of the self-similarity sensu stricto, the result of an affine projection of the original pattern in the case of self-affine sets, and the pattern "statistically indistinguishable" from the original pattern in the case of random fractals (Falconer, 1990). Behind all of these definitions is, however, the idea of scale invariance. This idea has been originally related to the problem of the measurement of the length of shoreline (Richardson, 1961) which apparently depends on the resolution of the scale used for this measurement. In planar terminology, the measured size of any real area depends on the resolution of the scale used, because finer resolutions necessarily lead to respecting more and more details. We are therefore looking for a measure of area which is independent of the scale used – i.e. is scale invariant. Scale invariance sensu stricto is thus a property of the way in which we measure geometrical objects rather than a necessary property of the objects themselves.

When attempting to fulfill the requirement of scale invariance, it is necessary to obey the formal condition that the measured area of the whole must be equal the sum of measured areas of particular patches (see Fig. 5.1). To meet this condition, we have to treat the term *area* more generally than it is in Euclidean space. This can be done as follows.

Let the whole be an $i$th square patch at any level of aggregation. The Euclidean area of the whole equals $L_i^2$ where $L_i$ is the length of the edge of this patch; the Euclidean area calculated using the finer information on the structure of the patches at the subsequent level of aggregation equals $\sum_{j=1}^{n_i} l_{i,j}^2$ where $n_i$ is the number of subpatches within the $i$th patch and $l_{i,j}$ are the lengths of their edges. As we can see, the equality of the areas calculated using coarse and fine scale is

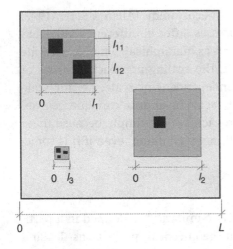

**Figure 5.1** Three levels of aggregation of the most common random fractal. While the Euclidean area at the coarsest scale equals $L^2$, it equals $l_1^2 + l_2^2 + l_3^2$ for the following level and $\sum l_{i,j}^2$ through all possible combinations of $i,j$ for the bottom level of aggregation.

met only if patches at the subsequent level of aggregation completely cover the whole. This can occur only if the *similar copy of the original pattern* is identical to the whole, and the topological dimension is 2. However, if the similar copy of the original pattern is patchy, and we are still going to meet the requirement of the scale invariance of area, we have to change the dimension of the set. In other words, we have to change the definition of area. The formal condition of self-similarity is then

$$L_i^D = \sum_{j=1}^{n_i} l_{i,j}^D.$$  (5.1)

To be accurate – if there is such $D \geq 0$ that

$$\sum_{j=1}^{n_i} \lambda_{i,j}^D = 1 \text{ where } \lambda_{i,j} = l_{i,j}/L_i$$  (5.2)

for all $i$ and all levels of aggregation, then we call the set *fractal* and $D$ its *fractal/Hausdorff* dimension (the definition adapted from Falconer, 1990).

It can be seen that a pair "a patch and its replacement" has always $D \geq 0$, and the Eq. (5.2) is thus always met. However, this $D$ could potentially vary from patch to patch within a particular level of aggregation, as well as between subsequent levels. In the case of fractals, however, we have to keep this dimension stable through all the set to meet the condition of scale invariance. This can be realized in several ways. The simplest is the case of proper schoolbook fractals – the $\lambda_{i,j}$ are the same for all $i,j$, and they are also in the same number for all $i$. For example, in Fig. 5.2 $\lambda$ equals to 1/3 and $n$ is 5. Thus, $\sum_{j=1}^{n_i} \lambda_{i,j}^D = 5\left(\frac{1}{3}\right)^D = 1$ and the $D$ is necessarily $\frac{\ln 5}{\ln 3} \approx 1.46$.

For self-similar sets as they are usually defined (i.e. where "similar" refers to the proportional lessening of the original pattern), both the number of

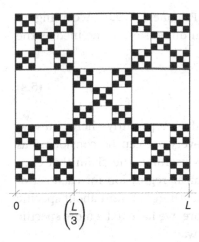

0    $\left(\dfrac{L}{3}\right)$    L

**Figure 5.2** Classical regular fractal. In this case, the fractal dimension, $D$, remains the same for all subsequent levels of aggregation and for all chosen patches. $D$ for the first two subsequent levels of aggregation is the solution of equation $L^D = 5\left(\frac{L}{3}\right)^D$, for the following pair of levels it is the solution of $5\left(\frac{L}{3}\right)^D = 25\left(\frac{L}{9}\right)^D$, etc. The fractal area of this set is thus $L^D$.

subpatches, $n_i$, and their proportional sizes, $\lambda_{i,j}$, are constant for all replacements (i.e. for all $i$). Consequently, $D$ is kept through the whole set and the set is fractal (it is scale invariant). This is also valid for those random fractals that keep the number and sizes of subpatches and where the randomness consists just in the random shuffling of particular patches. For more irregular structures, e.g. the patterns that vary in the number of subpatches for a particular replacement, or in the vector of $\lambda_{i,j}$, the fractality, however, represents very strong and very restrictive condition. Namely, the condition of scale invariance (Eq. 5.2) implies that for each subpatch $k$ of a patch $i$, the equality

$$\lambda_{i,k} = \sqrt[D]{1 - \sum_{\substack{j=1 \\ j \neq k}}^{n_i} \lambda_{i,j}^D} \qquad (5.3)$$

must be met. This means that the area of at least one of the subpatches must depend on the areas of other subpatches and that all subpatches must fall into a particular range of possible sizes. This condition is derived purely from the aforementioned requirement of the independency of the area measurement from the scale used (Eq. 5.1), and thus it is entirely a matter of how we measure areas. There is no reason why this should be met in nature, because there is no reason (in a metaphorical sense) why nature should take care of our problems of measurement. A more realistic view seems to be that there is some other way in which the number and sizes of the subpatches are related. For instance, relative Euclidean area of subpatches, instead of fractal area, could be kept constant – $\sum_{j=1}^{n_i} \lambda_{i,j}^2 = const.$ In the next step, we will try to generalize the idea of fractals with the aim of releasing it from the mentioned restrictive conditions.

One way to generalize the idea of fractals would be to adopt the classical (albeit a bit extreme) interpretation of random fractals which says that the fractal is almost any spatial structure (Falconer, 1990). According to this definition, a fractal is each set with fractal dimension, $D$, defined as the root of

$$E\left(\sum_{j=1}^{n_i} \lambda_{i,j}^D\right) = 1, \tag{5.4}$$

where $E(x)$ is the expectation of $x$, i.e. its mean value. Apparently, there is always such a $D$ that obeys this equation, and thus every set can be considered as (random) fractal. This approach, however, is as useful as the claim that each curve is a line because of the existence of a linear regression for each set of points ($N > 1$), and consequently it cannot say anything relevant about specific properties of particular self-similar sets. Therefore, we have to be more specific in the attempt to generalize fractals in a useful way.

## Generalized fractals

As we have shown, self-similarity is a general concept of aggregated geometrical structures which can be applied for any mechanism that forms species spatial distributions. Fractality is, by contrast, the result of the postulate of scale invariance of our measurement, which imposes very special conditions on the process of spatial clustering. Such a process, for example, would have to cause the negative correlation between the number of patches and the proportional area occupied, $\sum_{j=1}^{n_i} \lambda_{i,j}^2$, for all levels of aggregation (the larger is the fractal dimension, the stronger would necessarily be this correlation). Therefore, we have to broaden the concept of fractality to release its narrow and – at least for ecological systems – apparently unrealistic restrictions. We call the broader concept *generalized fractals*, which we define as structures that originate by replacing patches of the original pattern with any pattern formed by any process. The only condition on this process is that it has to remain essentially the same for all levels of aggregation, though it could vary in its parameters. Note that the process can be very broadly defined – it can be either entirely random or constrained in some aspects, as shown below.

To be accurate, we can define generalized fractals as follows. Each spatial structure which can be decomposed into several patches and their subpatches is a generalized fractal if there is a number of subpatches within the $i$th patch, $n_i$, and if there is a $r_i$ ($0 < r_i \leq 1$) such that

$$F\left(\lambda_1^2, \lambda_2^2, \cdots, \lambda_{n_i}^2\right) = r_i \tag{5.5}$$

for all $i$, where $F$ is any function of the vector $\vec{\lambda}^2$. Note that for our purposes the general form of $F$ can be replaced with the sum of particular functions, $f$, which yields

$$\sum_{j=1}^{n_i} f\left(\lambda_j^2\right) = r_i.$$ (5.6)

In nature, various processes can form spatially aggregated structures, and these processes will in fact probably differ between different levels of aggregation. However, we can expect that some very general statistical regularity should apply universally, across different levels of aggregation, so that real spatial distributions can be modeled using the universal assumptions (say, macro-assumptions) concerning these regularities. There are several possibilities:

1. We can assume scale invariance in the strict sense, which leads to $f(x) = x^{\frac{D}{2}}$ and $r_i = 1$ for all $i$ (which leads to true fractals). We have shown that this requirement is probably biologically meaningless, and thus we have to set up other assumptions that could be more biologically relevant – or at least more easily interpretable.
2. Total proportion of area occupied within any patch is kept within each level and through all levels of aggregation, whereas the number, the sizes of individual patches, and their location are random.
3. Total proportion of occupied area of all subpatches within any patch is kept within each level of aggregation, but it varies randomly between these levels.
4. Everything is random. There is preference neither in number of subpatches nor in their sizes. Apparently, this is a null model for generalized fractals.
5. The probability distribution (but not the parameters of this distribution) that controls the randomness of the proportion of occupied area within patches is independent of the total area considered and is universal for all taxa. This can seem quite a special assumption, but it is actually the most general one, as will be explained in detail later (see also Appendix 5.I). Simply said, this assumes an existence of processes that are actually independent of scale, and that do not depend even on our choice of the "zero" level of aggregation.

## Generating generalized fractals – models of more or less random multiscale aggregation

To explore the properties of spatial distributions characterized as generalized fractals, we constructed models of spatial distributions differing in the assumptions mentioned above, and compared their features. Model realizations were in all cases based on the modified percolation model (Falconer, 1990; Lennon et al., this volume), the algorithm being identical in all cases. The models thus differ only in their parameters, and thus they are comparable to one another. The basic pattern was square, i.e. not only the total area considered (the zero level of aggregation) was square-shaped, but also all patches and their subpatches were squares. The models are as follows.

## M1    *The fractal model*

In the first step, the fractal dimension, $D$ $(0 < D \leq 2)$, was drawn from the distribution of fractal dimensions observed for spatial distributions of bird species within the Czech Republic (see below). Then the square was overlapped with a grid of a randomly chosen number of square-shaped cells, drawn from a regular distribution between $2 \times 2$ and $5 \times 5$. In the next step, $n$ squares smaller than one grid cell were randomly located within randomly chosen (yet unoccupied) grid cells, $n$ being drawn from a regular distribution between 1 and the total number of the grid cells (so that each grid cell could be finally either empty or occupied by just one square of random size and random position within the cell). The only condition was that the sum of proportional fractal areas of these squares, $\sum_{i=1}^{n} \lambda_i^{D}$, was equal to 1 (see Eq. 5.2). This process was applied repeatedly for each level of aggregation (i.e. for each new square), keeping $D$ for all squares within all levels of aggregation. We stopped the process when reaching the fifth level of aggregation. Note that whereas in an ideal case the distribution of subpatches should be entirely random, here it is quasi-random because their location is constrained by the grid used, i.e. by locations of grid cells. This is the case of all following models as well, and the reason is that otherwise the process would be too excessively time-consuming, as large already located patches would too strongly constrain possible locations of the other patches in the case of large $D$.

## M2    *The model of stable proportion of occupied area among levels*

In the first step, the proportional area occupied, $r$ $(0 < r < 1)$, was drawn from regular distribution and then the same procedure as for the fractal model was used. The only difference between these two models was in their parameters. While we used $D$ as an exponent and 1 as the sum of areas in the previous case, we used 2 as the exponent and $r$ as the sum of areas, respectively, in the case of this model. Therefore, this model did not keep the fractal dimension across all levels of aggregation, keeping instead $r$ for each patch across all levels of aggregation and changing the number of subpatches within each patch.

This model can be biologically interpreted as the model of habitat hierarchy where a species occurrence is restricted to some portion of respective level of habitat hierarchy, and this portion remains the same across all levels and all patches. Species can differ in this proportion (as $r$ can vary among species), but each species has some ability to be potentially present in a part of available habitats regardless of the level of habitat hierarchy, and this ability can be determined, for example by its niche width (i.e. specialists would potentially occupy smaller portion of habitat on each level).

**M3    *The model of stable proportion of area within levels***
This model is similar to the previous one except that the proportion of occupied area r is set up separately for each level of aggregation (but remains the same for different patches within one level). This is actually more biologically reasonable than the previous model, as it is probable that each level of aggregation (say, level of habitat hierarchy) is very different and thus the proportion of patches where species occurrence is allowed varies from level to level.

**M4    *The random proportion model***
Here we set up the r separately (and randomly) not only for each level of aggregation, but also for each patch. This model can thus be regarded as an entirely null model, as nothing is kept stable during the process of the emergence of respective spatial structure.

**M5    *The area- and taxa-invariance model***
The main idea behind this model is that the previous model is not as "null" as it looks, because the rules comprising individual patches cannot be equally applied to the basic squares of all sizes (see Appendix 5.I). Therefore, the model M4 in fact assumes that there is some basic level (the zero level of aggregation) which is given, and which cannot itself represent a part of some larger area. Model M5 ensures that the same rules can be applied for basic squares of all possible sizes, i.e. it is independent of the scale we start with. In practice this means that the process is the same as in the previous model (M4), but r is not chosen from the uniform distribution but from the distribution which had been proven to be indeed independent of scale (for details see Appendix 5.I and Fig. 5.8). The parameters of this distribution were generated randomly, but since this process allowed too wide a range of possible patterns, we selected the set of simulations with the distribution of fractal dimensions equal to the observed distribution of D.

## Model properties and tests
We explored statistical properties of all the models, choosing properties which are biologically relevant and have been studied previously. These are the ability of the models (1) to predict the scale–occupancy relationship, or more accurately the relationship between area and the probability of species occurrence, (2) to predict the species–area relationship and (3) to predict the distribution of occupied Euclidean area, which we assume to be proportional to the species abundance distribution. We compared these model properties between models M1–M5 and also with respective patterns of species distributions and abundances in central European birds. Species distribution data comprised quadrat-based distributional atlases of breeding birds of the Czech Republic (Šťastný, Bejček & Hudec, 1996) and Europe (Hagemeijer & Blair, 1997), from which we

used squares of $16 \times 16$ quadrats (see Šizling & Storch, 2004 for details). Data on abundance distributions were obtained from BirdLife International/EBCC (2000), comprising estimated abundances of breeding birds from 33 European countries excluding Russia and Turkey. These abundance data represent probably the only suitable set for this type of comparison, because they are at the same time large scale and reasonably accurate, containing information on abundances across a large range of magnitudes, from one breeding pair to several million. Abundances were calculated as a geometrical mean of the upper and lower estimate for each country if the lower estimate was not zero; if it was, the abundance was calculated as an arithmetical mean.

## The relationship between area and probability of occurrence

The relationship between the area of grid cell and the probability of occurrence within cells of respective area (hereafter p–area relationship) is a very important measure of scaling of spatial distribution. It potentially provides a way to estimate species occupancies or even abundances within fine scales from coarse-scale censuses (Kunin, 1998; Kunin, Hartley & Lennon, 2000; He & Gaston, 2000; He & Condit, this volume; note, however, that these authors were not dealing with the probability of occurrence but with relative occupancy; nevertheless, these measures converge in the limit as area approaches zero). The knowledge of p–area functions is sufficient for the construction of species–area curves simply by summing p–area functions for individual species (Coleman, 1981; Ney-Nifle & Mangel, 1999; Šizling & Storch, 2004). The p–area relationship is generally assumed to be the power law in the case of fractals (i.e. it should be linear in the log-log scale, although see He & Condit, this volume), and for this reason we tested the linearity of the growing part of these relationships for the observed data and models. As a measure of linearity we used the maximal correlation coefficient between log(area) and log(probability of occurrence) obtained by rotating axes. This correlation coefficient does not depend on the slope of the regression line and reflects purely the linearity of the relationship. The curvilinearity of this relationship may, however, generally depend on species rarity – the rarer the species, the less linear it is (He & Condit, this volume). For this reason we plotted the maximum correlation against the calculated fractal dimension of respective spatial distribution (assuming that $D$ tightly correlates with both abundance and occupancy) to have comparison across different rarity classes.

All the models have apparently equal ability to predict the shape of the p–area relationship (Fig. 5.3). When using the Nachman's and logistic models instead of the power law (He & Condit, this volume), i.e. using $-\ln(1-p)$ and $\frac{p}{1-p}$, respectively, instead of the logarithm of probability of occurrence $\ln p$, we obtained smaller correlations with the logarithm of area, i.e. larger curvilinearity, for both models and observed data – but again, all the models were indistinguishable from each other and also from the observed p–area relationships.

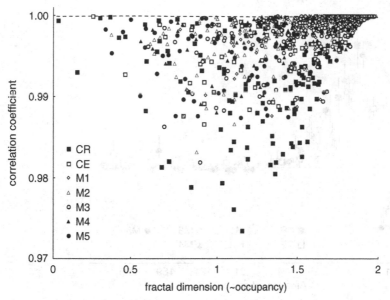

**Figure 5.3** Maximum correlation coefficient (see the text) of the growing part of the p–area relationship in the log-log scale, plotted against the fractal dimension of the spatial distribution. The correlation coefficient is a measure of the linearity of the p–area relationship in the logarithmic scale (i.e. how close it is to the power law) and the fractal dimension correlates with species occupancy (and abundance). Note that all correlation coefficients are quite high, and correlations for different models fill approximately the same space in the plot. This indicates that all models, as well as the observed data, provide the p–area relationship which is very close to the power law. CR, Czech Republic; CE, central Europe; for details of the data see Šizling & Storch (2004).

Another possibility for comparing the models in terms of their ability to predict the p–area relationship is to compare the p–area relationships produced by the models with an "ideal" power-law relationship. In this case, we compared the probability of occurrence for each area predicted by each model with the probability predicted by the power-law relationship obtained by approximating the modeled relationship with the regression line in the log-log scale up to the point of saturation (i.e. up to the point where the probability of occurrence was 1; see Šizling & Storch, 2004). All the models, including the fractal one (M1), as well as observed spatial distributions, apparently deviate from the power-law p–area relationship (Fig. 5.4) but the mean deviation of all the models is relatively low and – more importantly – approximately the same for all models and observations for all areas. Notably, the highest deviation was revealed by the observed spatial distributions of birds within the Czech Republic, and also by the area- and taxa-invariance model (M5) whose parameters were obtained from these observed distributions. All the other models are effectively

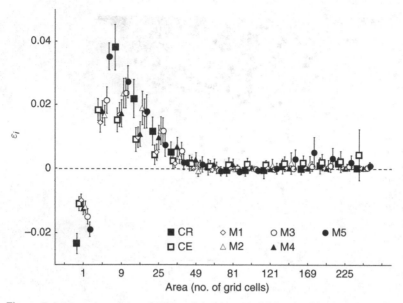

**Figure 5.4** Mean (marks) and $CI_{0.05}$ of the mean (whiskers) of deviations, $\varepsilon$, from the finite area model for assemblages of 200 species in the cases of individual models, and for observations of 142 and 193 bird species within the Czech Republic (CR) and central Europe (CE), respectively. The $\varepsilon$ was calculated for each area as the difference between the probability of occurrence calculated by the finite area model (i.e. the power law bounded by the point of saturation) and the probability predicted by each model or observation.

indistinguishable from one another in terms of their mean deviation from the power-law p–area relationship.

## The species–area relationship

The species–area relationship (hereafter SAR) can be exactly predicted using the knowledge of spatial distribution of individual species, because mean number of species occurring within a plot of area $A$ is exactly equal to the sum of probabilities of occurrence in this area across all species (Coleman, 1981; Ney-Nifle & Mangel, 1999; Lennon, Kunin & Hartley, 2002; Šizling & Storch, 2004). Therefore, we can construct the SAR simply by summing the p–area curves for all species. We constructed 200 realizations (i.e. 200 randomly generated "species") of each model, and compared resulting SARs with one another and also with SARs observed for birds in the Czech Republic and central Europe (after normalizing the species numbers and areas). We have previously shown that the fractal model (M1) produces SARs which are indistinguishable from those observed, provided that the distribution of fractal dimensions used in the model is the same as the observed distribution of measured fractal dimensions (Šizling & Storch, 2004). Also, it is not surprising that the model M5 gives the SAR which is very close to the observed one, as this model was also based on

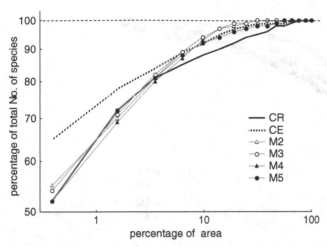

**Figure 5.5** Species–area curves for individual models (marked thin lines) and observed avifauna within the Czech Republic (bold full line) and central Europe (bold dashed line). The prediction of the fractal model (M1) is not shown, as this model needs a parameterization by some distribution of fractal dimensions, when it has been shown to exactly follow the observed SARs (Šizling & Storch, 2004). Note that the curvilinearity and the associated deviation of modeled species numbers from those observed for large areas could be potentially due to the fact that the construction of generalized fractals was not entirely random (see the section headed "Generalized fractals"), and this quasi-randomness apparently affected large areas more strongly.

an observed distribution of fractal dimensions. Much more surprisingly, the other models which were not dependent on any ad-hoc parameterization produced SARs which were also very close to observed SARs, and individual models predicted SARs very similar to each other (Fig. 5.5). The species-specific properties which must have been adjusted to give exact prediction of the SAR in the case of the fractal model (i.e. fractal dimensions) thus emerged from the other models themselves. Indeed, the distributions of fractal dimensions (calculated by standard box-counting method) predicted by the models closely followed the observed distributions (Fig. 5.6). The shape of the SAR is therefore very well predicted by several models of generalized fractals without any assumptions concerning parameters of species spatial distributions. Note also that the slope of the linearly increasing part of predicted SARs is approximately 0.17, which is very close to the generally observed mean slope of mainland SARs (0.15; Rosenzweig, 1995).

## Frequency distribution of the occupied Euclidean area

So far, we have shown that particular generalized fractals (including the scale invariant sets in the original meaning) have similar abilities to predict the p–area relationships for individual species, as well as the species–area relationships.

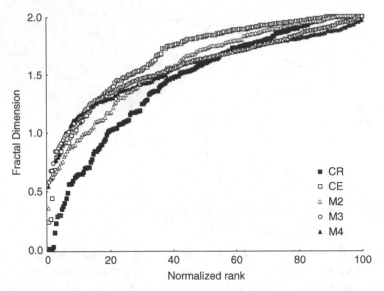

**Figure 5.6** The distribution of fractal dimensions that emerged from models M2–M4, expressed as the rank–dimension relationship (the rank was rescaled to obtain comparable curves for observations and predictions). Fractal dimensions were extracted from 200 independent simulations of species spatial distributions (open diamonds, circles, and closed triangles for M2, M3 and M4, respectively) and the observed distributions of fractal dimensions of bird spatial distributions within the Czech Republic (CR, full squares) and central Europe (CE, open squares). The results of models M1 and M5 are not shown, as in these cases the frequency distribution of fractal dimensions was the input parameter and was set to be equal to the distribution observed for the avifauna of the Czech Republic. Note that the distributions predicted by the models fall between the distributions observed for CR and CE, with the distribution produced by the model M2 falling exactly in the middle.

Consequently, it is no wonder that most published studies showed that species spatial distributions are more or less close to fractal, even if they were not true fractals at all. To show the differences between particular self-similar models, we have had to test the property in which they should differ, and this is the distribution of the Euclidean areas they produce. Each such area corresponds to the area potentially occupied by an individual species and should be in some level of aggregation proportional to species abundance. The strong proportionality would be expected if the spatial requirements of individuals were equal for all species, otherwise the area divided by the mean individual's spatial requirement (i.e. mean home range) should be proportional to abundance.

The distributions of the Euclidean areas occupied, $P$, obey formulae

$$P_n = L^2 r^n, \qquad\qquad\qquad\qquad (M2)(5.7)$$

$$P_n = L^2 \prod_{j=1}^{n} r_j \qquad \text{(M3)(5.8)}$$

and

$$P_n = L^2 0.5^{n-1} r, \qquad \text{(M4)(5.9)}$$

where $r$ is a random number between 0 and 1 (drawn from the regular distribution), $n$ is the number of levels of aggregation and $L^2$ is the area of the original patch, in the case of M2, M3 and M4, respectively. The area occupied is in these cases independent from any parameter but $r$ (for details see Appendix 5.II). In the cases of the other two models (M1 and M5), the distribution of area occupied depends on an external parameter such as the distribution of fractal dimensions, and this cannot be expressed so easily. We calculated these distributions numerically for various levels of aggregation using the models depicted above.

To compare the distributions of areas occupied for the individual models with observed distributions of species abundances, we extracted the variance and normalized skewness of the distribution of their logarithmically (base 2) transformed values from both the model predictions (for various levels of aggregation) and the abundance distributions of birds in European countries. Only two models fitted the data well: the model of the stable proportion of area within levels (M3) and the area- and taxa-invariance model (M5). In the case of the model M5 it is not too surprising, as this model always provides almost lognormal distribution of areas, fitting even better than the lognormal model to observed distributions (using Kolmogorov–Smirnov statistics; Šizling & Storch, unpublished manuscript). The fit of model M3 is more interesting (Fig. 5.7). Note that we should not expect a perfect fit, as the areas occupied on $n$th level of aggregation cannot be exactly proportional to the abundances, considering that individuals from different species have different spatial requirements (home ranges). Indeed, when we included an assumption of different home range sizes, assuming an approximately lognormal distribution, the fit of the model M3 improved, and even the model of the stable proportion of occupied area among levels (M2) provided good predictions of species abundance distributions. Therefore the spatial distribution characterized by generalized fractals is likely to lie behind observed species abundance distributions.

## Discussion and conclusions

Our results show that spatial structures that are effectively indistinguishable from true fractals can emerge by simple random hierarchical processes taking place on several spatial scales. Such processes can be modeled in several ways, differing in the constraints on the randomness. Quite intriguingly, the models which best fitted the observed data were those where the proportion of area potentially occupied within the lower level of aggregation was kept constant throughout space within

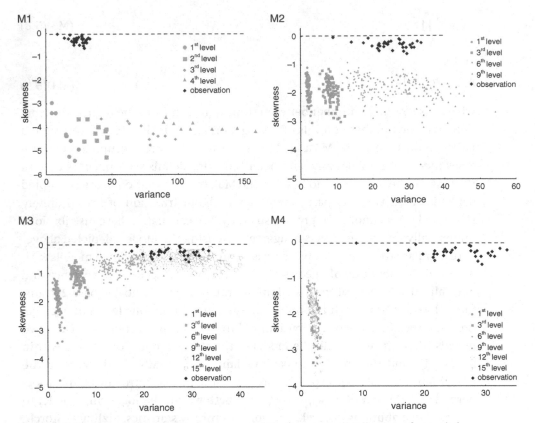

**Figure 5.7** Variance and normalized skewness of the frequency distribution of occupied areas for models M1, M2, M3 and M4 (grey marks; the number of species for each assemblage/point was 200; the number of assemblages/points for each setting was 10 in M1 and 100 in M2–M4), and corresponding parameters for logarithmized abundance distributions of avifaunas of European countries (black marks). The parameters for different levels of aggregation are marked with different shapes (see legends inside the figures). Note that with the exception of the model M4, the more levels of aggregation, the higher is the variance of the respective distribution. The frequency distribution of fractal dimensions used for the fractal model (M1) was extracted from the observed central European avifauna data set (see text). Only in the case of model M3 did the parameters of observed and modeled distributions overlap, albeit only for relatively high levels of aggregation.

each level of aggregation (M3) or even among different levels of aggregation (M2), although in the latter case the occupancy/abundance distributions fitted only when accounting for different spatial requirements of individuals, i.e. assuming particular nonequal distribution of home ranges (unpublished simulations). The real pattern of species spatial distribution can in fact lie somewhere between these two models. Anyway, regardless of which model is closer to nature, all the models produce structures that are similar to fractals in most properties, although they are not true fractals, and are in fact much more directly interpretable biologically.

Different levels of modeled spatial aggregation can represent different levels of habitat association (macrohabitat – mesohabitat – resource patches) and/or of spatial population dynamics (e.g. range dynamics – local metapopulation dynamics – behavioral decision-driven changes in occurrence). Various propor- tions of area selected at each scale that ultimately lead to interspecific differ- ences in the distribution and abundance can then be related to species-specific ecological properties such as body size, niche width, mean dispersal distance or competitive ability. Therefore, although we assume entirely random processes, they can in fact refer to particular biologically relevant mechanisms, and their "randomness" is just a way to treat different processes in one framework – or, in other words, it is a way to ensure that different spatial scales and processes taking place within them can be related to each other in a formal manner.

The finding that our model of random aggregation does not only produce spatial structures which are very close to observed fractal-like distributions, and predicts realistic species–area curves, but also gives the distributions of occupied area which are close to observed species abundance distributions, deserves atten- tion. There are plenty of models of abundance distributions within species assemblages (for reviews see Tokeshi, 1999; Gaston & Blackburn, 2000), some of them based on niche divisions among species (Sugihara, 1980; Tokeshi, 1996), some on nonlinearities in population dynamics (Bell, 2000; Hubbell, 2001). Recently it has become clear that a successful model of the species abundance distribution within larger scales should take space seriously, as abundance always has an inherent spatial dimension. Therefore, good models must be implicitly or explicitly spatial. The most prominent of these models is Hubbell's neutral theory of biodiversity, according to which the distribution of species abundance is the result of "community drift" and processes of random colonization, extinction, migration and speciation (see also He, 2005; Borda-de-Água et al., this volume). However, this theory assumes that individual species do not differ ecologically, which is apparently an extremely restrictive assumption. Interspecific niche differences are almost surely as important as space, and a successful theory should comprise them as well. There are models that comprise both space and interspecific niche differences (Marquet, Keymer & Cofré, 2003), and our model can be treated as one of them. Arguably, our model is the null model of species abundance distribution, because it does not assume any particular way in which niches are divided among species, neither any sort of interspecific interactions (either in evolutionary or ecological time). It is entirely individualistic (i.e. community-level properties emerge purely from species-level spatial processes) and ecological differences between species are assumed implicitly, as these contribute to the process of hierarchical random aggregation.

Generally, there are two major approaches which attempt to treat most macroecological patterns in species distribution and diversity within one uni- versal framework. One of them is the above-mentioned Hubbell's neutral theory of biodiversity and biogeography (Hubbell, 2001; see also Bell, 2001; Chave, 2004). The second one is the HEAP (Hypothesis of Equal Allocation Probabilities) approach which attempts to derive most patterns from basic statistical assumptions (Harte *et al.*, 2005; Harte, this volume). Both approaches have, however, some limitations. Hubbell's theory does not rely only on the restrictive assumption of species per-capita ecological identity mentioned above, but also assumes complete biotic saturation, i.e. that total number of individuals per unit area remains constant, which leads to strong interspecific competition on space, albeit the outcome of this competition is not given a priori. By contrast, Harte's HEAP model represents a rather statistical description, whose biological interpretation is still unclear (see Harte, this volume). Moreover, although HEAP predicts many patterns in species distribution and diversity, it needs the abundance distribution of the whole assemblage as an input. On the contrary, our model of hierarchical random aggregation does not need any assumption concerning interspecific relationships or other community-level constraints, nor any external parameters to predict realistic patterns of species abundance distribution (the abundance distribution being one of its outputs).

It is not yet clear whether our theory is able to predict as wide a range of spatial ecological phenomena as those predicted either by Hubbell's neutral theory or the HEAP. However, since our theory predicts realistic spatial scaling of species distribution and diversity with a minimal set of assumptions and without free parameters, and is at the same time biologically reasonable, it can be treated as a null hypothesis of spatial scaling of ecological patterns.

## Acknowledgments

We are grateful to László Hajnal for his mental support in discussions between biologists and mathematicians, and to Stephen Hartley for his useful comments on the manuscript. The study was supported by the Grant Agency of the Academy of Sciences of the CR (KJB6197401), Grant no. CC06073 of the Czech Ministry of Education, and the Research Program CTS MSM0021620845.

## Appendix 5.I    The area- and taxa-invariant distribution

As mentioned above, the random proportion model (M4) is not simultaneously applicable for all sizes of patch area, and thus is not "scale invariant" even in the most general sense. Assuming, for example, its validity for an area of $500 \times 500 \, \text{km}^2$, we cannot simultaneously assume its validity for any larger or smaller area. The reason is that this model assumes a regular distribution of proportional areas within each patch, $r$, through all of $S$ simulations (i.e. for an assemblage of $S$ species). However, if we do assume it, for example for the mentioned area $500 \times 500 \, \text{km}^2$, we obtain an irregular distribution of $r$ for an area composed from several such areas (Fig. 5.8). The area of $500 \times 500 \, \text{km}^2$ is thus in this case privileged and must be considered as basal.

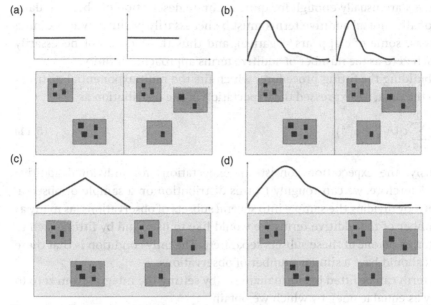

**Figure 5.8** Top: the frequency distributions of the proportion of occupied area used for the construction of spatial distributions within the left and the right plots in the case of (a) the random proportion model (M4) and (b) the area- and taxa-invariance model (M5). Below: the resulting distributions of the proportion of occupied area when joining the left and right plots for models M4 (c) and M5 (d). While in the case of the regular distribution (a) the joining of the two areas yields a roof-shaped distribution (c), in the case of the multiexponential distribution (b) the distribution of joined plots remains multiexponential (d).

To build a model that is really independent of "scale" we have to find a distribution that conserves its form when enlarging the basal area (see Fig. 5.8). Since area is always positive, the distribution must allow only positive random values, and also should attain zero, as we never know how many species are absent on the modeled area. The distribution that obeys these conditions is independent of area chosen as the basal area (zero level of aggregation) and of the set of considered species, and we thus call it the area- and taxa-invariant distribution. We found that this distribution can be expressed using the multi-exponential form

$$f(x) = \sum_{i=1}^{\infty} c_i \left( e^{-A_i x} - e^{-\alpha_i x} \right), \tag{5.10}$$

where $A_i$ and $\alpha_i$ are positive and $c_i$ is any real number (Šizling & Storch, manuscript in preparation). The number of additive terms, $c_i \left( e^{-A_i x} - e^{-\alpha_i x} \right)$, does not have to be necessarily infinite – it is defined as infinite because it can vary unlimitedly as it arises whenever any two areas are joined. However, three or four terms are usually enough for quite accurate description of observed data. Additionally, not all additive terms must be necessarily positive (when joining two areas, some of $c$ appears negative), and thus the $c_i$ does not necessarily approach zero as the number of additive terms approaches infinity.

For building the fitting procedure, which fits the multiexponential distribution to the data, we expressed the expectation of the distribution as

$$E(x) = \sum_{i=1}^{\infty} c_i \left( A_i^{-2} - \alpha_i^{-2} \right).$$  (5.11)

Obviously, the expectation consists of expectations for individual additive terms. Therefore, we can roughly fit this distribution on a sample of observations just by dividing the sample into several subsets of observations (as many as the number of the additive terms we would like to use), and by fitting each of these terms on one of these subsets separately. The only condition is that these subsets should have a similar number of observations.

One term can be fitted by normalizing it (by setting the integral from zero to infinity as equal to one), by which we obtain

$$E_i(x) = A_i^{-1} + \alpha_i^{-1}.$$  (5.12)

If $\alpha_i > A_i$, the expected value can vary between $A_i^{-1}$ and $2A_i^{-1}$. Estimating the expectations as a mean, $M$, we can estimate the parameters as

$$A_i = \frac{2 - \kappa/(1 + \kappa)}{M_i} \text{ and } \alpha_i = (1 + \kappa)A_i \text{ where } \kappa > 0.$$  (5.13)

The vector of parameters of proportionality, $c_i$, was estimated as the best fitted vector from 200 vectors calculated as $c_i = \frac{random}{E_i(x)}$ where $random$ is a random number between 0 and 1. The term "best fitted" refers to the vector for which the Kolmogorov–Smirnov statistics (i.e. the maximal deviation between two cumulative distribution functions) between the analytical form and the fitted data was minimal. The estimation is not too sensitive to the choice of $\kappa$ but in an attempt to minimalize numerical errors we set it as $10^{99}$.

## Appendix 5.II   Calculating the distribution of occupied areas

To set up the general form for the total areas occupied we used the proportional areas, $\lambda^2$, for each patch within each level of aggregation. For two levels of aggregation, for example, we can write

$$P_2 = L^2 \begin{pmatrix} \lambda^2_{i_1=1} \left( \lambda^2_{i_1=1,i_2=1} + \lambda^2_{i_1=1,i_2=2} + \cdots + \lambda^2_{i_1=1,i_2=k_{i_1=1}} \right) + \\ +\lambda^2_{i_1=2} \left( \lambda^2_{i_1=2,i_2=1} + \lambda^2_{i_1=2,i_2=2} + \cdots + \lambda^2_{i_1=2,i_2=k_{i_1=2}} \right) + \\ \cdots \\ +\lambda^2_{i_1=k} \left( \lambda^2_{i_1=k,i_2=1} + \lambda^2_{i_1=k,i_2=2} + \cdots + \lambda^2_{i_1=k,i_2=k_{i_1=k}} \right) \end{pmatrix}$$  (5.14)

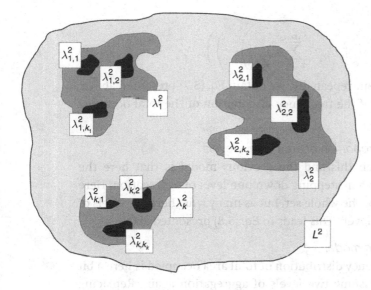

**Figure 5.9** Three levels of aggregation with the labels indicating areas of individual patches and subpatches. Using these areas, total occupied area within respective level of aggregation can be calculated using Eq. (5.14). Note that the calculation is actually independent of the exact shape of individual patches, and the $L$ and $\lambda$ can be imaginary values (because they are the square roots of areas of the patches).

where $P_2$ is the total area occupied by patches at the second level of aggregation, $L^2$ is the total area of the area of origin, and indexes $i_1$ and $i_2$ refer to the order of a particular patch within the first and second level of aggregation, respectively. So, for instance, $\lambda^2_{i_1=m,i_2=n}$ means the proportional area of $n$th patch within the $m$th patch at the second level of aggregation (see Fig. 5.9; note that the indices are simplified in this figure so that $\lambda^2_{i_1=m,i_2=n}$ is replaced with $\lambda^2_{m,n}$, for example).

Making the form (5.14) more compact, we can write

$$P_2 = L^2 \sum_{i_1=1}^{k} \left( \lambda^2_{i_1} \sum_{i_2=1}^{k_{i_1}} \lambda^2_{i_1,i_2} \right) \tag{5.15}$$

in the case of two levels of aggregation, and generally

$$P_n = L^2 \sum_{i_1=1}^{k} \left( \lambda^2_{i_1} \sum_{i_2=1}^{k_{i_1}} \left( \lambda^2_{i_1,i_2} \sum_{i_3=1}^{k_{i_1,i_2}} \left( \lambda^2_{i_1,i_2,i_3} \cdots \left( \lambda^2_{i_1 K i_{n-1}} \sum_{i_n=1}^{k_{i_1} K i_{n-2}} \lambda^2_{i_1 \cdots i_n} \right) \cdots \right) \right) \right) \tag{5.16}$$

for $n$ of those levels. This relatively complicated general form can be simplified in the cases of individual models as follows.

### M2  *The model of stable proportion of occupied area between levels*

In this case, the proportional areas occupied, $r$, were kept constant through the whole set. In general, considering the form Eq. (5.16) and replacing all proportional areas at the lowest level with $r$, we obtain

$$P_n = L^2 \sum_{i_1=1}^{k} \left( \lambda^2_{i_1} \sum_{i_2=1}^{k_{i_1}} \left( \lambda^2_{i_1,i_2} \sum_{i_3=1}^{k_{i_1,i_2}} \left( \lambda^2_{i_1,i_2,i_3} \cdots \sum_{i_{n-1}=1}^{k_{i_1} K i_{n-2}} \left( \lambda^2_{i_1 K i_{n-1}} r \right) \right) \cdots \right) \right). \tag{5.17}$$

After simplifying

$$P_n = L^2 r \sum_{i_1=1}^{k} \left( \lambda_{i_1}^2 \sum_{i_2=1}^{k_{i_1}} \left( \lambda_{i_1,i_2}^2 \sum_{i_3=1}^{k_{i_1,i_2}} \left( \lambda_{i_1,i_2,i_3}^2 \cdots \sum_{i_{n-1}=1}^{k_{i_1}K_{i_{n-2}}} \lambda_{i_1 K_{i_{n-1}}}^2 \right) \cdots \right) \right), \tag{5.18}$$

and applying this replacement repeatedly, we obtain Eq. (5.7) presented above, which is the simplest form of the frequency distribution of the total occupied area.

## M3   *The model of stable proportion of area within levels*

The only difference between this and the previous model is that here the proportional area changes when stepping down one level of aggregation. Here there is not the only one $r$ for the whole set, but as many $r_j$ as there are levels of aggregation (one $r_j$ for each level). This leads to Eq. (5.8) presented above.

## M4   *The random proportion model*

The calculation of the frequency distribution of total area occupied is here a bit more complicated. Let us assume two levels of aggregation again. Replacing each sum of proportional areas occupied at the second level of aggregation with its average value, 0.5, plus its deviation, $\varepsilon$, we obtain

$$P_2 = L^2 \begin{pmatrix} \lambda_{i_1=1}^2 (0.5 + \varepsilon_1) + \\ +\lambda_{i_1=2}^2 (0.5 + \varepsilon_2) + \\ \cdots \\ +\lambda_{i_1=k}^2 (0.5 + \varepsilon_k) \end{pmatrix}. \tag{5.19}$$

After simplifying,

$$P_2 = L^2 0.5 \left( \lambda_{i_1=1}^2 + \lambda_{i_1=2}^2 + \cdots + \lambda_{i_1=k}^2 \right) + L^2 \left( \lambda_{i_1=1}^2 \varepsilon_1 + \lambda_{i_1=2}^2 \varepsilon_2 + \cdots + \lambda_{i_1=k}^2 \varepsilon_k \right). \tag{5.20}$$

Obviously, the area is given by the area at the higher level of aggregation and an error term. The error term is a number drawn from a unimodal distribution (nearly Gaussian) which has average value of zero (because all $\varepsilon_i$ follow the distribution with the mean of zero).

Replacing the proportional area of the first level with $r_1$, we obtain

$$P_2 = L^2 0.5 r_1 + L^2 \varepsilon \tag{5.21}$$

in the case of two levels of aggregation, and using this algorithm repeatedly we obtain

$$P_n = L^2 0.5^{n-1} r_1 + L^2 \varepsilon \tag{5.22}$$

in general. The $n$ is the number of levels of aggregation and $r_1$ is the proportional area occupied at the first level of aggregation. Since the average value of the error term, $L^2 \varepsilon$, is zero, for larger samples we obtain Eq. (5.9) presented above.

This formula could be criticized, however, for allowing an unrealistic extent of areas. For instance, the area of $L^2$ is not allowed by this form, although, according to the model, it is principally possible (all levels of aggregation having $r$ equal to one for all subpatches). The areas larger than $L^2 0.5^{n-1}$ are, by contrast, very improbable, so that Eq. (5.9) can be used for nearly any number of species (spatial distributions). This was verified comparing the outputs from a numerical model ($N = 50$; 4 levels of aggregation) with the analytical form derived.

## References

Allen, T. F. H. & Starr, T. (1982). *Hierarchy: Perspectives for Ecological Complexity*. Chicago: University of Chicago Press.

Bell, G. (2000). The distribution of abundance in neutral communities. *American Naturalist*, **155**, 606–617.

Bell, G. (2001). Neutral macroecology. *Science*, **293**, 2413–2418.

BirdLife International/European Bird Census Council (2000). *European Bird Populations: Estimates and Trends*. Cambridge: BirdLife International.

Chave, J. (2004). Neutral theory and community ecology. *Ecology Letters*, **7**, 241–253.

Coleman, D. B. (1981). On random placement and species-area relations. *Mathematical Biosciences*, **54**, 191–215.

Condit, R., Ashton, P. S., Baker, P., *et al.* (2000). Spatial patterns in the distribution of tropical tree species. *Science*, **288**, 1414–1418.

Falconer, K. J. (1990). *Fractal Geometry: Mathematical Foundations and Applications*. Chichester: John Wiley.

Gaston, K. J. & Blackburn, T. M. (2000). *Pattern and Process in Macroecology*. Oxford: Blackwell Science.

Hagemeijer, W. J. M. & Blair, M. J. (1997). *The EBCC Atlas of European Breeding Birds*. London: T. & A. D. Poyser.

Halley, J. M., Hartley, S., Kallimanis, S. A., Kunin, W. E., Lennon, J. J. & Sgardelis, S. P. (2004). Uses and abuses of fractals in ecology. *Ecology Letters*, **7**, 254–271.

Harte, J., Kinzig, A. & Green, J. L. (1999). Self-similarity in the distribution and abundance of species. *Science*, **284**, 334–336.

Harte, J., Conlisk, E., Ostling, A., Green, J. L. & Smith, A. B. (2005). A theory of spatial structure in ecological communities at multiple spatial scales. *Ecological Monographs*, **75**, 179–197.

Hartley, S., Kunin, W. E., Lennon, J. J. & Pocock, M. J. O. (2004). Coherence and continuity in the scaling of species' distribution patterns. *Proceedings of the Royal Society of London, Series B*, **271**, 81–88.

Hastings, H. M. & Sugihara, G. (1993). *Fractals, a User's Guide for the Natural Sciences*. Oxford: Oxford University Press.

He, F. L. (2005). Deriving a neutral model of species abundance from fundamental mechanisms of population dynamics. *Functional Ecology*, **19**, 187–193.

He, F. L. & Gaston, K. J. (2000). Estimating species abundance from occurrence. *American Naturalist*, **156**, 553–559.

Hubbell, S. P. (2001). *The Unified Theory of Biodiversity and Biogeography*. Princeton: Princeton University Press.

Kunin, W. E. (1998). Extrapolating species abundances across spatial scales. *Science*, **281**, 1513–1515.

Kunin, W. E., Hartley, S. & Lennon J. J. (2000). Scaling down: on the challenge of estimating abundance from occurrence patterns. *American Naturalist*, **156**, 560–566.

Lennon, J. J., Kunin, W. E. & Hartley, S. (2002). Fractal species distributions do not produce power-law species-area relationships. *Oikos*, **97**, 378–386.

Marquet, P. A., Keymer, J. E. & Cofré, H. (2003). Breaking the stick in space: of niche models, metacommunities and patterns in the relative abundance of species. In *Macroecology: Concepts and Consequences*, ed. T. M. Blackburn & K. J. Gaston, pp. 64–81. Oxford: British Ecological Society and Blackwell Science.

Ney-Nifle, M. & Mangel, M. (1999). Species-area curves based on geographic range and occupancy. *Journal of Theoretical Biology*, **196**, 327–342.

Richardson, L. F. (1961). The problem of contiguity: an appendix of statistics of deadly quarrels. *General Systems Yearbook*, **6**, 139–187.

Rosenzweig, M. L. (1995). *Species Diversity in Space and Time*. Cambridge: Cambridge University Press.

Šizling, A. L. & Storch, D. (2004). Power-law species-area relationships and self-similar species distributions within finite areas. *Ecology Letters*, **7**, 60–68.

Šťastný, K., Bejček, V. & Hudec, K. (1996). *Atlas of Breeding Bird Distribution in the Czech Republic 1985–1989*. Jihlava: Nakladatelství a vydavatelství H & H, in Czech.

Sugihara, G. (1980). Minimal community structure: an explanation of species abundance pattern. *American Naturalist*, **116**, 770–787.

Tokeshi, M. (1996). Power fraction: a new explanation for species abundance patterns. *Oikos*, **75**, 543–550.

Tokeshi, M. (1999). *Species Coexistence: Ecological and Evolutionary Perspectives*. Oxford: Blackwell Science.

Ulrich, W. & Buszko, J. (2003). Self-similarity and the species-area relation of Polish butterflies. *Basic and Applied Ecology*, **4**, 263–270.

Virkkala, R. (1993). Ranges of northern forest passerines: a fractal analysis. *Okois*, **67**, 218–226.

# CHAPTER SIX

# Toward a mechanistic basis for a unified theory of spatial structure in ecological communities at multiple spatial scales

JOHN HARTE

*University of California, Berkeley*

## Introduction

Macroecology, the search to identify and understand the origin of patterns in the distribution and abundance of species is a major focus of ecology (Gaston & Blackburn, 2000). Knowledge of such patterns is central to formulating local, national and global conservation and land use policies, as well as to the effort to understand the principles governing ecosystem function and temporal dynamics. Many mathematical models have been proposed and tested against specific macroecological patterns (e.g. He & Legendre, 2002) but few have been tested against the wide array of spatial metrics that can be derived from spatially explicit census data. Moreover, many of these models contain adjustable parameters whose values are difficult to determine a priori, and it is often unclear whether fitting parameterized models to data yields predictive insight into ecosystems. By testing highly constrained theory against a variety of metrics, as opposed to testing parameter-laden theory against a small number of metrics, the search for plausible underlying pattern-generating mechanisms may be expedited.

Two types of spatial metric are of interest here – those that characterize the distributions of individual species and those that characterize spatial structure in a community of species. Table 6.1 lists and defines a diverse set of spatial metrics of both types. The metrics are defined in terms of a scale label, $i$, which is explained in Box 6.1. That box also illustrates the definitions of the spatial metrics using a simple example.

In a previous paper (Harte *et al.*, 2005), we showed that starting only with the observed set of species abundances $\{n_0\}$ at some largest spatial scale of area $A_0$, and with no adjustable parameters, a new theory of spatial structure (HEAP) predicts at each smaller scale the explicit form of all but two (see below) of the metrics in Table 6.1. We tested the theory using spatially explicit census data across a wide range of spatial scales from three vegetation communities. Two are at tropical forest sites: the BCI 50-ha plot in Panama (Hubbell & Foster, 1983; Condit *et al.*, 1996) and a $\sim$10-ha plot in dry forest at San Amelio, Costa Rica

*Scaling Biodiversity*, ed. David Storch, Pablo A. Marquet and James H. Brown. Published by Cambridge University Press. © Cambridge University Press 2007.

**Table 6.1** *Spatial metrics*

**Species-level metrics**

| | | |
|---|---|---|
| $P_i^{(n_0)}(n)$ | Species-level spatial abundance distribution | Probability that $n$ individuals of a species with total abundance $n_0$ in $A_0$ are found in cell of area $A_i$. |
| $R_i^{(n_0)}$ | Range–area relationship (RAR) | Box-counting measure of occupancy for a species with $n_0$ individuals in $A_0$: relates range size of a species ($=$ number of occupied cells $\times$ cell area) to cell area $A_i$. |
| $\chi^{(n_0)}(A_i, D_j)$ | Species-level commonality function | Probability a species with total abundance $n_0$ in $A_0$ is found in two $A_i$ cells separated by the $j$th bisection but not the $j-1$st bisection. |
| $\Omega_i^{(n_0)}$ | Measure of aggregation | Density of conspecifics at distance $A_i^{1/2}$ from average individual, relative to random distribution for a species with $n_0$ individuals in $A_0$. |

**Community-level spatial metrics**

| | | |
|---|---|---|
| $S_i$ | Species–area relationship (SAR) | Relates number of all species occurrences in a census cell to area $A_i$ of that cell. |
| $E_i$ | Endemics–area relationship (EAR) | Relates number of species unique to a cell to area $A_i$ of that cell. |
| $\chi(A_i, D_j)$ | Community-level commonality function | Fraction of all species in common to two cells $A_i$ separated by the $j$th bisection but not the $j-1$st bisection. |
| $\Phi_i(n)$ | Species-abundance distribution | Fraction of all possible species occurrences with $n$ individuals in cells of area $A_i$. |
| $F_i(N)$ | Community-level spatial-abundance distribution | Probability that $N$ individuals from all species are in cell $A_i$. |

(Enquist *et al.*, 1999); the third is a $64\,m^2$ serpentine meadow plot in the McLaughlin Natural Reserve in California (Green, Harte & Ostling, 2003). While the theoretically predicted metrics are generally consistent with the data, a systematic discrepancy was shown to arise. In particular, Harte *et al.* (2005) show that the theory overpredicts the level of aggregation for the more abundant species in each data set, but that the discrepancies generally decrease at finer spatial scales. I argue below that in the search for a mechanistic understanding of the HEAP model, this pattern of discrepancy provides important clues.

The two metrics in Table 6.1 that were not discussed in Harte *et al.* (2005) were the species- and community-level "commonality functions" describing spatial turnover of species occurrences. After summarizing the essential ideas and findings of HEAP, I present a new result: a pair of coupled recursion relations that determine both the species- and community-level spatial commonality

## Box 6.1

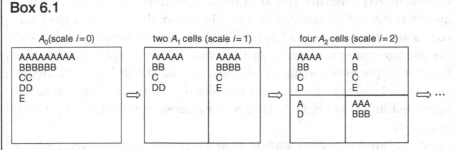

**Figure 6.1** Explanation of scale label, $i$, and selected spatial metrics in Table 6.1. Five species (A, B, C, D, E) are shown, with total abundances 9, 6, 2, 2, 1 respectively. An area $A_0$ (scale $i = 0$) is bisected once to create two $A_1$ cells (scale $i = 1$); the second bisection yields four $A_2$ cells (scale $i = 2$). Examples of numerical values of the spatial metrics in Table 6.1 are given below.

### Species level metrics

**Spatial abundance distribution $P_i^{(n_0)}(n)$:** For species A at scale $i = 2$, there are 4, 3, 1, and 1 individuals, so $P_2^{(9)}(4) = \frac{1}{4}$, $P_2^{(9)}(3) = \frac{1}{4}$, $P_2^{(9)}(1) = \frac{1}{2}$.

**Range area relationship $R_i^{(n_0)}$:** For species B at scale $i = 2$, there are 3 occurrences $\times$ area $A_2 = 3A_2$.

**Commonality function $\chi^{(n_0)}(A_i, D_j)$:** For species B, with 6 individuals in $A_0$ the probability of occurrence in two $A_2$ cells ($i = 2$) separated by the second but not the first bisection ($j = 2$) is the average of 0 (B is *not* found in both the upper left and lower left $A_2$ cells) and 1 (the species *is* found in both the upper right and the lower right $A_2$ cells). Thus $\chi^{(6)}(A_2, D_2) = (0 + 1)/2 = \frac{1}{2}$.

**Aggregation measure $\Omega_i^{(n_0)}$:** This metric cannot be illustrated at the coarse scale of resolution shown above, but for a detailed explanation of how it is calculated and tested within our bisection formalism, see Ostling, Harte and Green (2000).

### Community-level metrics

**Species–area relationship $S_i$:** $S_0 = 5$; $S_1 = (4 + 4)/2 = 4$; $S_2 = (4 + 4 + 2 + 2)/4 = 3$.

**Endemics–area relationship $E_i$:** At the largest scale $i = 0$, all five species are defined to be endemic so $E_0 = 5$. At scale $i = 1$, one species (D) is found only in the left-hand $A_1$ cell, and one species (E) is found only in the right-hand cell, so $E_1 = (1 + 1)/2 = 1$. At scale $i = 2$, no species are unique to the upper left cell, 1 species (E) is unique to the upper right cell, and no species are unique to either of the lower cells, so $E_2 = (0 + 1 + 0 + 0)/4 = \frac{1}{4}$.

**Commonality function** $\chi(A_i, D_j)$: Consider the fraction of species in common to two $A_2$ cells separated by the $j = 2$ bisection: the fraction of species in common to the two left-hand $A_2$ cells is $2/3$ (2 are in common, A and D, and the average number of species in the two cells is $(4+2)/2 = 3$), while the fraction of species in common to the two right-hand cells is also $2/3$. Hence $\chi(A_2, D_2) = 2/3$. For $j = 2$, we do not consider the fraction in common to the upper left and lower right $A_2$ cells because those are separated by a $j = 1$ bisection.

**Species-abundance distribution** $\Phi_i(n)$: At scale $i = 0$, the five species have abundances 9, 6, 2, 1, and 1, so $\Phi_0(9) = 1/5$, $\Phi_0(6) = 1/5$, $\Phi_0(2) = 2/5$, and $\Phi_0(1) = 1/5$. At scale $i = 2$ there are potentially $2^2 S_0 = 20$ species occurrences or nonoccurrences in the 4 quadrants. In fact, there are 8 nonoccurrences (0 individuals), 8 occurrences with 1 individual, 1 with 2 individuals, 2 with 3 individuals, and 1 with 4 individuals. So $\Phi_2(0) = 8/20$, $\Phi_2(1) = 8/20$, $\Phi_2(2) = 1/20$, $\Phi_2(3) = 2/20$, $\Phi_2(4) = 1/20$.

**Community-level spatial-abundance distribution** $F_i(N)$: At scale $i = 0$, $F_0(N) = 1$ for $N = 20$ and 0 otherwise. At scale $i = 1$, there are 10 individuals in the left-hand $A_1$ cell and 10 in the right-hand cell, so $F_1(N) = 1$ for $N = 10$ and 0 otherwise. At scale $i = 2$, in the four quadrats there are 8, 6, 4, and 2 individuals, so $F_2(8) = F_2(6) = F_2(4) = F_2(2) = \frac{1}{4}$.

functions on patch size and interpatch distance. I also discuss potential applications of this result to the estimation, from presence–absence data, of species richness and species abundances at spatial scales so large that only patchy censusing, rather than complete censusing, is possible.

I originally interpreted HEAP as a kind of null model, in the sense that random placement (Coleman, 1981) is a null model. The failure of such a null model would imply the existence of some dynamical mechanism to explain the observed patterns. I adopt a different interpretation here for the following reason. The HEAP model can be shown to be a special case within a continuum of models that are characterized by a single parameter, $\theta$ (Eq. 6.8 below). The continuum spans the range from random placement ($\theta = 0$) to maximally aggregated ($\theta = \infty$; every individual is located in a single grid cell at every spatial scale), with HEAP corresponding to the special value $\theta = 1$. The systematic pattern of discrepancy noted above between HEAP and census data can be thought of as a systematic variation of $\theta$ with abundance and scale; thus it may be a mechanistically regulated parameter. Here I show, using a very simple dynamical model based on the assumption of dispersal/recruitment limitation, that from species to species the value of $\theta$ depends upon scale, abundance, and dispersal distribution in an explicit and testable manner. This mechanistic model is highly simplified and is thus presently just a heuristic device to illustrate the possibility of a dynamical explanation for the value of $\theta$ and therefore of the conditions under which HEAP adequately describes macroecological spatial patterns.

## Some formalities

In any theory of spatial pattern, an exact mathematical relationship can be shown (Harte, Blackburn & Ostling, 2001) to exist between two of the patterns listed in Table 6.1: the species–area relationship (SAR) and the set of range–area relationships (RARs) for the species. The SAR describes the dependence of species richness on area of sampled cell, while the RAR is defined for each species and describes the dependence of a species' occupancy (number of cells occupied by that species) on cell area. To understand the relationship between these two metrics, we can introduce a scale label, $i$, as defined in the caption to Fig. 6.1 in Box 6.1: at the largest scale, $i = 0$ and thus $A_0$ is the area of the entire ecosystem or biome being studied; at finer spatial scale, $A_i$ cells have area $A_i = A_0/2^i$. A formal shape-preserving procedure for this bisection process exists (Harte, Kinzig & Green, 1999a; Plotkin et al., 2000; Ostling et al., 2004) and a consistent procedure for avoiding potentially unrealistic, artifactual consequences has been described (Ostling et al., 2004). We can then introduce a community-level species-richness scaling parameter, $a_i$, defined by

$$a_i = S_i/S_{i-1},\tag{6.1}$$

where $S_i$ is the average number of species found in the $A_i$ cells. Over a scale range such that $a_i$ is independent of $i$ (and thus scale independent in that scale range) it can be shown that the SAR obeys a power-law behavior (Harte et al., 1999a; Ostling et al., 2003). For each species, we can define an analogous set of parameters, $\alpha_i^{(n_0)}$, defined by

$$\alpha_i^{(n_0)} = R_i^{(n_0)}/R_{i-1}^{(n_0)},\tag{6.2}$$

where the superscript $(n_0)$ is a species label such that $n_0$ is the number of individuals of the species in $A_0$, and $R_i^{(n_0)}$ is the product of cell area, $A_i$, times the number of $A_i$ cells occupied by the species.

From the definition of $R_i$, and the fact that we are only considering species that are present in $A_0$ so that $R_0 = A_0$, the $\alpha_i^{(n_0)}$ can be interpreted in terms of occupancy probabilities. In particular, $\alpha_1^{(n_0)}$ is the probability the species $(n_0)$ is present in an arbitrary (i.e. randomly chosen) $A_1$ cell, $\alpha_1^{(n_0)}\alpha_2^{(n_0)}$ is the probability the species is present in a randomly chosen $A_2$ cell, and in general $\prod_{j=1}^{i} \alpha_j^{(n_0)}$ is the probability the species is present in a randomly chosen $A_i$ cell.

To simplify notation, we define

$$\lambda_i^{(n_0)} = \prod_{j=1}^{i} \alpha_j^{(n_0)},\tag{6.3}$$

so that $\lambda_i^{(n_0)}$ is the probability that the species with abundance $n_0$ in $A_0$ is present in a randomly chosen $A_i$ cell. In terms of the species-level spatial abundance distribution $P_i^{(n_0)}(n)$ in Table 6.1, we can therefore express $\lambda_i^{(n_0)}$ as

$$\lambda_i^{(n_0)} = 1 - P_i^{(n_0)}(0). \tag{6.4}$$

We have derived the following exact relationship between the community parameters $a_i$ and the $\lambda_i^{(n_0)}$ parameters (Harte et al., 2001; Ostling et al., 2003):

$$\prod_{j=1}^{i} a_j = <\lambda_i^{(n_0)}>_{\text{species}} . \tag{6.5}$$

In Eq. (6.5) and below, the notation $<x>$ refers to the average of x, and the subscript "species" informs the reader that this particular average is taken over all the species in $A_0$.

Equation (6.5) has the interesting consequence that it is impossible for both the $a_i$ and all the $\alpha_i^{(n_0)}$ to be scale independent over *any* scale range unless the $\alpha_i^{(n_0)}$ are identical for all species. In other words, unless the counterfactual condition that all the species have the same fractal dimension and thus identical RARs holds, it is impossible for both the SAR and the RARs for all species to simultaneously exhibit power-law behavior. For that reason we have called Eq. (6.5) the "impossibility theorem". Further implications of Eq. (6.5) have been discussed by Lennon, Kunin and Hartley (2002) and Šizling and Storch (2004).

HEAP is, as must be the case, consistent with the impossibility theorem, but HEAP also leads to an explicit decision regarding the choice between whether the SAR or the RARs can be scale independent. In particular, in Harte et al. (2005) we showed that for *every* species and over any scale range, HEAP forbids scale independence and associated power-law behaviors for the range–area relationship $R_i^{(n_0)}$. In other words, the $\alpha$'s are intrinsically scale dependent over any scale interval, under HEAP. Moreover, HEAP yields an exact power-law SAR only over a limited scale range and only under constrained conditions on the species–abundance distribution. Thus HEAP does not describe fractal patterns of species spatial distributions. We shall see further evidence of this below when we examine the relationship under HEAP between the mean and the variance of the spatial distribution.

## Statistical formulations of HEAP

There are two ways to formulate the HEAP model and to generate its predictions (Harte et al., 2005), both within the framework of the cell-bisection approach defined above. The first, inspired by the statistical mechanics of indistinguishable particles (Ruhla, 1992), builds on the assumption that all numerically distinct allocations of indistinguishable individuals between the two halves of any cell are equally likely. This is the origin of the acronym HEAP, which stands for Hypothesis of Equal Allocation Probabilities.

The meaning of HEAP can best be illustrated by contrasting HEAP with the way in which classical statistical mechanics describes the allocation of classical (not quantum mechanical) molecules to the left and right halves of a room. Because classical molecules are treated as distinguishable, the counting rule for allocation leads to a binomial distribution. Thus, if two molecules, labeled a and b, are to be allocated, the probabilities of each of the following assignments is equally likely: [none, ab], [a, b], [b, a], [ab, none]. Because there are two ways to place one molecule in each half, and only one way to place both molecules on the left-hand side, the probability is twice as high that a molecule will be in each half than that the left half will be empty. With a large number of molecules, this allocation rule, which is the basis of classical statistical mechanics, leads to the result that it is overwhelmingly more likely that molecules will be evenly divided across the room than that there will be far more in one half or the other.

Under HEAP, in contrast, with two objects to allocate, the options of [a, b] and [b, a] are not distinct because a and b are identical. Thus there is a 1/3 probability of there being none on the left, one on each side, and none on the right. All numerically distinct allocations are equally likely. With a larger number of objects (i.e. of individuals within a species), the distinct allocations are still equally likely, so that for example with 100 objects, the probabilities of the two options [none, 100] and [50, 50] are equally likely and each has probability 1/101. Once an allocation has been made at a largest scale, then the rule is iterated at finer scale, so that for example, if [20, 80] obtains at the first alloca-tion, then the 80 individuals on the right-hand side are allocated according to HEAP between the two halves of the right-hand side. Clearly this rule results in spatial distributions that are more aggregated than in the standard random placement model that results in a binomial distribution.

I emphasize that the HEAP allocation rule is posited to hold at all scales, but the distributions that this scale-invariant rule generates are not themselves scale independent and thus the theory will not lead to fractal spatial distributions. The theory can be thought of as a neutral theory at the intraspecific level, but at least currently not neutral at the interspecific level. It is neutral at the intra-specific level because individuals within a species are treated as statistically indistinguishable. It is currently not neutral at the interspecific level because the different abundances of species are assumed at the outset, and this results in differently shaped spatial distributions (different degrees of aggregation) for species of differing abundance. In a more unified theory of ecology in which the abundance distribution is generated by an assumed set of processes, then it is the nature of those processes that will determine if the theory is neutral at the interspecific level (e.g. Hubbell, 2001; Borda-de-Água et al., this volume).

Because genetic and other differences between individuals are ignored in HEAP, in the real world we would expect to see corrections that reflect the distinctions across individuals within a species. Thus we do not claim that it will fully explain empirical spatial patterns. The issue becomes: which is a better null random theory of spatial allocation, HEAP or the standard random placement model? We have demonstrated elsewhere (Harte *et al.*, 2005) that HEAP provides a better null theory for understanding spatial patterns in ecology.

As shown in Harte *et al.* (2005), the HEAP allocation rule leads directly to the following recursion relation for the species-level spatial abundance distribution $P_i^{(n_0)}$ defined in Table 6.1:

$$P_i^{(n_0)}(n) = \sum_{q=n}^{n_0} \frac{P_{i-1}^{(n_0)}(q)}{(q+1)}. \tag{6.6}$$

Box 6.2 provides an explanation of how Eq. (6.6) follows from the allocation rule.

The solutions to Eq. (6.6) uniquely generate the predictions for most of the other species- and community-level metrics listed in Table 6.1 (see Appendix 6.I). Some representative tests of these metrics are shown in Figs. 6.3–6.5; these are excerpted from a much more extensive set of published comparisons (Harte *et al.*, 2005). The community-level spatial abundance distribution, $F_i(N)$, is generated from the solutions to Eq. (6.6) for each species in the community only if we make the additional assumption that the species are distributed independently of each other within $A_0$. Making that assumption, we test the HEAP prediction for $F_i(N)$ in Fig. 6.6.

The second formulation of the theory may provide a better basis for developing a mechanistic understanding of it. In particular, Eq. (6.6) and the HEAP statistical rule from which the recursion relation is derived are mathematically equivalent (see Appendix 6.II) to the following "assembly" or "colonization" rule. Consider the individuals of a single species being allocated to the two halves of a cell in which the species is known to exist. Assume the individuals are allocated, one individual at a time until all the individuals have been allocated using the following sequential colonization rule:

$$\beta(\text{left}|l, r) = (l+1)/(l+r+2), \tag{6.7}$$

where $\beta$ is the probability that if there are $l$ and $r$ individuals in the left and right halves of the cell, then the next individual is allocated to the left half. Symmetrically, individuals are allocated to the right with probability $\beta(\text{right}|l,r) = (r+1)/(l+r+2)$. This assembly rule can be applied successively to generate spatial distributions at finer and finer scale. Thus, if $n_0$ individuals are known to exist in an $A_0$, then Eq. (6.7) generates a division of those individuals into the two $A_1$ cells that comprise $A_0$. Continuing in this way, the individuals in each of the two $A_2$ cells comprising each $A_1$ cell can be assembled. This process can be continued to arbitrarily large values of the scale index $i$.

Note that the assembly rule given by Eq. (6.7) promotes aggregation; at any stage in the assembly process, the half that has more individuals has a greater than 50% probability of attracting the next individual. For example, if $l = 5$ and

**Box 6.2**

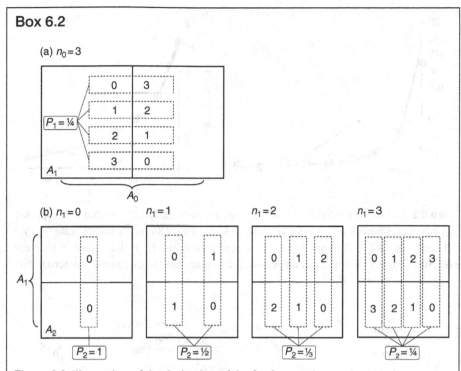

(a) $n_0 = 3$

(b) $n_1 = 0$      $n_1 = 1$      $n_1 = 2$      $n_1 = 3$

**Figure 6.2** Illustration of the derivation of the fundamental recursion relation.

Given a species with $n_0 = 3$ in $A_0$, and under the hypothesis of equal allocation probabilities (HEAP), the four allocation options for the two $A_1$'s (panel a of Figure 6.2) are each associated with equal probabilities of ¼. That is, considering the left $A_1$, and using the notation $P_1$ to denote the probability of any particular number $n_1 \leq n_0$ of individuals being in that left $A_1$, then $P_1 = 1/(n_0 + 1)$.

Further subdividing the left $A_1$ into two $A_2$ halves, the allocation options for $A_2$ are illustrated in panel (b) for each outcome of the left $A_1$. The associated probabilities are now labeled by $P_2$; for the top $A_2$ and each $n_1$, $P_2 = 1/(n_1 + 1)$. $P_2^{(n_0)}(n)$ is then calculated by multiplying the conditional probabilities for the particular cases of allocation to $A_1$ and $A_2$, and summing terms. Thus,

$$P_2^{(3)}(1) = P_1^{(3)}(1).1/2 + P_1^{(3)}(2).1/3 + P_1^{(3)}(3).1/4,$$

or:

$$P_2^{(3)}(n) = \sum_{q=n}^{n_0} \frac{P_1^{(3)}(q)}{(q+1)}.$$

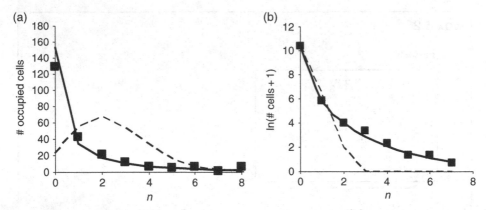

**Figure 6.3** Test of the predicted species-level spatial distribution, $P_i^{(n_0)}(n)$ for a BCI species with $n_0 = 621$. Comparisons are for (a) scale $i = 8$ (cell area = 50 ha/$2^8$) and (b) scale $i = 15$ (cell area = 50 ha/$2^{15}$). The solid lines are the predicted values from HEAP; dashed lines are predictions from a random placement model (Coleman, 1981). The squares are actual data.

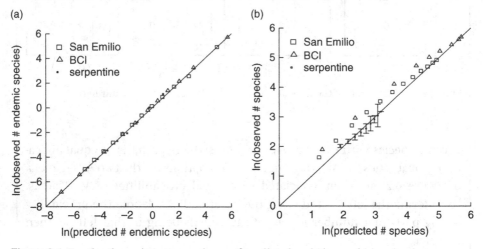

**Figure 6.4** For the three sites, comparisons of predicted and observed (a) endemic species richness, and (b) total species richness. In both, straight lines are 1:1 lines.

$r = 4$, then the probability that the 10th individual is added to the left half is $(5 + 1)/(5 + 4 + 2) = 6/11 > \frac{1}{2}$. In contrast under random assembly, the probability that a new individual is added to the left half is always exactly $\frac{1}{2}$.

Equation (6.7) can be seen as a special case of the more general allocation rule:

$$\beta(\text{left}|l, r) = (l\theta + 1)/(l\theta + r\theta + 2). \tag{6.8}$$

When $\theta = 0$, the rule is equivalent to the random-placement model (Coleman, 1981), while $\theta = \infty$ yields a maximally aggregated distribution in which, at every scale $i$, all individuals of each species are located in just one of the $2^i A_i$ cells. Within a range of negative values of $\theta$, Eq. (6.8) yields a distribution of

(a)

(b)

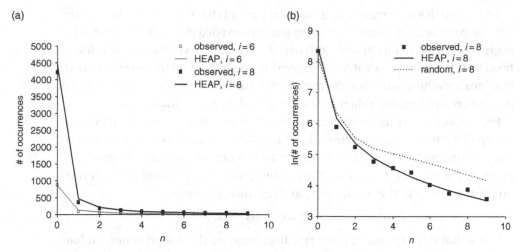

**Figure 6.5** Observed and predicted values of the scale-dependent species abundance distribution, $\Phi_i(n)$, for the serpentine site. (a) Comparison of predicted and empirical species–abundance distribution $\Phi_i(n)$ for $i = 6$ (lower curve and data) and $i = 8$ (upper curve and data) for the serpentine plot. (b) Comparison of HEAP and the random model predictions for the $i = 8$ data, with $\ln(\Phi_i(n))$ plotted to better highlight the differences at small $\Phi_i(n)$; a random model prediction is shown for comparison.

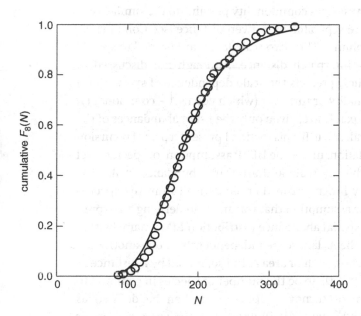

**Figure 6.6** Test of the prediction for the community-level spatial abundance probability distribution, $F_i(N')$ for the BCI site. The solid line is the HEAP prediction for the cumulative distribution (sum of $F_i(N')$ from $N' = 0$ to $N' = N$) and the open circles are BCI data at scale $i = 8$.

individuals that is more uniform than random. The value $\theta = 1$ corresponds to HEAP. Not all spatial distributions are generated by repeated application of Eq. (6.8); e.g. the negative binomial distribution and a pure fractal or self-similar distribution do not appear to correspond to any value of $\theta$.

Because such a wide variety of distributions are all characterized by the value of a single parameter, $\theta$, likelihood testing is readily carried out without concern for degrees-of-freedom adjustment. In Harte *et al.* (2005) we conducted such likelihood tests for each species at our three census sites and found that the likelihood-maximizing value of $\theta$ tends to decrease from 1 (the HEAP value) or larger, toward 0 (the random placement value), as species abundance in $A_0$ increases.

Harte *et al.* (2005) presented the relationship between the spatial variance and the spatial mean of $n$, at arbitrary scale $i$, under the HEAP assumption for the spatial distribution $P_i^{(n_0)}(n)$ (that is, under the assumption that the distribution is given by the solution to Eq. 6.6). The variance, $(\sigma_i^{(n_0)})^2$, is the sum of two terms, one that is linear in the mean, $<n_i>$, and one that is quadratic:

$$(\sigma_i^{(n_0)})^2 = [(4/3)^i - 1] <n_i>^2 + [1 - (2/3)^i] <n_i>.$$

I note that this expression is intermediate between that found under random placement ($\sigma^2 \sim <n>$) and that found under the assumption of self-similarity ($\sigma^2 \sim <n>^2$) as derived in Banavar *et al.* (1999). In this sense the HEAP spatial distributions are more aggregated than under random placement but less aggregated than under the assumption of self-similarity or fractality.

## Species turnover or commonality

The concept of scale-dependent species commonality pertains to the similarity of patches of a given area that are separated by a given distance (see Condit *et al.*, 2002, and Gaston *et al.*, this volume). Thus two scale labels are needed to specify commonality: patch size and interpatch distance. Although not discussed in Harte *et al.* (2005), HEAP uniquely predicts the scale dependence of species-level and community-level commonality or turnover (which equals 1 − commonality) on interpatch distance and on patch size, given only the list of abundances of the species at the largest spatial scale, $i = 0$. In this section I present a pair of recursion relationships that allow calculation, under the HEAP assumption, of species-level commonality function for arbitrary scale and arbitrary abundance in $A_0$. The community-level commonality function can then be derived from the species-level functions under the same assumption that was made in deriving an expression for the community-level spatial abundance distribution $F_i(N)$ – namely, that the species are distributed on the $A_0$ landscape independently of one another.

Consider two censused patches, each of area $A$ and separated by a distance $D$. I define a similarity measure, $\Psi(A,D)$, to be the number of species in common to the two patches. A measure of turnover, $T(A,D)$, can then be defined as $T(A,D) = 1 - \chi(A,D)$, where $\chi(A,D)$ equals $\Psi(A,D)$ divided by the average number of species, $S(A)$, in the two patches. I refer to $\chi(A,D)$ as the community-level commonality function. I can also define species-level commonality functions, $\chi^{(n_0)}(A,D)$, as the probability that a species with $n_0$ individuals in $A_0$ is found in two cells of area $A$ separated by the distance $D$.

Because our theory is formulated on a landscape that is repeatedly bisected in alternately perpendicular directions to yield the $A_j$ cells, a discrete definition of distance $D$ is required to connect theoretical predictions to the real world. Toward that end, and following Ostling et al. (2004), we denote the bisection of the $A_0$ cell that creates two $A_1$ cells a first-order bisection. The two second-order bisections yields four $A_2$ cells. There are four third-order bisections and together they yield eight $A_3$ cells, etc. The distance $D_j$ is defined to be the average distance between two $A_i$ cells that are separated by the $j$th, but not the $j - 1$st, bisection, where $1 \leq j \leq i$ (Ostling et al., 2004).

An exact pair of coupled recursion relationships for each of the $\chi^{(n_0)}$ can be derived from HEAP (see Appendix 6.III). The first is:

$$\chi^{(n_0)}(A_i, D_j) = (n_0 + 1)^{-1} \sum_{m=2}^{n_0} \chi^{(m)}(A_{i-1}, D_{j-1}). \qquad (6.9)$$

Repeated application of Eq. (6.9) will lead to an expression for $\chi^{(n_0)}(A_i, D_j)$ in terms of the set of functions $\chi^{(n_0)}(A_{i-j+1}, D_j)$. A second relationship determines the $\chi^{(n_0)}(A_{i-j+1}, D_j)$:

$$\chi^{(n_0)}(A_i, D_1) = (n_0 + 1)^{-1} \sum_{m=1}^{n_0-1} \lambda_{i-1}^{(m)} \lambda_{i-1}^{(n_0-m)}, \qquad (6.10)$$

where the $\lambda_i^{(n_0)}$ expressions are given by Eq. (6.4).

Equations (6.9) and (6.10) determine the species level commonality functions in terms of the $\lambda$'s, which in turn are determined by HEAP using Eqs. (6.4) and (6.6). Assuming HEAP applies independently to all species, the community-level similarity measure, $\Psi(A_i, D_j)$, is then given by a sum over species of the $\chi^{(n_0)}(A_j, D_k)$ and the community-level commonality function, $\chi(A_i, D_j)$ is then given by

$$\chi(A_i, D_j) = \sum_{\text{species}} \chi^{(n_0)}(A_i, D_j) / \sum_{\text{species}} \lambda_i^{(n_0)}. \qquad (6.11)$$

Understanding the dependence of the commonality function on the $\lambda$'s is of practical importance because the shape of the species–area relationship is entirely determined by the $\lambda$'s (Eq. 6.20). If measurements of species-level commonality functions at large values of interpatch separation $D_j$ (small $j$-values) can provide estimates of the $\lambda_j$'s for each species, then in principle at these large spatial scales the number of species in biomes that are too large to census completely can be determined from large-distance (small $j$) commonality estimates of the $\lambda_j$-values.

In earlier work, we assumed power-law behavior for the SAR over a scale range for which commonality values could be extracted from patchy census data, and then tested whether we could predict species richness at large spatial scales from the commonality data. For example, using data on tree species commonality among pairs of 48 0.25 ha plots in the Western Ghats of India, we successfully predicted species richness in a 60 000 km² biome (Krishnamani, Kumar & Harte, 2004). Additional tests and applications have been carried out for montane meadow plants (Harte *et al.*, 1999b) and for microbial diversity in Sturt National Park, Australia (Green *et al.*, 2004). See also Green and Bohannan in this volume.

It is not clear from Eqs. (6.9–6.11) how the commonality metric relates to the SAR under HEAP; this is an ongoing area of study. Because the $\lambda$'s determine the SAR (Eq. 6.20), one approach is to find a scaling relation for $\chi$ in terms of the $\lambda$'s. Toward that end, and based on earlier analysis of the scaling behavior of the commonality function in self-similar models (Harte *et al.*, 1999b), I had postulated that

$$\chi^{(n_0)}(A_i, D_j) \approx c(\lambda_i^{(n_0)})^2 / \lambda_j^{(n_0)}. \tag{6.12}$$

The motivation for this postulate derived from analysis (Harte *et al.*, 1999b) of self-similar models in which the conditional probability $\chi^{(n_0)}(A_i, D_j)/(1 - P_i^{(n_0)}(0)) = \chi^{(n_0)}(A_i, D_j)/\lambda_i^{(n_0)}$ scales as $(A_i/D_j^2)^{y'} = 2^{(j-i)y'}$ where $y' = -\log_2(\alpha^{(n_0)})$. Because we had assumed that $\alpha^{(n_0)}$ is scale independent, $2^{-iy'} = (\alpha^{(n_0)})^i = \lambda_i^{(n_0)}$ and $2^{jy'} = 1/(\alpha^{(n_0)})^j = 1/\lambda_j^{(n_0)}$. Hence, it appeared reasonable to postulate more generally, even when the $\alpha$'s are not scale independent, that:

$$\chi^{(n_0)}(A_i, D_j)/\lambda_i^{(n_0)} \approx \prod_{k=1...i} \alpha_k^{(n_0)} / \prod_{k=1...j} \alpha_k^{(n_0)} = c\lambda_i^{(n_0)}/\lambda_j^{(n_0)} \tag{6.13}$$

from which Eq. (6.12) follows. To test this, I compare in Fig. 6.7 the exact value of $\chi^{(100)}$ calculated numerically from the recursion relations (Eqs. 6.9, 6.10), and the value of the right-hand side of Eq. (6.13) calculated from an exact recursion relation for the $\lambda$'s that was derived in Harte *et al.* (2005). The apparent good agreement is *not* an identity because for $i \sim j$ the scaling rule works poorly and for many $i \gg j$ combinations there are discrepancies of a few percent. Figure 6.7 indicates that the constant $c$ in Eq. (6.13) is numerically very close to 1.

A closer examination of the "data" in Fig. 6.7 indicates, however, that the high $R^2$ value (0.9994) is illusory and the scaling relationship (Eq. 6.12) requires modification. In particular, if the exact solutions to the recursion relations are compared with Eq. (6.12) at a large but fixed value of the patch-scale index $i$, and plotted as a function of $j$, then a large discrepancy shows up (Fig. 6.8). Figure 6.7 only appeared to confirm Eq. (6.13) because the range of the index $i$ is much greater than the scale range of $j$ and therefore the $i$-dependence of $\chi^{(n_0)}$ dominates the $R^2$ value. Thus Fig. 6.7 confirms the scaling dependence of $\chi^{(n_0)}$ on $(\lambda_i^{(n_0)})^2$ as in Eq. (6.13), but the $j$-dependence (i.e. distance dependence) of species-level commonality does *not* scale like $1/\lambda_j^{(n_0)}$.

To examine this further, I plot in Fig. 6.9 the slope of the graph of the exact numerical value (from Eqs. 6.9 and 6.10) of $\log_2(\chi^{(n_0)}(A_i, D_j))$ versus $j$ for

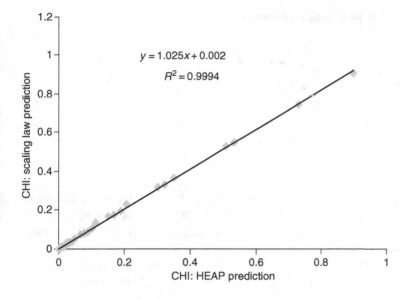

Figure 6.7 Test of the theoretical scaling behavior of $\chi^{(100)}(A_i, D_j)$ for $j = 1, \ldots, 5$ and $i = j+3, \ldots, 15$. The $y$-axis is the value of $\chi$ calculated from Eq. (6.12), using the exact HEAP values for the $\lambda$'s; the $x$-axis is the exact solution to the recursion relations, Eqs. (6.9) and (6.10).

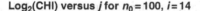

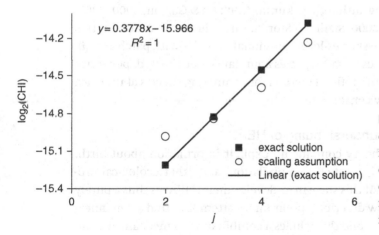

Figure 6.8 A more detailed comparison of the scaling relation (Eq. 6.12) and the exact solution for the commonality function at fixed $i$ and $n_0$ as a function of interpatch scale label $j$.

increasing values of $i$ and for three values of $n_0$: 10, 100, and 1000. As $i$ increases ($A_i$ shrinks), the slope asymptotically approaches a constant value of ~0.415 (which is, inexplicably and perhaps coincidentally, exceedingly close to $\log_2(4/3)$), and the approach to that asymptotic value is faster for smaller $n_0$. Further analysis of the dependence of $\chi^{(n_0)}(A_i, D_j)$ on $\lambda_j^{(n_0)}$ under the assumption of HEAP could provide a means of more accurately predicting species richness at biome scale using sparse commonality data from small patches scattered throughout the biome.

Another potential application of HEAP in conjunction with commonality data is to the problem of estimating the abundances of species from sparse

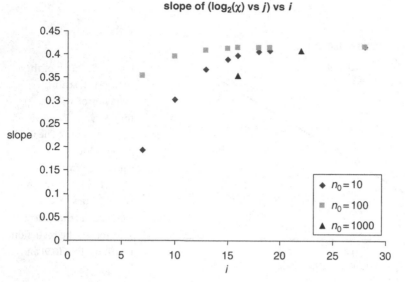

**slope of $(\log_2(\chi)$ vs $j)$ vs $i$**

**Figure 6.9** The slope of the graph of $\log_2(\chi^{(n_0)}(i,j))$ versus $j$, as a function of patch scale $i$ and abundance $n_0$.

presence–absence data on patches scattered throughout a biome. This problem has been discussed by many authors (e.g. Kunin, 1998; He & Gaston, 2000, 2003; Kunin, Hartley & Lennon, 2000; Šizling & Storch, this volume; He & Condit, this volume). Knowledge of how species-level commonality scales with patch area ($i$), interpatch distance ($j$), and especially species abundance (see the $n_0$-dependence in Fig. 6.9) may lead to a more refined method for estimating species abundance at large scales from patchy census data.

## Towards a mechanistic understanding of HEAP

In its current form, the theory contains no explicit information about birth, death, migration, dispersal, competition, predation, and other ecological processes that exist in nature. At this stage in its development, HEAP is thus a purely statistical null theory. I now describe a preliminary attempt to find a dynamical modeling framework that explicitly includes a combination of mechanisms and from which spatial distributions resembling those that result from the family of generalized HEAP allocation rules (Eq. 6.8) might follow. With such a model, the conditions under which any particular value of $\theta$ arises for a particular species and at a particular spatial scale could be identified and related to meaningful ecological variables such as properties of the dispersal distribution. Here I describe progress toward that end, with the focus on a single species rather than an entire community.

I assume that the addition of new individuals into a population is, for each species, limited by some combination of seed dispersal, and germination and seedling establishment (for plants) or dispersal and successful rearing of young (for animals). Rather than treating seed dispersal and germination (or hatching and growth to maturity) as distinct processes, however, I simply consider the combined process of establishment of offspring that will grow to become reproducing adults. I denote the distribution of distances between offspring (at the time of their maturity) and their parent (at the time of their reproductive activity) as the "spatial reproduction distribution" (SRD). This distribution plays a central role in the model developed here.

Consider the population dynamics of an arbitrary species in an arbitrary cell of area $A$ imbedded within a much larger area $A_R$, where $A_R$ is the geographic range of the particular species. By focusing on an arbitrary cell, I avoid having to deal with artificialities that result from the bisection scheme described above (Ostling $et\ al.$, 2004). I assume there are $N_R$ individuals of that species in $A_R$ and $n$ individuals in $A$, values which of course may change over time. The area that we denoted $A_0$ in the formulation of HEAP could be larger or smaller than $A_R$ but it is larger than $A$.

Suppose the species happens to contain abundances $n_L$ and $n_R$ in the left and right halves of $A$. Note, then, that Eq. (6.7), and thus HEAP, is obtained if $dn_L/dt = c(n_L + 1)$ and $dn_R/dt = c(n_R + 1)$ where $c$ is independent of abundance but may depend on $A$. The reason this would result in HEAP is that according to Eq. (6.7), a HEAP distribution results if the probability of the next individual being added to the left-hand side of a cell that happens to have $n_L$ and $n_R$ in the left and right hand sides, respectively, is $(n_L + 1)/[(n_L + 1) + (n_R + 1)]$, which is guaranteed if $dn_L/dt = c(n_L + 1)$ and $dn_R/dt = c(n_R + 1)$.

Because $A$ was arbitrary, a sufficient condition from which the allocation rule in Eq. (6.7) would result is that for $any$ cell of any area, the occupancy of the cell changes according to $dn/dt = c(n + 1)$. I remind the reader that the reason for the term "+1" in the expression for this time derivative is because HEAP corresponds to a value of $\theta = 1$; more generally, from Eq. (6.8) we would write $dn/dt = c(n + \theta^{-1})$. Our task then is to find a mechanism that guarantees that assembly occurs at a rate $dn/dt = c(n + 1)$ where $n$ is the abundance in the cell at an arbitrary time. At large $n$ this might be modified with a density-dependent loss rate, but for purposes of this exploratory model we ignore that here.

I now make two major approximations. The first is that the growth of each species is independent of the existence and distribution of all other species. In a future extension of the single species analysis carried out here, a zero-sum rule imposed on the entire community would generate effective interspecies dependence, but here we ignore that. The second approximation is that environmental heterogeneity plays no explicit role in determining where a species exists or at what rate its individuals are born, grow, reproduce, or die. Then, for our arbitrary species, we can write $dn/dt = G(n, N_R)$ where $G$ is the sum of two functions: the first, $G_1(n)$, describes the rate at which individuals of the species in cell $A$ contribute to the rate of change of $n$; the second, $G_2(N_R - n)$, describes the rate at which individuals in the rest of $A_R$ contribute to the rate of change of the abundance $n$ in the cell $A$. $G_1$ and $G_2$ may contain parameters that are unique to the species we are considering (for example, a reproductive rate constant or a dispersal distance) but the functions are independent of the characteristics of all the other species.

Ignoring density dependence, the first function will be proportional to $n$ and the second to $N_R - n$. The SRD is not well characterized for most species, but as a first, clearly oversimplified, case, I take the SRD to be uniform within a disk of area $D^2$ centered around each parent. The value of $D$ may differ from species to species, but I assume $D$ is a constant for each species and thus does not depend on location of parents within $A_R$.

I examine two limiting cases: $A \ll D^2$ and $A \gg D^2$, but in both cases I assume $A_R \gg A$, $N_R \gg n$ and $A_R \gg D^2$. If $A \ll D^2$, then $G_1 = rnA/D^2$, where $r$ is a per-capita reproductive rate constant for the selected species. This results from the assumption of uniformity of the SRD within $D^2$, from which it follows that $A/D^2$ is the fraction of offspring of an individual in $A$ that will be found in $A$. Similarly, $G_2 = r(N_R - n)[D^2/(A_R - A)][A/D^2]$, which also follows from our assumption about the uniformity of the SRD; the factor $(D^2/(A_R - A))$ is the fraction of individuals in $A_R$, but not in $A$, whose offspring could "land" in an area $D^2$ that includes the cell $A$, provided $A \ll D^2$, while $(A/D^2)$ is the fraction of those offspring that have landed in $D^2$ that will more specifically land in $A$. Because I am ignoring density dependence, I take $r$ in these expressions to be a constant. Note that we are ignoring geometric factors of order $\pi$ or 4.

Using $A_R \gg A$ and $N_R \gg n$, the contribution to offspring in $A$ from parents outside of $A$ becomes $G_2 \sim r(N_R)(A/A_R)$. Hence $dn/dt = G = G_1 + G_2 \sim r[nA/D^2 + N_R A/A_R] = rA/D^2[n + N_R D^2/A_R]$. This can be rewritten in the form $dn/dt = c(n + b)$ if we set $b = N_R D^2/A_R$ and set $c = rA/D^2$. Comparing this expression for $dn/dt$ with Eq. (6.8), we see that the term $\theta$ in Eq. (6.8) can be identified with $b^{-1}$. Moreover, we obtain

$$dn/dt \sim c(n + 1) \quad (\text{for } A \ll D^2) \tag{6.14}$$

and thus HEAP $(\theta = b^{-1} = 1)$ if

$$N_R \sim A_R/D^2. \tag{6.15}$$

In words, in the absence of density dependence and at spatial scales $A \ll D^2$ a sufficient condition for HEAP is that the density of individuals within the geographic range of the species is such that there is on average one individual in each area $D^2$. If there is density dependence, so that the rate constant $r$ is no longer constant, then other options are possible but I do not pursue those here. As the abundances $n$ and $N_R$ grow, this implies that for fixed $\theta$ the geographic range $A_R$ must increase in proportion to $N_R$ because $D^2$ is fixed in this simple model. In reality, as abundance grows, some combination of the following could occur: density dependence alters the value of $r$, the value of $\theta$ changes, and the geographic range of the species increases. Just how these factors will interplay will require fully spatially explicit simulations that go beyond the mean-field discussion given here.

If $A$ is sufficiently large so that $A \gg D^2$, then the result is different. In this case, $G_1 \sim rn$ because nearly all offspring of a parent in $A$ will "land" in $A$. To calculate $G_2$ we again have to estimate how many parents living in $A_R$ but not in $A$ happen to reside near enough to $A$ so that their offspring will land in $A$. Those parents will reside in an annulus of diameter $\sim A^{1/2}$ and width $\sim D^{1/2}$. Thus the area of the annulus is $\sim (AD^2)^{1/2}$ and the fraction of individuals that are located there is then $\sim N_R(AD^2)^{1/2}/A_R$. Here again we have implicitly assumed that $A_R \gg A$ and $N_R \gg n$ and we are again ignoring geometric factors of order $\pi$ or 4. Because roughly half of the offspring of those individuals land in $A$, we obtain $G_2 \sim rN_R(AD^2)^{1/2}/A_R$. Hence, for sufficiently large $A$, $G \sim r[n + N_R(AD^2)^{1/2}/A_R]$. Recalling that the quantity we defined as $b$ is given by $b = N_R D^2/A_R$, we can rewrite this as $dn/dt = G = r[n + b(A/D^2)^{1/2}]$. If Eq. (6.15) is satisfied, so that $b = 1$, then this becomes

$$dn/dt \sim r[n + (A/D^2)^{1/2}] \quad (A \gg D^2). \tag{6.16}$$

We note that for $A \gg D^2$, the second term in the brackets is greater than 1, and thus if we compare Eq. (6.16) with Eq. (6.8), in this limit of large $A$ the effective value of $\theta$ is less than 1. More generally, as $A$ increases to a value $A \gg D^2$, the effective value of $\theta$ decreases from $b^{-1}$ to $b^{-1}(D^2/A)^{1/2}$. If $b = 1$, so that HEAP ($\theta = 1$) results at spatial scales such that $A \ll D^2$, then as we look at larger scales this model predicts that $\theta$ decreases to values $<1$. Such values imply a more random distribution than HEAP, with less aggregation. More generally, in this simple model:

$$\theta \sim (D^2/A)^{1/2} A_R/(N_R D^2). \tag{6.17}$$

Hence the model predicts that as scale, characterized by $A$, increases, the spatial distributions in this model become increasingly more random ($\theta$ decreases) than is predicted by HEAP. This is important because it corrects the most apparent failing of HEAP, which is to overpredict the degree of aggregation in the higher-abundance species at larger spatial scales. In other words, without introducing density dependence explicitly, this model yields the same qualitative effect that density dependence would have on aggregation, and it does so in a scale-dependent manner that is in at least qualitative accord with observations (Harte et al., 2005).

The above results derive from a model that is based on highly simplified assumptions, but this initial model may point the way to a more refined analysis. First, the assumption that the SRD is uniform in a disk centered around each parent is clearly oversimplified; investigation of the effect on model output of more realistic distributions (see for example Borda-de-Água et al., this volume) is an obvious next step. Because of the central role played by the SRD in this modeling approach, it will be critical to test, for particular species, whatever predicted relationship emerges among density, the shape of the SRD, and the parameter $\theta$. Second, the effect of explicit density dependence, either at the level of each species or at the community level in the form of an overall resource constraint, on model output is worthy of study. Finally, the model described above utilized a mean-field approximation to single out a single cell of area $A$, which was treated distinctly from the pool of individuals in $A_R$; the mean-field model needs to be extended to a more comprehensive and satisfying one in which all individuals and cells are treated comparably and simultaneously.

## Conclusion

HEAP is a statistical theory of spatial structure, across multiple spatial scales, in ecosystems. Starting only with the list of abundances of the species in a community in some area $A_0$, the theory predicts the general shape of a large variety of spatial metrics at both species and community levels. Considering its absence of adjustable parameters, it provides a reasonable phenomenological description of the dominant spatial patterns in three ecosystems for which there are spatially explicit data on the locations of all individual plants. Its predictions tend to break down for the most abundant species, especially at larger spatial scales.

I have derived here the HEAP predictions for the dependence of the species-level and community-level commonality functions on cell size and intercell distance. At species level, these functions are determined by solving a set of coupled recursion relations (Eqs. 6.9 and 6.10), and the community-level function is determined from them (Eq. 6.11). These predictions remain to be tested and the scaling properties of the commonality functions remain to be derived. Understanding those scaling properties may allow estimation of species richness and species abundances at large spatial scales, using presence–absence data from which the species commonality metric can be estimated between multiple pairs of small, widely separated, census patches.

Because the HEAP allocation rule results in aggregation relative to the standard random placement model (Coleman, 1981), it is not surprising that HEAP generally outperforms the standard random model of spatial structure in ecology (see e.g. Fig. 6.3). The statistical assembly rule (Eq. 6.7), or the equivalent equal allocation rule illustrated in Box 6.2, can be viewed as an alternative to the coin-flipping rule that generates the binomial distribution and thus the traditional random placement model. Based on this, I originally interpreted HEAP as a null model that, like the random placement model, could be used to determine if observed spatial patterns implied the existence of some dynamical mechanism. With the realization that HEAP was a special case ($\theta = 1$) within a continuum of models that are characterized by a single parameter $\theta$ (Eq. 6.8), and that likelihood testing suggested that the optimum $\theta$ systematically varied with species abundance and spatial scale (Harte *et al.*, 2005), a search for a mechanism that generates the distributions within this continuum appeared warranted. Preliminary results from that search have been presented here.

In particular, I have hypothesized a possible mechanistic origin for the continuum of $\theta$-models in a simple dynamical framework in which reproduction and dispersal rather than niche limitations constrain population dynamics. The model suggests that the HEAP model ($\theta = 1$) derives from an explicit relationship, Eq. 6.15, between abundance, range size, and the spatial reproduction distribution describing the distribution of viable offspring from their parent. The relationship asserts that within very large areas such as the entire geographic range of a species, the abundance of a species is comparable in order of magnitude to the geographic range size divided by the effective area characterized by the spatial reproduction distribution. Deviations from that relationship lead to deviations from the value $\theta = 1$, with the predicted pattern of deviation at least in qualitative agreement with observation. Future tasks include refining the dynamical model by using more realistic spatial reproduction distribution functions, examining the role of explicit density dependence, and going beyond the mean-field approximation that led to Eqs. (6.15–6.17).

## Acknowledgments

I thank the Editors of this volume for their constructive suggestions on improving the manuscript, all the participants at the Prague Workshop for stimulating discussions, and Erin Conlisk for thoughtful advice. Funding from the US National Science Foundation is gratefully acknowledged.

## Appendix 6.I    Relating the spatial metrics in Table 6.1 to the $P_i^{(n_0)}(n)$

Each of the spatial metrics in Table 6.1 can be expressed in terms of the $P_i^{(n_0)}(n)$ or more specifically the $\lambda_i^{(n_0)}$. The appropriate expressions are given here for all but the species-level and community-level commonality functions, $\chi$, which are expressed in the form of recursion relations in Eqs. (6.9–6.11) and discussed further in Appendix 6.III.

Using Eqs. (6.2) and (6.3), the range–area relationship can be simply expressed as

$$R_i^{(n_0)} = \lambda_i^{(n_0)} A_0, \tag{6.18}$$

where the $\lambda$'s are given in terms of the $P$'s by Eq. (6.4).

The aggregation statistic, $\Omega_i^{(n_0)}$, can also be directly related to the $\lambda$ parameters (Ostling *et al.*, 2000):

$$\Omega_i^{(n_0)} = \frac{2}{\lambda_i^{(n_0)}} - \frac{1}{\lambda_{i+1}^{(n_0)}}. \tag{6.19}$$

The average number of species in cells of scale $i$ (that is, $A_i$ cells) can be expressed as the sum over the occupancy probabilities at scale $i$, and thus the species–area relationship can be written as

$$S_i = \sum_{n_0} [1 - P_i^{(n_0)}(0)] = \sum_{n_0} \lambda_i^{(n_0)}. \tag{6.20}$$

A species $(n_0)$ is endemic to a cell of area $A_i$ only if all the individuals of that species that are found in $A_0$, which we are denoting by $k$, are found in that particular cell. Hence, the endemics–area relationship for the average number of species unique to a cell of area $A_i$ takes the form

$$E_i = \sum_{\text{species}} P_i^{(n_0)}(n_0). \tag{6.21}$$

But from Eq. (6.5) it is straightforward to show that

$$P_i^{(n_0)}(n_0) = \frac{1}{(n_0 + 1)^i}. \tag{6.22}$$

and hence the EAR takes the simple form

$$E_i = \sum_{\text{species}} \frac{1}{(n_0 + 1)^i}. \tag{6.23}$$

I remind the reader that our definition of endemism is such that all species in $A_0$ are considered endemic at that scale, and that endemism at finer scales is defined relative to the distribution within $A_0$. Note, also, that because $E_i$ and $S_i$ are defined to be averages across cells, their values can be less than 1 and in fact except at the largest scales $E_i$ is often less than 1.

The scale-dependent species-abundance distribution $\Phi_i(n)$, which is the distribution of species occurrences at scale $i$ with abundance $n$, is then expressed by the sum over species of the probabilities of abundance $n$, normalized to the number of species:

$$\Phi_i(n) = \frac{\sum\limits_{\text{species}} P_i^{(n_0)}(n)}{S_0}. \tag{6.24}$$

Finally, the community-level spatial abundance distribution is given by

$$F_i(N) = \sum_{\forall n_{(k)}} \prod_{\text{species}} P_i^{(n_{j0})}(n_j) \; \delta(N, \textstyle\sum_j n_j) \tag{6.25}$$

where $\delta(a,b)$ is 1 if $a = b$ and is 0 if $a \neq b$. Here $n_j$ is an abundance variable for the $j$th species, and the equation simply states that the probability of a total of $N$ individuals in an $A_i$ cell is given by the sum over the joint probabilities for all the various combinations of individual species abundances that add up to the value $N$. The symbol $\sum_{\forall n_{(k)}}$ refers to the sum over all such combinations, and $\prod_{\text{species}}$ refers to the product over species.

## Appendix 6.II    Derivation of HEAP from an assembly function

Here I show how to derive the HEAP recursion relation (Eq. 6.6) in terms of the assembly function $\beta(1|l, r)$ in Eq. (6.7). I first write a set of quite general expressions for the $P_i^{(n0)}(n)$ in terms of the assembly functions and then re-express them in the form of two coupled recursion relations. All definitions and notations below are exactly as defined following Eq. (6.7) (for the $\beta$'s) and in Table 6.1 (for the $P_i^{(n_0)}$).

Recalling the definition of $\beta$, and focusing on the spatial abundance distribution for the left-hand $A_1$:

$$P_1^{(1)}(0) = \beta(0|0,0) \tag{6.26a}$$

$$P_1^{(1)}(1) = \beta(1|0,0) \tag{6.26b}$$

$$P_1^{(2)}(0) = \beta(0|0,0)\beta(0|0,1) \tag{6.26c}$$

$$P_1^{(2)}(1) = \beta(1|0,0)\beta(0|1,0) + \beta(0|0,0)\beta(1|0,1) \tag{6.26d}$$

$$P_1^{(2)}(2) = \beta(1|0,0)\beta(1|1,0) \tag{6.26e}$$

$$P_1^{(3)}(0) = \beta(0|0,0)\beta(0|0,1)\beta(0|0,2) \tag{6.26f}$$

etc.

Without loss of generality, consider the spatial abundance distribution of the upper left $A_2$ cell, and replace "up" and "down" for "left" and "right" in the definition of $\beta$, we have

$$\begin{aligned} P_2^{(1)}(0) &= \beta(0|0,0) + \beta(1|0,0)\,\beta(0|0,0) \\ &= P_1^{(1)}(0) + P_1^{(1)}(1)\,\beta(0|0,0) \end{aligned} \tag{6.27a}$$

(note that this last equation says that the probability that there are no individuals in the upper left quadrant is equal to the probability that there is none on the left plus the probability that there is one on the left but that it is allocated to the lower left).

Similarly,

$$P_2^{(1)}(1) = P_1^{(1)}(1)\,\beta(1|0,0) \tag{6.27b}$$

$$P_2^{(2)}(0) = P_1^{(2)}(0) + P_1^{(2)}(1)\beta(0|0,0) + P_1^{(2)}(2)\,\beta(0|0,0)\,\beta(0|0,1) \tag{6.27c}$$

$$\begin{aligned} P_2^{(2)}(1) &= P_1^{(2)}(1)\beta(1|0,0) + P_1^{(2)}(2)\{\beta(1|0,0)\beta(0|1,0) \\ &\quad + \beta(0|0,0)\beta(1|0,1)\} \end{aligned} \tag{6.27d}$$

$$P_2^{(2)}(2) = P_1^{(2)}(2)\,\beta(1|0,0)\beta(1|1,0) \tag{6.27e}$$

etc.

For $i = 3$,

$$P_3^{(2)}(0) = P_2^{(2)}(0) + P_2^{(2)}(1)\beta(0|0,0) + P_2^{(2)}\beta(0|0,0)\beta(0|0,1) \tag{6.28}$$

etc.

It is straightforward but tedious to show that the extension of these equations to all scales and all values of $n_0$ and $n$ imply

$$\sum_{n=0}^{n_0} P_i^{(n_0)}(n) = 1 \tag{6.29}$$

and that $<n>$, the average value of $n$, is given by

$$<n> = n_0/2^i. \tag{6.30}$$

Quite generally, the above equations can be encapsulated in the following pair of coupled recursion relationships for $i > 0$:

$$P_i^{(n_0)}(n) = \sum_{q=n}^{n_0} P_{i-1}^{(n_0)}(q)P_1^{(q)}(n). \tag{6.31}$$

Equation (6.31) says that for there to be $n$ individuals in an $A_i$ cell, there has to be at least $q \geq n$ individuals in the $A_{i-1}$ cell containing it, and that of those $q$ individuals, $n$ are in the $A_i$ cell.

A second recursion relation also follows from this $\beta$-framework; this one determines the $P_1$:

$$P_1^{(n_0)}(n) = P_1^{(n_0-1)}(n)\beta(0|n, n_0 - n - 1) + P_1^{(n_0-1)}(n-1)\beta(1|n-1, n_0 - n). \tag{6.32}$$

This equation states that the probability that there are $n$ individuals in, say, the left-hand $A_1$ cell, for a species with $n_0$ individuals in $A_0$, is equal to the probability that a species with $n_0 - 1$ individuals in $A_0$ has $n$ individuals in the left-hand $A_1$ cell and that the $n_0$th individual is placed in the right-hand $A_1$ cell plus the probability that it has $n - 1$ individuals in the left-hand cell and that the $n_0$th individual is placed in the left-hand $A_1$ cell.

Equation (6.5) follows directly from Eqs. (6.31) and (6.32). This is most easily seen inductively, starting with the $i = 1$ recursion relation (Eq. 6.32) and the identity $P_1^{(0)}(n) = \delta_{n,0}$, from which the general result $P_1^{(n_0)}(n) = (n_0 + 1)^{-1}$ follows. Equation (6.31) and straightforward algebra then lead to Eq. (6.6).

## Appendix 6.III    Recursion relations for species turnover in HEAP

We sketch here the derivation of the recursion relations for the species level commonality functions, $\chi^{(n_0)}$, as given in Eqs. (6.9) and (6.10).

Equation (6.9) is an immediate consequence of the scaling property of the HEAP allocation rule discussed in the text, with the factor $(n_0 + 1)^{-1}$ in front of the summation equal to the probability that if there are $n_0$ individuals in $A_0$, then there are $n$ individuals in a particular $A_1$ cell.

Equation (6.10) can be derived by first noting that a species with $n_0$ individuals in $A_0$ will be found in a pair of $A_i$ cells, one on each side of the first order bisection, and with $q_L$ individuals in the left-hand $A_i$ cell and $q_R$ individuals in the right-hand side $A_i$ cell, with probability

$$P(n_0, q_L, q_R, i) = (n_0 + 1)^{-1} \sum_{m=1}^{n_0} P_{i-1}{}^{(m)}(q_L) P_{i-1}{}^{(n_0-m)}(q_R). \tag{6.33}$$

The factor $(n_0 + 1)^{-1}$ is the probability from HEAP that $m$ individuals are in the left-hand $A_1$ cell and $n_0 - m$ individuals are in the right-hand $A_1$ cell. $P_{i-1}{}^{(m)}(q_L)$ is the probability that if there are $m$ individuals in $A_0$ then there are $q_L$ individuals in an $A_{i-1}$ cell; but equivalently, because of the scale invariance of the HEAP rule, it is the probability that if there are $m$ individuals in the left-hand $A_1$ cell, then there are $q_L$ individuals in a particular $A_i$ with that $A_1$ cell, and similarly for $P_{i-1}{}^{(n_0-m)}(q_R)$. The sum over $m$ then yields the desired probability $P(n, q_L, q_R, i)$. Then summing $P(n_0, q_L, q_R, i)$ over all $q_L$ and $q_R$ from 1 to $m$ and 1 to $n_0 - m$ respectively, and using the fact that

$$\lambda_{i-1}{}^{(n_0)} = 1 - P_{i-1}{}^{(n_0)}(0) = \sum_{q=1}^{n_0} P_{i-1}{}^{(n_0)}(q) \tag{6.34}$$

yields Eq. (6.10).

Equations (6.9) and (6.10) determine the species-level commonality functions in terms of the $P$'s, which in turn are determined by HEAP. Assuming HEAP applies independently to all species, then its definition, $\Psi(A_i, D_j)$, is given by a sum over species of the $\chi^{(n_0)}(A_i, D_j)$ and thus the community-level similarity measure $\chi(A_i, D_j)$ is given by

$$\chi(A_i, D_j) = \sum_{\text{species}} \chi^{(n_0)}(A_i, D_j) / \sum_{\text{species}} \lambda_i^{(n_0)}. \tag{6.35}$$

## References

Banavar, J. R., Green, J. L., Harte, J. & Maritan, A. (1999). Finite size scaling in ecology. *Physical Review Letters*, **83**, 4212–4214.

Coleman, B. (1981). On random placement and species-area relations. *Journal of Mathematical Biosciences*, **54**, 191–215.

Condit, R., Hubbell, S. P., LaFrankie, J. V., *et al.* (1996). Species-area and species-individual relationships for tropical trees: a comparison of three 50-ha plots. *Journal of Ecology*, **84**, 549–562.

Condit, R., Pitman, N., Leigh Jr., E. G., *et al.* (2002). Beta-diversity in tropical forest trees, *Science*, **295**, 666–669.

Enquist, B. J., West, G. B., Charnov, E. L. & Brown, J. H. (1999). Allometric scaling of production and life history variation in vascular plants. *Nature*, **401**, 907–911.

Gaston, K. & Blackburn, T. (2000). *Pattern and Process in Macroecology*. Oxford: Blackwell Scientific.

Green, J., Harte, J. & Ostling, A. (2003). Species richness, endemism and abundance patterns: tests of two fractal models in a serpentine grassland. *Ecology Letters*, **6**, 919–928.

Green, J. L., Holmes, A. J., Westoby, M., *et al.* (2004). Spatial scaling of microbial eukaryote diversity. *Nature*, **432**, 747–750.

Harte, J., Kinzig, A. & Green, J. (1999a). Self similarity in the distribution and abundance of species. *Science*, **284**, 334–336.

Harte, J., McCarthy, S., Taylor, K., Kinzig, A. & Fischer, M. (1999b). Estimating species-area relationships from plot to landscape scale using species spatial-turnover data. *Oikos*, **86**, 45–54.

Harte, J., Blackburn, T. & Ostling, A. (2001). Self similarity and the relationship between abundance and range size. *American Naturalist*, **157**, 374–386.

Harte, J., Conlisk, E., Ostling, A., Green, J. & Smith, A. (2005). A theory of spatial-structure in ecological communities at multiple spatial scales. *Ecological Monographs*, **75**(2), 179–197.

He, F. & Gaston, K. (2000). Estimating species abundance from occurrence. *American Naturalist*, **156**, 553–559.

He, F. & Gaston, K. (2003). Occupancy, spatial variance, and the abundance of species. *American Naturalist*, **162**, 366–375.

He, F. & Legendre, P. (2002). Species diversity patterns derived from species area models. *Ecology*, **83**, 1185–1198.

Hubbell, S. (2001). *The Unified Neutral Theory of Biodiversity and Biogeography*. Monographs in Population Biology 32. Princeton: Princeton University Press.

Hubbell, S. P. & Foster, R. B. (1983). Diversity of canopy trees in a neotropical forest and implications for conservation. In *Tropical Rain Forest: Ecology and Management*, ed. S. L. Sutton, T. C. Whitmore & A. C. Chadwick, pp. 25–41. Oxford: Blackwell Scientific Publications.

Krishnamani, R., Kumar, A. & Harte, J. (2004). Estimating species richness at large spatial scales using data from small discrete plots. *Ecography*, **27**, 637–642.

Kunin, W. E. (1998). Extrapolating species abundance across spatial scales. *Science*, **281**, 1513–1515.

Kunin, W. E., Hartley, S. & Lennon, J. (2000). Scaling down: on the challenge of estimating abundance from occurrence patterns. *American Naturalist*, **156**, 553–559.

Lennon, J., Kunin, W. & Hartley, S. (2002). Fractal species distributions do not produce power-law species-area relationships. *Oikos*, **97**, 378–386.

Ostling, A., Harte, J. & Green, J. (2000). Self similarity and clustering in the spatial distribution of species. *Science*, **290**, 671. (Technical Comment: www.sciencemag.org/cgi/content/full/290/5492/671a)

Ostling, A., Harte, J., Green, J. & Kinzig, A. (2003). A community-level fractal property produces power-law species-area relationships. *Oikos*, **103**, 218–224.

Ostling, A., Harte, J., Green, J. & Kinzig, A. (2004). Self similarity, the power law form of the species-area relationship, and a probability rule: a reply to Maddux. *American Naturalist*, **63**, 627–633.

Plotkin, J., Potts, M., Leslie, N., Manokaran, N., LaFrankie, J. & Ashton, P. (2000). Species-area curves, spatial aggregation, and habitat specialization in tropical forests. *Journal of Theoretical Biology*, **207**, 81–99.

Ruhla, C. (1992). *The Physics of Chance*. Oxford: Oxford University Press.

Šizling, A. L. & Storch, D. (2004). Power-law species-area relationships and self-similar species distributions within finite areas. *Ecology Letters*, **7**, 60–68.

# PART II

# Alternative measures of biodiversity: taxonomy, phylogeny, and turnover

# CHAPTER SEVEN

# Biodiversity scaling relationships: are microorganisms fundamentally different?

JESSICA GREEN
*University of California, Merced*
BRENDAN J. M. BOHANNAN
*University of Oregon*

## Introduction

One of the key goals of ecology is to understand the spatial scaling of species diversity. Spatial patterns of species diversity provide important clues about the underlying mechanisms that regulate biodiversity and are central in the development of biodiversity theory (MacArthur & Wilson, 1967; Rosenzweig, 1995; Brown, 1995; Gaston & Blackburn, 2000; Hubbell, 2001; Holyoak, Leibold & Holt, 2005). Assumptions regarding the spatial scaling of biodiversity are a fundamental component of conservation biology and are frequently used to identify local- and global-scale priority conservation areas (Ferrier *et al.*, 2004; Desmet & Cowling, 2004) and to predict extinction risk due to climate change (Thomas *et al.*, 2004) and habitat loss (Gaston, Blackburn & Goldewijk, 2003). Although scaling patterns have been documented in hundreds of studies of plant and animal diversity, such patterns in microbial species (i.e. bacteria, archaea, and single-celled eukarya) have not been well documented. This is a serious omission, given that microorganisms may comprise much of Earth's biodiversity (Whitman, Coleman & Wiebe, 1998; Torsvik, Ovreas & Thingstad, 2002) and play critical roles in biogeochemical cycling and ecosystem functioning (Balser, 2000; Wardle, 2002; Morin & McGrady-Steed, 2004). Furthermore, microbial biodiversity is a major source of novel pharmaceuticals and other compounds of industrial importance, and an understanding of the scaling of microbial biodiversity is crucial to the search for such compounds (Bull, 2004).

There are both technical and conceptual reasons for our lack of understanding of the scaling of microbial biodiversity. Technically, it has been very challenging to quantify microbial biodiversity. Prokaryotic and many eukaryotic microorganisms cannot be identified morphologically, and must either be identified using traits that require culture in the laboratory (e.g. the utilization of specific substrates) or identified via biochemical markers extracted from environmental samples (e.g. phospholipid fatty acids or DNA sequences from indicator genes (O'Donnell, Goodfellow & Hawksworth, 1994). Even at small scales it

*Scaling Biodiversity*, ed. David Storch, Pablo A. Marquet and James H. Brown. Published by Cambridge University Press. © Cambridge University Press 2007.

has proven impractical to inventory microbial communities exhaustively. Conceptually, it has long been assumed that microorganisms have cosmopolitan distributions (Bass-Becking, 1934; Fenchel & Finlay, 2004). The small size and high abundance of microbes (as well as other aspects of their biology) have been assumed to increase the rate and geographic distance of dispersal to levels where dispersal limitation is essentially nonexistent. It has been argued that such continuous large-scale dispersal would result in fundamentally different biodiversity scaling relationships for microbes, relative to those observed for other forms of life (Fenchel & Finlay, 2004).

Should microbes have cosmopolitan distributions? Do they have cosmopolitan distributions? In this chapter, we discuss the evidence for cosmopolitan distributions of microbes. We argue that the assumption of a lack of dispersal limitation among microbes is based on a confusion of hypotheses for facts, and that the actual evidence for microbial cosmopolitanism is mixed, often misinterpreted, and likely an artifact of broad taxonomic definitions for microorganisms.

## Should microbes have cosmopolitan distributions?

It has been argued that due to their unique biology, organisms smaller than 1 mm in diameter should have cosmopolitan distributions. These biological differences include very large population sizes, a high capacity for dispersal, and low extinction rates (Table 7.1). Although these differences have been assumed to be universally characteristic of microbes, the evidence for this is scant, as described below.

### Population sizes of microbes

The most commonly claimed mechanism underlying a cosmopolitan distribution of microbes is that their large population sizes result in high rates of

**Table 7.1** *Differences assumed by some microbiologists to exist between macroorganisms and microorganisms*

These differences are unproven hypotheses, although they are often treated as facts.

| Characteristic | Plants and animals | Microorganisms |
|---|---|---|
| Species abundance | Low | High |
| Migration rate | Low | High |
| Speciation rate | High | Low |
| Extinction rate | High | Low |
| Relative number of endemics | High | Low |
| Global number of species | High | Low |
| Local:global species richness | Low | High |

Modified from Finlay and Esteban (2004).

dispersal (Fenchel & Finlay, 2004). The probability of chance dispersal (e.g. via an accidental vector such as a bird or mammal) is increased when abundance is high. Certainly microbes are abundant. A gram of soil may contain $10^9$ individual bacteria and perhaps ten thousand ciliates (Torsvik *et al.*, 2002; Fenchel & Finlay, 2004). Overall abundance, however, does not necessarily suggest that the population sizes of individual species of microbes are large; what matters is how these abundant individuals are distributed among taxa. The size of a given species population will depend on how one defines "species" (or whatever taxonomic classification is used). A broader definition of a taxon will result in a larger estimated taxon population. For example, if one defined a taxon as "all plants" that definition would result in a very large estimate of taxon population size, a large potential rate of dispersal, and a high probability of cosmopolitanism (which is what we observe).

How are taxa usually defined? For many eukaryotic microorganisms, an approach is used that is roughly similar to that used for the taxonomy of macroorganisms. Morphological traits are used to group individuals into species, with the underlying assumption that shared morphological traits reflect interbreeding, although this is rarely tested. It is unclear whether microbial species defined via morphological traits are comparable in genetic diversity, evolutionary relatedness or ecological breadth to macroorganism species. In general, the smaller the organism, the more limited the morphological information. It has been argued that some protists present as many morphological traits as macroorganisms (Fenchel & Finlay, 2004) but this is debatable (Foissner, 1999; Coleman, Finlay & Fenchel, 2002; Hedlund & Staley, 2004). It is certainly not true for some protists (such as amoebae and flagellates) nor for bacteria or archaea, which have very few morphological features, even when magnified with electron microscopy. It is likely that due to reduced morphological information, microbial morphospecies represent a coarser taxonomic resolution than plant or animal species (Hedlund & Staley, 2004).

Phenotypic traits other than morphology (such as the utilization of specific substrates) have been used historically to identify microorganisms that lack sufficient morphological traits. Determining such phenotypic traits usually requires that the organism be cultured in the laboratory. It has become apparent that the vast majority of prokaryotic microorganisms (as well as many eukaryotic microorganisms) cannot yet be cultured (Amann *et al.*, 1995) and thus an alternative approach is needed.

One alternative approach is to use biochemical markers to define taxa. The most common of these techniques use ribosomal gene sequences as indicators of microbial diversity, although other genes, including protein-coding genes, have also been used. The use of these molecular techniques and their drawbacks and biases has been reviewed in detail elsewhere (e.g. Wintzingerode, Göbel & Stackebrandt, 1997). These approaches have enabled the detection of nonculturable species and allowed a more complete and detailed picture of bacterial communities (reviewed in Head, Saunders & Pickup, 1998; Mlot, 2004). Taxa are usually defined as sequence similarity groups using this approach. For bacteria and archaea, 97% DNA sequence similarity of 16S rDNA is the most common definition of taxa and is considered to approximate the species level of resolution defined using culture-dependent methods (Stackebrandt & Rainey, 1995). Taxa defined using such approaches are likely not comparable to macroorganism species. If this definition was applied to animals, all the primates (from lemurs to humans) would be considered the same species (and would be cosmopolitan; Staley, 1997). A number of studies have demonstrated that substantial ecological diversity is often hidden within taxa defined in this manner (Moore, Rocap & Chisholm, 1998; Ward et al., 1998).

Even if it was possible to define "species" of microbes in a manner comparable to macroorganisms, we would still not be able to predict the dispersal rates of microbes without an understanding of the taxon–abundance relationships among microbes. If we could determine that the abundance of bacteria was distributed among a limited number of species (defined in some way comparable to that of plants and animals) this would not necessarily suggest that population sizes were universally large unless we also knew that the taxon–abundance relationship was very even (i.e. that individuals were distributed relatively evenly among taxa). Little is known about microbial rank-abundance relationships, and both highly skewed and very even distributions have been reported (Dunbar et al., 2002; Zhou et al., 2002).

It is not reasonable to claim that microbes have larger population sizes than macroorganisms if different definitions of taxa are used for microbes and macroorganisms, and without an understanding of taxon–abundance relationships. Finding an equivalent taxon definition for both microbes and macroorganisms may not be possible, rendering this claim (and the debate over microbial cosmopolitanism) meaningless. It is more interesting (and tractable) to ask: at what level of taxonomic resolution does cosmopolitanism break down for microbes? And what is the ecological relevance of this level of taxonomy (e.g. can we detect differences among groups of this resolution in ecological function, environmental optima, or response to environmental change)? Although these questions were essentially suggested over a decade ago (Tiedje, 1993), they are just beginning to be addressed by microbial ecologists (Cho & Tiedje, 2000; Whitaker, Grogan & Taylor, 2003; Horner-Devine et al., 2004b).

### High capacity for dispersal

In addition to high rates of dispersal from source populations, the capacity to disperse over long distances is also necessary for cosmopolitan distributions. If microbes have cosmopolitan distributions it may ultimately be due to a high capacity for dispersal. Many microbes can be dispersed passively through the environment due to their small size (Lighthart, 1997; McNair, Newbold & Hart, 1997; Leff, McArthur & Shimkets, 1998; Gage, Isard & Colunga, 1999), and many have the ability to form resistant and dormant life stages that allow them to survive long dispersal distances (Roberts & Cohan, 1995). It is not known how widespread dispersal adaptations are among microbes, and few studies have been able to quantify the dispersal patterns of individual microbial taxa. A number of studies have demonstrated that many protist (Finlay, 2002; Fenchel & Finlay, 2004; Finlay & Esteban, 2004) and bacterial (Glöckner et al., 2000; Brandao, Clapp & Bull, 2002; Ward & O'Mullan, 2002; Zwart et al., 2002) taxa have worldwide distributions, suggesting a high capacity for dispersal. There is also evidence that some microbial taxa have restricted geographic distributions, and that this pattern is due to dispersal limitation, implying that not all microorganisms have the capacity to disperse globally (reviewed in Papke et al., 2003; Martiny et al., 2006).

**Low rates of extinction and speciation**
Another common a-priori argument for microbial cosmopolitanism is a low extinction rate in comparison to macroorganisms. The argument for lower extinction rates is based on the assumption that microbes have larger population sizes than macroorganisms, which makes stochastic extinction events less likely (Dykhuizen, 1998; Cohan, 2001; Fenchel & Finlay, 2004). Also, some microbes have the ability to develop hardy life stages (spores) which may reduce the probability of local extinction following catastrophic environmental changes. There are no direct measures of microbial extinction rates in the natural environment, rendering it difficult to assess the degree to which these mechanisms influence global extinction rates over geological timescales.

It has also been argued that microbes have low rates of speciation and that such low rates contribute to cosmopolitanism by reducing local diversification. The primary argument for lower speciation rates is based on the idea that microbes have a high capacity for dispersal, and that this lack of dispersal barriers would prevent the geographic isolation necessary for allopatric speciation (Finlay & Fenchel, 2004). Recent studies have begun to reveal evidence for physical isolation in microbial populations across a variety of habitats, highlighting the importance of genetic drift and allopatric speciation in microbial evolution (Papke & Ward, 2004).

Another mechanism that could result in relatively low speciation rates for microbes is parasexuality. Some eukaryotic microbes and many prokaryotic microbes are "parasexual"; i.e. they exchange genetic material "rarely but promiscuously" through a variety of mechanisms (Ochman, Lawrence & Groisman, 2000; Gogarten, 2003). Such exchange, if it occurs at a high rate, could lower the rate of speciation by acting as a homogenizing force, spreading key innovations among a number of different microbial lineages. However, if exchange occurs at or below the rate of mutation (rates typical of many bacteria; Cohan, 2002) it can have the opposite effect, increasing the rate of speciation by introducing genetic novelty. Despite these claims, there are no direct measures of microbial speciation rates in the field.

## Do microbes have cosmopolitan distributions?

The discussion above suggests that there is not strong evidence that microbes *should* have cosmopolitan distributions. But do they? In the discussion below we provide an overview of the direct evidence for microbial cosmopolitanism. We focus on three spatial patterns of microbial biodiversity often cited as evidence for cosmopolitanism: the distance–decay relationship (how community composition changes with geographic distance), the taxa–area relationship, and the local/global taxa richness ratio.

### Distance–decay relationship

The assumption of global microbial dispersal by a combination of randomizing forces (e.g. wind, water, animal vectors, etc.) would lead to random primary spatial distributions, followed by subsequent population growth in nonrandom spatial niches. According to this cosmopolitan view of the microbial world, spatial patterns of microbial diversity are primarily driven by environmental heterogeneity. Thus, one might expect to find similar microbial communities in similar habitats, and differentiated microbial communities along an environmental gradient. One approach for testing the assumption of global dispersal is through analysis of how similarity in community composition between sites changes with the geographic distance separating sites, or the "distance–decay relationship" (Nekola & White, 1999). When coupled with environmental data, the distance–decay relationship offers a means to assess the relative importance of environmental heterogeneity and dispersal history in controlling the spatial scaling of biodiversity. Although it is widely accepted that plant and animal community composition decays with increasing distance between samples (Condit *et al.*, 2002; Tuomisto, Ruokolainen & Yli-Halla, 2003; Qian, Ricklefs & White, 2005), little is known about microbial community turnover rates.

To our knowledge, Hillebrand and colleagues (Hillebrand *et al.*, 2001) were the first to report on the relationship between microbial taxa similarity and geographic distance. They gathered morphospecies data on diatoms, ciliates, corals and polychaetes sampled from similar habitats and environmental conditions (e.g. temperature, light, salinity) that were separated by distances ranging from 1 km to 1000 km. For each group of organisms, they estimated the similarity of species composition between samples in terms of the widely used Jaccard index, which is based on presence/absence data. Finally, for each group they quantified the rate at which similarity decayed with increasing distance between samples, or the slope of the "distance–decay relationship" (Nekola & White, 1999). They found that for all groups, species similarity decayed significantly with distance, which contradicts the hypothesis of ubiquitous dispersal. However, metazoan species were characterized by substantially steeper slopes than the diatom and ciliate species, suggesting that body size may influence spatial biodiversity patterns.

The first report we are aware of that discusses a distance–decay relationship for prokaryotes is that of Franklin and Mills (2003). They determined the composition of bacterial communities from soil samples taken in a nested design, with sample distances ranging from 2.5 cm to 11 m apart. They assessed community composition using AFLP analysis, a molecular fingerprinting method. They observed a significant distance–decay relationship, with a scale-dependent slope which decreased in magnitude at larger scales. Franklin and Mills argued that because the scale of sampling was relatively small, the observed distance–decay relationship was due only to environmental heterogeneity, rather than dispersal limitation. However, this assertion was not tested.

More recent analyses that utilize molecular approaches provide further evidence that the spatial scaling of microbial communities may be influenced by dispersal history. In a study of *Sulfobolus* strains across the spatial scales ~6 km to 6000 km, Whittaker *et al.* (2003) found that genetic divergence was explained by geographic distance rather than environmental sources. Across the scales 1 m to ~100 km, Green *et al.* (2004) also found that geographic distance was a more useful predictor for ascomycete fungi community turnover than habitat (classified by soil and vegetation type) (Fig. 7.1). In contrast, bacterial communities studied at smaller spatial scales (3 cm to 300 m) have shown that environmental heterogeneity is the primary factor controlling microbial biogeography (Horner-Devine *et al.*, 2004a). These studies suggest that the spatial scaling of microbes is likely influenced by both environmental heterogeneity and dispersal history, with dispersal history becoming increasingly important at larger spatial scales (see review Martiny *et al.*, 2006).

## Taxa–area relationship

The relationship between species richness and sampled area – the "species–area relationship" (SAR), is one of the most widely cited and studied patterns in ecology. Evidence that the number of species tends to increase with increasing area was reported as early as 1855 (DeCandolle, 1855). In his dissertation, Olof Arrhenius was the first to propose a mathematical description of the SAR, which he later simplified to a general power law of the form:

$$S = cA^z, \tag{7.1}$$

where $S$ is species number, $A$ is area, and $z$ and $c$ are constants (Arrhenius, 1921). Although many functional forms of the SAR have been proposed (Connor & McCoy,

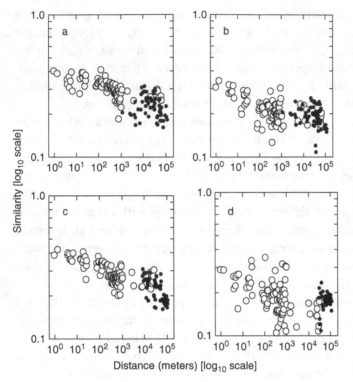

**Figure 7.1** The similarity–geographic distance relationship for microbial fungi. Shown are the average Sørensen similarity values for within land system data (open circles) and between land system data (closed circles). Data correspond to different desert land systems (a) Pulgamurtie – stony foothills below silcrete ridges, (b) Rodges – sand plains with dominant mulga trees (*Acacia aneura*), (c) Olive Downs – stone covered rolling downs, and (d) Corner – sand dunes with scattered sandhill wattle. From Green *et al.* (2004).

1979; He & Legendre, 1996), the power-law form has withstood the test of time relatively well (May, 1975; Rosenzweig, 1995). Empirical evidence suggests that for large organisms (i.e. plants and animals) within continental habitat patches, $z$ is generally in the range of 0.1–0.3. There is evidence for slightly steeper SARs between islands in archipelagos ($0.25 < z < 0.35$) and the steepest SARs when whole biotas are compared ($0.5 < z < 1.0$) (Rosenzweig, 1995).

Advocates of microbial cosmopolitanism have suggested that microbes should be characterized by relatively flat species–area (or more accurately, taxa–area) curves, with $z$ values lower than those reported for macroorganisms. Taxa–area relationships (TARs) have only recently been studied for microbes and consequently few have been published, rendering comparison with larger organisms difficult. Of these few existing microbial studies, most report $z < 0.1$; however, there are recent reports of higher $z$ values consistent with those of macroorganisms (Fig. 7.2).

A central challenge in TAR studies is estimating the true number of taxa in large areas where it is not possible to sample completely. For microbes, detailed distribution maps are unavailable, and relying on observed counts of taxa richness may result in biased $z$ values. For example, reported patterns for diatoms ($z = 0.066$) and ciliates ($z = 0.077$) are based on the cumulative species richness observed in noncontiguous sample points covering large areas. If the true

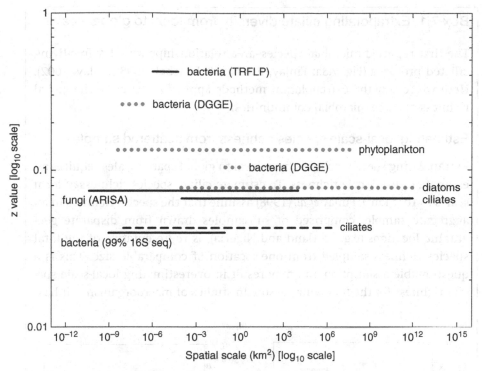

**Figure 7.2** TAR z values for published microbial biogeography studies. Dotted lines pertain to studies of discrete areas of increasing size (Bell *et al.*, 2005; Reche *et al.*, 2005; Smith *et al.*, 2005), solid lines are for contiguous TARs within nested areas in a single region (Azovksy, 2002; Green *et al.*, 2004; Horner-Devine *et al.*, 2004a; Noguez *et al.*, 2005), and dashed line is a noncontiguous TAR that estimates the increase in taxa richness from local to global scales (Finlay *et al.*, 1998; Finlay, 2002). TRFLP, terminal restriction fragment length polymorphism; DGGE, denaturing gradient gel electrophoresis; ARISA, automated ribosomal intergenic spacer analysis. Ciliates, diatoms and phytoplankton identified by morphology.

number of species at the largest scales (i.e. synopses of whole seas) is greater than that observed from sampling a small fraction of these large areas, then the observed SAR slope *z* will underestimate the true slope. Understanding microbial TARs will require creative approaches for estimating the total number of taxa in particular localities and methods for extrapolating richness to larger scales using sparse sample data (Cam *et al.*, 2002; Bohannan & Hughes, 2003; Green *et al.*, 2005).

One approach to extrapolating microbial taxa richness is to make assumptions about microbial species–abundance distributions and how they vary with spatial scale. This type of approach has been used to extrapolate ciliate (Box 7.1) and bacterial (Curtis, Sloan & Scannell, 2002) diversity. Little is currently known about the spatial scaling of microbial species–abundance relationships, and it is thus difficult to assess the validity of projected extrapolations. An alternative

## Box 7.1 Extrapolating ciliate diversity from local to global scales

The first reported microbial species–area relationships were for free-living ciliated protozoa (Fig. 7.3a; Finlay, Esteban & Fenchel, 1998; Finlay, 2002). Here we review the extrapolation methods applied to estimate the global richness of these microbial communities.

### Estimating local-scale species richness from scattered samples

Extrapolating species richness from local to global spatial scales requires an estimate of local-scale richness. To estimate ciliate species richness at local scales ($\sim 10^{-8}\,\mathrm{km^2}$), Finlay et al. (1998) assume that the species richness in an aggregate sample, comprised of subsamples drawn from disparate geographic locations (e.g. Scotland and Nigeria), is representative of the total species richness sampled from one location of comparable size. This is a questionable assumption and may result in overestimating local-scale species richness for the following reason. In studies of macroorganisms, it has

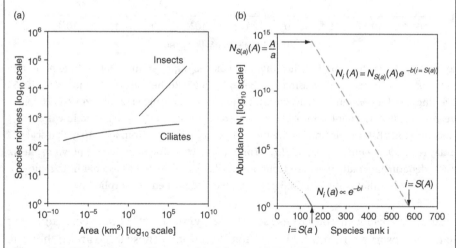

Figure 7.3 Extrapolating ciliate species richness. (a) The ciliate species–area relationship is deduced by extrapolating rank-abundance curves as shown in (b), and assuming that at any given spatial scale the species with the largest rank has one individual. This technique yields an estimated species–area relationship for ciliates that is relatively flat compared with the pattern found in insects sampled from various regions of the world (Finlay, 2002). (b) The assumed scaling of rank-abundance curves: species are ranked from most to least abundant along the horizontal axis. The functional form and slope of the terminal component of the rank-abundance curve at large (dashed line) and small (solid line) spatial scales are assumed to be equivalent. For this example, $a = 87\,\mathrm{cm^2}$, $A = 2 \times 10^6\,\mathrm{km^2}$, $b = 0.0338$, $S(a) = 151$, and $S(A) = 576$ (parameters estimated from ciliate marine interstitial data in Finlay et al., 1998).

long been established that the number of species counted in scattered sub-plots will generally exceed the number of species surveyed in one contiguous subplot of equivalent area (Gleason, 1922; Rosenzweig, 1995). One potential consequence of overestimating local-scale species richness is underestimating the rate at which species richness increases with sampling area.

## Estimating global-scale species richness from rank–abundance plots

The observed rank–abundance plot is used to extrapolate ciliate species richness (Fig. 7.3b). Data for the rare ciliate species ($N < 20$) fit an exponential rank–abundance curve of the form $N_i \propto e^{-bi}$, where $N_i$ is the number of individuals in the $i$th species, and $b$ is the slope of the curve. The exponential rank–abundance curve corresponds to a geometric series species–abundance distribution (Magurran, 2004). Extrapolating species richness requires four assumptions:

- The observed rank–abundance curve, sampled from disparate geographic locations, is representative of the species–abundance pattern in one contiguous area $a$.
- The unobserved species at larger spatial scales $A$ are described by an exponential rank–abundance curve with equivalent slope $b$, or

$$\log N_i(A) = \log N_{S(a)}(A) - b[i - S(a)].\tag{7.2}$$

Here, $N_i(A)$ is the abundance of the $i$th species in some large region $A$, and $S(a)$ is the assumed species richness at a smaller spatial scale $a$.

- The abundances of the rare species ($N < 20$) in $a$ increase linearly with spatial scale. This allows one to assume $N_{S(a)}(A) = \frac{A}{a} N_{S(a)}(a)$.
- The least abundant species has one individual at each spatial scale, or $N_{S(a)}(a) = N_{S(A)}(A) = 1$. Applying these assumptions to Eq. (7.2) yields a log-arithmic species–area relationship of the form:

$$S(A) = S(a) + \frac{1}{b}\log\left[\frac{A}{a}\right].\tag{7.3}$$

A plot of $S(A)$ versus $\log[A]$ will yield a linear relationship with slope $\frac{1}{b}$, and $\log[S(A)]$ versus $\log[A]$ will yield a curvilinear relationship, as illustrated in Fig. 7.3a.

Little is known about the spatial scaling of rank–abundance curves for either macroorganisms or microorganisms. If the species–abundance distribution shifted from the geometric series to a more dominant (or less even) distribu-tion at larger scales, then the extrapolation technique discussed above would yield higher species richness estimates. Further investigation on patterns in the spatial distribution and abundance of microbes is needed to better under-stand the scaling of ciliate species richness.

approach is to use the slope of the distance–decay relationship to estimate the slope of the taxa–area relationship (Krishnamani, Kumar & Harte, 2004). The advantage of this approach is that it only requires sampling localities spatially in such a way that the decline in similarity with distance can be measured. This method was recently applied to estimate the spatial scaling of microbial diversity at local (Horner-Devine *et al.*, 2004a) and regional (Green *et al.*, 2004) scales. While both of these studies show that microbes are characterized by a relatively flat taxa–area relationship, testing the hypothesis of global dispersal will require further analyses of distance–decay patterns at global scales.

Theoretically, the TAR slope *z* should vary with taxonomic resolution, and this must be taken into account when comparing the biodiversity scaling of microorganisms and macroorganisms (Box 7.2). The analysis of Green *et al.* (2004) was based on taxa defined using automated ribosomal RNA intergenic

---

### Box 7.2 The influence of taxonomic resolution on spatial biodiversity patterns

Recent analyses of microbial data suggest that observed spatial biodiversity patterns are sensitive to taxon definitions. Here we show that the slope of the taxa–area relationship can either increase or decrease with increasing taxonomic resolution. For clarity we examine the slope of the taxa–area relationship for species versus genera, but our analysis can be applied to any two levels of taxonomic resolution, such as 99% versus 95% 16S rDNA sequence similarity.

Consider a study region of area $A$ with $S_A$ species, and let $S_a$ denote the expected number of species in patches of size $a$, where $a < A$. The patches of size $a$ may be nested within $A$, implying a "mainland" species–area relationship, or biologically isolated, implying an "island" species–area relationship. Now assume that the $S_A$ species within $A$ are classified into $G_A$ genera, and let $G_a$ equal the expected number of genera in patches of size $a$.

Due to the hierarchical structure of phylogenetic trees, the number of genera in any given patch $a$ may never exceed the number of species in that patch, and thus

$$G_a \leq S_a \qquad (7.4)$$

for $a \leq A$. Likewise, with increasing patch area $a$, the addition of a new genus requires the addition of at least one new species. Thus the rate of genera accumulation at increasing spatial scales must be less than or equal to the rate of species accumulation, or

$$\frac{dG_a}{da} \leq \frac{dS_a}{da}. \qquad (7.5)$$

This implies that when considering the taxa–area relationship on a linear-linear scale, the slope of the genera–area relationship must be less than or equal to the slope of the species–area relationship.

A common practice in ecology is to model the species–area relationship as a power law of the form:

$$S_a = ca^z, \tag{7.6}$$

where $c$ and $z$ are empirically derived constants, and $0 \leq z \leq 1$. As a consequence, ecologists often plot species–area relationships on log-log axes, and report the slope of the power-law relationship $z$. Analogous to the power-law species–area relationship, a power-law genera–area relationship takes the form:

$$G_a = ba^y, \tag{7.7}$$

where $b$ and $y$ are empirically derived constants, and $0 \leq y \leq 1$.

Although the rate of genera accumulation at increasing spatial scales must be less than or equal to the rate of species accumulation on a linear scale, this is not necessarily true on a logarithmic scale. The condition $y \leq z$ is equivalent to $\dfrac{d \log G_a}{d \log a} \leq \dfrac{d \log S_a}{d \log a}$, or

$$\frac{1}{G_a}\frac{dG_a}{da} \leq \frac{1}{S_a}\frac{dS_a}{da}. \tag{7.8}$$

Equation (7.8) may be violated despite the constraints given by Eqs. (7.2) and (7.3). In conclusion, while it is impossible for genera richness to accumulate more rapidly than species richness, it is possible for $y \geq z$. These findings highlight the need to further develop analytical tools to understand how taxonomic resolution influences observed biodiversity patterns.

spacer analysis (ARISA), a commonly used DNA-based community fingerprinting method (Yannarell & Triplett, 2005). It is not clear how such taxa compare with traditionally defined species for plants and animals, although it is likely that ARISA-defined taxa are of coarser resolution. The analyses of Horner-Devine et al. (2004a) found that the slope of the TAR relationship $z$ varied with taxonomic resolution, ranging from $z = 0.019$ at 95% sequence similarity to $z = 0.040$ at 99% sequence similarity. Their data clearly indicate that spatial biodiversity patterns depend on the defined taxonomic resolution (Fig. 7.4).

The taxa–area patterns described above were documented for contiguous areas. Studies of plants and animals have shown that the scaling of biodiversity can be different in discontinuous areas (i.e. "islands" of habitat surrounded by inhospitable territory). For example, the TAR slope $z$ tends to be higher when

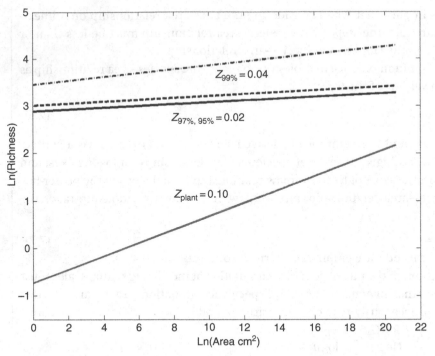

**Figure 7.4** The taxa–area relationships for salt marsh bacteria varied with taxonomic resolution. From Horner-Devine *et al.* (2004a).

measured across islands (reviewed in Rosenzweig, 1995). Three recent studies have documented "island" patterns in microbial biodiversity. In one study, van der Gast *et al.* (2005) studied bacterial communities colonizing metal-cutting fluids from machines of increasing sump tank size, assuming these to be analogous to islands of variable size. Similarly, Bell *et al.* (2005) studied bacterial communities in water-filled tree holes of varying volume. Both studies estimated bacterial taxonomic richness as the number of unique ribotypes detected using Denaturing Gradient Gel Electrophoresis (DGGE) of 16S rDNA. These studies found that the number of taxa detected increased significantly with increasing volume, and that the rate of increase was similar to that reported for plants and animals ($z = 0.245$ to $0.295$ for sump tanks, $z = 0.26$ for tree holes). Reche *et al.* (2005) used a similar approach to study bacterial communities in lakes of varying size. They observed that taxonomic richness (estimated using techniques similar to those of Bell *et al.*, 2005; van der Gast *et al.*, 2005) increased significantly with lake area, with an estimated $z$ value of 0.104. These studies differ from traditional island-biogeography studies of macroorganisms because bacterial taxa richness was quantified in equal volumes sampled from islands assumed to be relatively well mixed, which is analogous to randomly sampling an equal number of individuals from every island. In contrast, island $z$ values reported for plants and animals (Rosenzweig, 1995) are commonly based on estimates from surveys or atlases that tally species sited over multiple years. The relationship between $z$ estimated from equal-sized random samples per island versus a cumulative survey of an archipelago will depend on several factors, including population aggregation patterns, the rank–abundance curve on each island, and the sampling effort per survey.

## Local/global taxa richness ratio

If microorganisms are cosmopolitan, they will show a higher relative local taxa richness compared with the global taxa pool than larger organisms. In other words, for a specified habitat type, microbes should have a higher local/global taxa richness ratio than macroorganisms. The most compelling evidence of this pattern comes from research on protist morphospecies. In a study of the flagellate genus *Paraphysomonas*, 80% of the known global species were found in <0.1 cm$^2$ of sediment collected from Priest Pot, a 1-ha freshwater pond in England (Finlay & Clarke, 1999). Data compiled by Fenchel and Finlay across a wide range of eukaryotic taxonomic groups (e.g. amoebae, diatoms, mollusks, etc.) in Priest Pot suggest a more general relationship between body size and global distribution (Fenchel & Finlay, 2004). They found that the local/global species ratio, expressed as a percentage of the global number of freshwater species, consistently decreased with mean body size. A parallel analysis of data collected from Nivå Bay, a 2-ha marine shallow-water habitat in Denmark, revealed the same pattern, indicating that small organisms (less than 1 mm in length) tend to have a cosmopolitan distribution (Fenchel & Finlay, 2004). Data on polar surveys for testate amoeba assemblages also support this hypothesis (Wilkinson, 2001).

These studies are potentially misleading for at least two reasons. First, they assume that for a given habitat type, the magnitude of microbial eukaryote global species richness is known, or as least as well known as that of macro-organisms. Some researchers claim that for particular groups of microbial eukaryotes, such as ciliated protozoa, the number of described species globally is unlikely to increase in the future (Finlay *et al.*, 1996), while others claim that a large number remain undiscovered (Foissner, 1997). Due to unequal relative sampling effort, the probability of underestimating species richness at the global scale is significantly higher than the probability of underestimating species richness in a local sample. Underestimating global species richness will inflate projected local/global species ratios, and hence distort reported patterns of microbial eukaryote biogeography.

A second point to consider is that almost all data on protist species richness rely on morphological species concepts (as described above). The proposed cosmopolitan distribution of microbes based on morphospecies has been repeatedly criticized (Foissner, 1999; Hillebrand *et al.*, 2001; Coleman *et al.*, 2002; Hedlund & Staley, 2004). A major question is whether the resolution of morphospecies is poorer for smaller than for larger organisms. It has been suggested (although see Finlay & Fenchel, 2004) that at some body size or morphological complexity limit more sensitive and less subjective taxonomic criteria (e.g. criteria based on genetic similarity) may be more appropriate (Hedlund & Staley, 2004). Higher resolution taxonomic criteria for microbial eukaryote species would likely lead to increased global species pool estimates and decreased local/global species ratio estimates.

As discussed above, studies using molecular techniques to examine spatial patterns of prokaryote diversity suggest that the observed spatial distribution of microbes depends on the taxonomic criteria used. Studies using a wide array of methods including 16S rDNA sequencing, pairwise DNA/DNA hybridization, repetitive extragenic palindromic (REP) genomic fingerprinting, and amplified ribosomal DNA restriction analysis (ADRA) suggest that prokaryotic genera are widely distributed in their respective habitats (Fulthorpe, Rhodes & Tiedje, 1998; Staley & Gosink, 1999; Hagstrom, Pinhassi & Zweifel, 2000; Hedlund & Staley, 2004). However, when methods offering finer genetic resolution are employed, bacteria appear to have endemic geographical distributions (Fulthorpe *et al.*, 1998; Cho & Tiedje, 2000; Papke *et al.*, 2003; Whittaker *et al.*, 2003).

## Conclusions

How biodiversity scales with space is a central question in ecology. It has long been assumed that microorganisms have cosmopolitan distributions, and that this results in fundamentally different biodiversity scaling relationships for microbes, relative to those observed for other forms of life. The evidence, however, is inconclusive. The fundamental processes assumed to underlie microbial cosmopolitanism (large populations sizes, low extinction rates, etc.) are hypotheses, although they are frequently assumed to be facts, and there is little direct evidence that these are universal attributes of microbial life. Although some microbial taxa appear to have cosmopolitan distributions, microbial spatial patterns are sensitive to how taxa are defined, and there is evidence that microbial taxa as they are now defined are of much lower resolution than the typical plant or animal species (Tiedje, 1993; Staley, 1997; Fuhrman & Campbell, 1998; Moore *et al.*, 1998; Hedlund & Staley, 2004). If this is true, then many observations of microbial cosmopolitanism may be merely the result of taxonomic "lumping" of microorganisms.

We suggest, as have others (Tiedje, 1993; Hedlund & Staley, 2004), that the debate over microbial cosmopolitanism be recast. Rather than ask the unanswerable question "do microbes have fundamentally different scaling relationships from those of plants and animals?" we suggest that the debate focus instead on the question "is there a spatial scale and a level of taxonomic resolution at which microbial biodiversity scaling relationships approach those of macroorganisms?" This is a tractable question, and one that avoids the impossible task of identifying equivalent taxonomic definitions for microbes and macroorganisms. To answer this question, microbial ecologists would need to use multiple taxonomic definitions based on a variety of genetic markers (and biochemical and morphological traits if accessible). Such a polyphasic approach to studies of microbial biogeography is just beginning to be applied.

Biodiversity scaling rules have been suggested to be universal to all life. The universality of such rules has been called into question by the conclusion of some microbiologists that microbial biodiversity obeys fundamentally different rules. Determining rigorously the validity of this conclusion will not only increase our understanding of microbial ecology, but it will also provide ecologists with a true understanding of the universality of spatial scaling rules.

## References

Amann, R. I., Ludwig, W., Schleifer, K. H., Torsvik, V. & Goksoyr, J. (1995). Phylogenetic identification and *in situ* detection of individual microbial-cells without cultivation. *Microbiological Reviews*, **59**, 2019–2027.

Arrhenius, O. (1921). Species and area. *Journal of Ecology*, **9**, 95–99.

Azovksy, A. I. (2002). Size-dependent species-area relationships in benthos: is the world more diverse for microbes? *Ecography*, **25**, 273–282.

Balser, T. C. (2000). *Linking Microbial Communities and Ecosystem Functioning*. Berkeley: University of California.

Bass-Becking, L. G. M. (1934). *Geobiologie of Inleiding to de Milieukunde*, The Hague: W. P van Stockum & Zoon N. V.

Bell, T., Ager, D., Song, J.-I., *et al.* (2005). Larger islands house more bacterial taxa. *Science*, **308**, 1884.

Bohannan, B. J. M. & Hughes, J. (2003). New approaches to analyzing microbial bio-diversity data. *Current Opinion in Microbiology*, **6**, 282–287.

Brandao, P. F. B., Clapp, J. P. & Bull, A. T. (2002). Discrimination and taxonomy of geo-graphically diverse strains of nitrile-metabolizing actinomycetes using chemometric and molecular sequencing techniques. *Environmental Microbiology*, **4**, 262–276.

Brown, J. H. (1995). *Macroecology*, Chicago: University of Chicago Press.

Bull, A. T. (2004). How to look, where to look. In *Microbial Diversity and Bioprospecting*, ed. A. T. Bull, Washington D.C.: American Society for Microbial Press.

Cam, E., Nichols, J. D., Hines, J. E., Sauer, J. R., Alpizar-Jara, R. & Flather, C. H. (2002). Disentangling sampling and ecological explanations underlying species-area relationships. *Ecology*, **83**, 1118–1130.

Cho, J.-C. & Tiedje, J. M. (2000). Biogeography and degree of endemicity of fluorescent *Pseudomonas* strains in soil. *Applied and Environmental Microbiology*, **66**, 5448–5456.

Cohan, F. M. (2001). Bacterial species and speci-ation. *Systematic Biology*, **50**, 513–524.

Cohan, F. M. (2002). What are bacterial species? *Annual Review of Microbiology*, **56**, 457–487.

Coleman, A. W., Finlay, B. J. & Fenchel, T. (2002). Microbial eukaryote species. *Science*, **297**, 337.

Condit, R., Pitman, N., Leigh Jr., E. G., *et al.* (2002). Beta-diversity in tropical forest trees. *Science*, **295**, 666–669.

Connor, E. F. & McCoy, E. D. (1979). The statistics and biology of the species-area relationship. *American Naturalist*, **113**, 791–833.

Curtis, T. P., Sloan, W. T. & Scannell, J. W. (2002). Estimating prokaryotic diversity and its limits. *Proceedings of the National Academy of Sciences of the United States of America*, **99**, 10494–10499.

DeCandolle, A. (1855). *Géographie Botanique Raisonnée; ou exposition des faits principaux et des lois concernant la distribution géograhique des plates de l'époque actuelle.* Paris: Maisson.

Desmet, P. & Cowling, R. (2004). Using the species-area relationship to set baseline targets for conservation. *Ecology and Society*, **9**, 11.

Dunbar, J., Barns, S. M., Ticknor, L. O. & Kuske, C. R. (2002). Empirical and theoretical bacterial diversity in four Arizona soils. *Applied and Environmental Microbiology*, **68**, 3035–3045.

Dykhuizen, D. E. (1998). Santa Rosalia revisited: Why are there so many species of bacteria? *Antonie van Leeuwenhoek*, **73**, 25–33.

Fenchel, T. & Finlay, B. J. (2004). The ubiquity of small species: patterns of local and global diversity. *BioScience*, **54**, 777–784.

Ferrier, S., Powell, G. V. N., Richardson, K. S., *et al.* (2004). Mapping more of terrestrial biodiversity for global conservation assessment. *BioScience*, **54**, 1101–1109.

Finlay, B. J. (2002). Global dispersal of free-living microbial eukaryote species. *Science*, **296**, 1061–1063.

Finlay, B. J. & Clarke, K. J. (1999). Ubiquitous dispersal of microbial species. *Nature*, **400**, 828.

Finlay, B. J. & Esteban, G. (2004). Ubiquitous dispersal of free-living microorganisms. In *Microbial Diversity and Bioprospecting*, ed. A. T. Bull, Washington D.C.: American Society for Microbiology Press.

Finlay, B. J. & Fenchel, T. (2004). Cosmopolitan metapopulations of free-living microbial eukaryotes. *Protist*, **55**, 237–244.

Finlay, B. J., Corliss, J. O., Esteban, G. & Fenchel, T. (1996). Biodiversity at the microbial level: the number of free-living ciliates in the biosphere. *Quarterly Review of Biology*, **71**, 221–237.

Finlay, B. J., Esteban, G. V. & Fenchel, T. (1998). Protozoan diversity: converging estimates of the global number of free-living ciliate species. *Protist*, **149**, 29–37.

Foissner, W. (1997). Global scale ciliate (Protozoa, Ciliophora) diversity: a probability-based approach using large sample collections from Africa, Australia and Antartica. *Biodiversity and Conservation*, **6**, 1627–1638.

Foissner, W. (1999). Protist diversity: estimates of the near-imponderable. *Protist*, **150**, 363–368.

Franklin, R. B. & Mills, A. L. (2003). Multi-scale variation in spatial heterogeneity for microbial community structure in an eastern Virginia agricultural field. *FEMS Microbiology Ecology*, **44**, 335–346.

Fuhrman, J. & Campbell, L. (1998). Microbial microdiversity. *Nature*, **393**, 410–411.

Fulthorpe, R. R., Rhodes, A. N. & Tiedje, J. M. (1998). High levels of endemicity of 3-chlorobenzoate-degrading soil bacteria. *Applied and Environmental Microbiology*, **64**, 1620–1627.

Gage, S. H., Isard, S. A. & Colunga, G. M. (1999). Ecological scaling of aerobiological dispersal processes. *Agricultural and Forestry Meteorology*, **30**, 249–261.

Gaston, K. & Blackburn, T. (2000). *Pattern and Process in Macroecology*, Oxford: Blackwell Science.

Gaston, K. J., Blackburn, T. M. & Goldewijk, K. K. (2003). Habitat conversion and global avian biodiversity loss. *Proceedings of the Royal Society of London: Biological Sciences*, **270**, 1293–1300.

Gleason, H. A. (1922). On the relation between species and area. *Ecology*, **71**, 213–225.

Glöckner, F. O., Zaichikov, E., Belkova, N., *et al.* (2000). Comparative 16S rRNA analysis of lake bacterioplankton reveals globally distributed phylogenetic clusters including an abundant group of Actinobacteria. *Applied and Environmental Microbiology*, **66**, 5053–5065.

Gogarten, J. P. (2003). Gene transfer: gene swapping craze reaches eukaryotes. *Current Biology*, **13**, R53–R54.

Green, J. L., Holmes, A. J., Westoby, M., *et al.* (2004). Spatial scaling of microbial eukaryote diversity. *Nature*, **432**, 747–750.

Green, J. L., Hastings, A., Arzberger, P., *et al.* (2005). Complexity in ecology and conservation: mathematical, statistical, and computational challenges. *Bioscience*, **55**, 501–510.

Hagstrom, A., Pinhassi, J. & Zweifel, U. L. (2000). Biogeographical diversity among marine bacterioplankton. *Aquatic Microbial Ecology*, **21**, 231–244.

He, F. & Legendre, P. (1996). On species-area relations. *American Naturalist*, **148**, 719–737.

Head, I. M., Saunders, J. R. & Pickup, R. W. (1998). Microbial evolution, diversity, and ecology: a decade of ribosomal RNA analysis of uncultivated organisms. *Microbial Ecology*, **35**, 1–21.

Hedlund, B. P. & Staley, J. T. (2004). Microbial endemism and biogeography. In *Microbial Biodiversity and Bioprospecting*, ed. A. T. Bull, Washington D.C.: ASM Press.

Hillebrand, H., Watermann, F., Karez, R. & Berninger, U. (2001). Differences in species richness patterns between unicellular and multicellular organisms. *Oecologia*, **126**, 114–124.

Holyoak, M., Leibold, M. A. & Holt, R. D. (2005). *Metacommunities: Spatial Dynamics and Ecological Communities*, Chicago: University of Chicago Press.

Horner-Devine, M., Lage, M., Hughes, J. & Bohannan, B. (2004a). A taxa-area relationship for bacteria. *Nature*, **432**, 750–753.

Horner-Devine, M. C., Carney, K. M. & Bohannan, B. J. M. (2004b). An ecological perspective on bacterial biodiversity. *Proceedings of the Royal Society of London, Series B*, **271**, 113–122.

Hubbell, S. P. (2001). *The Unified Neutral Theory of Biodiversity and Biogeography*. Princeton: Princeton University Press.

Krishnamani, R., Kumar, A. & Harte, J. (2004). Estimating species richness at large spatial scales using data from small discrete plots. *Ecography*, **27**, 637–642.

Leff, L. G., McArthur, J. V. & Shimkets, L. J. (1998). Persistence and dissemination of introduced bacteria in freshwater microcosms. *Microbial Ecology*, **36**, 202–211.

Lighthart, B. (1997). The ecology of bacteria in the alfresco atmosphere. *FEMS Microbiology Ecology*, **23**, 263–274.

MacArthur, R. H. & Wilson, E. O. (1967). *The Theory of Island Biogeography*. Princeton: Princeton University Press.

Magurran, A. E. (2004). *Measuring Biological Diversity*. Malden, MA: Blackwell Science.

Martiny, J. B. H., Bohannan, B. J. M., Brown, J. H., *et al.* (2006). Microbial biogeography: putting microorganisms on the map. *Nature Reviews Microbiology*, **4**, 102–112.

May, R. M. (1975). Patterns of species abundance and diversity. In *Ecology and Evolution of Communities*, ed. M. L. Cody & J. M. Diamond. Cambridge: Harvard University Press.

McNair, J. N., Newbold, J. D. & Hart, D. D. (1997). Turbulent transport of suspended particles and dispersing benthic organisms: how long to hit bottom? *Journal of Theoretical Biology*, **188**, 29–52.

Mlot, C. (2004). Microbial diversity unbound: what DNA-based techniques are revealing about the planet's hidden biodiversity. *Bioscience*, **54**, 1064–1068.

Moore, L. R., Rocap, G. & Chisholm, S. W. (1998). Physiology and molecular phylogeny of coexisting *Prochlorococcus* ecotypes. *Nature*, **393**, 464–467.

Morin, P. J. & McGrady-Steed, J. (2004). Biodiversity and ecosystem functioning in aquatic microbial systems: a new analysis of temporal variation and species richness-predictability relations. *Oikos*, **104**, 458–466.

Nekola, J. C. & White, P. S. (1999). The distance decay of similarity in biogeography and ecology. *Journal of Biogeography*, **26**, 867–878.

Noguez, A. M., Arita, H. T., Escalante, A. E., Forney, L. J., Garcia-Oliva, F. & Souza, V. (2005). Microbial macroecology: highly structured prokaryotic soil assemblages in a tropical deciduous forest. *Global Ecology and Biogeography*, **14**, 241–248.

Ochman, H., Lawrence, J. G. & Groisman, E. A. (2000). Lateral gene transfer and the nature of bacterial innovation. *Nature*, **405**, 299–304.

O'Donnell, A. G., Goodfellow, G. & Hawksworth, D. L. (1994). Theoretical and practical aspects of the quantification of biodiversity among microorganisms. *Philosophical Transactions of the Royal Society of London, Series B*, **345**, 65–73.

Papke, R. T. & Ward, D. M. (2004). The importance of physical isolation to microbial diversification. *FEMS Microbiology Ecology*, **48**, 293.

Papke, R. T., Ramsing, N. B., Bateson, M. M. & Ward, D. M. (2003). Geographical isolation in hot spring cyanobacteria. *Environmental Microbiology*, **5**, 650–659.

Qian, H., Ricklefs, R. E. & White, P. S. (2005). Beta diversity of angiosperms in temperate floras of eastern Asia and eastern North America. *Ecology Letters*, **8**, 1–15.

Reche, I., Pulido-Villena, E., Morales-Baquero, R. & Casamayor, E. O. (2005). Does ecosystem size determine aquatic bacterial richness? *Ecology*, **86**, 1715–1722.

Roberts, M. S. & Cohan, F. M. (1995). Recombination and migration rates in natural populations of *Bacillus subtilis* and *Bacillus mojavensis*. *Evolution*, **49**, 1081–1094.

Rosenzweig, M. L. (1995). *Species Diversity in Space and Time*. Cambridge: Cambridge University Press.

Smith, V. H., Foster, B. L., Grover, J. P., Holt, R. D., Leibold, M. A. & Denoyelles, F. (2005). Phytoplankton species richness scales consistently from laboratory microcosms to the world's oceans. *Proceedings of the National Academy of Sciences of the United States of America*, **102**, 4393–4396.

Stackebrandt, E. & Rainey, F. A. (1995). Partial and complete 16S rDNA sequences, their use in generation of 16S rDNA phylogenetic trees and their implications in molecular ecological studies. In *Molecular Microbial Ecology Manual*, ed. A. D. L. Akkermans, J. D. Van Elsas & F. J. De Bruijn. Dordrecht: Kluwer Academic Publishers.

Staley, J. T. (1997). Biodiversity: are microbial species threatened? Commentary. *Current Opinion in Biotechnology*, **8**, 340.

Staley, J. T. & Gosink, J. J. (1999). Poles apart: biodiversity and biogeography of sea ice bacteria. *Annual Review of Microbiology*, **53**, 189–215.

Thomas, C. D., Cameron, A., Green, R. E., *et al.* (2004). Climate change and extinction risk. *Nature*, **427**, 145–148.

Tiedje, J. (1993). Approaches to the comprehensive evaluation of prokaryotic diversity of a habitat. In *Microbial Diversity and Ecosystem Function*, ed. D. Allksopp, R. R. Colwell & D. L. Hawksworth. Wallingford, UK: CAB International.

Torsvik, V., Ovreas, L. & Thingstad, T. F. (2002). Prokaryotic diversity – magnitude, dynamics, and controlling factors. *Science*, **296**, 1064–1066.

Tuomisto, H., Ruokolainen, K. & Yli-Halla, M. (2003). Dispersal, environment, and floristic variation of western Amazonian forests. *Science*, **999**, 241–244.

van Der Gast, C. J., Lilley, A. K., Ager, D. & Thompson, I. P. (2005). Island size and bacterial diversity in an archipelago of engineering machines. *Environmental Microbiology*, **7**, 1220–1226.

Ward, B. B. & O'Mullan, G. D. (2002). Worldwide distribution of *Nitrosococcus oceani*, a marine ammonia-oxidizing {gamma}-proteobacterium, detected by PCR and sequencing of 16 S rRNA and amoA genes.

*Applied and Environmental Microbiology*, **68**, 4153–4157.

Ward, D. M., Ferris, M. J., Nold, S. C. & Bateson, M. M. (1998). A natural view of microbial biodiversity within hot spring cyanobacterial mat communities. *Microbiology and Molecular Biology Reviews*, **62**, 1353–1370.

Wardle, D. A. (2002). *Communities and Ecosystems: Linking Aboveground and Belowground Components*. Princeton: Princeton University Press.

Whitaker, R. J., Grogan, D. W. & Taylor, J. W. (2003). Geographic barriers isolate endemic populations of hyperthermophilic archaea. *Science*, **301**, 976–978.

Whitman, W. B., Coleman, D. C. & Wiebe, W. J. (1998). Prokaryotes: the unseen majority. *Proceedings of the National Academy of Sciences of the United States of America*, **95**, 6578–6583.

Wilkinson, D. M. (2001). What is the upper size limit for cosmopolitan distribution in free-living microorganisms? *Journal of Biogeography*, **28**, 285–291.

Wintzingerode, F. V., Göbel, U. B. & Stackebrandt, E. (1997). Determination of microbial diversity in environmental samples: pitfalls of PCR-based rRNA analysis. *FEMS Microbiology Reviews*, **21**, 213–229.

Yannarell, A. C. & Triplett, E. W. (2005). Geographic and environmental sources of variation in lake bacterial community composition. *Applied and Environmental Microbiology*, **71**, 227–239.

Zhou, J., Xia, B., Treves, D. S., et al. (2002). Spatial and resource factors influencing high microbial diversity in soil. *Applied and Environmental Microbiology*, **68**, 326–334.

Zwart, G., Crump, B. C., Agterveld, M. P. K. V., Hagen, F. & Han, S. K. (2002). Typical freshwater bacteria: an analysis of available 16S rRNA gene sequences from plankton of lakes and rivers. *Aquatic Microbial Ecology*, **28**, 141–155.

CHAPTER EIGHT

# The importance of phylogenetic structure in biodiversity studies

JÉRÔME CHAVE
*Université Paul Sabatier, Toulouse*
GUILLEM CHUST
*Université Paul Sabatier, Toulouse*
CHRISTOPHE THÉBAUD
*Université Paul Sabatier, Toulouse*

## Introduction

A central goal of biodiversity research is to understand processes of species coexistence at different spatial and temporal scales. Much empirical research has revolved around documenting patterns of species abundance and distribution with sound sampling techniques and statistics (May, 1975; Magurran, 1988; Krebs, 1998). Such data are of tremendous importance not only for documenting current biological diversity patterns, but also for testing fundamental ecological theories (Ricklefs & Schluter, 1993; Brown, 1995; Hubbell, 2001). A common feature of these approaches is the emphasis placed on species as the appropriate currency for quantifying biological diversity. However, documenting species diversity often represents a considerable practical challenge. First, no one exactly knows the total number of extant species on Earth (Erwin, 1982; May, 1994; Novotný *et al.*, 2002; Alroy, 2002). Second, in any given sample, a sizeable fraction of the individuals may represent previously undescribed species, as is especially the case for lesser known groups, like plants in tropical forests, insects or protists. Third, species recognition usually relies upon a set of morphological cues which are not always observable. Thus, many individuals within a sample cannot be reliably assigned to previously described species. This is obvious in microbial communities, where different operational taxonomic units (OTUs) can only be distinguished by DNA screening or other molecular methods (e.g. see Suau *et al.*, 1999 for a study of the microbial diversity of the human gut, and Green & Bohannan, this volume). This issue is also serious in macroscopic organisms. For example, in spite of enormous efforts by botanists, as many as 40% of South American herbarium specimens may be improperly identified (M. J. Hopkins, personal communication). In general, there is considerable uncertainty concerning the quality of diversity surveys, and a consistent definition of OTUs is lacking.

*Scaling Biodiversity*, ed. David Storch, Pablo A. Marquet and James H. Brown. Published by Cambridge University Press. © Cambridge University Press 2007.

These technical difficulties hamper reliable estimation of the local species diversity in ecological communities, and regional maps of local species diversity are likely to suffer from these limitations. This clearly is a limitation in conservation biology when ecosystems are valued proportionally to their local species richness (Faith, 1994). Assessing landscape-scale diversity – or beta diversity (*sensu* Whittaker, 1972) – is even more difficult than alpha diversity. Beta diversity measures the turnover in species composition – or species overlap – among sites and within a landscape (Gaston *et al.*, this volume). Species overlap is meaningful only if the taxa are consistently delimited across the landscape. To circumvent such problems, some tropical forest plant researchers have limited their investigations to better-known taxonomic groups, such as palms (Kahn & Meija, 1991; Clark *et al.*, 1995; Vormisto *et al.*, 2004), ferns and fern allies (Tuomisto & Poulsen, 2000; Tuomisto, Ruokolainen & Yli-Halla, 2003), in the hope that these groups are good indicators of diversity.

Another approach to this problem is to consider that the diversity represented by species richness and species overlap is only part of the overall evolutionary diversity in communities. Species are of uneven importance in view of their place in the tree of life, if only because they may represent variable amounts of evolutionary history (Vane-Wright, Humphries & Williams, 1991; Faith, 1994; Nee & May, 1997). One simple way of measuring this taxonomic diversity is to compute species-to-genera ratios: if the ratio is high, then on average every genus is represented by many species and the loss of any one species should not result in any important evolutionary loss. However, species-to-genera ratios may not appropriately summarize the phylogenetic information if the corresponding phylogenetic tree is unbalanced (Yule, 1925; Mooers & Heard, 1997; Webb & Pitman, 2002), and because they are dependent on sample size (Gotelli & Colwell, 2001). Extensions of this approach consist in making full use of phylogenetic tree topology in measures of biological diversity and of overlap. For instance, methods have been developed to assess the conservation value of species (Faith, 1994; Nee & May, 1997; Pavoine, Ollier & Dufour, 2005). More recently, it has been realized that measures of phylogenetic diversity could be used to evaluate the evolutionary originality of a whole community (Webb, 2000; Webb *et al.*, 2002) and to test fundamental biodiversity theories. For instance if a community is made of species randomly drawn from a regional species pool – as should be the case if the neutral theory of biodiversity (Hubbell, 2001) holds – then they should evenly represent the clades of the regional phylogeny. By contrast, if limiting similarity is predicted because of competitive exclusion of closely allied species, then the species should be overdispersed on the phylogeny (Webb *et al.*, 2002; Webb & Pitman, 2002). Thus integrating the evolutionary dimension into biodiversity research goes beyond a simple refinement of diversity indices. It provides new tests for comparing ecological processes.

Here, we define a simple and consistent measure of phylogenetic diversity, based on existing population genetics theory, and which has several mathematical advantages. Then we explore how making use of information on evolutionary relationships among species may aid in understanding why biodiversity varies within and across localities. To illustrate the use of the measures, we use data on South American plant communities assembled by A. H. Gentry (1982, 1988) and phylogenetic information from the Angiosperm Phylogeny Group (henceforth APG) consortium. Specifically, we address the following questions: (1) Is the phylogenetic measure of diversity well predicted by nonphylogenetic measures based on species diversity? (2) Does the phylogenetic structure have an influence on biodiversity patterns in these communities? (3) What is the spatial structure of phylogenetic diversity, and what are the determinants in its variation? Thus, our overall goal is to examine to what extent phylogenetics is informative to central questions of community ecology, and the interplay between ecological versus evolutionary explanations of biodiversity patterns (Ricklefs, 2004). We do not address the biogeographical implications of our analysis (Gentry, 1988; Prance, 1994), a topic deferred to a forthcoming publication.

## Theory

Population genetics has been instrumental in developing statistics characterizing population substructure (Wright, 1931; Ewens, 1972; Watterson, 1974; Nei, 1987; Lande, 1996). We first summarize common measures of diversity in population genetics, then establish the correspondence with diversity measures in community ecology. Let us consider $K$ distinct populations, and $x_{ki}$, the relative abundance of the $i$th allele in population $k$ for one locus having $S$ alleles. Then classical population genetics theory (e.g. Nei, 1987) utilizes the following measure of diversity between populations $k$ and $l$:

$$\overline{D}_{kl} = 1 - \sum_{i=1}^{S} x_{ki} x_{li}. \tag{8.1}$$

The basic measure of local gene diversity is the heterozygosity, the probability that, in a randomly mating population, two individuals have different alleles at the same polymorphic locus, or $\overline{D}_{kk} = 1 - \sum (x_{ki})^2 = \sum_{i,j,i \neq j} x_{ki} x_{kj}$. Nei (1973) showed that a measure of diversity between two populations, excluding intrapopulation diversity, would be

$$\overline{H}_{kl} = \overline{D}_{kl} - \frac{\overline{D}_{kk} + \overline{D}_{ll}}{2} = \frac{1}{2} \sum_{i=1}^{S} (x_{ki} - x_{li})^2. \tag{8.2}$$

This quantity may be best thought of as proportional to the squared Euclidean distance between site $i$ and site $k$. The total diversity across all populations can then be defined as

$$\overline{D}_T = \langle \overline{D}_{kk} \rangle_k + \langle \overline{H}_{kl} \rangle_{k,l} = 1 - \sum_{i=1}^{S} \left( \langle x_{ki} \rangle_k \right)^2, \tag{8.3}$$

where in general $\langle Y_k \rangle_k = \frac{1}{K} \sum_{k=1}^{K} Y_k$ is the mean of variable $Y_k$ over $k$ ($\langle \overline{H}_{kl} \rangle_{k,l}$ is the mean over both $k$ and $l$). $\overline{H}_{kl}$ is defined by Eq. (8.2).

Lande (1996) already pointed out that this formalism could be ported from population genetics into biodiversity studies. Specifically, he suggested that if $x_{ki}$ is now interpreted as being the relative abundance of taxon $i$ in habitat $k$, then Eqs. (8.1) to (8.3) define measures of local and spatial diversity. To follow the terminology of community ecology, $\overline{D}_{kk}$ is usually called the Simpson index, and is a measure of alpha diversity, and $\overline{H}_{kl}$ is a measure of beta diversity (Whittaker, 1972). At the community level Eq. (8.3) can be interpreted as an *additive* partition of diversity into a within-locality (alpha-diversity) component $\overline{D}_\alpha = \langle \overline{D}_{kk} \rangle_k$ and a between-locality (beta-diversity) component $\overline{D}_\beta = \langle \overline{H}_{kl} \rangle_{k,l}$.

Our goal is to extend this formalism to the study of phylogenetically structured communities. A simple generalization of formula (8.1) for genetically structured populations is

$$D_{kl} = \sum_{i=1}^{S} \sum_{j=1}^{S} t_{ij} x_{ki} x_{lj}. \tag{8.4}$$

In the present work, $t_{ij}$ denotes the divergence time between taxon $i$ and taxon $j$, such that the maximal divergence time is set to unity. In population genetic theory, $t_{ij}$ denotes the fraction of nucleotide substitutions between haplotypes $i$ and $j$ (Nei, 1987). Haplotype refers here to a set of closely linked alleles inherited as a unit. The above formulas (8.1–8.3) correspond to the limiting case where the divergence time is assumed to take the maximal value ($t_{ij} = 1$) for each $i \neq j$, which is also called a "star-shaped" phylogeny (every pair of distinct taxa is equidistant). To generalize the above formulas, we also define the matrix $P_{ij} = 1 - t_{ij}$, such that $P_{ij}$ for each $i \neq j$ and 1 otherwise. In this case, $D_{kl} = 1 - \sum_{i=1}^{S} \sum_{j=1}^{S} P_{ij} x_{ki} x_{lj}$. Note that Pavoine *et al.* (2005) recently called this quantity the "quadratic entropy", based on some earlier work in statistics.

In (8.4) and subsequent formulas, $D$ and $H$ now refer to measures of phylogenetic diversity taking into account the distribution of divergence times between species pairs. Throughout the text, nonphylogenetic measures of diversity are distinguished from phylogenetic measures by the bar over the symbol. We can write the companion of Eq. (8.2):

$$H_{kl} = D_{kl} - (D_{kk} + D_{ll})/2 = \frac{1}{2}\sum_{i=1}^{S}\sum_{j=1}^{S}(x_{ki} - x_{li})P_{ij}(x_{kj} - x_{lj}) \qquad (8.5)$$

and of Eq. (8.3):

$$D_T = \langle D_{kk}\rangle_k + \langle H_{kl}\rangle_{k,l} = 1 - \sum_{i=1}^{S}\sum_{j=1}^{S}\langle x_{ki}\rangle_k P_{ij}\langle x_{kl}\rangle_k, \qquad (8.6)$$

where $\omega_k$ is defined as in Eq. (8.3). At the community level this formula can still be interpreted as an additive partition of phylogenetic diversity into alpha and beta diversity $D_T = D_\alpha + D_\beta$.

In principle, the term $t_{ij}$ could still be interpreted as a measure of among-species divergence in DNA sequence data. This is most convenient in microbiology, where the OTUs are directly defined by a DNA sequence (Martin, 2002; Green & Bohanann, this volume). Because of differences in rate of molecular evolution among species in most groups of organisms, dissimilarity in molecular sequences is not a consistent measure of evolutionary divergence across taxa. Divergence time estimation from DNA sequence data often requires calibration points using independent evidence, such as dates of unambiguous evolutionary splits inferred from fossil or biogeographic data (Arbogast *et al.*, 2002). Thus, in the present work, we shall interpret the term $t_{ij}$ as a divergence time, assuming problems associated with variance in rate of nucleotide substitutions have been dealt with using appropriate approaches (e.g. Sanderson, 1997, 2002). The term $t_{ij}$ hence denotes the age of the most recent common ancestor of taxon $i$ and $j$, divided by the age of the most recent common ancestor of the whole set of taxa; that is, $t_{ij}$ is between 0 and 1. A simple measure of among-locality differentiation (Nei, 1973; Slatkin, 1991) can be defined as

$$F_{ST} = \frac{D_\beta}{D_T}, \qquad (8.7)$$

where this variable is defined by analogy to the $F_{ST}$ in population genetics and measures community turnover instead of population genetic differentiation.

## Data and statistical analyses

To test the relevance of our approach we used a large tropical plant census collected by A. H. Gentry (Gentry, 1982, 1988; Phillips & Miller, 2002), which was made available online by the Missouri Botanical Garden (www.mobot.org/MOBOT/Research/gentry/transect.shtml). For the purpose of this work, we used only the data for the 124 South American sites. Each site consists of 10 randomly placed transects $2 \times 50$ m in size, totaling roughly 0.1 ha in area. In these plots all woody ferns, trees, lianas and monocots above 2.5 cm in diameter (originally, 1 inch) were identified to the species, or sorted into morphospecies (*c.* 95% of the individuals were identified at least at the species or genus level, see below). For each site, an elevation was recorded (range 10–3050 m a.s.l.) as well as annual rainfall for 123 of the 124 sites (range 400–9000 mm/yr).

The data set contained a total of 44 114 stems. To minimize the number of spelling errors in the data set we matched the genus names to a list of all plant genera maintained by the Royal Botanic Gardens at Kew (www.rbgkew.org.uk/web.dbs/genlist.html), and corrected typos. We then verified that the family names matched the most recent molecular-based plant phylogeny, based on the work of the Angiosperm Phylogeny Group (APG, 2003), and on Soltis *et al.* (2002) for more ancestral nodes (tracheophytes). In total, the data set we used contained 4471 morphospecies. Of these, 1094 taxa were described only to the genus level (38.7% of the individuals) and 56 to the family level (6.2% of the individuals). For instance, 732 individuals were grouped into 16 morphospecies of the difficult genus *Miconia* (Melastomataceae). Only 115 individuals could not be identified even to the family level (0.2%). It is important to emphasize that although many papers have made use of the Gentry data set, not all have achieved the same effort of data standardization. Also, many voucher specimens of the Gentry collection are continuously being identified by the specialists of the Missouri Botanical Garden. Thanks to their dedication, the data set used here is considerably improved over that used a decade ago (for an overview, see, e.g. Phillips & Miller, 2002).

Next, we obtained a phylogeny for the species included in this data set by using a method inspired from that of Webb (2000). A super-tree containing the full APG II phylogeny (APG, 2003), plus other literature sources, were assembled by C. O. Webb (Webb & Donoghue, 2004; www.phylodiversity.net), updated for the present work, and pruned accordingly. In the tree, terminal nodes always correspond to species, branching off from genus-level nodes. The most ancestral node corresponds to the origin of vascular plants (euphyllophytes). We empha-size that our phylogenetic hypothesis has many issues, being unevenly resolved across clades, being the result on a "grafting" of the phylogeny of selected families onto the APG phylogeny. Thus our quantitative results are likely to be altered when better phylogenetic hypotheses are made available. However, we are confident that the present hypothesis faithfully reflects the current stage of knowledge in plant phylogenetics.

Finally, we "dated" the phylogeny using a calibration produced by Wikström, Savolainen & Chase (2001), who combined fossil data and existing molecular-based data on angiosperms to date divergence times for over 400 interior nodes, mostly families and orders. Nodes above the family level used all angiosperm families, so we could define the age of the nodes as the maximal age between two taxa within the clade. The family level nodes were more difficult to resolve, as they were based on a small subsample of the total number of genera. For instance, if only two genera of a genus-rich family were included in the phylogeny, then the divergence time between these two genera would likely underestimate the true age of the family. We further discuss this issue in the Appendix. We postulated an age of 450 Myr for the origin of euphyllophytes (the most ancestral node in our phylogeny), and 166 Myr for the origin of Cyatheaceae (tree ferns). Soltis *et al.* (2002) showed that divergence times of tree ferns tend to be underestimated using molecular-based techniques, so we privileged the estimate based on fossil information. This tree enabled us to construct a matrix $t_{ij}$, representing divergence times between species $i$ and species $j$. For instance, the cucumber family and the beech family diverged 84 Myr ago, so the relative divergence time between *Cucurbita maxima* and *Fagus sylvatica* would be $84/450 = 0.187$. The divergence time of any two distinct genera within the same family was estimated by the divergence time of the family, as inferred in the Appendix. For instance, the divergence between *Iryanthera sagotiana* and *Virola calophylla*, both in the Myristicaceae, was taken to be 46 Myr, so $t_{ij} = 46/450 = 0.1$. Because the species level was not resolved in our phylogenetic hypothesis, we assumed that the divergence between two congeneric species was equal to the estimated genus age.

We contrasted results obtained by using this distance matrix, to a star-shaped phylogeny, such that $t_{ij} = 1$ for all $i \neq j$, and $t_{ii} = 0$, from which we computed the nonphylogenetic diversity indices $\overline{D}_\alpha, \overline{D}_\beta$ (we remind the reader that nonphylogenetic measures of diversity are distinguished from phylogenetic measures by the bar over the symbol).

First, we tested whether the addition of a phylogenetic structure significantly modified measures of biodiversity. A simple approach to this question is to ask whether the alpha diversity, as measured by $D_\alpha$, and the among-site differentiation, as measured by $F_{ST}$, significantly differ from a null expectation. A direct comparison between the phylogenetic measure $D$ and the nonphylogenetic measure $\overline{D}$ is not straightforward given the different scaling of times (however, the dimensionless $F_{ST}$ may be compared). Instead, we constructed a randomization test by which we kept the species lists unchanged in the sites, but reshuffled the species location across the phylogeny (Slatkin, 1991). Hence, the tree structure remains unchanged: only the labels of the tip nodes are permuted. For each randomized phylogeny, we computed $D_\alpha$ and $F_{ST}$, and we compared the observed value with the null expectation by means of a simple Student's $t$-test.

To test for spatial variation in diversity, we compared the diversity matrices with environmental or geographical distance matrices, using the Mantel test. The Mantel test compares two similarity or distance matrices computed for the same sites (Legendre & Legendre, 1998). The Mantel statistic $r_M$ is a measure of the correlation between the two matrices, and behaves like a correlation coefficient. It is usually tested by a nonparametric permutational test as the assumption of independence between values of the variable is not fulfilled in similarity or distance matrices.

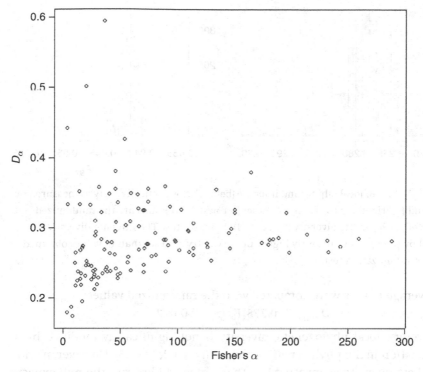

**Figure 8.1** Scatter plot of $D_\alpha$ against Fisher's $\alpha$, a measure of local species diversity controlling for sample size.

## Results

First, we asked if nonphylogenetic diversity is a suitable approximation of phylogenetic diversity. Figure 8.1 illustrates a comparison between the measure of phylogenetic alpha diversity $D_\alpha$ and a commonly used measure of alpha diversity, Fisher's alpha (see e.g. ter Steege *et al.*, 2003). Except at low diversity values, there was no significant relationship between these two measures: the plots with highest species diversity were not necessarily those with largest phylogenetic diversity. We also compared the phylogenetic and nonphylogenetic measures of beta diversity. Specifically, we performed a Mantel test to compare the phylogenetic diversity matrix $H$ with the nonphylogenetic diversity matrix $\overline{H}$. Mantel's correlation coefficient was found to be $r_M = 0.66$, and the significance level, obtained by permutations was $P = 0.001$. Thus, nonphylogenetic beta diversity is significantly correlated with phylogenetic beta diversity.

Second, we compared the mean phylogenetic diversity to that measured with randomized phylogenetic trees. In so doing, we also tested for the presence of phylogenetic structure in the data. Mean local phylogenetic diversity and phylogenetic beta diversity were equal to

$$D_\alpha = 0.283, F_{ST} = 0.059.$$

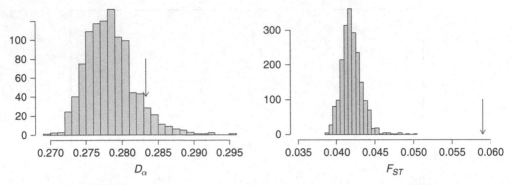

**Figure 8.2** Values of local (alpha) and intersite (beta) phylogenetic diversity as measured by $D_\alpha$ (left) and $F_{ST}$ (right) for the Gentry data set (arrows). Histograms are the randomized measures of phylogenetic diversity (based on 1000 replicates). The intersite diversity as measured by the $F_{ST}$ is significantly higher in the Gentry data set than in values obtained from the randomization test.

These average figures were compared with the randomized values:

$$D_\alpha|_{rand} = 0.278, F_{ST}|_{rand} = 0.042.$$

Thus, average local phylogenetic diversity is not significantly modified by a randomization in the phylogenetic structure ($t = 0.62$, $P > 0.5$). However, phylogenetic beta diversity as measured by the $F_{ST}$ does differ from the null expectation ($t = 12.6$, $P < 0.001$). This test is further illustrated in Fig. 8.2. Cross-plot local phylogenetic diversity $D_\alpha$ varied from 0.17 for Puyeyhue (Ecuador) to 0.59 for Alto de Mirador (Colombia) while the randomized measure of local diversity varied from 0.19 to 0.37. The randomization test summarized in Fig. 8.3 also shows that 26 plots are significantly less phylogenetically diverse locally than the null expectation, and 24 plots are more phylogenetically diverse (*t*-test, $P < 0.05$). Measures of phylogenetic beta diversity were also tested individually: 24% of the values were significantly greater than the randomized value, while 14% were significantly smaller (*t*-test, $P < 0.05$). Two sites were outliers in this analysis, having very high local phylogenetic diversities: Alto de Mirador ($D_\alpha = 0.59$) and Alto de Sapa ($D_\alpha = 0.50$), both from the highlands of Colombia. This is explained by the abundance of ancient plant groups that were rare in the other plots (e.g. tree ferns, *Cyathea* spp.). Excluding these two sites, however, we found $D_\alpha = 0.279$, $F_{ST} = 0.055$, and the significance tests for $D_\alpha$ and $F_{ST}$ were not modified. Hence, our results are not driven by outliers.

Third, we used a correlative approach to relate observed patterns of phylogenetic alpha and beta diversity. For alpha diversity, we used a linear model to correlate $D_\alpha$ with elevation and rainfall. Both rainfall and (rainfall)$^2$ were significant predictors of local diversity, and they explained 22% of the total variance. This contrasts with the nonphylogenetic measure of local diversity $\bar{D}_\alpha$ in which we found only a weak signal: only rainfall was significant

**Table 8.1** *Linear regression of phylogenetic and nonphylogenetic measures of local (alpha) diversity against elevation, and annual rainfall*
Numbers represent the partial $R^2$ for the variables. We also report the best regression model.

|  | Phylogenetic local diversity $D(A, A)$ | Nonphylogenetic local diversity $\bar{D}(A, A)$ |
|---|---|---|
| Elevation | $0.127, P < 10^{-4}$ | $0.0282, P = 0.062$ |
| Rainfall | $0.151, p < 10^{-4}$ | $0.0708, P = 0.003$ |
| (Rainfall)$^2$ | $0.075, P = 0.001$ | $0.0178, P = 0.129$ |
| Variables of regression model | Rainfall, (Rainfall)$^2$ | Rainfall |
| Predicted $R^2$ for regression model | $R^2 = 0.226$ | $R^2 = 0.0708$ |

**Table 8.2** *Mantel correlations ($r_M$) and significance levels (based on 999 permutations) for both phylogenetic and nonphylogenetic diversity matrices H (a measure of beta diversity), compared with geographical distance (GD), logarithmically transformed geographical distance, elevation, and annual rainfall*

|  | Phylogenetic diversity $H(A, B)$ | Nonphylogenetic diversity $\bar{H}(A, B)$ |
|---|---|---|
| $\bar{H}(A, B)$ | $0.6604, P = 0.001$ |  |
| Geographical distance ($GD$) | $0.2606, P = 0.001$ | $0.3015, P = 0.001$ |
| ln($GD$) | $0.1908, P = 0.001$ | $0.2144, P = 0.001$ |
| Elevation | $0.2264, P = 0.001$ | $0.1273, P = 0.037$ |
| Annual rainfall | $0.0026, P = 0.371$ | $0.0458, P = 0.491$ |
| Variables of regression model | Elevation, $GD$ | Elevation, $GD$ |
| Predicted $R^2$ for regression model | $R^2 = 0.133$ | $R^2 = 0.131$ |

(Table 8.1). For the phylogenetic and nonphylogenetics beta-diversity matrices $H$ and $\bar{H}$, we used Mantel tests. We correlated them with environmental and geographical distance matrices. The results are displayed in Table 8.2. Geographical distance was the best descriptor of both phylogenetic and non-phylogenetic diversity ($r_M = 0.261$, and $r_M = 0.301$, respectively). Elevation was also a significant predictor in both cases, but phylogenetic diversity was better predicted by this variable than nonphylogenetic diversity ($r_M = 0.226$, and $r_M = 0.127$, respectively).

## Discussion

We showed that incorporating phylogenetic information affects both the local and regional biodiversity patterns observed in neotropical plant communities. We detected a strong phylogenetic signal on estimation of mean beta-diversity

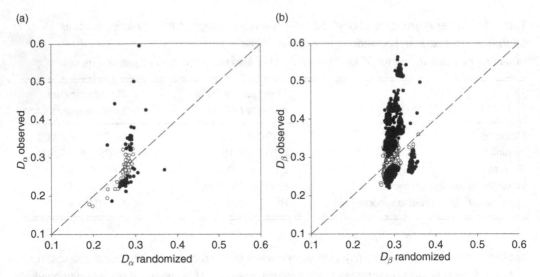

**Figure 8.3** (a) Observed values of $D_\alpha$ for the 124 Gentry plots, against the null expectation (mean $D_\alpha$ obtained with the randomization test). (b) Observed values of $D_\beta$ for pairs of Gentry plots plotted against the randomized value. Both panels evidence the large range in diversity within and across plots. Black dots refer to values significantly lower or higher than the null expectation.

$F_{ST}$; a site-by-site analysis, as reported in Fig. 8.3, also revealed a strong local phylogenetic signal in 50 sites out of 124. This shows that phylogenies encapsulate an information that is not summarized in species-based measures of diversity, both for local diversity (at least in a large fraction of the sites) and for beta diversity. In other words, species diversity does not accurately reflect overall evolutionary diversity, a central message of the present work.

Why are some sites significantly more phylogenetically diverse than expected by chance? A closer inspection at the species assemblages in these sites reveals that they had a greal deal of species belonging to ancient clades, like tree ferns or basal dicot species, in the Magnoliales and in the Laurales. They were predominantly montane species, which supports the often discussed biogeographic pattern of an origin of the angiosperms in the montane tropics (Axelrod, 1952; Takhtajan, 1969). Other sites were less phylogenetically diverse than expected by chance, due to the overrepresentation of single families or orders. This high degree of phylogenetic clustering is compatible with two alternative ecological mechanisms. It could either be that sites are overrepresented by a single species, which might be a poor disperser. This clumping effect would then be an indirect evidence for dispersal limitation in tropical floras. Alternatively, species of most clades but one might have been filtered out by the environment, suggesting that the species co-occurring in the site would have been selected for a biological feature not shared by the species of other clades.

For example, the hyperabundance of palm species in neotropical swamps prob-ably reflects a special adaptation of this clade to the anaerobic growth of the root system. It would be interesting to explore further such patterns of phylogenetic clustering or overdispersion over large spatial scales. Notably, besides elevation, only geographical distance stood out as a significant predictive factor of the phylogenetic diversity matrix H.

So far, conservation planning at the regional scale has almost exclusively focused on species count data. We have shown here that for neotropical plants, species richness does not predict phylogenetic diversity. While Prance (1994) found that diversity above the species level exhibited considerably smoother variation than species level patterns in neotropical plant communities, our results suggest that reservoirs for phylogenetic history cannot always be deduced from patterns of local species richness. Thus, it is clearly important to incorporate phylogenetic information, when available, in planning conser-vation strategies or in identifying areas of high biodiversity. Also, it should be pointed out here that consideration of phylogenetic structure does not circum-vent the problem of first documenting species diversity. In view of the limi-tations of such protocols, discussed in the Introduction, one might wonder why this refinement is at all a useful step forward. A first practical answer to this question is that, within the formalism of phylogenetic diversity developed above, one can easily accommodate heterogeneous taxonomic censuses. For instance, if a fraction of the taxa are known only to the family level or to the genus level, it is still possible to explore their relatedness to other taxa. Thus measures of phylogenetic diversity are less sensitive to the issue of sorting taxa into morphospecies. Further, phylogenetic diversity has a natural connection to the rapidly expanding field of DNA bar coding. This technique largely bypasses classical taxonomic identification by sequencing universal genes, which are sufficiently variable to show a significant level of interspecific signal (Hebert *et al.*, 2004; see however Moritz & Cicero, 2004). While unable to resolve deep nodes of the phylogeny, such markers could be used to develop an individual-based phylogeny of an ecological community, within which species would be considered as monophyletic clades. This would partially circumvent the problem of taxonomic identification and at the same time would provide a method for assessing the total amount of divergence within an ecological community.

Our analysis is a first attempt to relate concepts of evolutionary diversity and empirical data both for alpha diversity and beta diversity. While quantifying biodiversity using phylogenetic information is, at least conceptually, an obvious improvement over traditional approaches, the present attempt still suffers from a number of limitations. Despite our efforts to use well-resolved phylogenies and to calibrate the resulting super-tree, our estimates of evolutionary diversity are not devoid of possible bias. In the case of flowering plants, a number of important nodes remain poorly supported, and the branch lengths as well as the tree topology remain indicative, particularly below the family level (see Saladin *et al.*, 2005, for recent developments). For instance, in one important order for neotropical woody plant species, the Malpighiales, it has been shown that Wikström *et al.* (2001)'s estimate of the ages in this clade was considerably underestimated (Davis *et al.*, 2005), a common situation when fossil evidence is limited or controversial. It may be argued that diversity measures based on nucleotide differences (the basis for the construction of phylogenetic trees), rather than on divergence times would produce estimates that would be less dependent on assumptions on diversification rates. However, we contend that our measure is more biologically relevant, as it directly relates to the evolutionary history of the species assemblages under study. For instance, our result that the minimum local diversity is $D_\alpha = 0.17$ may be reinterpreted as follows: on average two randomly chosen individuals in the community come from lineages that diverged 76.5 Myr ago. Clarke and Warwick, in a series of recent reports (Clarke & Warwick, 2001; Warwick & Clarke, 2001) defined very similar measures of phylogenetic diversity, in which branch lengths measure taxonomic levels (species, genus, family, suborder, order, and so forth). This measure of "taxonomic diversity" gives an equal weight to recent and to old lineages (e.g. the fairly recent Chrysobalanaceae and the very ancient Piperaceae), but should provide a good approximation to phylogenetic diversity in cases where no reliable phylogeny is available, or for historical species lists, as pointed out by Clarke and Warwick (2001).

## Acknowledgments

This work was based on the invaluable data set collected by the late A. H. Gentry, and made available through the Missouri Botanical Garden website. We thank Vincent Savolainen and Cam Webb for discussions, Steve Hubbell, David Storch, and Pablo Marquet for useful critiques on the manuscript, Monique Gardes for pointing out the reference Martin (2002), and Sandrine Pavoine for spotting an error in Eq. (8.5).

## Appendix 8.I  Maximum likelihood estimation of the age of a family from an incomplete sampling

For each family, Wikström *et al.* (2001) listed the maximal possible age, $T_{max}$ (divergence time to the sister family), the minimal age $T_{min}$ (age of the most recent ancestral node if more than one genus is present; zero otherwise), $k$ the number of sampled genera. Moreover, $K$, the total number of genera in each family, is available. An estimate of $T$, the true age of the family, is a function of these four parameters:

$$T = f(T_{min}, T_{max}, k, K).$$

**Table 8.3** *Estimation of the family age for the most represented families in the Gentry data set* $T_{min}$ is the age of the most ancestral genus in the family, $T_{max}$ the divergence time to the sister family, $k$ the number of sampled genera within the family. All three parameters are reported in Wikström *et al.* (2001). $K$ is the total number of extant genera in this family after the Kew checklist of plant genera (in parentheses, after Smith *et al.* 2004), and $N$, the number of sampled individuals in the Gentry data set. The sampling parameter $\beta$ is estimated from Eq. (8.1) if $k > 1$ or set to 1 if $k = 1$ (uniform prior sampling distribution). $T$ is the estimated family age.

| Family name | $N$ | $T_{min}$ | $T_{max}$ | $k$ | $K$ | $\beta$ | $T$ |
|---|---|---|---|---|---|---|---|
| Annonaceae | 954 | 63 | 82 | 2 | 125(135) | 0.98 | 81 |
| Apocynaceae | 732 | 18 | 45 | 2 | 496(250–550) | 2.82 | 41 |
| Araceae | 547 | 98 | 124 | 2 | 109(105) | 0.92 | 123 |
| Arecaceae | 2387 | 73 | 99 | 7 | 205(189) | 1.81 | 94 |
| Asteraceae | 588 | 44 | 50 | 5 | 1511(1535) | 1.009 | 50 |
| Bignoniaceae | 2024 | 38 | 47 | 3 | 111(120) | 1.05 | 46 |
| Burseraceae | 571 | 0 | 51 | 1 | 18(18) | 1 | 48 |
| Celastraceae | 522 | 42 | 58 | 5 | 92(76) | 1.66 | 55 |
| Clusiaceae | 917 | 0 | 45 | 1 | 47(36) | 1 | 44 |
| Euphorbiaceae | 1670 | 0 | 69 | 1 | 333(300) | 1 | 69 |
| Fabaceae | 3762 | 56 | 79 | 3 | 677(650–700) | 1.41 | 78 |
| Lauraceae | 1397 | 34 | 80 | 2 | 49(52) | 2.61 | 64 |
| Lecythidaceae | 530 | 65 | 88 | 3 | 25(20) | 1.3 | 81 |
| Malvaceae | 876 | 34 | 54 | 8 | 273(245)[a] | 2.54 | 49 |
| Melastomataceae | 1691 | 0 | 41 | 1 | 194(155) | 1 | 41 |
| Meliaceae | 1088 | 30 | 40 | 2 | 51(50) | 1.04 | 39 |
| Moraceae | 1474 | 23 | 36 | 2 | 37(37) | 1.42 | 33 |
| Myristicaceae | 840 | 23 | 113 | 2 | 18(19) | 6.35 | 46 |
| Polygonaceae | 536 | 26 | 37 | 2 | 49(45) | 1.19 | 36 |
| Rubiaceae | 2844 | 56 | 64 | 4 | 623(650) | 0.83 | 64 |
| Salicaceae | 646 | 40 | 53 | 5 | 82(–) | 1.52 | 50 |
| Sapindaceae | 1020 | 36 | 56 | 5 | 138(147) | 2.71 | 48 |
| Sapotaceae | 860 | 0 | 54 | 1 | 59(53) | 1 | 53 |
| Urticaceae | 503 | 22 | 42 | 2 | 55(46–58)[a] | 1.95 | 37 |
| Violaceae | 642 | 0 | 51 | 1 | 20(25) | 1 | 48 |

[a] Sum of number of genera considered as different families in Smith *et al.* (2004)'s treatment.

We constructed the following probabilistic model. By definition, the age $T$ of a family is the maximal age of all genera within the family. Let $\{x_1, x_2, \ldots, x_K\}$ be the sequence of ages of the $K$ genera within a family. Then:

$$T = \max_{i \leq K}(x_i),$$

where, for all $i$, $x_i < T_{max}$.

The simplest model consists in assuming that the genus ages are Poisson-distributed between 0 and $T_{max}$, and to estimate $T$ for $K$ draws using extreme value theory. However, we already know that $k$ genera were sampled, out of the total of $N$ genera. Let us assume that the genus ages $x_i$ are distributed according to a beta probability density function $P(x) = A(T_{max} - x)^{\beta - 1}$, with $0 < x < T_{max}$, and $A = \beta / T_{max}^{\beta}$. If $\beta > 1$, values of $x$ close to $T_{max}$ are less likely, hence the situation corresponds to a family with genera that all tend to be younger than $T_{max}$. The extreme value probability density function of this process is given by

$$F_k(x) = kP(x) \left( \int_0^x P(y)dy \right)^{k-1}.$$

This is the probability that in $k$ trials, all $k$ but one are below the value $x$. In our case, we define a likelihood function

$$L(\beta|k, T_{min}, T_{max}) = F_k(T_{min}).$$

The maximal likelihood estimator of $\beta$ is defined implicitly by

$$\beta \left( 1 - \frac{k-1}{(1-\tau)^{-\beta}-1} \right) + \frac{1}{\ln(1-\tau)} = 0, \tag{8.8}$$

with $\tau = \frac{T_{min}}{T_{max}}$.

The expected age of the family can be estimated as the first moment of $F_K(x)$:

$$T = T_{max} \left[ 1 - \int_0^1 \left( 1 - x^\beta \right)^K dx \right] = T_{max} \left[ 1 - \frac{B(K+1, 1/\beta)}{\beta} \right]. \tag{8.9}$$

For each family, we first computed parameter $\beta$ as a function of $k$ and $\tau$ by solving iteratively Eq. (8.8). Then we used this parameter together with $K$, the total number of genera in the family, to provide an estimate of the family age. This procedure is illustrated in Table 8.3 for the most abundant families in the Gentry data set.

## References

Alroy, J. (2002). How many named species are valid? *Proceedings of the National Academy of Sciences of the USA*, **99**, 3706–3711.

Angiosperm Phylogeny Group [APG]. (2003). An update of the Angiosperm Phylogeny Group classification for the orders and families of flowering plants: APG II. *Botanical Journal of the Linnean Society*, **141**, 399–436.

Arbogast, B. S., Edwards, S. V., Wakeley, J., Beerli, P. & Slowinksi, J. J. (2002). Estimating divergence times from molecular data on phylogenetic and population genetic time-scales. *Annual Review of Ecology and Systematics*, **33**, 707–740.

Axelrod, D. I. (1952). A theory of angiosperm evolution. *Evolution*, **4**, 29–60.

Brown, J. H. (1995). *Macroecology*. Chicago: University of Chicago Press.

Clark, D. A., Clark, D. B., Sandoval, R. M. & Castro Vinicio, M. C. (1995). Edaphic and human effects on landscape-scale distributions of tropical rain forest palms. *Ecology*, **76**, 2581–2594.

Clarke, K. R. & Warwick, R. M. (2001). A further biodiversity index applicable to species lists: variation in taxonomic distinctness. *Marine Ecology Progress Series*, **216**, 265–278.

Davis, C. C., Webb, C. O., Wurdack, K. J., Jaramillo, C. A. & Donoghue, M. J. (2005). Explosive radiation of Malpighiales supports a mid-Cretaceous origin of modern tropical rain forests. *American Naturalist*, **165**, E36–E65.

Erwin, T. L. (1982). Tropical forests: their richness in coleopteran and other arthropod species. *Coleopterists Bulletin*, **36**, 74–75.

Ewens, W. J. (1972). The sampling theory of selectively neutral alleles. *Theoretical Population Biology*, **3**, 87–112.

Faith, D. P. (1994). Phylogenetic pattern and the quantification of organismal diversity. *Philosophical Transactions of the Royal Society of London, Series B*, **345**, 45–58.

Gentry, A. H. (1982). Patterns of Neotropical plant species diversity. *Evolutionary Biology*, **15**, 1–84.

Gentry, A. H. (1988). Changes in plant community diversity and floristic composition on environmental and geographical gradients. *Annals of the Missouri Botanical Garden*, **75**, 1–34.

Gotelli, N. J. & Colwell, R. K. (2001). Quantifying biodiversity: procedures and pitfalls in the measurement and comparison of species richness. *Ecology Letters*, **4**, 379–391.

Hebert, P. D., Stoeckle, M. Y., Zemlak, T. S. & Francis, C. M. (2004). Identification of birds through DNA barcodes. *PLoS Biology*, **2-e**, 312.

Hubbell, S. P. (2001). *A Unified Neutral Theory of Biodiversity and Biogeography*. Princeton, NJ: Princeton University Press.

Kahn, F. & Mejia, K. (1991). The palm communities of two "terra firme" forests in Peruvian Amazonia. *Principes*, **35**, 22–26.

Krebs, C. J. (1998). *Ecological Methodology*, 2nd edn. Reading, MA: Addison-Welsey.

Lande, R. (1996). Statistics and partitioning of species diversity, and similarity among multiple communities. *Oikos*, **76**, 5–13.

Legendre, P. & Legendre, L. (1998). *Numerical Ecology*, 2nd English edition. Amsterdam: Elsevier Science.

Magurran, A. E. (1988). *Ecological Diversity and its Measurement*. London: Chapman and Hall.

Martin, A. P. (2002). Phylogenetic approaches for describing and comparing microbial communities. *Applied and Environmental Microbiology*, **68**, 3673–3682.

May, R. M. (1975). Patterns of species abundance and diversity. In *Ecology and Evolution of Communities*, ed. M. L. Cody & J. M. Diamond, pp. 81–120. Cambridge, MA: Belknap Press of Harvard University Press.

May, R. M. (1994). Conceptual aspects of the quantification of the extent of biological diversity. *Philosophical Transactions of the Royal Society of London, Series B*, **345**, 13–20.

Mooers, A. O. & Heard, S. B. (1997). Inferring evolutionary process from phylogenetic tree shape. *Quarterly Review of Biology*, **72**, 31–54.

Moritz, C. & Cicero, C. (2004). DNA barcoding: promise and pitfalls. *PLoS Biology*, **2-e**, 279.

Nee, S. & May, R. M. (1997). Extinction and the loss of evolutionary history. *Science*, **278**, 692–694.

Nei, M. (1973). Analysis of gene diversity in subdivided populations. *Proceedings of the National Academy of Sciences of the USA*, **70**, 3321–3323.

Nei, M. (1987). *Molecular Evolutionary Genetics*. New York: Columbia University Press.

Novotný, V., Basset, Y., Miller, S. E., et al. (2002). Low host specificity of herbivorous insects in a tropical forest. *Nature*, **416**, 841–844.

Pavoine, S., Ollier, S. & Dufour, A. B. (2005). Is the originality of a species measurable? *Ecology Letters*, **8**, 579–586.

Phillips, O. L. & Miller, J. (2002). *Global Patterns of Plant Diversity: Alwyn H. Gentry's Forest Transect Data Set*. St. Louis, MO: Missouri Botanical Garden.

Prance, G. T. (1994). A comparison of the efficacy of higher taxa and species numbers in the assessment of biodiversity in the Neotropics. *Philosophical Transactions of the Royal Society of London, Series B*, **345**, 89–99.

Ricklefs, R. E. (2004). A comprehensive framework for global patterns in biodiversity. *Ecology Letters*, **7**, 1–15.

Ricklefs, R. E. & Schluter, D. (eds) (1993). *Species Diversity in Ecological Communities: Historical and Geographical Perspectives*. Chicago: University of Chicago Press.

Saladin, N., Hodkinson, T. R. & Savolainen, V. (2005). Towards building the tree of life: a simulation study for all angiosperm genera. *Systematic Biology*, **54**, 183–196.

Sanderson, M. J. (1997). A nonparametric approach to estimating divergence times in the absence of rate constancy. *Molecular Biology and Evolution*, **14**, 1218–1231.

Sanderson, M. J. (2002). Estimating absolute rates of molecular evolution and divergence times: a penalized likelihood approach. *Molecular Biology and Evolution*, **19**, 101.

Slatkin, M. (1991). Inbreeding coefficients and coalescent times. *Genetic Research*, **58**, 167–175.

Smith, N., Mori, S. A., Henderson, A., Stevenson, D. W. & Heald, S. V. (2004). *Flowering plants of the Neotropics*. Princeton: Princeton University Press.

Soltis, P. S., Soltis, D. E., Savolainen, V., Crane, P. E. & Barraclough, T. G. (2002). Rate heterogeneity among lineages of tracheophytes: integration of molecular and fossil data and evidence for molecular living fossils. *Proceedings of the National Academy of Sciences of the USA*, **99**, 4430–4435.

Suau, A., Bonnet, R., Sutren, M., *et al.* (1999). Direct analysis of genes encoding 16S rRNA from complex communities reveals many novel molecular species within the human gut. *Applied and Environmental Microbiology*, **65**, 4799–4807.

Takhtajan, A. (1969). *Flowering Plants: Origin and Dispersal*. Edinburgh: Oliver & Boyd.

ter Steege, H., Pitman, N., Sabatier, D., *et al.* (2003). A spatial model of tree alpha-diversity and tree density for the Amazon. *Biodiversity and Conservation*, **12**, 2255–2277.

Tuomisto, H. & Poulsen, A. D. (2000). Pteridophyte diversity and species composition in four Amazonian rain forests. *Journal of Vegetation Science*, **11**, 383–396.

Tuomisto, H., Ruokolainen, K. & Yli-Halla, M. (2003). Dispersal, environment, and floristic variation of Western Amazonian forests. *Science*, **299**, 241–244.

Vane-Wright, R. I., Humphries, C. J. & Williams, P. H. (1991). What to protect? Systematics and the agony of choice. *Biological Conservation*, **55**, 235–254.

Vormisto, J., Svenning, J. C., Hall, P. & Balslev, H. (2004). Diversity and dominance in palm (Arecaceae) communities in terra firme forests in the western Amazon basin. *Journal of Ecology*, **92**, 577–588.

Warwick, R. M. & Clarke, K. R. (2001). Practical measures of marine biodiversity based on relatedness of species. *Oceanography and Marine Biology*, **39**, 207–231.

Watterson, G. A. (1974). Models for the logarithmic species abundance distributions. *Theoretical Population Biology*, **6**, 217–250.

Webb, C. O. (2000). Exploring the phylogenetic structure of ecological communities: an example for rain forest trees. *American Naturalist*, **156**, 145–155.

Webb, C. O. & Donoghue, M. J. (2004). Phylomatic: tree retrieval for applied phylogenetics. *Molecular Ecology Notes*, **5**, 181–183.

Webb, C. O. & Pitman N. C. A. (2002). Phylogenetic balance and ecological evenness. *Systematic Biology*, **51**, 898–907.

Webb, C. O., Ackerly, D. D., McPeek, M. A. & Donoghue, M. J. (2002). Phylogenies and community ecology. *Annual Review of Ecology and Systematics*, **33**, 475–505.

Whittaker, R. H. (1972). Evolution and measurement of species diversity. *Taxon*, **21**, 213–251.

Wikström, N., Savolainen, V. & Chase, M. W. (2001). Evolution of the angiosperms: calibrating the family tree. *Proceedings of the Royal Society of London, Series B*, **268**, 2211–2220.

Wright, S. (1931). Evolution in Mendelian populations. *Genetics*, **16**, 97–159.

Yule, G. U. (1925). A mathematical theory of evolution based on the conclusions of Dr J. C. Willis. *Philosophical Transactions of the Royal Society of London, Series B*, **213**, 21–87.

# CHAPTER NINE

# On the quantification of local variation in biodiversity scaling using wavelets

TIMOTHY H. KEITT

*University of Texas at Austin*

## Introduction

It is obvious to even the most casual naturalist that community composition varies through space and that this variation is related in some way to environmental gradients. Yet the problem of understanding in detail patterns of species turnover in space remains a difficult and unsolved challenge in spatial ecology. How do we relate spatial turnover in community composition to the underlying biological processes regulating the origin and maintenance of biological diversity in landscapes? The basic components are simple. If each species is restricted to a unique set of preferred environmental conditions and the environment varies spatially, then in a deterministic world, spatial variation in community composition simply reflects environmental variation. If rates of environmental change are constant, we should find a highly regular and simple pattern of species turnover. The complicating factors are of course ecology, history and variation in the "texture" of the physical environment. Species unable to track a temporally changing environment will be present in suboptimal conditions and missing from the preferred environment (Vetaas, 2002). The vagaries of extinction-recolonization dynamics imply that some fraction of species which could occur in some particular local environment will be missing solely for historical reasons (Hanski & Gyllenberg, 1997). Species may also be absent from preferred habitats because of competitive exclusion or absence of an obligate mutualist (Caley & Schluter, 1997). Further complicating the picture are lags in species responses to changing conditions simply owing to long life span or because of the length of time required for indirect ecological interactions to propagate through a community (Ives, 1995). In addition, rates of environmental change are highly variable through space and so we may predict that patterns of species turnover also are highly variable. We are led logically to the somewhat uncomfortable conclusion that spatial patterns in biodiversity depend strongly on conditions unique to particular locations. How then can we understand the pattern without being overwhelmed by its inherent complexity?

Community ecologists seem to have approached this question from two opposite ends of a spectrum. A long tradition in ecology has been content to

*Scaling Biodiversity*, ed. David Storch, Pablo A. Marquet and James H. Brown. Published by Cambridge University Press. © Cambridge University Press 2007.

document the enormous variation in communities, fortunately so, as we would have few data to debate were it not for the dedicated efforts of field ecologists. At the other extreme, ecologists have attempted to characterize spatial turnover with a single number, the exponent of a power law relating number of species to sample area. Species–area analysis makes considerable sense in the context of island biogeography where analysis is constrained to species lists from islands of different size (MacArthur & Wilson, 1967). Ocean waters buffer island climate resulting in reduced local environmental variation and the separation of islands means they can reasonably be treated as point samples. Both properties lend themselves to species–area analysis. Application of species–area analysis to regional- to continental-scale landscapes seems far less appropriate, despite heroic efforts to predict the species–area exponent from paired island-like samples embedded in the larger landscape (Harte, Kinzig & Green, 1999). The difficulty is that for reasons stated above, rates of species turnover are likely to be highly variable from location to location, implying that a considerable amount of information is lost by taking a global average of this behavior. A far more compelling approach is to embrace this variation and attempt to explain the pattern in terms of local environmental contexts and the general principles of habitat selection (Pulliam & Danielson, 1991) and isolation-by-distance effects (Slatkin, 1993) that generate and redistribute biodiversity on the landscape. Allowing for localized variation also avoids a tautological conclusion (Klvana, Berteaux & Cazelles, 2004): if scaling patterns are invariant, we can have greater confidence if scale invariance is not a fundamental assumption as is the case when assuming a power-law form of the species–area relationship.

As an initial step towards a functional understanding of biodiversity scaling, it is desirable to identify methods that can capture local variation in species turnover without overwhelming the analyst with the full detail of the raw data. We present here a method of quantifying local turnover in community composition at multiple scales based on the wavelet transform (Daubechies, 1992). The wavelet transform arose in the context of signal processing and was designed precisely to optimize the trade-off between estimating global patterns and adapting to local variation (Mallat, 1999). Wavelets achieve this optimum by measuring local fluctuations in increasingly coarse-grained or locally averaged representations of the original signal (Walker, 1999). In this sense, wavelets are similar to block-quadrat methods developed in vegetation science (Dale, 1999) (see also Gaston et al., this volume). However, unlike more heuristic methods, concepts of pattern and scale have precise mathematical definitions within the wavelet framework facilitating interpretation of results and comparisons among systems. In the remainder of this chapter, we briefly describe the wavelet transform and construct a measure of scale-dependent community dissimilarity in the wavelet domain. We then apply this method to spatial turnover in breeding bird community composition within the State of Texas, USA.

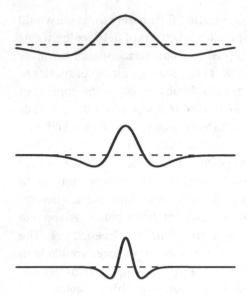

**Figure 9.1** The Difference-of-Gaussians wavelet at three different scales. The narrower wavelets extract fine-scale information, whereas the wider wavelets extract broad-scale information.

## Wavelets

Wavelets (Daubechies, 1992) were used to extract scale-specific information from the bird community data. Wavelets like the Fourier transform and other harmonic methods allow one to isolate variation at specific frequencies in data. One can imagine the pitch controls on a high fidelity stereo system. If we wish to hear only the low-frequency sounds we turn up the bass and turn down the midrange and treble controls. Wavelets operate in a similar manner – by tuning the width of a chosen wavelet (see Fig. 9.1), we can isolate and analyze separately low-frequency, midrange or high-frequency components of a signal. The Fourier transform is ideal when analyzing a pure stationary sinusoidal signal, such as that produced when a single note is played on a piano, because sine and cosine functions form the basis of the Fourier transform. For signals that have sharp transients – e.g. the sound wave produced by a snare drum – or where the dominant frequency changes over time, the Fourier transform is not ideal because it requires a complex superposition of sine and cosine function such that they cancel in precisely the right way to capture the transient nature of the signal. The interference between sines and cosines fitted to different parts of the signal leads to a large number of extraneous values being returned from the transform. For transient nonstationary patterns, the wavelet transform is preferred because wavelets rapidly decay to zero at longer distances and can thus capture localized behavior without interfering with other wavelets applied to the signal at other points in time or space.

Wavelets come in a wide variety of shapes, some more suited to capturing transient behavior and others more suitable for extracting regular oscillations.

Wavelets can further be classified as either continuous or discrete. For this study, the two-dimensional continuous wavelet transform (Antoine, 1999) was used, defined mathematically by

$$(T^{wav}f)(a,b,s) = \frac{1}{h(s)} \int\limits_{-\infty}^{+\infty}\int\limits_{-\infty}^{+\infty} \psi\left(\frac{x-a}{s},\frac{y-b}{s}\right)f(x,y)\mathrm{d}x\mathrm{d}y,$$

(9.1)

where $f(x,y)$ represents the spatial pattern of interest and $\psi\left(\frac{x-a}{s},\frac{y-b}{s}\right)$ is a wavelet with width $s$ centered at $a,b$. The function $h(s)$ is a normalization that standardizes the variance of the transform across scales. The dominant scale of analysis is governed by the scale parameter $s$. For the wavelet used in this study, patterns repeating every $s$ distance units were highlighted by the transform. Variation at scales much larger or smaller than $s$ distance units was suppressed by the wavelet filter. We used an adaptive "Difference-of-Gaussians" (DoG) wavelet (Fig. 9.1). Further details are given in the Appendix.

## Community dissimilarity in the wavelet domain

Wavelet-based Euclidean distances were used to examine changes in community composition as a function of scale within localized contexts. Given lists of species abundances from two sample areas, recall that the Euclidean distance between the samples is simply the root sum of squared differences in abundance computed species by species. The DoG wavelet used for analysis (see Appendix) was computed by taking the difference between two nested samples, one with a narrow radius and another with a broader radius, both centered on the point of interest. Let $f_i(x, y)$ be the density of the $i$th species selected from a pool of $N$ species, then

$$D_{a,b}^{wav}(s) = \sqrt{\sum_{i=1}^{N}[(T^{wav}f_i)(a,b,s)]^2}$$

(9.2)

is "wavelet dissimilarity" computed as the Euclidean distance between the nested samples centered at $a,b$ and highlights community turnover occurring over $s$ distance units (Fig. 9.2).

This measure of community dissimilarity is similar to other methods of measuring beta diversity across scales. An alternative approach, used by for example Condit et al. (2002), would be to plot spatial separation between samples versus a measure of distance between community composition and then examine the decay of similarity (or increase of dissimilarity) as a function of increasing spatial separation between samples. In this case, the pairwise differences are accumulated and then averaged within distance bins or fit directly from theory or regression. The power of this approach is in modeling the specific form of the decay curve. What is different is that community similarity is always computed at the sample plot level – the relationship between distance

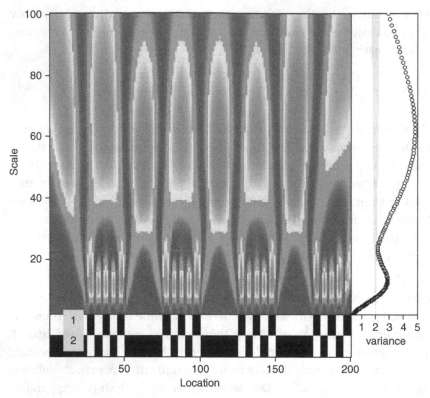

**Figure 9.2** Illustration of wavelet dissimilarity applied to simulated data. The 10 species were divided into two communities labeled 1 and 2. The communities alternate along a linear transect according to the black and white sequences at the bottom with white indicating the presence of that community and black the absence. The color plot shows the output of the wavelet transform with blue indicating small values of community dissimilarity and red colors indicating large values. The average behavior is shown to the right as a function of scale. (For color version see Plate 3.)

and similarity is modeled in a second step, typically by averaging within small distance bins. Using wavelets, the averaging and differencing steps are combined into a single operation. To increase scale, the wavelet smoothly averages community composition over increasing regions and then computes differences between these increasingly larger average species pools. The result of computing differences on spatially averaged data is that the measure is quite stable, even at a single location, thus allowing one to look at community turnover as a function of scale at a particular location. With species–area and similarity-by-distance methods, results are generally averaged across the entire landscape. The wavelet method is not unlike breaking a sample transect into increasingly larger blocks and then computing differences between pooled communities in neighboring blocks (so called "block-quadrat" methods in plant ecology). Dale

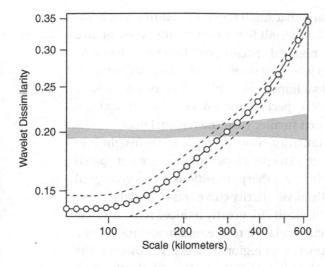

**Figure 9.3** Community turnover in BBS data measured at different scales using wavelets. The shaded area bounds 95% of 1000 bootstrap randomizations of the data. Open circles are the spatial average of dissimilarity computed at each route. Dotted lines are ±1 standard error.

(1999) has pointed out that this procedure is essentially a Haar wavelet transform and so is conceptually aligned to the method applied here. However, the Haar wavelet has certain undesirable properties, particularly in the case of irregular spatial sampling (Daubechies, 1992), hence our preference for the less abrupt DoG wavelet. A further advantage we see of the wavelet method is the natural interpretation of linear regression models on wavelet transformed data (Keitt & Urban, 2005) which would allow, for example, one to test the relationship between spatial turnover in environmental data and spatial turnover in species composition.

## Application to community data

Data from the North American Breeding Bird Survey (BBS) were used to study spatial variation in community turnover. The BBS is a census spanning much of North America conducted each spring and was designed to track changes in population sizes of breeding bird species. Once per year, trained observers take point counts at regular intervals along 39-km sampling "routes". Data analyzed here are route totals for each species and locations given are for the route midpoints. Additional details can be found in Peterjohn and Sauer (1993). The full BBS data set was subsetted to include only those routes falling within the State of Texas, USA.

Spatially averaged results of the wavelet dissimilarity analysis are shown (on logarithmic scales) in Fig. 9.3. The pattern of wavelet dissimilarity deviated strongly from a null model where route totals for each species were randomly assigned to route locations. Average dissimilarity was much less than for the null model at scales below 300 km, indicating greatly reduced species turnover at these scales. The likely explanation is that small regions constitute much less environmental variability and therefore permit fewer community types relative to a purely random sampling of the regional species pool. However, the direction of causality is not necessarily clear. If species distributions are strongly clustered, perhaps because of dispersal limitation or other factors unrelated to environmental turnover, then one still expects to see reduced community turnover as local species pools will be much smaller than the regional pool.

Fortunately, the slope of the dissimilarity curve provides some insight into potential processes regulating diversity. Steeper slopes indicate greater spatial patterning and changes in slope can indicate sharp transitions across ecological boundaries. Notice that the slope of the dissimilarity curve was essentially flat at the finest scales analyzed (50–100 km), albeit still greatly reduced relative to the null model. Again, the overall reduction relative to the null model indicates a sharply reduced local species pool relative to regional diversity. However, the flat slope, paralleling the null model, indicates little or no spatial pattern in community composition across the landscape at the finest scales. This could result from spatially uncorrelated observer errors obscuring the pattern of community turnover, or could result from localized random dispersal events that effectively blur community boundaries. Above 100 km in scale, the curve begins to slope upward, indicating greater patterning and the emergence of distinct community types.

At scales greater than 300 km, dissimilarity greatly exceeds that of the null model. This is likely the result of broad environmental gradients, such as moisture availability and temperature, that are well-known features of the Texas climate. There also appears to be a slight increase in the slope of the dissimilarity curve around 400 km in scale. This is the scale at which one begins to cross a major divide between a wetter, forested east Texas and a dry desert west Texas.

We assessed spatial variation in biodiversity scaling by computing a local community dissimilarity exponent. This was done by computing the median of $\Delta \log D_{a,b}^{\mathrm{wav}}(s)/\Delta \log s$ across 25 scale increments spaced between the minimum and maximum scales analyzed. (Note that smaller exponents should generally correspond to larger species–area exponents, although the relationship is not exact.) These results are plotted in Fig. 9.4. A wide range of scaling exponents was observed, suggesting considerable local variation in biodiversity scaling. No strong spatial patterning was apparent. There did appear to be a band of higher exponents running from the eastern border through central Texas towards the Big Bend region in lower west Texas; however, the pattern is not sufficiently robust to warrant further interpretation. More important appears to be the local variation in dissimilarity scaling. A thorough understanding of the local variation would require detailed environmental data and likely field studies and is beyond the scope of this chapter.

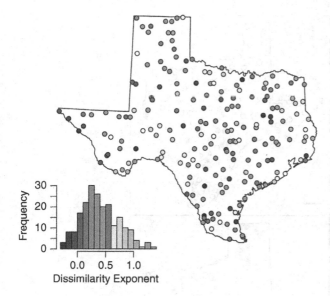

**Figure 9.4** Spatial variation in biodiversity scaling across the Texas BBS data set. The inset shows a frequency histogram of values. (For color version see Plate 4.)

Somewhat more insight can be obtained through examination of the pattern of turnover "hot spots" (locations with significantly greater dissimilarity in comparison with the null model at a particular scale) and "cold spots" (locations with significantly reduced dissimilarity in comparison with the null model at a particular scale). These results are plotted in Fig. 9.5.

At the finer scales (75 km–150 km), many routes showed significantly less turnover than the randomized null model ($\alpha = 0.05$). Three areas did, however, show up as turnover hot spots with larger wavelet dissimilarity values than expected at random. One of the hot spots includes several routes in east Texas located just south and east from Dallas, a major metropolitan area. It is difficult to ascertain why these routes are hot spots without field data. However, one can speculate that these routes have been engulfed by suburban sprawl since their initiation and are now sampling a large pool of invasive bird species, such as European Starling (*Sturnus vulgarus*) and House Sparrow (*Passer domesticus*), not present in neighboring survey routes.

Another area includes several routes in the southern panhandle region (northwest quadrant) located between the cities of Midland-Odessa and Lubbock. Again, it seems likely that this is an anthropogenic hot spot driven by extensive irrigation for agriculture. (Green irrigation circles are readily apparent in satellite pictures of this area available at http://maps.google.com/.) The high productivity, increased humidity and anthropogenic disturbance in this area must contrast sharply with neighboring semidesert habitats, possibly leading to high rates of species turnover.

Another hot spot occurred in southern Texas along the Mexican border. This area is well known to ornithologists as a region of high species diversity and rapid

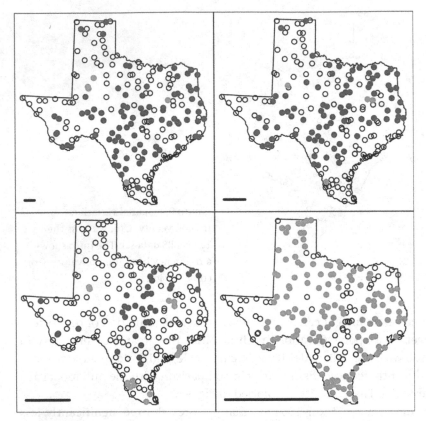

**Figure 9.5** Hot and cold spots for community dissimilarity plotted at four scales. Open circles correspond to BBS routes that were not significantly different from the result of 1000 bootstrap randomizations of the data. Blue-filled circles showed significantly ($\alpha = 0.05$) less turnover at that scale and red-filled circles significantly more. The horizontal bar at the lower left of each panel indicates the scale of analysis. (For color version see Plate 5.)

community turnover. A large number of bird species whose primary affinities are tropical reach their northern range limit along lower Rio Grande valley. There is a rapid transition as one moves northward to a more temperate bird fauna and this likely accounts for the high wavelet dissimilarity indices in this region.

At the largest scales (>600 km) most routes showed significantly higher turnover than expected at random. At these distances, local environments range from subtropical to temperate grasslands and from southeastern pine forests to southwestern deserts. It is thus unsurprising that species turnover is quite large at these scales.

## Discussion
The current results illustrate the applicability of wavelets to problems in pattern detection and analysis in biology and environmental sciences. The flexibility of

wavelet methods combined with their ability to represent local variation at different scales makes them ideal for probing complex, spatially and temporally varying patterns, such as patterns of species turnover in landscapes.

Despite the fact that scaling patterns can be powerfully characterized using wavelets (Arneodo, Grasseau & Holschneider, 1988; Muzy, Bacry & Arneodo, 1991, 1993; Ivanov et al., 1996), we did not find strong evidence for a single scaling exponent for the biodiversity data analyzed here. We believe this is the result of the many complex interacting factors that influence community composition and species turnover in space. Our view is that quantification of scaling properties is most useful in cases where the pattern of dynamics may be governed by a small number of key variables. For example, Keitt et al. (2002) examined time-invariant scaling properties of breeding bird populations across North America. They hypothesized that scaling in the data was a consequence of a few simple factors: the size of a species' geographic range and the pattern of subdivision of the range into independently fluctuating subpopulations (see also Marquet et al., this volume). Is such a result likely in community data? We feel it is unlikely. Compositional turnover in communities across space is likely to be determined by a large array of factors, including evolutionary history. Historical isolating barriers and zones of rapid change in the physical environment should generate spatially varying and scale-dependent patterns in diversity. Instead, it may be more fruitful to attempt to understand why beta diversity patterns are nonstationary and why some areas are turnover hot spots and why hot spots appear and disappear at different scales of analysis.

We see a number of interesting avenues for future studies. It would be quite interesting to incorporate environmental covariates into our analysis of community turnover. Keitt and Urban (2005) discuss wavelet transformation of ordinary linear regression models. One could easily add additional layers of information such as temperature, precipitation, etc. and then model the dependence of observed wavelet dissimilarity measures on local rates of environmental changes (also modeled with wavelets). On a more methodological level, we note that the smoothing functions used here (see Appendix) are equivalent to the intercept of a local linear regression (Silverman, 1986). Some bias reduction near boundaries might be achieved using higher-order local linear estimators (Hastie & Loader, 1993), or perhaps even semiparametric smoothers (Ruppert, Wand & Carroll, 2003) could be used to partial out influences of nuisance covariates.

## Acknowledgments

The author acknowledges the kind invitation of the workshop organizers, insights and helpful comments from workshop participants, Keitt Lab members and several anonymous reviewers, and the generous support of the David and Lucile Packard Foundation.

## Appendix 9.1

We implemented an adaptive "second generation" wavelet filter conceptually derived from Sweldens' "lifting scheme" (Sweldens, 1998). Second generation wavelets are built upon the idea that variation at a particular scale can be quantified by fitting increasingly smooth functions to input data and then examining changes in the lack-of-fit between successive smoothers. If the input signal contains a great deal of variation at a particular scale then a smooth function fit to the data at that scale will leave behind a large amount of residual variation. If the input signal is quite smooth at a particular scale, then the smoothing function will give a close fit and little residual variation will remain. The magnitude of the variation not explained by a smooth function fitted at a particular scale therefore estimates the intensity of pattern present in the data at that scale. Because second generation wavelets are built piecewise from locally smooth function, they have the advantage of adapting their shape near sampling gaps and boundaries. As a result, artificial boundary adjustments, such as periodic wrapping of the data, are not needed. Most previous applications have involved the discrete wavelet transform in which the scale of analysis jumps by powers of two at each level of the transform. For our purposes, the continuous wavelet transform is far more informative as the scale of analysis can take any value within the limits imposed by the grain and extent of the data.

Our construction of a second-generation continuous wavelet transform is based on the subtraction of local Gaussian-kernel regression estimators producing an adaptive "Difference-of-Gaussians" wavelet (Muraki, 1995). Let the local smoother centered at $a,b$ take the form

$$\eta_{a,b}^s(x,y) = \frac{k\left(\frac{x-a}{s}, \frac{y-b}{s}\right)}{\sum\limits_{(u,v)\in\Omega} k\left(\frac{u-a}{s}, \frac{v-b}{s}\right)}, \tag{9.3}$$

where $\Omega = \{(u_1, v_1), (u_2, v_2), (u_3, v_3), \ldots (u_n, v_n)\}$ is the set of sampling points and $k(x,y) = e^{-(x^2+y^2)/2}$. We can then define the adaptive wavelet filter

$$\psi_{a,b}^s(x,y) = \eta_{a,b}^s(x,y) - \eta_{a,b}^{\beta s}(x,y), \tag{9.4}$$

where $\beta > 1$. Variance transmitted by the adaptive DoG wavelet at frequencies $\omega_x$, $\omega_y$ is asymptotically given by

$$\left(T^{\text{Fourier}}\,\psi_{a,b}^s\right)(\omega_x, \omega_y) = e^{-s^2\left(\omega_x^2+\omega_y^2\right)/2} - e^{-\beta^2 s^2\left(\omega_x^2+\omega_y^2\right)/2}, \tag{9.5}$$

which has a maximum at

$$\omega_x^2 + \omega_y^2 = \frac{4\ln\beta}{s^2(\beta^2 - 1)}. \tag{9.6}$$

For convenience, we chose $\beta = 1.87$ such that the maximum frequency solution was reduced to $\omega_x^2 + \omega_y^2 = s^{-2}$. The result was that for any scaling $x, y \rightarrow (x, y)/s$, the dominant scale of analysis was $s$ distance units.

We can then define the adaptive wavelet transform as

$$(T^{wav}f)(a, b, s) = \frac{1}{h_{a,b}(s)} \sum_{(u,v) \in \Omega} \psi_{a,b}^s(u, v) f(u, v),$$ (9.7)

where

$$h_{a,b}(s) = \sqrt{\sum_{(u,v) \in} \left[ \psi_{a,b}^s(u, v) \right]^2}$$ (9.8)

ensures that wavelet variances are comparable across all locations and scales.

For statistical analysis, species counts were randomly assigned to route locations in repeated Monte Carlo trials. The wavelet transform and any subsequent statistics based on the wavelet coefficients were computed for each trial. Confidence regions were constructed to bound 95% of the Monte Carlo results falling closest to the median of the bootstrap ensemble. Observed values falling outside the confidence region were deemed statistically significant.

## References

Antoine, J. P. (1999). The 2-D wavelet transform, physical applications and generalizations. In *Wavelets in Physics*, ed. J. C. Van den Berg, chapter 2, pp. 23–32. Cambridge: Cambridge University Press.

Arneodo, A., Grasseau, G. & Holschneider, M. (1988). Wavelet transform of multifractals. *Physical Review Letters*, **61**, 2281–2284.

Caley, M. J. & Schluter, D. (1997). The relationship between local and regional diversity. *Ecology*, **78**, 70–80.

Condit, R., Pitman, N., Leigh Jr., E. G., *et al.* (2002). Beta-diversity in tropical forest trees. *Science*, **295**, 666–669.

Dale, M. R. T. (1999). *Spatial Pattern Analysis in Plant Ecology*. Cambridge: Cambridge University Press.

Daubechies, I. (1992). *Ten Lectures On Wavelets*. CBMS-NSF Regional Conference Series in Applied Mathematics. Philadelphia: Society for Industrial and Applied Mathematics.

Hanski, I. & Gyllenberg, M. (1997). Uniting two general patterns in the distribution of species. *Science*, **275**, 397–400.

Harte, J., Kinzig, A. & Green, J. (1999). Selfsimilarity in the distribution and abundance of species. *Science*, **284**, 334–336.

Hastie, T. & Loader, C. (1993). Local regression: automatic kernel carpentry. *Statistical Science*, **8**, 120–129.

Ivanov, P. C., Rosenblum, M. G., Peng, C. K., *et al.* (1996). Scaling behavior of heartbeat intervals obtained by wavelet-based time-series analysis. *Nature*, **383**, 323–327.

Ives, A. R. (1995). Predicting the response of populations to environmental change. *Ecology*, **76**, 926–941.

Keitt, T. H. & Urban, D. L. (2005). Scale-specific inference using wavelets. *Ecology*, **86**, 2497–2504.

Keitt, T. H., Amaral, L. A. N., Buldyrev, S. V. & Stanley, H. E. (2002). Scaling in the growth of geographically subdivided populations: invariant patterns from a continent-wide biological survey. *Philosophical Transactions of the Royal Society of London, Series B*, **357**, 627–633.

Klvana, I., Berteaux, D. & Cazelles, B. (2004). Porcupine feeding scars and climatic data show ecosystem effects of solar cycle. *American Naturalist*, **164**, 283–297.

MacArthur, R. H. & Wilson, E. O. (1967). *Island Biogeography*. Princeton: Princeton University Press.

Mallat, S. (1999). *A Wavelet Tour of Signal Processing*, 2nd edn. New York: Academic Press.

Muraki, S. (1995). Multiscale volume representation by a DOG wavelet. *IEEE Transactions on Visualization and Computer Graphics*, **1**, 109–116.

Muzy, J. F., Bacry, E. & Arneodo, A. (1991). Wavelets and multifractal formalism for singular signals: application to turbulence data. *Physical Review Letters*, **67**, 3515–3518.

Muzy, J. F., Bacry, E. & Arneodo, A. (1993). Multifractal formalism for fractal signals: the structure-function approach versus the wavelet-transform modulus-maxima method. *Physical Review E*, **47**, 875–884.

Peterjohn, B. G. & Sauer, J. R. (1993). North American breeding bird survey annual summary 1990–1991. *Bird Populations*, **1**, 1–15.

Pulliam, H. R. & Danielson, B. J. (1991). Sources, sinks, and habitat selection: a landscape perspective on population dynamics. *American Naturalist*, **137**, S50–S60.

Ruppert, D., Wand, M. P. & Carroll, R. J. (2003). *Semiparametric Regression*. Cambridge Series in Statistical and Probabilistic Mathematics. Cambridge: Cambridge University Press.

Silverman, B. W. (1986). *Density Estimation for Statistics and Data Analysis*. London: Chapman and Hall.

Slatkin, M. (1993). Isolation by distance in equilibrium and non-equilibrium populations. *Evolution*, **47**, 264–279.

Sweldens, W. (1998). The lifting scheme: a construction of second generation wavelets. *SIAM Journal on Mathematical Analysis*, **29**, 511–546.

Vetaas, O. R. (2002). Realized and potential climate niches: a comparison of four rhododendron tree species. *Journal of Biogeography*, **29**, 545–554.

Walker, J. S. (1999). *A Primer on Wavelets and Their Scientific Applications*. New York: Chapman and Hall.

CHAPTER TEN

# The scaling of spatial turnover: pruning the thicket

KEVIN J. GASTON
*University of Sheffield*
KARL L. EVANS
*University of Sheffield*
JACK J. LENNON
*The Macaulay Institute, Aberdeen*

## Introduction

The level and pattern of spatial variation in the similarity (or dissimilarity) in composition of local or regional species assemblages is striking. Some pairs of areas have similar levels of richness but share no individual species in common (e.g. some local assemblages existing under similar environmental conditions on different continents), others have markedly different levels of richness but all the species in the less speciose area also occur in the other (e.g. some habitat patch or island systems), and there are all shades of patterns in between.

Such spatial turnover in species identities, or beta diversity (we will use the two terms interchangeably), lies at the heart of many important ecological issues and phenomena, including the magnitude of regional and global diversities, the determinants of those diversities, likely biotic responses to climate change, and the design of protected area networks (Cody, 1986; Magurran, 1988, 2004; Harrison, Ross & Lawton, 1992; Harrison, 1993; Oliver, Beattie & York, 1998; Groves, 2003; Koleff, Gaston & Lennon, 2003a). And yet, historically, spatial turnover has received notably less attention than has spatial variation in raw species numbers (i.e. species richness). Even then, most of that attention has been in the less direct terms of local–regional richness relationships (plots of the numbers of species in a locality versus the numbers in the region in which that locality is embedded; e.g. Cornell & Lawton, 1992; Caley & Schluter, 1997; Bini *et al.*, 2000), species–area relationships (SARs; e.g. Connor & McCoy, 1979; Rosenzweig, 1995; Crawley & Harral, 2001; Stevens & Willig, 2002; Diniz-Filho, Rangel & Hawkins, 2004), and nested-subset analyses (explorations of the extent to which less speciose assemblages are composed of subsets of the species occurring in more speciose assemblages; e.g. Wright & Reeves, 1992; Worthen, 1996).

This relative paucity of attention is changing, however, with a dramatic resurgence of interest in spatial turnover and beta diversity per se since the

*Scaling Biodiversity*, ed. David Storch, Pablo A. Marquet and James H. Brown. Published by Cambridge University Press. © Cambridge University Press 2007.

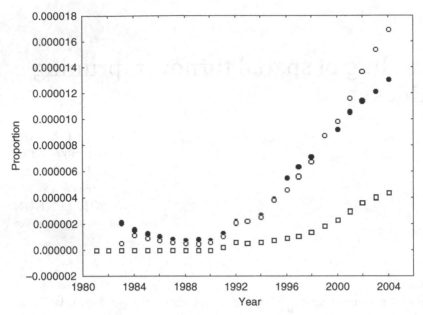

**Figure 10.1** Temporal trends in the proportions of science papers listed on ISI Web of Science that include in their title, keywords or abstract the terms alpha diversity (closed circles), beta diversity (open circles), and/or gamma diversity (open squares) (data for 2004, as of April 9, 2004). Note that whereas numerous publications addressing issues of local and regional diversity do not include the terms alpha diversity or gamma diversity, respectively, in their title, keywords or abstract, and hence are markedly underestimated here, this tends not to be true of publications concerned with beta diversity.

early 1990s (Fig. 10.1). This has included reappraisals of the measurement of beta diversity, the development of new theory to predict its patterns, and a stream of recent empirical papers that directly or indirectly test those predictions (see literature cited below). In this chapter, we provide an overview of the present understanding of selected issues in the scaling of spatial turnover, a topic central to a firm understanding of beta diversity in general, and particularly with regard to scaling with spatial grain, species richness, distance and environmental variation. We place emphasis on definitions and approaches to the measurement of spatial turnover, and predicted and observed patterns in that turnover. In so doing, we seek to make some sense of what Rosenzweig (1995, p. 33) then saw for beta diversity as "only a growing thicket of observations", and what Lawton (2000, p. 407) observed to be "no progress in untangling and discovering useful rules and generalizations about what determines its magnitude".

Throughout, we concentrate on the more traditional and widely used approaches to thinking about spatial turnover and beta diversity, based on the presence/absence of species across areas. We largely ignore those based on ordination and those that address issues of variation in abundance (e.g. Økland, Eliertsen & Økland, 1990; Plotkin & Muller-Landau, 2002; Williams, Marsh & Winter, 2002; Pélissier *et al.*, 2003; Chao *et al.*, 2005). Whereas ultimately the incorporation of abundance is vital, at present, particularly at larger geographic scales, there is vastly more information available about where species occur than about the numbers in which they do so.

## Definitions and approaches

Much confusion has surrounded the literature on spatial turnover. Foremost, this is because of a marked lack of consistency in the use of this term and that of beta diversity (for discussion see Vellend, 2001; Whittaker, Willis & Field, 2001; Koleff *et al.*, 2003a; Novotny & Weiblen, 2005). Some of this confusion has centered on the spatial scales at which the concept is intended to pertain (for discussion see Whittaker, 1972; Cody, 1975, 1993; Whittaker *et al.*, 2001; Koleff & Gaston, 2002). However, we take the view that spatial turnover can be addressed at any spatial scale of interest, although it is obviously necessary to be explicit about that scale (see also Loreau, 2000; Vellend, 2001; Arita & Rodríguez, 2002; Veech *et al.*, 2002); this is consistent with the view that ecologists should abandon circumscribed concepts of local communities (Loreau, 2000; Ricklefs, 2004). Throughout, we distinguish between local and regional scales, with the sole inference that the former is smaller (at a finer resolution) than the latter. Of greater concern is the variety of ways that have been employed purportedly to measure spatial turnover, which reveals a fundamental lack of agreement as to the nature of this property. Here, we focus on three different approaches to measuring beta diversity, and some of the connections to local–regional richness relationships and SARs (the two of which themselves are related).

### Whittaker's beta

The earliest, and consistently the most commonly employed, measure of beta diversity is that of Whittaker (1960, 1972), who expressed this as the proportion by which the species richness of a region exceeds the average richness of a single locality within that region:

$$\beta_w - \frac{S}{\bar{s}_i},\tag{10.1}$$

where $S$ is the overall number of species across all of the local areas being considered (gamma diversity) and $s_i$ is the number of species in local area $i$ (alpha diversity). Whittaker presented this measure both without Eq. (10.1) and with a '$-1$' correction ($\beta_w = \frac{S}{\bar{s}_i} - 1$), which simply rescales the index. One or other version, often alongside other measures, has continued to be employed in many recent empirical studies (e.g. Weiher & Boylen, 1994; Blackburn &

Gaston, 1996; Griffiths, 1997; Davis, Scholtz & Chown, 1999; Clarke & Lidgard, 2000; Ellingsen, 2001; Felfili & Felfili, 2001; Moreno & Halffter, 2001; Ellingsen & Gray, 2002; Lorance, Souissi & Uiblein, 2002).

Bivariate plots of local versus regional species richness (typically with local richness as the dependent variable) have become a popular tool for exploring the structuring of species assemblages (e.g. Ricklefs, 1987; Cornell & Lawton, 1992; Caley & Schluter, 1997; Srivastava, 1999; Cornell, 1999), although their use for this purpose may in some cases have been overly simplistic (Srivastava, 1999; Hillebrand & Blenckner, 2002; Mouquet *et al*., 2003; He *et al*., 2005). Here, a constant slope with an intercept of zero on untransformed axes implies a proportional sampling of regional richness by local areas and identical values of $\beta_w$ for all local–regional pairs (the slope should be $\frac{1}{1+\beta_w}$, after the '−1' correction to $\beta_w$), while a saturating (curvilinear) relationship implies an increase in $\beta_w$ with increasing regional richness (Srivastava, 1999; Arita & Rodríguez, 2002).

The fundamental components of spatial turnover are the matching/mis-matching components $a$, $b$ and $c$, where (i) $a$ is the total number of species shared by two areas; (ii) $b$ is the number of species present in the other area but not in the focal one, and (iii) $c$ is the number of species present in the focal area but absent from the other one. The $a$ component is thus the species in common for a pair of areas (we term this continuity), while the $b$ component measures species gain and the $c$ component species loss relative to the focal area.

For a pairwise comparison of areas, the basic unit of the vast majority of analyses of spatial turnover, $\beta_w$ can be re-expressed as

$$\beta_w = \frac{a+b+c}{(2a+b+c)/2} - 1. \tag{10.2}$$

If there is a large difference in the richness between areas, then $\beta_w$ will clearly tend to be large.

Viewed another way, and ignoring for a moment the '−1' correction, $\beta_w$ is the ratio of the overall number of areas considered to the number of those areas occupied on average by a species (Routledge, 1977; Schluter & Ricklefs, 1993; Leitner & Rosenzweig, 1997; Vellend, 2001; Arita & Rodríguez, 2002), or the reciprocal of the average proportion of the overall number of areas occupied by a species (Rodríguez & Arita, 2004), such that for a pair of areas

$$\beta_w = \frac{2}{(2a+b+c)/(a+b+c)}. \tag{10.3}$$

If species richness can be characterized by a power-function SAR (Arhennius, 1921) with constant slope and intercept, when areas are physically nested there is a direct link between $\beta_w$ and that slope, such that species turnover is invariant between areas differing in size by a constant proportion (Arita & Rodríguez, 2002). Thus, if

$$s = CA^z$$ (10.4)

and

$$S = C(2A)^z,$$ (10.5)

where $S$ is the number of species in an area comprised of two subareas each containing $s$ species in an area of size $A$ (i.e. the SAR is perfect), and $z$ is the slope of the power-function SAR and $C$ the intercept, then

$$\frac{S}{s} = \frac{C2^z A^z}{CA^z} = 2^z$$ (10.6)

and, following from Eq. (10.1),

$$z = \frac{\log(\beta_w)}{\log 2}.$$ (10.7)

This reflects the link between the average occupancy of areas by species and both the SAR (Leitner & Rosenzweig, 1997; Ney-Nifle & Mangel, 1999; Storch, Šizling & Gaston, this volume) and $\beta_w$. Inserting Eq. (10.3) into (10.7) and rearranging, gives

$$z = 1 - \frac{\log((2a+b+c)/(a+b+c))}{\log 2}$$ (10.8)

(Koleff et al., 2003a). This emphasizes why, unless further assumptions are made (see below), the SAR is rather uninformative about the details of spatial turnover. It says nothing about the relative pattern of gains and losses, only about the net change in species numbers. Likewise, on average

$$b \text{ or } c = (1 - 2^{-z})S$$ (10.9)

and

$$a = (2(2^{-z}) - 1)S$$ (10.10)

(Harte & Kinzig, 1997).

In practice, $z$ often changes with spatial scale (size of area), generating a triphasic species–area relationship as one proceeds from local to global scales, although the exact pattern of scale dependence is debated (Palmer & White, 1994; Rosenzweig, 1995; Crawley & Harral, 2001; Hubbell, 2001; Palmer, this volume).

Since Whittaker's (1960, 1972) original suggestion that beta diversity should be measured as the ratio of the species richness of a region to the average richness of a single locality within that region, numerous measures have been proposed that constitute, often rather important, variations on this theme (Table 10.1; for recent reviews see Koleff et al., 2003a; Magurran, 2004). Indeed, a formidable array of ways of combining the matching components $a$, $b$ and $c$ have been employed to measure beta diversity (Table 10.1). Inevitably, many of these capture different facets of spatial turnover and exhibit different properties. This has led to much confusion as different measures

Table 10.1 *Measures of species spatial turnover*

The expressions in terms of matching components are based principally on Koleff *et al.* (2003a), who provide various caveats on the interpretation of the original sources, and may not reflect the precise form of a measure used in the empirical studies listed. In some cases, these expressions are identical for particular pairs of measures, although this may not be so under other circumstances.

| Abbr. | Expression | Original source | Examples of additional empirical studies |
|---|---|---|---|
| **Measures of continuity and loss** | | | |
| $\beta_{rlb}$ | $\dfrac{a}{a+c}$ | Ruggiero *et al.* (1998) | |
| **Measures of species richness gradients** | | | |
| $\beta_{gl}$ | $\dfrac{2\lvert b-c \rvert}{2a+b+c}$ | Lennon *et al.* (2001) | |
| **Measures of continuity ('broad-sense' turnover)** | | | |
| $\beta_{j}$ | $\dfrac{a}{a+b+c}$ | Jaccard (1912) | Scheiner & Rey-Benayas (1994), Clarke & Lidgard (2000), Rivadeneira *et al.* (2002), McGill & Collins (2003) |
| $\beta_{sor}$ | $\dfrac{2a}{2a+b+c}$ | Dice (1945), Sørenson (1948) | Southwood *et al.* (1979), Poynton & Boycott (1996), Price *et al.* (1999), Plotkin & Muller-Landau (2002) |
| $\beta_{wb}$ | $\dfrac{b+c}{2}$ | Weiher & Boylen (1994) | |
| $\beta_{c}$ | $\dfrac{b+c}{2}$ | Cody (1975) | |
| $\beta_{l}$ | $b+c$ | Allan (1975) | See text |
| $\beta_{cc}$ | $\dfrac{b+c}{a+b+c}$ | Colwell & Coddington (1994) | Ellingsen (2001) |

| Measure | Formula | Reference | |
|---|---|---|---|
| $\beta_g$ | $\dfrac{b+c}{a+b+c}$ | Gaston et al. (2001) | Gaston et al. (2001) |
| $\beta_{sr}$ | $\dfrac{a+b+c}{2a+b+c}$ | Garcillán & Ezcurra (2003) | Schluter & Ricklefs (1993) |
| $\beta_w$ | $\dfrac{a+b+c}{(2a+b+c)/2} - 1$ | See text | Whittaker (1960) |
| $\beta_{-1}$ | $\dfrac{a+b+c}{(2a+b+c)/2} - 1$ | Blackburn & Gaston (1996), Arellano & Halffter (2003) | Harrison et al. (1992) |
| $\beta_{hk}$ | $1 - \dfrac{2a}{2a+b+c}$ | | Harte & Kinzig (1997) |
| $\beta_t$ | $\dfrac{b+c}{2a+b+c}$ | Willig & Sandlin (1991), Mourelle & Ezcurra (1997), Willig & Gannon (1997), Naranjo et al. (1998) | Wilson & Shmida (1984) |
| $\beta_{me}$ | $\dfrac{b+c}{2a+b+c}$ | | Mourelle & Ezcurra (1997) |
| $\beta_m$ | $(2a+b+c)\left(1 - \dfrac{a}{a+b+c}\right)$ | | Magurran (1988) |
| $\beta_z$ | $1 - \dfrac{\log((2a+b+c)/(a+b+c))}{\log 2}$ | | Lennon et al. (2001) |

***Measures of gain and loss ('narrow-sense' turnover)***

| Measure | Formula | Reference |
|---|---|---|
| $\beta_{co}$ | $1 - \dfrac{a(2a+b+c)}{2(a+b)(a+c)}$ | Cody (1993) |
| $\beta_r$ | $\dfrac{(a+b+c)^2}{(a+b+c)^2 - 2bc}$ | Routledge (1977) |
| $\beta_l$ | $\log(2a+b+c) - \left(\dfrac{1}{2a+b+c}\,2a\log 2\right)$ $-\left(\dfrac{1}{2a+b+c}((a+b)\log(a+b) + (a+c)\log(a+c))\right)$ | Routledge (1977) |

(cont.)

**Table 10.1** (*cont.*)

| Abbr. | Expression | Original source | Examples of additional empirical studies |
|---|---|---|---|
| $\beta_e$ | $\exp(\beta_l) - 1$ | Routledge (1977) | |
| $\beta_{rs}$ | $\dfrac{bc + 1}{((a + b + c)^2 - (a + b + c))/2}$ | Williams (1996) | |
| $\beta_{-2}$ | $\dfrac{\min(b, c)}{\max(b, c) + a}$ | Harrison et al. (1992) | Blackburn & Gaston (1996), Clarke & Lidgard (2000) |
| $\beta_{-3}$ | $\dfrac{\min(b, c)}{a + b + c}$ | Harrison et al. (1992) | |
| $\beta_{sim}$ | $\dfrac{\min(b, c)}{\min(b, c) + a}$ | Lennon et al. (2001) | See text |

are frequently a priori predicted to exhibit different spatial patterns, making it difficult if not impossible to compare the outcomes of many published empirical studies.

## Broad-sense and narrow-sense measures

Vellend (2001) argues that $\beta_w$, and many of the measures derived from or related to it, do not truly reflect the concept of spatial turnover, in as much as their values are independent of any spatial or environmental structure in species distributions, and that therefore beta diversity and spatial turnover should not be used interchangeably. Koleff *et al.* (2003a) express a different viewpoint, reflecting a somewhat more generic approach to what constitutes turnover and the difficulty, after such a long history of their frequent synonymous usage, of treating spatial turnover and beta diversity as two distinct issues. Acknowledging that a wide variety of measures can be employed to explore patterns with or without respect to spatial structure and environment (e.g. along gradients), they differentiate between two important groups of measures, which they term "broad-sense" and "narrow-sense" (Table 10.1). By definition, gradients in species numbers produce spatial turnover, in as much as the identities of species present change between two areas. Broad-sense turnover implicitly incorporates differences in composition attributable to such richness gradients, but ignores the relative magnitude of species gains and losses. Whittaker's measure ($\beta_w$) is one example (see Table 10.1 for others). The effect of local richness gradients on $\beta_w$ can be approximated for a pair of areas by subtracting the proportional difference in richness between the two (elsewhere termed $\beta_g$)

$$\beta_g = \frac{a+b+c}{(2a+b+c)/2} - \frac{2|b-c|}{2a+b+c} \tag{10.11}$$

(Lennon *et al.* 2001).

Narrow-sense turnover focuses on the relative magnitude of the species gains and losses, and as such captures the notion that turnover is high when the proportion of species shared between two areas is low and the proportions lost and gained moving from one to the other are similar. To focus on compositional differences, Lennon *et al.* (2001) introduced a narrow sense turnover index, effectively a symmetric form of Simpson's (1943) asymmetric index, which takes the form

$$\beta_{sim} = \frac{1}{n}\sum_{i=1}^{n}\left(1 - \left(\frac{a_i}{a_i + \min(b_i, c_i)}\right)\right), \tag{10.12}$$

where $n$ is the number of pairwise comparisons. For a single pair of areas

$$\beta_{sim} = \frac{\min(b,c)}{\min(b,c)+a} \tag{10.13}$$

Lennon *et al.* (2001) verified that $\beta_{sim}$ is not strongly influenced by local differences in richness, and it was subsequently shown to have a number of other desirable statistical properties and to perform as well as or better than other narrow-sense measures (Koleff *et al.*, 2003a). It has been employed in a variety of empirical studies (Lennon *et al.*, 2001; Koleff & Gaston, 2002; Koleff, Lennon & Gaston, 2003b; Bonn, Storch & Gaston, 2004; van Rensburg *et al.*, 2004).

## Multiplicative and additive partitions

Whittaker's measure of beta diversity and many others that have followed (including $\beta_{sim}$) are multiplicative partitions of diversity, and are dimensionless. Although they also have a long history in the ecological literature, additive partitions of diversity have recently come to the fore when exploring spatial patterns of diversity (Loreau, 2000; Wagner, Wildi & Ewald, 2000; Veech *et al.*, 2002; Crist *et al.*, 2003; Gering, Crist & Veech, 2003; Summerville *et al.*, 2003a, 2003b). Here,

$$\beta_1 = S - \bar{s} \tag{10.14}$$

(Allan, 1975; Lande, 1996; Lande, Engen & Sæther, 2003); Koleff *et al.* (2003a) employed the '1' subscript in acknowledgment of Lande's use of this measure, and we retain the convention here although this measure was proposed much earlier by others. Beta diversity is then expressed in terms of numbers of species, making it possible to calculate the relative contributions to regional species richness both of local species richness and of the turnover in that richness. Here, a local versus regional species richness relationship with a constant slope, passing through the origin on untransformed axes, implies an increase in $\beta_1$ for local–regional pairs with increasing regional richness (for discussion of local–regional relationships and $\beta_1$, see Gering & Crist, 2002).

Again, re-expressing in terms of matching components for a pair of areas

$$\beta_1 = \frac{b + c}{2} \tag{10.15}$$

(Koleff *et al.*, 2003a).

While $\beta_1$ has been termed a measure of beta diversity, it is plainly capturing something rather different from $\beta_w$ and $\beta_{sim}$, and will be highly influenced by local species richness gradients, which generate high values of $b$ and/or $c$. Multiplicative and additive partitions should thus be regarded as complementary rather than competing approaches to understanding patterns of diversity (Veech *et al.*, 2002).

If species richness can be characterized by a semilog SAR (Gleason, 1922) with constant slope and intercept, when areas are physically nested there is a direct link between $\beta_1$ and that slope, such that species turnover is invariant between areas differing in size by a constant proportion. Thus, if

$$s = K + m \log A \tag{10.16}$$

and

$$S = K + m \log 2A, \tag{10.17}$$

where $S$ is the number of species in an area comprised of two subareas each containing $s$ species in an area of size $A$, and $m$ is the slope and $K$ the intercept of the semilog SAR then

$$S - s = K + m \log A + m \log 2 - K - m \log A = m \log 2 \tag{10.18}$$

(Lennon et al., 2001).

## Theory and predictions

Theory to predict the form of patterns in scaling of spatial turnover, however measured, remains remarkably scant. At present there are three principal general frameworks: dispersal limitation, niche limitation and SARs. We consider each of these in turn, focusing particularly on the first two and deriving predictions for these regarding four major issues in the scaling of spatial turnover (Table 10.2). First, we consider the effects of variation in spatial grain, given that spatial turnover in species composition has been evaluated for many different units of study (spatial grain), from a few square meters (e.g. Whittaker, 1960; Routledge, 1977; Wilson & Shmida, 1984; Pharo, Beattie & Binns, 1999) to tens, hundreds and thousands of square kilometers (e.g. Cody, 1986; Willig & Sandlin, 1991; Harrison et al., 1992; Blackburn & Gaston, 1996; Williams, 1996; Poyton & Boycott, 1996; Price, Keeling & O'Callaghan, 1999; Clarke & Lidgard, 2000; Koleff & Gaston, 2001). Second, we address the effects of variation in species richness, with the suggestion having repeatedly been made, particularly in the context of latitudinal gradients in richness, that higher regional species richness is attained through greater local spatial turnover in species identities (e.g. Major, 1988; Stevens, 1989; Gaston & Williams, 1996; Brown & Lomolino, 1998; Willig, Kaufman & Stevens, 2003). The third scaling issue considered is that associated with distance-decay (sensu Nekola & White, 1999) relationships between the spatial distance by which local assemblages are separated and their similarity or dissimilarity of species composition. Finally, we address scaling with what is widely considered to be the fundamental driver of spatial turnover, namely environmental variation.

In the main, we focus on the theoretical predictions made with regard to three measures of beta diversity that capture the three main concepts behind this term: broad-sense turnover ($\beta_w$), narrow-sense turnover ($\beta_{sim}$), and additive partitioning ($\beta_1$).

**Table 10.2** *Predictions of dispersal limitation and niche limitation concerning the change in spatial turnover in species composition with regard to (i) spatial grain of analyses (the sizes of the areas being compared), (ii) variation in species richness, (iii) distance between areas, and (iv) environmental gradients*

| | $\beta$ | Expression | Spatial grain | Species richness | Distance | Environmental gradients |
|---|---|---|---|---|---|---|
| Dispersal limitation | $\beta_w$ | $\dfrac{a+b+c}{(2a+b+c)/2} - 1$ | Decline with coarser grain, and decline greater than for other measures | Any trend possible | Increase with distance | No relationship[a] |
| | $\beta_{sim}$ | $\dfrac{\min(b,c)}{\min(b,c)+a}$ | Decline with coarser grain | Any trend possible | Increase with distance[b] | No relationship[a] |
| | $\beta_l$ | $\dfrac{b+c}{2}$ | Decline with coarser grain | Any trend possible | Increase with distance | No relationship[a] |
| Niche limitation | $\beta_w$ | $\dfrac{a+b+c}{(2a+b+c)/2} - 1$ | Decline with coarser grain, and decline greater than for other measures | Any trend possible | Increase with distance[c] | Increase with environmental difference |
| | $\beta_{sim}$ | $\dfrac{\min(b,c)}{\min(b,c)+a}$ | Decline with coarser grain | Any trend possible | Increase with distance[b,c] | Increase with environmental difference[b] |
| | $\beta_l$ | $\dfrac{b+c}{2}$ | Decline with coarser grain | Any trend possible | Increase with distance[c] | Increase with environmental difference |

[a] Detecting such patterns may be in practice be difficult due to correlations between distance and the magnitude of environmental difference between two sites.

[b] At some distance and degree of environmental difference between two sites there will be no species common to these sites; that is, component a will be zero, and $\beta_w$ and $\beta_{sim}$ will thus remain constant, as will $\beta_l$ if the two sites have equal numbers of species.

[c] Assuming that habitat differences increase with distance, otherwise there should be no relationship.

### Dispersal limitation

At one extreme, the distributions of individual species can be considered to be purely dispersal limited, at the other limited purely by traits that influence the conditions in which they can survive and successfully reproduce (niche limitation). Although both influences doubtless play some role in structuring most assemblages, in considering the patterns in spatial turnover that theory predicts it is useful to contrast these two extremes. In a similar vein, the neutral theory of biodiversity and biogeography, in which species distributions are dispersal limited, has proven valuable in predicting the expected form of many ecological and evolutionary patterns in the absence of niche limitation (Hubbell, 1979, 1997, 2001; Borda-de-Água et al., this volume).

Under dispersal limitation, the distributions of individual species tend to be aggregated. Increasing amounts of aggregation will increase species turnover (Ney-Nifle & Mangel, 1999; Plotkin et al., 2000; Green & Ostling, 2003). This can also be thought of in terms of the relationship between local and regional richness. Assuming that the number of individuals and species in a region is constant, increasing the degree of aggregation will reduce local measures of richness (Veech, Crist & Summerville, 2003), thus reducing the slopes of local–regional richness plots (where local richness is the dependent variable and relationships pass through the origin). This influence of aggregation on turnover aids the development of predictions regarding the nature of patterns in the scaling of species turnover that should arise under dispersal limitation.

*Spatial grain*

Under dispersal limitation, continuity (matching component $a$), will increase with spatial grain as (i) larger areas have more species, and (ii) larger areas reduce the extent to which species distributions are aggregated (i.e. many species occur in many of the areas rather than only in some of them). As grain increases, the second effect may also reduce species gain/loss (matching components $b$ and $c$). All three measures of turnover ($\beta_w$, $\beta_{sim}$ and $\beta_l$) will thus tend to decline with increasing spatial grain. It is likely, however, that the magnitude of change in species continuity with increasing grain will be greater than the number of species gained/lost and this will result in $\beta_{sim}$ being less sensitive to change in spatial grain than $\beta_w$.

*Species richness*

When comparing turnover measures between a focal local assemblage with a species richness that is high, similar, or low compared with that of its neighboring local assemblage, the influence of absolute species richness of the focal assemblage on turnover will depend on the contrasting nature of species distributions between the pair of assemblages. Three main broad scenarios may arise. First, species may form perfectly nested distributions in which all species present in species-poor assemblages are present in richer ones. If the focal assemblage is the more species rich then as species richness of focal areas increases continuity may increase, decrease or remain constant, species gain will always be zero and species loss may be constant, increase or decrease. If the neighboring assemblage is more species rich then continuity will increase, species gain may exhibit any trend or be constant and species loss will be zero. Second, at the other extreme, none of the species present in one assemblage may be present in the other. Regardless of whether the focal area has lower or higher richness than the neighbor then as the richness of the focal area increases continuity will be zero, species gain may increase, decrease or remain constant and species loss will increase. If area pairs contain an equal number of species then under this scenario an increase in focal species richness will give rise to increasing species gain/loss while continuity remains zero. In the third scenario, some species may be present in both assemblages. In this situation, regardless of whether the focal or neighboring area contains more species, as richness of the focal area increases then continuity, species gain and species loss may all remain constant, increase or decrease.

Clearly a multitude of trends in continuity and gain/loss may arise when species richness increases from one focal assemblage to another. Regardless of how species richness changes in relation to focal and neighboring assemblages, if focal richness increases certain combinations of trends in continuity and loss/gain are not possible, i.e. if continuity remains constant or decreases then species loss must increase. However, sufficient plausible combinations remain for $\beta_w$, $\beta_{sim}$ and $\beta_l$ to exhibit increases, decreases or stability while focal species richness increases.

As pure dispersal limitation means that all species have the potential to occur everywhere (having no niche limitation), although they cannot reach many places, perfectly nested species distributions (scenario one) are unlikely to arise. That all species may occur everywhere also restricts the probability that two assemblages will not share any species (scenario two), and although such situations may arise for any one pair of assemblages it is unlikely generally to be true. By default the third scenario, partially nested distributions, is the most likely to arise under dispersal limitation, which thus rather unhelpfully predicts that trends in all three measures of beta diversity ($\beta_l$, $\beta_w$, $\beta_{sim}$) may exhibit any pattern as species richness of the focal area increases.

*Distance*
Because local dispersal creates nonuniform species distributions, the similarity between assemblages will decrease with distance (Bell, 2001; Hubbell, 2001; Chave & Leigh, 2002; Condit *et al.*, 2002). The exact form of such patterns will, however, be particularly sensitive to the pattern of dispersal distances assumed. Regardless, continuity will decrease with distance and thus gain/loss will

increase, leading to $\beta_w$, $\beta_{sim}$ and $\beta_l$ increasing with distance. At some unspecified distance, continuity will become zero and thus $\beta_{sim}$ will remain at unity with further increases in distance.

## Environment

Pure dispersal limitation models assume that species do not exhibit traits that influence their ability to exist in a given habitat type. They thus predict that environmental factors will not exert a direct influence on species turnover. However, in nature environmental factors typically change with distance and the dispersal limitation prediction that turnover changes with distance may thus lead to observations that turnover changes along environmental gradients in a manner that may frequently be indistinguishable from niche-based predictions (Gilbert & Lechowicz, 2004).

## Niche limitation

Predictions about spatial turnover in species composition are most frequently rooted in niche theory (for a recent review of this theory see Chase & Leibold, 2003). This differs critically from disperal limitation in that it assumes that species possess traits that influence the range of biotic and abiotic conditions in which they can survive and successfully reproduce, i.e. different species occur in different environments. It thus assumes that assemblage composition will change along environmental gradients as a result of species-specific differences in evolved adaptive responses.

## Spatial grain

Niche limitation suggests that changing spatial grain is likely to change spatial patterns in beta diversity, in as much as it amounts to changing the scale at which the heterogeneity of the interactions between organisms and their environment is manifested (Loreau, 2000). All else being equal, the level of spatial turnover in composition is expected to decrease as spatial grain becomes coarser and fine-scale heterogeneity is averaged out (e.g. Mac Nally et al., 2004). In terms of matching components, continuity will increase with spatial grain as larger areas have more species and because, all else being equal, pairs of larger areas will have greater similarity in their habitat type than pairs of smaller areas, with the latter effect reducing both species gain and loss at larger grains. Patterns in the scaling of turnover with spatial grain arising from niche limitation thus match those arising from dispersal limitation.

## Species richness

The manner in which spatial turnover scales with species richness under niche limitation depends on which of the aforementioned scenarios regarding the pattern of species distributions are likely to arise. One explanation for spatial variation in species richness is that speciose assemblages contain a greater number of specialist species, while species poor assemblages consist of generalists. Generalists, by definition, can occur everywhere and thus nested species distributions may arise. However, evidence for increasing specialization in speciose assemblages is equivocal (Hillebrand, 2004; Vázquez & Stevens, 2004), and while many studies document some degree of nested species distributions these are rarely, if ever, perfect, and thus under niche limitation scenario one appears unlikely. Niche theory suggests that some species are much more generalist and thus more widespread than others (Gregory & Gaston, 2000); therefore, it is likely that, at least within a given bioregion, most pairs of local assemblages will have some species in common. It thus appears that scenario three, partially nested distributions, is the most likely to arise under niche, as well as dispersal, limitation. Under this scenario species continuity, gain and loss may exhibit a plethora of trends with increasing richness of the focal area (see above) and all three measures of beta diversity ($\beta_w$, $\beta_l$, $\beta_{sim}$) may increase, decrease or remain stable as species richness increases.

### Distance

Niche limitation suggests that species prefer different environments. As, on average, localities that are closer together have more similar habitats than ones further apart, niche limitation predicts that spatial turnover in assemblage composition will increase with distance – although such patterns should not occur if there is no relationship between habitat and distance (Gilbert & Lechowicz, 2004). Assuming that one samples increasingly different habitats as the distance between sites increases then continuity will decrease while species loss or gain will increase with distance and beta diversity will scale with distance in a similar manner under both dispersal limitation and niche limitation.

### Environment

Niche theory predicts that, because species exhibit habitat preferences, as the difference in environmental conditions between two sites increases continuity will decrease and species gain or loss will increase, thus elevating $\beta_w$, $\beta_{sim}$, and $\beta_l$. In addition, turnover estimates will be influenced by variation in mean species occupancy; other things being equal, higher occupancy reduces turnover. Thus, environmental factors that influence occupancy, in addition to the difference between environments, may affect turnover. For example, species population sizes may increase with resource availability (Wright, 1983; Kaspari, Yuan & Alonso, 2003; Evans, Warren & Gaston, 2004; Hurlbert, 2004; but see Srivastava & Lawton, 1998). As population size and range size are frequently positively correlated (Brown, 1984; Gregory & Blackburn, 1995; Gaston, Blackburn & Lawton, 1997; Gaston et al. 2000) the larger populations in resource-rich areas are likely to occupy more of that region, thus elevating mean species occupancy (Bonn *et al.*, 2004; Selmi & Boulinier, 2004; Storch, Šizling & Gaston, this volume). This increase in occupancy may increase the number of species shared between two areas within a region while decreasing species loss or gain and thus decreasing our three measures of beta diversity.

**Power SAR**

Although not an alternative framework to that of dispersal and niche processes, Harte and Kinzig (1997) derive predictions of patterns of spatial turnover based on a power SAR of constant slope (and no significant spatial gradients in species richness). These are framed in terms of a measure of the turnover in composition between two areas

$$\beta_{hk} = 1 - \frac{2a}{2a + b + c} \tag{10.19}$$

(i.e. 1-Sorensen's index), which is

$$\approx 1 - (2 - 2^z)\left(\frac{A}{d^2}\right), \tag{10.20}$$

where the areas are both of size $A$ with centers separated by distance $d$. Here, turnover is predicted to decrease as the surveyed area (spatial grain) increases and increase as the distance between areas increases. Related expressions could be derived for other measures of spatial turnover, and indeed the relationship between the power SAR and $\beta_w$ has already been remarked. Harte *et al.* (1999a) demonstrate how Eq. (10.20) can be expanded to accommodate spatial dependence in $z$, test its predictions using independently derived values for $z$, and also show how, conversely, estimates of turnover can be used to estimate $z$.

Revealing the links between turnover and the power SAR has been important. However, arguably, it is questionable how much per se this teaches about turnover. Where it occurs, the power SAR exists because of the patterns of turnover in species composition, rather than vice versa, and thus the approach has effectively been one of "reverse engineering". If power SARs were determined by self-similarity in the distributions of species this would give a more ultimate explanation of the determinants of spatial turnover, but the question of why species distributions are self-similar would remain. Debate continues around the extent and nature of any such self-similarity and the topic lies beyond the scope of this chapter (for discussion see Harte, Kinzig & Green, 1999b; Lennon, Kunin & Hartley, 2002; Green, Harte & Ostling, 2003; Ulrich & Buszko, 2003; Maddux, 2004; Ostling *et al.*, 2004; Šizling & Storch, 2004; Šizling & Storch, this volume). In addition, it should be noted that power SARs can readily be generated by the neutral model, a dispersal limitation model (Bell, 2001; Hubbell, 2001).

## Synthesis

Spatial grain, species richness, distance and environment are the four axes with which the literature has principally been concerned with scaling in spatial turnover. In some sense, pure dispersal limitation holds one of the axes constant, that of environment. Likewise, the power SAR framework arguably also holds one of the axes constant, in that it assumes an absence of species richness gradients. Although this enables some discrimination, the different theoretical frameworks are remarkably consistent in their qualitative predictions about the scaling of turnover. Differences in the quantitative predictions are difficult to derive, because these depend fundamentally on the particular parameter values assumed for the models.

## Empirical patterns

We now turn to the empirical evidence for predicted patterns in spatial turnover. We first test these predictions using one of the best distributional data sets available, that for breeding birds in Britain. In so doing, we make the first attempt simultaneously to assess diverse aspects of the nature of scaling in species turnover using the same assemblage. Second, we then place the results of these analyses in the context of empirical findings in the wider literature.

In analyzing data for the British avifauna we focus foremost on the three measures of beta diversity highlighted earlier, $\beta_w$, $\beta_{sim}$, and $\beta_l$. We used the summer (breeding) distribution of the avifauna recorded during April to July in 1988–91 in the British Trust for Ornithology/Scottish Ornithologists' Club/Irish Wildbird Conservancy atlas (Gibbons, Reid & Chapman, 1993). These data record species presence/absence at a resolution of $10\,km \times 10\,km$ quadrats on a continuous grid and were collated using an intensive sampling procedure. Therefore, the vast majority of species present in a quadrat are likely to have been recorded and we can in this case largely ignore concerns that undersampling biases turnover (Ricklefs & Lau, 1980; Wolda, 1981; Plotkin & Muller-Landau, 2002). We excluded marine species and many vagrants but retained established introductions and the more regular of the sporadic breeders. Our final data set comprised 196 species. Quadrats that contained less than 50% land were excluded, leaving a total of 2406 quadrats.

We estimated the matching components, measures of beta diversity, and species richness at a series of successively larger quadrat sizes (coarser scales), using a moving-window algorithm: a larger quadrat was positioned centrally over each base $10\,km$ quadrat and the values for each of these quantities determined (see Lennon *et al.*, 2001). The size of the window used increased from $10\,km \times 10\,km$ to $290\,km \times 290\,km$, in steps of $20\,km$, giving 15 data points. For present purposes, we focus foremost on quadrats at the $10\,km$, $30\,km$ and $90\,km$ scales.

For each $10\,km$ quadrat we obtained a variety of environmental data, which were then rescaled to provide data at coarser resolutions. Habitat diversity data were obtained from the land use classification of Fuller, Groom and Jones (1994), which is based on remote sensing. We amalgamated the 25 original land cover types into seven main habitat types (inland water, coastal, moor/heathland/bog, woodland, built, grassland, tilled land) and, for each quadrat, calculated the area covered by each of these. These were then used to calculate habitat diversity indices using the Shannon–Wiener information index (Ludwig & Reynolds, 1988). Mean altitude in each 10 km quadrat was calculated as the average of 400 equally spaced altitudes within the quadrat.

Much theory and empirical evidence suggest that assemblage structure is strongly influenced by environmental energy availability (Hawkins *et al.*, 2003; Evans *et al.*, 2004; Pimm & Brown, 2004). For assemblages such as the British avifauna, which have experienced little *in situ* evolution, such responses may occur through two pathways (Lennon, Greenwood & Turner, 2000; Evans *et al.*, 2004). First, increases in temperature may reduce the metabolic load on individuals, enabling them to divert resources away from thermogenesis and towards reproduction and thus population growth, size and viability. In accordance with this thermoregulatory load hypothesis, and following work documenting the form of the species–energy relationship in British birds (Turner, Lennon & Lawrenson, 1988; Lennon *et al.*, 2000; Evans & Gaston, 2005), we used mean summer temperature as our first measure of energy. This was calculated from the monthly averages for May, June and July using data that were derived from meteorological recording station readings for the period 1961–90 using surface interpolation techniques (Barrow, Hulme & Jiang, 1993). Second, assemblages may respond to resource availability, which in the case of consumers such as birds is ultimately determined by plant productivity. In accordance with this pathway we used Normalized Difference Vegetation Index (NDVI) data as a measure of resource availability. NDVI is strongly positively correlated with net primary productivity (Boelman *et al.*, 2003; Kerr & Ostrovsky, 2003) and an increasing number of studies have successfully used NDVI data in studies investigating how resource availability influences assemblage structure (e.g. Bonn *et al.*, 2004; Hawkins, 2004; Hurlbert, 2004). We obtained NDVI data from the NOAA/NASA Pathfinder AVHRR Land Data Set (see http://ciesin.columbia.edu/TG/RS/landpath.html). These data are at a spatial resolution of a 0.1° latitude/longitude grid, approximately equivalent to an 8 km quadrat in the UK. Daily readings are converted to maximum values for each ten-day period, which markedly reduces the effects of cloud cover. From these we calculated mean monthly NDVI values and then used a GIS to reproject these data at a 10 km resolution. We then calculated mean NDVI values during the summer (May, June and July) and the entire year. As well as these estimates of environmental conditions within a quadrat we obtained, for each variable, a measure of its "roughness", i.e. the mean difference between the value in the focal quadrat and each neighbor.

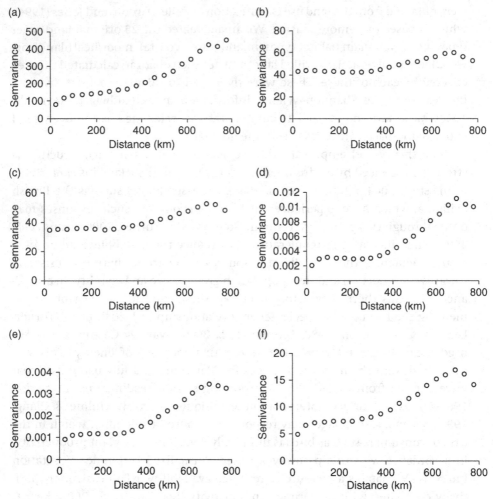

**Figure 10.2** Semivariograms, of mean semivariance and mean distance, for (a) species continuity, (b) species gain, (c) species loss, (d) $\beta_w$, (e) $\beta_{sim}$ and (f) $\beta_1$ for the breeding birds in Britain; turnover is assessed for each 10 km quadrat in comparison with its neighbors. Spatial correlation becomes negligible at the distance at which increases in semivariance are no longer marked, i.e. the semivariogram reaches a sill.

Spatial autocorrelation is inherent to many diversity patterns, and the moving-window algorithm increases this further (Fig. 10.2). This is dealt with using the SAS procedure "PROC MIXED" to implement spatial correlation models that fit a spatial covariance matrix to the data and use this to adjust test statistics accordingly (Littell *et al.*, 1996). Our spatial models assumed an exponential spatial covariance structure as, for each response variable, this gave a better fit to the null model than five alternative covariance structures: spherical, gaussian, linear, linear log and power. Comparing null spatial models to ones that assumed independent errors demonstrated that all our response variables were significantly spatially autocorrelated (likelihood ratio tests $P < 0.0001$ in all cases). In general, we constructed bivariate models, but when investigating the influence of environmental conditions on turnover we also constructed multiple regression models. We used a stepwise forwards selection process with the primary criterion for entry into the Minimum Adequate Model (MAM) being $P < 0.05$, we also ensured that the Akaike Information Criteria (AIC) value decreased, thus indicating a superior model fit.

## Spatial grain

For the breeding birds in Britain, continuity between neighboring quadrats increases with spatial grain, while species gain and loss remain approximately invariant, with average values of between 10 and 13 species across all scales (Fig. 10.3 and Fig. 10.4). While the latter pattern contrasts with our predictions this may arise because our smallest grain size is still a relatively large $100\,\mathrm{km}^2$. These trends result in $\beta_w$ and $\beta_{sim}$ declining with increasing grain, as predicted, while $\beta_l$ remains approximately constant (Fig. 10.4 and Fig. 10.5). That $\beta_w$ is scale dependent suggests that the slope of the power SAR is not spatially invariant (Arita & Rodríguez, 2002), which is indeed the case in this data set (Lennon et al., 2001).

Other empirical studies have also documented decreases in spatial turnover with increasing spatial grain. Similarity, assessed by Jaccard's index, increases with spatial grain for butterfly and bird assemblages in the Great Basin area of North America (Mac Nally et al., 2004), and among Mexican mammals $\beta_W$ declines with increasing scale (Arita & Rodríguez, 2002). In addition, Rivadeneira, Fernández and Navarrete (2002) show higher between-site values of 1-Jaccard's index than between latitudinal bands for intertidal invertebrate assemblages along a section of Chilean coastline encompassing 25° of latitude.

## Species richness

For the British birds, there are positive relationships between species richness and both continuity and species gain, and a negative relationship between species richness and species loss (Fig. 10.6a–c; and compare Figs. 10.3 and 10.7). All of these relationships weaken with increasing spatial grain, possibly because of an associated reduction in the ranges of the variables (Fig. 10.8). This results in negative relationships between species richness and all three beta diversity measures (Fig. 10.6d–e), which are highly significant across all spatial scales in the cases of $\beta_w$ and $\beta_l$, but are only strong at the finest spatial scale for $\beta_{sim}$ (Fig. 10.8). The decline in the strength of the relationship with increasing scale is particularly marked for $\beta_w$ and almost negligible for $\beta_l$, which is not surprising given that species gain and loss contrast in the direction of their relationships with species richness. Therefore, in general, where turnover is low species richness is high, particularly at fine spatial scales. The

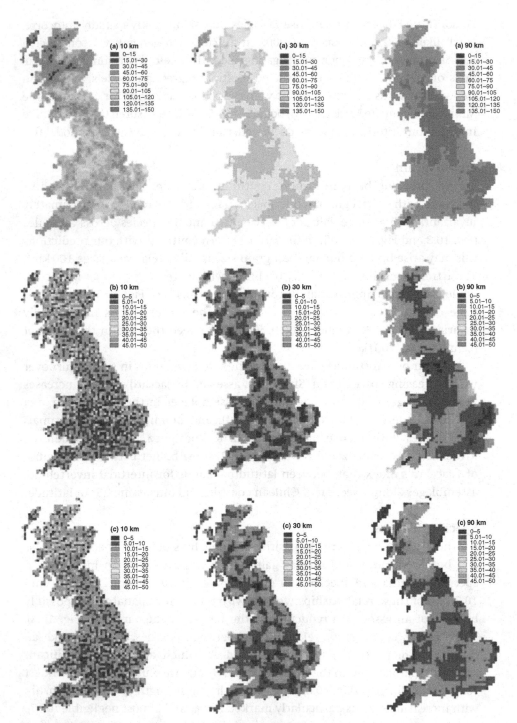

**Figure 10.3** Maps of the matching components at different spatial grains (from left to right, 10 km, 30 km, 90 km) for the breeding birds in Britain. Top row, species continuity; middle row, species gain; and bottom row, species loss. (For color version see Plate 6.)

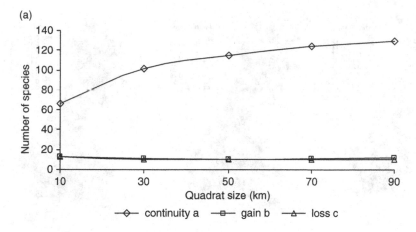

(a)

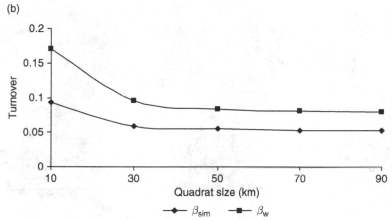

(b)

**Figure 10.4** Variation with coarsening scale of mean (a) species continuity, gain and loss and (b) $\beta_w$ and $\beta_{sim}$, for the breeding birds in Britain. Note that $\beta_1$ follows the pattern of species gain and loss as it equals half the sum of these components.

declines in turnover with richness concur with the predictions derived above for both dispersal and niche limitation, but given that our assemblages are partially nested these theories could also predict any other pattern.

The empirical evidence that higher regional species richness is attained through greater local spatial turnover in species identities is somewhat mixed (Willig & Gannon, 1997; Stevens & Willig, 2002; Koleff et al., 2003b; Okuda et al., 2004; Rodríguez & Arita, 2004). This may be influenced by a number of factors including the widespread use of measures of beta diversity that are heavily dependent on local richness gradients and confounding effects of variations in the area over which local or regional richness is measured at different latitudes (Koleff et al., 2003b) and the extent to which sampling is complete, with incomplete sampling leading to overestimates of turnover. The variety of results reported is, however, not surprising given theoretical predictions that increasing

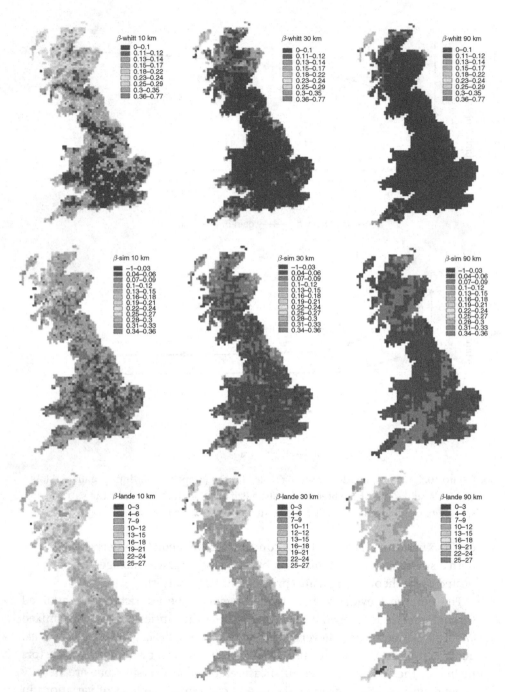

**Figure 10.5** Maps of beta diversity between neighboring quadrats at different spatial grains (from left to right, 10 km, 30 km, 90 km) for the breeding birds in Britain. Top row, $\beta_w$; middle row, $\beta_{sim}$; and bottom row, $\beta_l$. (For color version see Plate 7.)

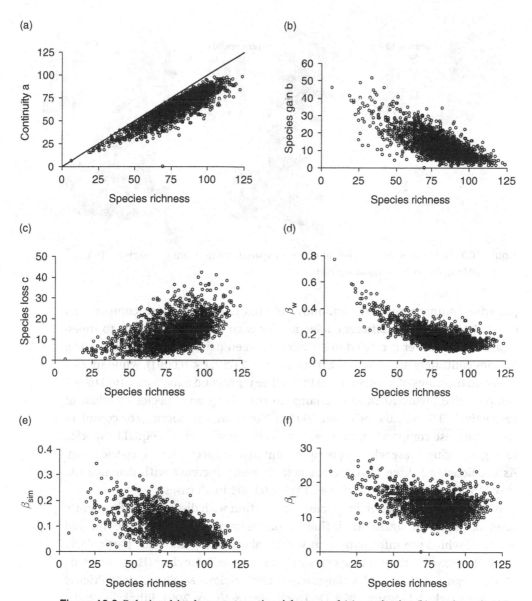

**Figure 10.6** Relationships between species richness and (a) continuity, (b) species gain, (c) species loss, (d) $\beta_w$, (e) $\beta_{sim}$ and (f) $\beta_1$ in 10 km quadrats, for the breeding birds in Britain. The line in plot (a) represents a 1:1 relationship.

species richness in focal assemblages can lead to beta diversity increasing, decreasing or remaining constant.

### Distance

We assessed turnover, in terms of its matching components and $\beta_w$, $\beta_{sim}$, and $\beta_1$, between each 10 km quadrat and all other quadrats (yielding almost 6 million

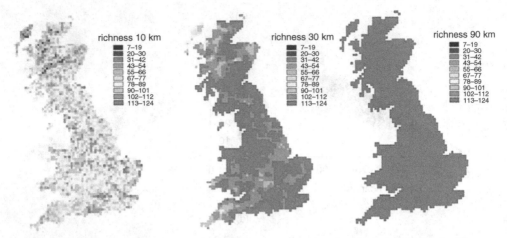

**Figure 10.7** Maps of species richness at different spatial grains (from left to right, 10 km, 30 km, 90 km). (For color version see Plate 8.)

pairwise comparisons). We randomly selected *c*. 0.5% of these comparisons ($n = 28\,744$), making a different selection for each response variable, to investigate how turnover is related to distance between pairs of quadrats (Fig. 10.9). Species continuity decreases with distance ($r^2 = 21.5\%$; $P < 0.0001$), while species loss/gain increases ($r^2 = 14.4\%$; $P < 0.0001$). The regression equations fitted to our samples give predicted rates of change in continuity and species gain/loss of respectively 3.7 and 2.6 species per 100 km. Note that, considering the complete set of pairwise comparisons between grid cells, species gain is equal to species loss, generating a case where $\beta_1$ is equivalent to half species loss or species gain. As predicted, all three measures of beta diversity increase with distance ($\beta_w$ $r^2 = 32.7\%$; $\beta_{sim}$ $r^2 = 37.7\%$; $\beta_1$ $r^2 = 41.1\%$; $P < 0.0001$ in all cases).

While increasing change in species composition with distance has frequently been documented, again the influence of the measure of change employed (some of which use information on species abundance), and thus particularly the influence of variation in species richness per se, is unclear (Harrison *et al.*, 1992; Gregory, Greenwood & Hagemeijer, 1998; Nekola & White, 1999; Price *et al.*, 1999; Clarke & Lidgard, 2000; De Troch, Fiers & Vincx, 2001; Ellingsen, 2001; Condit *et al.*, 2002; Duivenvoorden, Svenning & Wright, 2002; Ellingsen & Gray, 2002; Garcillán & Ezcurra, 2003; Tuomisto, Ruokolainen & Yli-Haila, 2003; Burnham, 2004; Gilbert & Lechowicz, 2004; Mac Nally *et al.*, 2004; Vormisto *et al.*, 2004; Qian, Ricklefs & White, 2005).

**Environmental gradients**

At the 10 km scale, the single best environmental predictor of $\beta_w$ and $\beta_{sim}$ is temperature, with species turnover being lower in areas with high temperatures (Table 10.3a; Fig. 10.10). In contrast, temperature roughness is the single best

(a)

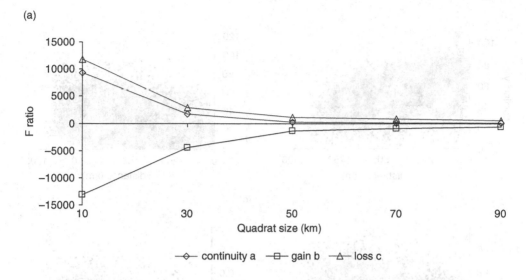

(b)

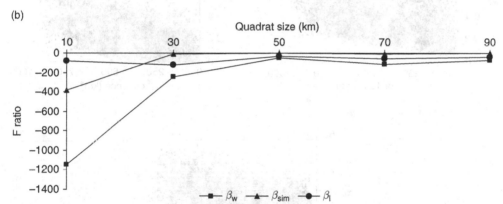

**Figure 10.8** The scale-dependency of relationships between species richness and (a) continuity, species gain, and species loss and (b) $\beta_w$, $\beta_{sim}$ and $\beta_l$, for the breeding birds in Britain. The sign of the F ratio indicates whether relationships were positive or negative. All relationships were highly significant ($P < 0.0001$) across the range of spatial scales analyzed except for $\beta_{sim}$, which is highly significant at the finest spatial scale but marginally significant at the 30 km ($P = 0.001$) and 70 km ($P = 0.006$) scales and nonsignificant ($P > 0.05$) at other scales.

predictor of $\beta_l$, with bigger differences in the temperature of the focal cell compared with its neighbors associated with greater species turnover. Multivariate models of the three beta diversity measures differ in terms of the exact nature of the predictor variables that they retain. In line with our predictions, beta diversity consistently correlates negatively with energy availability and positively with roughness in a range of environmental conditions (Table 10.4a).

At the 90 km scale, altitude roughness is the best single environmental predictor of species turnover, and in line with predictions such correlations are

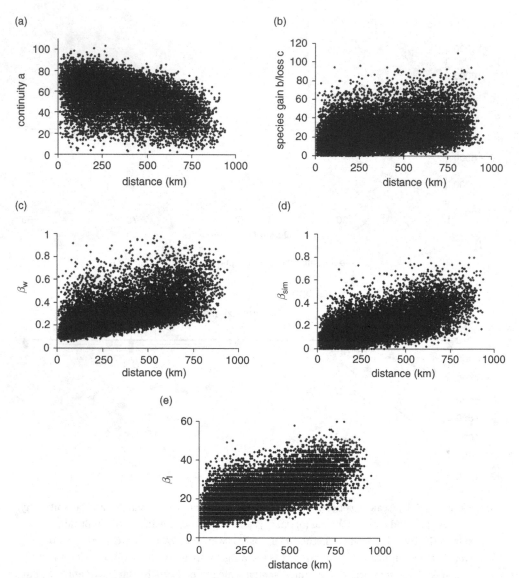

**Figure 10.9** Relationships between distance and (a) continuity, (b) species gain/loss, (c) $\beta_w$, (d) $\beta_{sim}$, and (e) $\beta_l$ for the breeding birds in Britain. Data represent a random selection (c. 0.5%, $n = 27\,844$) of all possible pairwise comparisons between 10 km quadrats.

positive (Table 10.3b; Fig. 10.10). Multivariate models retain fewer predictors compared with those relating to the 10 km scale (cf. Table 10.4); at coarser spatial scales there is inherently less information (reduced degrees of freedom) in spatial patterns and so statistical significance is harder to attain. In contrast to the results for the 10 km scale, at this 90 km scale only one measure of mean

**Table 10.3** *Bivariate relationships between environmental measures and continuity, species gain, species loss, $\beta_w$, $\beta_{sim}$ and $\beta_l$ for the breeding birds in Britain at scales of (a) 10 km and (b) 90 km.*

Figures given are the $F_{1,2404}$ ratios. The abbreviations used for each predictor variable are: species richness (spp. rich); mean annual NDVI (AnnNDVI); mean summer NDVI (SumNDVI); habitat diversity (Hdiv) and temperature (Temp); measures of roughness are indicated by the letter 'r' preceding the variable name.

|  | Continuity a | Gain b | Loss c | $\beta_w$ | $\beta_{sim}$ | $\beta_l$ |
|---|---|---|---|---|---|---|
| **(a)** | | | | | | |
| Spp.rich10 km | 9291.6 ++++ | 13130.8 ---- | 11802.0 ++++ | 1146.4 ---- | 381.1 ---- | 83.6 ---- |
| Spp.rich30 km | 53.7 ++++ | 2.4 ns | 20.0 ++++ | 0.0 ns | 0.5 ns | 62.9 ++++ |
| AnnNDVI10 km | 51.3 ++++ | 72.8 ---- | 7.3 ---- | 37.0 ---- | 15.1 ---- | 11.3 ---- |
| AnnNDVI30 km | 64.2 ++++ | 58.4 ---- | 17.9 --- | 40.4 ---- | 15.9 ---- | 8.1 -- |
| rAnnNDVI10 km | 7.4 - | 29.6 ++++ | 5.2 ++++ | 10.3 ++ | 10.4 ++++ | 16.2 ++++ |
| SumNDVI10 km | 35.6 ++++ | 79.4 ---- | 13.5 --- | 36.2 ---- | 20.3 --- | 13.4 --- |
| SumNDVI30 km | 59.8 ++++ | 71.6 ---- | 40.1 ---- | 52.9 ---- | 29.1 ---- | 11.0 ---- |
| rSumNDVI10 km | 8.3 --- | 25.6 ++++ | 5.3 + | 11.4 +++ | 6.0 + | 18.3 ++++ |
| Hdiv10 km | 328.1 ++++ | 311.1 ---- | 27.5 ++++ | 132.2 ---- | 59.1 ---- | 18.9 ---- |
| Hdiv30 km | 114.6 ++++ | 107.8 ---- | 20.2 ---- | 36.2 ---- | 24.5 ---- | 1.6 ns |
| rHdiv10 km | 6.6 - | 43.2 ++++ | 51.5 ++++ | 22.3 ++++ | 0.0 ns | 38.9 ++++ |
| Temp10 km | 226.6 ++++ | 217.3 ---- | 99.7 ---- | 196.5 ---- | 134.1 ---- | 50.6 ---- |
| Temp30 km | 53.9 ++++ | 160.3 ---- | 155.3 ---- | 79.4 ---- | 99.9 ---- | 20.9 ---- |
| rTemp10 km | 20.5 ---- | 93.9 ++++ | 67.5 ++++ | 59.4 ++++ | 15.7 ++++ | 91.5 ++++ |
| Altitude10 km | 125.0 ---- | 153.8 ++++ | 5.7 + | 110.3 ++++ | 50.5 ++++ | 34.0 ++++ |
| Altitude30 km | 30.0 ---- | 92.3 ++++ | 66.0 ++++ | 26.3 ++++ | 15.3 ++++ | 4.5 + |
| rAltitude10 km | 4.3 ---- | 65.7 ++++ | 69.7 ++++ | 26.7 ++++ | 10.3 ++++ | 47.2 ++++ |

*(cont.)*

Table 10.3 (cont.)

(b)

| | Continuity a | Gain b | Loss c | $\beta_w$ | $\beta_{sim}$ | $\beta_l$ |
|---|---|---|---|---|---|---|
| Spp.rich90 km | 57.6 ++++ | 697.6 ---- | 487.8 ++++ | 73.3 ---- | 3.5 ns | 43.9 ---- |
| Spp.rich270 km | 0.0 ns + | 17.7 ++++ | 1.0 + | 18.3 ++++ | 0.3 ns | 22.0 ++++ |
| AnnNDVI90 km | 10.7 ++ | 2.5 ns | 1.8 ns | 0.9 ns | 0.5 ns | 0.9 ns |
| AnnNDVI270 km | 1.9 ns | 0.4 ns | 0.1 ns | 0.5 ns | 0.1 ns | 0.4 ns |
| rAnnNDVI90 km | 1.7 ns | 10.2 ---- | 0.3 ns | 13.8 ---- | 2.3 ns | 11.3 --- |
| SumNDVI90 km | 21.5 ++++ | 1.9 ns | 0.7 ns | 2.2 ns | 2.6 ns | 2.6 ns |
| SumNDVI270 km | 9.4 ++ | 1.2 ns | 0.6 ns | 1.3 ns | 0.2 ns | 2.0 ns |
| rSumNDVI90 km | 2.8 ns | 13.1 ---- | 0.3 ns | 16.7 ---- | 1.9 ns | 13.9 --- |
| Hdiv90 km | 4.2 + | 22.1 ---- | 9.3 ++ | 5.4 - | 0.0 ns | 5.7 - |
| Hdiv270 km | 25.4 ++++ | 1.4 ns | 0.1 ns | 5.6 - | 0.3 ns | 7.8 -- |
| rHdiv90 km | 1.7 ns | 19.4 ++++ | 0.1 ns | 17.1 ++++ | 0.1 ns | 15.7 ++++ |
| Temp90 km | 3.5 ns | 1.7 ns | 0.2 ns | 3.4 ns | 0.0 ns | 4.0 - |
| Temp270 km | 3.2 ns | 0.1 ns | 3.6 ns | 3.5 ns | 0.7 ns | 6.3 - |
| rTemp90 km | 0.2 ns | 0.7 ns | 0.3 ns | 0.5 ns | 5.0 + | 0.3 ns |
| Altitude90 km | 0.00 ns | 1.5 ns | 1.4 + | 2.4 ns | 2.4 ns | 1.6 ns |
| Altitude270 km | 2.8 ns | 1.5 ns | 11.1 +++ | 1.2 ns | 9.9 ++ | 2.7 ns |
| rAltitude90 km | 0.6 ns | 30.5 ++++ | 2.3 ns | 17.6 ++++ | 11.7 +++ | 16.2 ++++ |

Significance levels: Positive effects ++++ $P < 0.0001$, +++ $P < 0.001$, ++ $P < 0.01$, + $P < 0.05$
Negative effects ---- $P < 0.0001$, --- $P < 0.001$, -- $P < 0.01$, - $P < 0.05$.

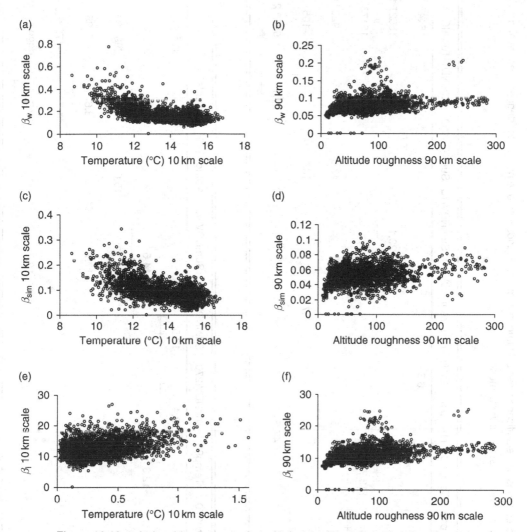

**Figure 10.10** Relationships between $\beta_w$ (a, b) $\beta_{sim}$ (c, d) and $\beta_l$, (e, f) and environmental conditions in the focal quadrat. Plots are presented for the best fitting predictor in univariate tests (see Table 10.3), at the 10 km (a, c and e) and 90 km scales (b, d and f).

environmental conditions is retained in the models: habitat diversity is negatively associated with $\beta_l$. Models contain a greater number of environmental roughness predictors. Roughness in summer NDVI is, counter to predictions, negatively correlated with $\beta_w$ and $\beta_l$. However, in line with predictions, altitudinal roughness is positively correlated with all three measures of beta diversity, and roughness in habitat diversity also correlates positively with $\beta_l$.

Much of the discussion of spatial turnover has concerned changes in species composition along environmental gradients. Our results, like those of the vast

**Table 10.4** *Relationships between environmental variables and various aspects of species spatial for the breeding birds in Britain at scales of (a) 10 km and (b) 90 km*

See Table 10.3 for a legend of predictor variable abbreviations and significance levels. Numbers indicate F ratios with one numerator degree freedom and denominator degrees freedom equal to 2405, minus the number of terms in the model.

(a)

| | Hdiv10 | Hdiv30 | rHdiv10 | Temp10 | Temp30 | rTemp10 | AnnNDVI10 | rAnnNDVI10 | SumNDVI10 | SumNDVI30 | rSumNDVI10 | AIC |
|---|---|---|---|---|---|---|---|---|---|---|---|---|
| Continuity a | 139.2 (++++) | | | 75.7 (++++) | | | 6.3 (+) | | | 17.6 (++++) | | 15445.4 |
| Gain b | 169.1 (++++) | 100.2 (++++) | 5.9 (+) | 56.0 (----) | 36.2 (++++) | | | | 23.1 (----) | | | 15527.1 |
| Loss c | 123.7 (++++) | 76.0 (----) | 41.3 (++++) | 68.8 (----) | 113.7 (----) | | | | | | | 15173.3 |
| $\beta_w$ | 47.0 (++++) | 13.6 (+++) | | 70.3 (----) | | 12.5 (+++) | | | 43.0 (----) | | | −9209.6 |
| $\beta_{sim}$ | 16.0 (----) | | | 82.8 (----) | | | | 7.7 (++) | | 10.8 (---) | | −10511.9 |
| $\beta_l$ | | | 33.9 (++++) | 22.8 (----) | | 47.5 (++++) | | | | | 21.1 (++++) | 9852.2 |

(b)

| | Hdiv90 | Hdiv270 | rHdiv90 | Temp270 | rTemp90 | AnnNDVI270 | SumNDVI90 | rSumNDVI90 | Altitude270 | rAltitude90 | AIC |
|---|---|---|---|---|---|---|---|---|---|---|---|
| Continuity a | 19.7 (++++) | | | | | 23.4 (----) | 13.5 (+++) | | | 32.1 (++++) | 15601.7 |
| Gain b | 14.1 (----) | | | | 12.3 (---) | | | 14.6 (++++) | | | 9964.9 |
| Loss c | 8.4 (++) | | | 4.4 (+) | | | | | 15.0 (++++) | | 8991.8 |
| $\beta_w$ | | | | | | | | 17.7 (----) | 18.6 (++++) | | −16195.9 |
| $\beta_{sim}$ | | | | | | | | | | 11.7 (+++) | −17294.9 |
| $\beta_l$ | | 12.2 (----) | 6.3 (+) | | | | | 12.4 (----) | | 10.8 (++++) | 6999.3 |

majority of studies, are compatible with the suggestion that species turnover is strongly influenced by environmental gradients (e.g. Whittaker, 1960, 1972; Routledge, 1977; Weiher & Boylen, 1994; Mourelle & Ezcurra, 1997; Harrison, 1999; Pharo *et al.*, 1999; Sweeney & Cook, 2001; Brehm, Homeier & Fiedler, 2003; Tuomisto *et al.*, 2003; Heegaard, 2004; Vormisto *et al.*, 2004; Qian *et al.*, 2005; but see Genner *et al.*, 2004 for a counter example). One carefully designed study has shown that such patterns are independent of the effects of distance and thus provides strong support for niche-based models over dispersal ones (Gilbert & Lechowicz, 2004).

Our results indicate that while differences in environmental conditions of the focal cell, relative to its neighbors, influence beta diversity the actual conditions within the focal cell can have equally important effects (presumably through their influences on average levels of occupancy). In this context, the negative association between energy availability and beta diversity is particularly marked at the 10 km scale, even in the case of $\beta_{sim}$, which is relatively insensitive to local species gradients. Such an influence concurs with studies reporting that turnover, measured by the slope of species–area relationships, is negatively related to energy availability (Pastor, Downing & Erickson, 1996), which is also the case in the British avifauna (Storch, Evans & Gaston, 2005). It is noteworthy that the exact nature of environmental predictors retained in the multivariate models varies with both scale and the manner in which beta diversity is measured. In particular, our demonstration of significant associations between turnover at one scale and mean environmental factors at the next coarser scale (e.g. 10 km turnover vs. 30 km environmental factors) show that at least some of this turnover is not driven locally, because by definition there is no environmental variation at the 10 km scale in a 30 km measure (Tables 10.3 and 10.4). To some extent these associations are explicable in statistical terms because of the positive correlation between the same factor measured at different scales. Nonetheless, it is likely that significant associations between mean environmental conditions and species turnover (Tables 10.3 and 10.4) indicate that the magnitude of difference in composition between local assemblages is partly driven by the average conditions experienced by these assemblages, and that geographical variation in these conditions in turn generates spatial variation in species turnover.

## Synthesis

In sum, the patterns of spatial turnover observed for breeding birds in Britain largely match those predicted from dispersal limitation and/or niche limitation. Turnover tends to decline with spatial grain and to increase with distance, as predicted by both theoretical frameworks. Neither framework makes a simple prediction as to how turnover should change with species richness, but it is observed to decline such that the regions of lowest turnover are those with highest richness, a scenario which is achievable from either framework. Finally, the degree of spatial turnover in species composition is associated with the environmental difference between areas as predicted by niche but not dispersal limitation.

## In conclusion

The "growing thicket of observations" on beta diversity on which Rosenzweig (1995) remarked has a number of origins. First, there has been persistent disagreement as to what constitutes beta diversity and spatial turnover. This should really constitute no significant obstacle to improving understanding, provided there is clarity of terminology.

Second, associated with these differences of opinion on definition there has been an ever-burgeoning number of approaches to measuring spatial turnover, as epitomized by the number of indices of beta diversity (Table 10.1). The solution here is to recognize that these are often measuring very different things (a recognition surprisingly lacking in the discussion sections of many empirical papers), and preferably to settle on a small number of such measures. We suggest that studies should focus on documenting variation in the matching components $a$, $b$ and $c$, which provide the fundamentals of turnover, and thence on three measures of turnover: $\beta_w$, due to its long history of frequent use, $\beta_{sim}$, due to its apparent relative independence from local species richness gradients, and $\beta_l$, as an example of an additive measure of beta diversity that focuses solely on loss and gain.

Third, the "thicket" has been further tangled by the lack of a theory of spatial turnover. This is now changing rapidly, which should enable some intelligent reappraisal of existing empirical results. However, a difficulty clearly looms in that different theoretical frameworks (e.g. dispersal limitation and niche limitation) may predict patterns in turnover that are extremely difficult to distinguish in the field. This may be particularly so given that the differences in predictions may be subtle and quantitative, rather than qualitative, and that patterns of turnover are sensitive to sampling inadequacies.

We see no reason why the "growing thicket of observations" should not shortly be severely pruned, and brought under some control.

## Acknowledgments

We are grateful to the editors for the invitation to write this chapter, to the many thousands of volunteers whose efforts in collecting the data made this work possible, to J. J. D. Greenwood and the British Trust for Ornithology for making the data available, and to S. L. Chown, S. Gaston, J. J. D. Greenwood, P. Koleff, M. McKnight, V. Novotný and D. Storch for comments and discussion. This work was supported by The Leverhulme Trust.

## References

Allan, J. D. (1975). Components of diversity. *Oecologia*, **18**, 359–367.

Arellano, L. & Halffter, G. (2003). Gamma diversity: derived from a determinant of alpha diversity and beta diversity. An analysis of three tropical landscapes. *Acta Zoologica Mexicana*, **90**, 27–76.

Arhennius, O. (1921). Species and area. *Journal of Ecology*, **9**, 95–99.

Arita, H. T. & Rodríguez, P. (2002). Geographic range, turnover rate and the scaling of species diversity. *Ecography*, **25**, 541–550.

Barrow, E., Hulme, M. & Jiang, T. (1993). *A 1961–90 baseline climatology and future climatic change scenarios for Great Britain and Europe. Part 1: 1961–90 Great Britain baseline climatology.* University of East Anglia Climatic Research Unit, Norwich.

Bell, G. (2001). Neutral macroecology. *Science*, **293**, 2413–2418.

Bini, L. M., Diniz-Filho, J. A. F., Bonfim, F. & Bastos, R. P. (2000). Local and regional species richness relationships in viperid snake assemblages from South America: unsaturated patterns at three different spatial scales. *Copeia*, **2000**, 799–805.

Blackburn, T. M. & Gaston, K. J. (1996). The distribution of bird species in the New World: patterns in species turnover. *Oikos*, **77**, 146–152.

Boelman, N. T., Stieglitz, M., Rueth, H. M., *et al.* (2003). Response of NDVI, biomass, and ecosystem gas exchange to long-term warming and fertilization in wet sedge tundra. *Oecologia*, **135**, 414–421.

Bonn, A., Storch, D. & Gaston, K. J. (2004). Structure of the species-energy relationship. *Proceedings of the Royal Society of London, Series B*, **271**, 1685–1691.

Brehm, G., Homeier, J. & Fiedler, K. (2003). Beta diversity of geometrid moths (Lepidoptera: Geometridae) in an Andean montane rainforest. *Diversity and Distributions*, **9**, 351–366.

Brown, J. H. (1984). On the relationship between abundance and distribution of species. *American Naturalist*, **124**, 255–279.

Brown, J. H. & Lomolino, M. V. (1998). *Biogeography*. Sunderland, MA: Sinauer Associates.

Burnham, R. J. (2004). Alpha and beta diversity of lianas in Yasuní, Ecuador. *Forest Ecology and Management*, **190**, 43–55.

Caley, M. J. & Schluter, D. (1997). The relationship between local and regional diversity. *Ecology*, **78**, 70–80.

Chao, A., Chazdon, R. L., Colwell, R. K. & Shen, T-J. (2005). A new statistical approach for assessing similarity of species composition with incidence and abundance data. *Ecology Letters*, **8**, 148–159.

Chase, J. M. & Leibold, M. A. (2003). *Ecological Niches: Linking Classical and Contemporary Approaches*. Chicago: University of Chicago Press.

Chave, J. & Leigh Jr., E. G. (2002). A spatially explicit neutral model of β-diversity in tropical forests. *Theoretical Population Biology*, **62**, 153–168.

Clarke, A. & Lidgard, S. (2000). Spatial patterns of diversity in the sea: bryozoan species richness in the North Atlantic. *Journal of Animal Ecology*, **69**, 799–814.

Cody, M. L. (1975). Towards a theory of continental species diversities: bird distributions over Mediterranean habitat gradients. In *Ecology and Evolution of Communities*, ed. M. L. Cody & J. M. Diamond, pp. 214–257. Cambridge, MA: Belknap Press of Harvard University.

Cody, M. L. (1986). Diversity, rarity, and conservation in Mediterranean-climate regions. In *Conservation Biology*, ed. M. E. Soulé, pp. 122–152. Sunderland, MA: Sinauer Associates.

Cody, M. L. (1993). Bird diversity components within and between habitats in Australia. In *Species Diversity in Ecological Communities: Historical and Geographical Perspectives*, ed.

R. E. Ricklefs & D. Schluter, pp. 147–158. Chicago: University of Chicago Press.

Colwell, R. K. & Coddington, J. A. (1994). Estimating terrestrial biodiversity through extrapolation. *Philosophical Transactions of the Royal Society of London, Series B*, **345**, 101–118.

Condit, R., Pitman, N., Leigh Jr., E. G., *et al.* (2002). Beta-diversity in tropical forest trees. *Science*, **295**, 666–669.

Connor, E. F. & McCoy, E. D. (1979). The statistics and biology of the species-area relationship. *American Naturalist*, **113**, 791–833.

Cornell, H. V. (1999). Unsaturation and regional influences on species richness in ecological communities: a review of the evidence. *Écoscience*, **6**, 303–315.

Cornell, H. V. & Lawton, J. H. (1992). Species interactions, local and regional processes, and limits to the richness of ecological communities: a theoretical perspective. *Journal of Animal Ecology*, **61**, 1–12.

Crawley, M. J. & Harral, J. E. (2001). Scale dependence in plant biodiversity. *Science*, **291**, 864–868.

Crist, T. O., Veech, J. A., Gering, J. C. & Summerville, K. S. (2003). Partitioning species diversity across landscapes and regions: a hierarchical analysis of $\alpha$, $\beta$, and $\gamma$ diversity. *American Naturalist*, **162**, 734–743.

Davis, A. L. V., Scholtz, C. H. & Chown, S. L. (1999). Species turnover, community boundaries and biogeographical composition of dung beetle assemblages across an altitudinal gradient in South Africa. *Journal of Biogeography*, **26**, 1039–1055.

De Troch, M., Fiers, F. & Vincx, M. (2001). Alpha and beta diversity of harpacticoid copepods in a tropical seagrass bed: the relation between diversity and species' range size distribution. *Marine Ecology Progress Series*, **215**, 225–236.

Dice, L. R. (1945). Measures of the amount of ecological association between species. *Ecology*, **26**, 297–302.

Diniz-Filho, J. A. F., Rangel, T. F. L. V. B. & Hawkins, B. A. (2004). A test of multiple hypotheses for the species richness gradient of South American owls. *Oecologia*, **140**, 633–638.

Duivenvoorden, J. F., Svenning, J-C. & Wright, S. J. (2002). Beta diversity in tropical forests. *Science*, **295**, 636–637.

Ellingsen, K. E. (2001). Biodiversity of a continental shelf soft-sediment macrobenthos community. *Marine Ecology Progress Series*, **218**, 1–15.

Ellingsen, K. E. & Gray, J. S. (2002). Spatial patterns of benthic diversity: is there a latitudinal gradient along the Norwegian continental shelf? *Journal of Animal Ecology*, **71**, 373–389.

Evans, K. L. & Gaston, K. J. (2005). People, energy and avian species richness. *Global Ecology & Biogeography*, **14**, 187–196.

Evans, K. L., Warren, P. H. & Gaston, K. J. (2004). Species-energy relationships at the macroecological scale: a review of the mechanisms. *Biological Reviews*, **79**, 1–25.

Felfili, M. C. & Felfili, J. M. (2001). Diversidade alfa e beta no cerrado *sensu stricto* da Chapada Pratinha, Brasil. *Acta Botanica Brasílica*, **15**, 243–254.

Fuller, R. M., Groom, G. B. & Jones, A. R. (1994). The land-cover map of Great Britain. An automated classification of Landsat Thematic Mapper data. *Photogrammetric Engineering and Remote Sensing*, **60**, 553–562.

Garcillán, P. P. & Ezcurra, E. (2003). Biogeographic regions and β-diversity of woody dryland legumes in the Baja California peninsula. *Journal of Vegetation Science*, **14**, 859–868.

Gaston, K. J. & Williams, P. H. (1996). Spatial patterns in taxonomic diversity. In *Biodiversity: a Biology of Numbers and Difference*, ed. K. J. Gaston, pp. 202–229. Oxford: Blackwell Science.

Gaston, K. J., Blackburn, T. M. & Lawton, J. H. (1997). Interspecific abundance-range size relationships: an appraisal of mechanisms. *Journal of Animal Ecology*, **66**, 579–601.

Gaston, K. J., Blackburn, T. M., Greenwood, J. J. D., Gregory, R. D., Quinn, R. M. & Lawton, J. H. (2000). Abundance-occupancy relationships. *Journal of Applied Ecology*, **37** (Suppl. 1), 39–59.

Gaston, K. J., Rodrigues, A. S. L., van Rensburg, B. J., Koleff, P. & Chown, S. L. (2001). Complementary representation and zones of ecological transition. *Ecology Letters*, **4**, 4–9.

Genner, M. J., Taylor, M. I., Cleary, D. F. R., Hawkins, S. J., Knight, M. E. & Turner, G. F. (2004). Beta diversity of rock-restricted cichlid fishes in lake Malawi: importance of environmental and spatial factors. *Ecography*, **27**, 601–610.

Gering, J. C. & Crist, T. O. (2002). The alpha-beta-regional relationship: providing new insights into local-regional patterns of species richness and scale dependence of diversity components. *Ecology Letters*, **5**, 433–444.

Gering, J. C., Crist, T. O. & Veech, J. A. (2003). Additive partitioning of species diversity across multiple spatial scales: implications for regional conservation of biodiversity. *Conservation Biology*, **17**, 488–499.

Gibbons, D. W., Reid, J. B. & Chapman, R. A. (1993). *The New Atlas of Breeding Birds in Britain and Ireland: 1988-1991*. London: Poyser.

Gilbert, B. & Lechowicz, M. J. (2004). Neutrality, niches, and dispersal in a temperate forest understorey. *Proceedings of the National Academy of Sciences of the U.S.A.*, **101**, 7651–7656.

Gleason, H. A. (1922). On the relation between species and area. *Ecology*, **3**, 158–162.

Green, J. L. & Ostling, A. (2003). Endemics-area relationships: the influence of species dominance and spatial aggregation. *Ecology*, **84**, 3090–3097.

Green, J. L., Harte, J. & Ostling, A. (2003). Species richness, endemism and abundance patterns: tests of two fractal models in a serpentine grassland. *Ecology Letters*, **6**, 919–928.

Gregory, R. D. & Blackburn, T. M. (1995). Abundance and body size in British birds:

reconciling regional and ecological densities. *Oikos*, **72**, 151–154.

Gregory, R. D. & Gaston, K. J. (2000). Explanations of commonness and rarity in British breeding birds: separating resource use and resource availability. *Oikos*, **88**, 515–526.

Gregory, R. D., Greenwood, J. J. D. & Hagemeijer, E. J. M. (1998). The EBCC atlas of European breeding birds: a contribution to science and conservation. *Biologia e Conservazione della Fauna*, **102**, 38–49.

Griffiths, D. (1997). Local and regional species richness in North American lacustrine fish. *Journal of Animal Ecology*, **66**, 49–56.

Groves, C. R. (2003). *Drafting a Conservation Blueprint: a Practitioner's Guide to Planning for Biodiversity*. Washington: Island Press.

Harrison, S. (1993). Species diversity, spatial scale, and global change. In *Biotic Interactions and Global Change*, ed. P. M. Kareiva, J. G. Kingsolver & R. B. Huey, pp. 388–401. Sunderland, MA: Sinauer.

Harrison, S. (1999). Native and alien species diversity at the local and regional scales in a grazed California grassland. *Oecologia*, **121**, 99–106.

Harrison, S., Ross, S. J. & Lawton, J. H. (1992). Beta diversity on geographic gradients in Britain. *Journal of Animal Ecology*, **61**, 151–158.

Harte, J. & Kinzig, A. P. (1997). On the implications of species-area relationships for endemism, spatial turnover, and food web patterns. *Oikos*, **80**, 417–427.

Harte, J., McCarthy, S., Taylor, K., Kinzig, A. & Fischer, M. L. (1999a). Estimating species-area relationships from plot to landscape scale using spatial-turnover data. *Oikos*, **86**, 45–54.

Harte, J., Kinzig, A. & Green, J. (1999b). Self-similarity in the distribution and abundance of species. *Science*, **284**, 334–336.

Hawkins, B. A. (2004). Summer vegetation, deglaciation and the anomalous bird diversity gradient in eastern North America. *Global Ecology and Biogeography*, **13**, 321–325.

Hawkins, B. A., Field, R., Cornell, H. V., *et al.* (2003). Energy, water and broad-scale geographic patterns of species richness. *Ecology*, **84**, 3105–3117.

He, F., Gaston, K. J., Connor, E. F. & Srivastava, D. S. (2005). The local-regional relationship: immigration, extinction and scale. *Ecology*, **86**, 360–365.

Heegaard, E. (2004). Trends in aquatic macrophyte species turnover in Northern Ireland – which factors determine the spatial distribution of local species turnover? *Global Ecology and Biogeography*, **13**, 397–408.

Hillebrand, H. (2004). On the generality of the latitudinal diversity gradient. *American Naturalist*, **163**, 192–211.

Hillebrand, H. & Blenckner, T. (2002). Regional and local impact on species diversity – from pattern to process. *Oecologia*, **132**, 479–491.

Hubbell, S. P. (1979). Tree dispersion, abundance, and diversity in a tropical dry forest. *Science*, **203**, 1299–1309.

Hubbell, S. P. (1997). A unified theory of biogeography and relative species abundance and its application to tropical rain forests and coral reefs. *Coral Reefs*, **16**, S9–S21.

Hubbell, S. P. (2001). *The Unified Neutral Theory of Biodiversity and Biogeography*. Princeton: Princeton University Press.

Hurlbert, A. H. (2004). Species-energy relationships and habitat complexity in bird communities. *Ecology Letters*, **7**, 714–720.

Jaccard, P. (1912). The distribution of the flora in the alpine zone. *New Phytologist*, **11**, 37–50.

Kaspari, M., Yuan, M. & Alonso, L. (2003). Spatial grain and the causes of regional diversity gradients in ants. *American Naturalist*, **161**, 459–477.

Kerr, J. T. & Ostrovsky, M. (2003). From space to species: ecological applications for remote sensing. *Trends in Ecology and Evolution*, **18**, 299–305.

Koleff, P. & Gaston, K. J. (2001). Latitudinal gradients in diversity: real patterns and random models. *Ecography*, **24**, 341–351.

Koleff, P. & Gaston, K. J. (2002). The relationships between local and regional species richness and spatial turnover. *Global Ecology and Biogeography*, **11**, 363–375.

Koleff, P., Gaston, K. J. & Lennon, J. J. (2003a). Measuring beta diversity for presence-absence data. *Journal of Animal Ecology*, **72**, 367–382.

Koleff, P., Lennon, J. J. & Gaston, K. J. (2003b). Are there latitudinal gradients in species turnover? *Global Ecology and Biogeography*, **12**, 483–498.

Lande, R. (1996). Statistics and partitioning of species diversity, and similarity among multiple communities. *Oikos*, **76**, 5–13.

Lande, R., Engen, S. & Sæther, B-E. (2003). *Stochastic Population Dynamics in Ecology and Conservation*. Oxford: Oxford University Press.

Lawton, J. H. (2000). Concluding remarks: a review of some open questions. In *The Ecological Consequences of Environmental Heterogeneity*, ed. M. J. Hutchings, E. A. John & A. J. A. Stewart, pp. 401–424. Oxford: Blackwell Science.

Leitner, W. A. & Rosenzweig, M. L. (1997). Nested species-area curves and stochastic sampling: a new theory. *Oikos*, **79**, 503–512.

Lennon, J. J., Greenwood, J. J. D. & Turner, J. R. G. (2000). Bird diversity and environmental gradients in Britain: a test of the species-energy hypothesis. *Journal of Animal Ecology*, **69**, 581–598.

Lennon, J. J., Koleff, P., Greenwood, J. J. D. & Gaston, K. J. (2001). The geographical structure of British bird distributions: diversity, spatial turnover and scale. *Journal of Animal Ecology*, **70**, 966–979.

Lennon, J. J., Kunin, W. E. & Hartley, S. (2002). Fractal species distributions do not produce power-law species-area relationships. *Oikos*, **97**, 378–386.

Littell, R. C., Milliken, G. A., Stroup, W. W. & Wolfinger, R. D. (1996). *SAS® system for mixed models*. Cary, USA: SAS Institute Inc.

Loreau, M. (2000). Are communities saturated? On the relationship between $\alpha$, $\beta$ and $\gamma$ diversity. *Ecology Letters*, **3**, 73–76.

Lorance, P., Souissi, S. & Uiblein, F. (2002). Point, alpha and beta diversity of carnivorous fish along a depth gradient. *Aquatic Living Resources*, **15**, 263–271.

Ludwig, J. A. & Reynolds, J. F. (1988). *Statistical Ecology*. New York: John Wiley.

Mac Nally, R., Fleishman, E., Bulluck, L. P. & Betrus, C. J. (2004). Comparative influence of spatial scale on beta diversity within regional assemblages of birds and butterflies. *Journal of Biogeography*, **31**, 917–929.

Maddux, R. D. (2004). Self-similarity and the species-area relationship. *American Naturalist*, **163**, 616–626.

Magurran, A. E. (1988). *Ecological Diversity and its Measurement*. London: Croom Helm.

Magurran, A. E. (2004). *Measuring Biological Diversity*. Oxford: Blackwell Publishing.

Major, J. (1988). Endemism: a botanical perspective. In *Analytical Biogeography: an Integrated Approach to the Study of Animal and Plant Distributions*, ed. A. A. Myers & P. S. Giller, pp. 117–146. London: Chapman & Hall.

McGill, B. & Collins, C. (2003). A unified theory for macroecology based on spatial patterns of abundance. *Evolutionary Ecology Research*, **5**, 469–492.

Moreno, C. E. & Halffter, G. (2001). Spatial and temporal analysis of $\alpha$, $\beta$ and $\gamma$ diversities of bats in a fragmented landscape. *Biodiversity and Conservation*, **10**, 367–382.

Mouquet, N., Munguia, P., Kneitel, J. M. & Miller, T. E. (2003). Community assembly time and the relationship between local and regional species richness. *Oikos*, **103**, 618–626.

Mourelle, C. & Ezcurra, E. (1997). Differentiation diversity of Argentine cacti and its relationship to environmental factors. *Journal of Vegetation Science*, **8**, 547–558.

Naranjo, S., Carballo, J. L. & García-Gómez, J. C. (1998). Towards a knowledge of marine boundaries using ascidians as indicators: characterizing transition zones for species distribution along Atlantic-Mediterranean shores. *Biological Journal of the Linnean Society*, **64**, 151–177.

Nekola, J. C. & White, P. S. (1999). The distance decay of similarity in biogeography and ecology. *Journal of Biogeography*, **26**, 867–878.

Ney-Nifle, M. & Mangel, M. (1999). Species-area curves based on geographic range and occupancy. *Journal of Theoretical Biology*, **196**, 327–342.

Novotny, V. & Weiblen, G. D. (2005). From communities to continents: beta diversity of herbivorous insects. *Annales Zoologici Fennici*, **42**, 463–475.

Økland, R. H., Eliertsen, O. & Økland, T. (1990). On the relationship between sample plot size and beta diversity in boreal coniferous forests. *Vegetatio*, **87**, 187–192.

Okuda, T., Noda, T., Yamamoto, T., Ito, N. & Nakaoka, M. (2004). Latitudinal gradient of species diversity: multi-scale variability in rocky intertidal sessile assemblages along the Northwestern Pacific coast. *Population Ecology*, **46**, 159–170.

Oliver, I., Beattie, A. J. & York, A. (1998). Spatial fidelity of plant, vertebrate, and invertebrate assemblages in multiple-use forest in eastern Australia. *Conservation Biology*, **12**, 822–835.

Ostling, A., Harte, J., Green, J. L. & Kinzig, A. P. (2004). Self-similarity, the power law form of the species-area relationship, and a probability rule: a reply to Maddux. *American Naturalist*, **163**, 627–633.

Palmer, M. W. & White, P. S. (1994). Scale dependence and the species-area relationship. *American Naturalist*, **144**, 717–740.

Pastor, J., Downing, A. & Erickson, H. E. (1996). Species-area curves and diversity-productivity relationships in beaver meadows of Voyageurs National Park, Minnesota, USA. *Oikos*, **77**, 399–406.

Pélissier, R., Couteron, P., Dray, S. & Sabatier, D. (2003). Consistency between ordination techniques and diversity measurements: two strategies for species occurrence data. *Ecology*, **84**, 242–251.

Pharo, E. J., Beattie, A. J. & Binns, D. (1999). Vascular plant diversity as a surrogate for bryophyte and lichen diversity. *Conservation Biology*, **13**, 282–292.

Pimm, S. L. & Brown, J. H. (2004). Domains of diversity. *Science*, **304**, 831–833.

Plotkin, J. B. & Muller-Landau, H. C. (2002). Sampling the species composition of a landscape. *Ecology*, **83**, 3344–3356.

Plotkin, J. B., Potts, M. D., Leslie, N., Manokaran, N., LaFrankie, J. & Ashton, P. S. (2000). Species-area curves, spatial aggregation, and habitat specialization in tropical forests. *Journal of Theoretical Biology*, **207**, 81–99.

Poynton, J. C. & Boycott, R. C. (1996). Species turnover between Afromontane and eastern African lowland faunas: patterns shown by amphibians. *Journal of Biogeography*, **23**, 669–680.

Price, A. R. G., Keeling, M. J. & O'Callaghan, C. J. (1999). Ocean-scale patterns of 'biodiversity' of Atlantic asteroids determined from taxonomic distinctness and other measures. *Biological Journal of the Linnean Society*, **66**, 187–203.

Qian, H., Ricklefs, R. E. & White, P. S. (2005). Beta diversity of angiosperms in temperate floras of eastern Asia and eastern North America. *Ecology Letters*, **8**, 15–22.

Ricklefs, R. E. (1987). Community diversity: relative roles of local and regional processes. *Science*, **235**, 167–171.

Ricklefs, R. E. (2004). A comprehensive framework for global patterns in biodiversity. *Ecology Letters*, **7**, 1–15.

Ricklefs, R. E. & Lau, M. (1980). Bias and dispersion of overlap indices: results of some Monte Carlo simulations. *Ecology*, **61**, 1019–1024.

Rivadeneira, M. M., Fernández, M. & Navarrete, S. A. (2002). Latitudinal trends of species diversity in rocky intertidal herbivore assemblages: spatial scale and the relationship between local and regional species richness. *Marine Ecology Progress Series*, **245**, 123–131.

Rodríguez, P. & Arita, H. T. (2004). Beta diversity and latitude in North American mammals: testing the hypothesis of covariation. *Ecography*, **27**, 547–556.

Rosenzweig, M. L. (1995). *Species Diversity in Space and Time*. Cambridge: Cambridge University Press.

Routledge, R. D. (1977). On Whittaker's components of diversity. *Ecology*, **58**, 1120–1127.

Ruggiero, A., Lawton, J. H. & Blackburn, T. M. (1998). The geographic ranges of mammalian species in South America: spatial patterns in environmental resistance and anisotropy. *Journal of Biogeography*, **25**, 1093–1103.

Scheiner, S. M. & Rey-Benayas, J. M. (1994). Global patterns of plant diversity. *Evolutionary Ecology*, **8**, 331–347.

Schluter, D. & Ricklefs, R. E. (1993). Species diversity: an introduction to the problem. In *Species Diversity in Ecological Communities: Historical and Geographical Perspectives*, ed. R. E. Ricklefs & D. Schluter, pp. 1–12. Chicago: Chicago University Press.

Selmi, S. & Boulinier, T. (2004). Distribution-abundance relationship for passerines breeding in Tunisian oases: test of the sampling hypothesis. *Oecologia*, **139**, 440–445.

Simpson, G. G. (1943). Mammals and the nature of continents. *American Journal of Science*, **241**, 1–31.

Šizling, A. L. & Storch, D. (2004). Power-law species-area relationships and self-similar species distributions within finite areas. *Ecology Letters*, **7**, 60–68.

Sørensen, T. A. (1948). A method of establishing groups of equal amplitude in plant sociology based on similarity of species content, and its application to analyses of the vegetation on Danish commons. *Kongelige Danske Videnskabernes Selskabs Biologiske Skrifter*, **5**, 1–34.

Southwood, T. R. E., Brown, V. K. & Reeder, P. M. (1979). The relationships of plant and insect diversities in succession. *Biological Journal of the Linnean Society*, **12**, 327–348.

Srivastava, D. S. (1999). Using local-regional richness plots to test for species saturation: pitfalls and potentials. *Journal of Animal Ecology*, **68**, 1–16.

Srivastava, D. S. & Lawton, J. H. (1998). Why more productive sites have more species, an experimental test of theory using tree-hole communities. *American Naturalist*, **152**, 510–529.

Stevens, G. C. (1989). The latitudinal gradient in geographical range: how so many species coexist in the tropics. *American Naturalist*, **133**, 240–256.

Stevens, R. D. & Willig, M. R. (2002). Geographical ecology at the community level: perspectives on the diversity of New World bats. *Ecology*, **83**, 545–560.

Storch, D., Evans, K. L. & Gaston, K. J. (2005). The species-area-energy relationship. *Ecology Letters*, **8**, 487–492.

Summerville, K. S., Boulware, M. J., Veech, J. A. & Crist, T. O. (2003a). Spatial variation in species diversity and composition of forest Lepidoptera in eastern deciduous forests of North America. *Conservation Biology*, **17**, 1045–1057.

Summerville, K. S., Crist, T. O., Kahn, J. K. & Gering, J. C. (2003b). Community structure of arboreal caterpillars within and among four tree species of the eastern deciduous forest. *Ecological Entomology*, **28**, 747–757.

Sweeney, B. A. & Cook, J. E. (2001). A landscape-level assessment of understorey diversity in upland forests of North-Central Wisconsin, USA. *Landscape Ecology*, **16**, 55–69.

Tuomisto, H., Ruokolainen, K. & Yli-Haila, M. (2003). Dispersal, environment, and floristic variation of western Amazonian forests. *Science*, **299**, 241–244.

Turner, J. R. G., Lennon, J. J. & Lawrenson, J. A. (1988). British bird distributions and the energy theory. *Nature*, **335**, 539–541.

Ulrich, W. & Buszko, J. (2003). Self-similarity and the species-area relation of Polish butterflies. *Basic and Applied Ecology*, **4**, 263–270.

van Rensburg, B. J., Koleff, P., Gaston, K. J. & Chown, S. L. (2004). Spatial congruence of ecological transition at the regional scale in South Africa. *Journal of Biogeography*, **31**, 843–854.

Vázquez, D. P. & Stevens, R. D. (2004). The latitudinal gradient in niche breadth: concepts and evidence. *American Naturalist*, **164**, E1–E19.

Veech, J. A., Summerville, K. S., Crist, T. O. & Gering, J. C. (2002). The additive partitioning of species diversity: recent revival of an old idea. *Oikos*, **99**, 3–9.

Veech, J. A., Crist, T. O. & Summerville, K. S. (2003). Intraspecific aggregation decreases local species diversity of arthropods. *Ecology*, **84**, 3376–3383.

Vellend, M. (2001). Do commonly used indices of β-diversity measure species turnover? *Journal of Vegetation Science*, **12**, 545–552.

Vormisto, J., Svenning, J-C., Hall, P. & Balslev, H. (2004). Diversity and dominance in palm (Arecaceae) communities in *terra firme* forests in the western Amazon basin. *Journal of Ecology*, **92**, 577–588.

Wagner, H. H., Wildi, O. & Ewald, K. C. (2000). Additive partitioning of plant species diversity in an agricultural mosaic landscape. *Landscape Ecology*, **15**, 219–227.

Weiher, E. & Boylen, C. W. (1994). Patterns and prediction of α and β diversity of aquatic plants in Adirondack (New York) lakes. *Canadian Journal of Botany*, **72**, 1797–1804.

Whittaker, R. H. (1960). Vegetation of the Siskiyou mountains, Oregon and California. *Ecological Monographs*, **30**, 279–338.

Whittaker, R. H. (1972). Evolution and measurement of species diversity. *Taxon*, **21**, 213–251.

Whittaker, R. J., Willis, K. J. & Field, R. (2001). Scale and species richness: towards a general, hierarchical theory of species diversity. *Journal of Biogeography*, **28**, 453–470.

Williams, P. H. (1996). Mapping variations in the strength and breadth of biogeographic transition zones using species turnover. *Proceedings of the Royal Society of London, Series B*, **263**, 579–588.

Williams, S. E., Marsh, H. & Winter, J. (2002). Spatial scale, species diversity, and habitat structure: small mammals in Australian tropical rain forest. *Ecology*, **83**, 1317–1329.

Willig, M. R. & Gannon, M. R. (1997). Gradients of species density and turnover in marsupials: a hemispheric perspective. *Journal of Mammalogy*, **78**, 756–765.

Willig, M. R. & Sandlin, E. A. (1991). Gradients of species density and species turnover in New World bats: a comparison of quadrat and band methodologies. In *Latin American Mammalogy: History, Biodiversity and Conservation*, ed. M. A. Mares & D. J. Schmidly, pp. 81–96. University of Oklahoma Press.

Willig, M. R., Kaufman, D. M. & Stevens, R. D. (2003). Latitudinal gradients of biodiversity: pattern, process, scale, and synthesis. *Annual Review of Ecology, Evolution and Systematics*, **34**, 273–309.

Wilson, M. V. & Shmida, A. (1984). Measuring beta diversity with presence-absence data. *Journal of Ecology*, **72**, 1055–1064.

Wolda, H. (1981). Similarity indices, sample size and diversity. *Oecologia*, **50**, 296–302.

Worthen, W. B. (1996). Community composition and nested-subset analysis: basic descriptors for community ecology. *Oikos*, **76**, 417–426.

Wright, D. H. (1983). Species-energy theory, an extension of species-area theory. *Oikos*, **41**, 496–506.

Wright, D. H. & Reeves, J. H. (1992). On the meaning and measurement of nestedness of species assemblages. *Oecologia*, **92**, 416–428.

# PART III

# Scaling of biological diversity with energy and the latitudinal biodiversity gradient

CHAPTER ELEVEN

# Climate and diversity: the role of history

ANDREW CLARKE

*British Antarctic Survey*

## Introduction

It has been known for over two centuries that the diversity of land plants, in the
familiar sense of species richness, is not distributed evenly over the surface of
the earth (von Humboldt, 1808). Similar patterns were soon established for
terrestrial animals (Wallace, 1876) but it was a long time before our knowledge
of marine organisms was sufficient to determine large-scale biogeographic
patterns in the sea. Although humans had long exploited the nearshore and
continental shelf seas for food and other resources, it was not until the pioneer-
ing oceanographic voyages of the late nineteenth and early twentieth century
that we began to determine similar global patterns of marine biogeography
(Angel, 1994, 1997). We now recognize that, as a broad generalization, diversity
on land and in the sea attains its highest values in the tropics and is lowest at the
poles, with temperate regions often intermediate (Gaston, 2000; Chown &
Gaston, 2000).

Although these global scale (macroecological) patterns in diversity are dramatic, we still lack an agreed explanation for their cause. We can correlate these
patterns with a range of environmental variables but ecology based solely on
correlations is incomplete. We might be able to use such correlations to make
predictions (Peters, 1983, 1991) but predictions without an underlying mechanistic understanding have limited usefulness because we lack knowledge of the
conditions under which those predictions might break down. Correlations are
thus a necessary but incomplete tool for obtaining a full understanding; however, in attempting to understand macroecological patterns of diversity, correlations are where we have to start.

The early naturalists identified the factors they believed to be driving speciation and extinction, and thus diversity. In the famous final paragraph of the
*Origin of Species*, Darwin (1859) draws a vivid picture of how competitive interactions lead to a struggle for existence and thereby selection for improved
phenotype. Here Darwin was focusing on ecological interactions on a local
scale, but elsewhere in the *Origin* he explicitly recognized a role for occasional
climatic extremes in limiting the overall number of species through extinction.
At about the same time Wallace (1876) had identified changes in sea level

*Scaling Biodiversity*, ed. David Storch, Pablo A. Marquet and James H. Brown. Published by Cambridge
University Press. © Cambridge University Press 2007.

driving vicariant speciation as an important factor in the high diversity he had observed in the Indo-West Pacific, Hooker had speculated in a letter to Darwin that fragmentation of a great southern continent might explain the disjunct distributions of plants such as *Nothofagus*, and Gulick (1872) had demonstrated the importance of vicariance in his seminal study of land snails in Hawaii. More than a century later we are still debating the mechanism(s) of speciation, but these early studies highlight two themes that remain important: the impact of climate on diversity through speciation and extinction, and the importance of spatial scale.

In this contribution I will examine the links between climate and diversity, and then set these in the context of spatial and temporal scale. I will concentrate in particular on processes taking place on timescales longer than the average generation time of the organisms involved. This covers a wide range of characteristic timescales, from moderate to the very long, but for convenience I will group them under the somewhat loose term of "history".

## Climate and diversity

Notions of the favorableness of climate as a factor driving diversity go back to the earliest naturalists, and temperature or broader climate-related factors have remained one of the favored explanations for global patterns of diversity. Although many of these hypotheses are couched in terms of energy, they differ in the extent to which a physical mechanism is described, and also in the nature of what is meant by energy.

### Temperature or energy?

The literature discussing the relationship between diversity and energy encompasses a number of different meanings of "energy". These may be summarized as follows:

1. Light, or more specifically photosynthetically active radiation (PAR), which is the fraction of the visible spectrum between 400 and 700 nm.
2. Temperature *sensu stricto*, or in combination with other factors that determine climate.
3. Gibbs free energy released from reduced organic compounds when they are oxidized during intermediary metabolism.

These are three quite distinct forms of energy, and confusion between them has led to a lack of clarity in the ecological debate over the role of energy in diversity (Wright, Currie & Maurer, 1993). Things are not helped by our inability to define energy other than as the ability to do work, but clear distinction needs to be maintained between thermal energy, light energy (photon flux) and chemical energy when discussing patterns of diversity. Allen, Gillooly and Brown (this volume) group light and temperature together under the term kinetic energy but I believe it is important to distinguish between electromagnetic and thermal energy in an ecological context. These distinctions are discussed in detail by Clarke and Gaston (2006).

Plants require light for photosynthesis. However, if sunlight were the only factor involved, plant diversity would be distributed far more evenly across the globe than we observe. Terrestrial plant diversity does show a classic symmetrical distribution about the equator at family level, albeit with very low values in desert areas (Francis & Currie, 2003), but at the species level angiosperm diversity is far more heterogeneous (Barthlott, Lauer & Placke, 1996; Kier et al., 2005).

The reason that patterns of terrestrial plant diversity do not map directly onto the global distribution of received solar energy is that for a plant to make use of the light it receives, it also needs water. In addition to providing the electron needed for photosynthesis, water is the solvent for biochemistry and is involved as reactant or product in all the major classes of chemical reaction that comprise physiology. Furthermore, it is movement of water that allows the plant to absorb nutrients and to distribute materials within its body. Plants transpire between 50% and 80% of the water they absorb, but typically utilize only ~0.2% of the incident light energy, so water availability is critical (Öpik & Rolfe, 2005).

Given the dependence of plant physiology on both solar energy and water availability, it is not surprising that many studies have documented strong correlations between terrestrial angiosperm plant diversity and climatic variables involving water. Currie (1991) and Francis and Currie (2003) have demonstrated strong correlations between angiosperm diversity and potential evapotranspiration (PET), a climate-related variable which involves temperature and atmospheric humidity. PET is a measure of the ability of the atmosphere to remove water from a plant through evaporation and transpiration, assuming no control on water supply. Actual evapotranspiration (AET) is the quantity of water actually removed; the difference between PET and AET thus reflects the availability of water to the plant. PET requires energy to drive the evaporation process, and much of this comes from the sun (with the wind influence on eddy diffusion also being important). Temperature affects PET through its influence on atmospheric relative humidity.

Whereas it is clear that habitats with freely available water and a warm temperature could support a larger biomass or abundance of plants, it is by no means clear how this translates to a higher plant diversity. The most frequent explanation is that the larger population size protects the species against stochastic extinction risk (the *more individuals hypothesis*), but other explanations have been suggested and none has unequivocal support (for a recent thorough review of this topic see Evans, Warren & Gaston, 2004). The widespread and strong correlation between climate and terrestrial plant diversity is thus underpinned by two quite distinct mechanisms: favorable conditions for plant production result in higher biomass and usually greater abundance, and this higher abundance is in turn distributed among more species.

## Higher trophic levels

The higher diversity of plants in warmer habitats with freely available water is almost universally accompanied by higher diversities at higher trophic levels. The explanation here is sometimes referred to as the *trophic cascade hypothesis* (Hawkins *et al.*, 2003, provide a succinct description of the history of this concept). The hypothesis is that herbivore diversity is limited by herbivore abundance, itself set by primary production (through the energy available to a herbivore from its food), and so on up the food chain. Limits to diversity are thus set by the amount of energy flowing through the food web (hence its alternative name of the *productivity hypothesis*; Wright *et al.*, 1993), though it necessarily includes elements of the *more individuals mechanism* through the link between abundance and diversity at each level of the food web. In this context, however, the energy is quite different from that which appears to be driving plant diversity. At higher levels in the food web, the energy transferred through trophic interactions is chemical energy (Gibbs free energy retained in the covalent bonds of reduced carbon compounds). Both the solar radiation used by plants and the chemical energy used by animals, be they herbivores, carnivores or parasites, may be viewed as resources which limit populations in some way, but it is important to recognize that they are fundamentally different forms of energy and they should not be confused (Clarke & Gaston, 2006; Allen *et al.*, this volume).

The distinction between light and chemical energy suggests that the mechanisms regulating plant diversity and animal diversity may be different. The two are, however, linked in that a greater diversity of plants tends to provide a more heterogeneous or structured environment, which can thereby support a greater diversity of animals (MacArthur, 1964; Pianka, 1967; Recher, 1969; Kerr & Packer, 1997), and hence to a widely observed correlation between AET and animal diversity (Currie, 1991). This linkage is primarily a feature of the terrestrial environment. In the sea, with the exception of shallow-water macroalgae and nearshore kelp forests, primary production is undertaken predominantly by a wide variety of phylogenetically distinct unicellular photoautotrophs (Quigg *et al.*, 2003), which do not influence herbivore diversity in the same way (Irigoien, Huisman & Harris, 2004). This intriguing emerging difference between the terrestrial and oceanic realms merits further investigation.

An extra factor that comes into play at consumer levels in the food web is the trophic specialization frequently evolved by herbivores or predators, or prey specializations evolved by parasites. These will provide a direct mechanistic link between one trophic level and the next, since a greater diversity of prey or hosts will support a greater variety of predators or parasites ("species are niches for species"; Whittaker, 1972). This is an ecological mechanism quite distinct from the energy-flow mechanisms discussed above.

### Climate and diversity: summary

There is a clear distinction between mechanisms influencing the diversity of primary producers, and that of herbivores and other consumers. The key energy source for plants is light and the diversity of land plants is highly correlated with water availability and temperature; however, the mechanistic link between more individuals and higher diversity remains unclear. The energy source for herbivores and other consumers is organic tissue, either plants or other animals. As with plants, a greater availability of resources allows a higher abundance, with diversity increasing as a result (again the mechanism is not entirely clear). However, at higher levels in the food web additional mechanisms come into play, such as habitat complexity or prey specialization. In the open ocean the relationship between plant and herbivore diversity appears to be quite different, though as yet we do not know why.

### Temperature and diversity

The hypotheses discussed above linking plant diversity to climate involve temperature either in isolation or in combination with other climatic variables. Because the marked global variability in atmospheric and seawater temperatures exhibits a global pattern somewhat similar to the global distribution of terrestrial and marine plant and animal diversity, ecologists have developed a number of different classes of explanation linking both plant and animal diversity to temperature. The two major of these are:

1.  Temperature affects diversity by influencing species coexistence over ecological timescales.
2.  Temperature affects diversity by determining rates of speciation and extinction over macroevolutionary timescales.

These two mechanisms differ in their characteristic time scales; they also differ in the extent to which they imply an equilibrium world.

  In considering the potential mechanisms by which temperature might influence diversity there is also an important distinction between direct and indirect effects of temperature. A direct effect is where temperature influences diversity mechanistically and without any intermediate processes being involved. A correlation between diversity and temperature is thus causal, and any change in temperature is necessarily accompanied by a change in diversity. An indirect effect is one where temperature affects some intermediate process, which in turn affects diversity. Here any relationship between temperature and diversity observed in the real world is correlative and not directly causal. These are, of course, simply extremes of what is in reality a continuum; indeed it is very difficult to conceive of a viable mechanism by which temperature could affect diversity directly (although such relationships are not infrequently inferred from correlations). The distinction is, however, a valuable one when considering the various theories linking organismal diversity to environmental temperature.

## Temperature and diversity: ecological time scales

Any hypothesis that temperature controls diversity directly (that is, mechanistically) leads to the simple and clear prediction that diversity will necessarily be higher where temperatures are warmer. This matches the intuitive feeling that warmer habitats are easier places to make a living than colder ones, and hence more species live there; this idea has been summarized succinctly by Currie (1991) as "benign conditions permit more species".

It may be true that the tropics are more amenable for endotherms in that a reduced differential between ambient and internal temperature will reduce the physiological workload involved in temperature regulation, and hence might be viewed as rendering warmer climes more amenable. Many mammals and bird groups do indeed tend to be more speciose in the tropics. An explanation based on apparently benign conditions promoting diversity in some way is, however, simplistic in that it ignores any role for structural, physiological or behavioral mechanisms for reducing the cost of maintaining a constant internal body temperature by shifting the thermoneutral zone. Lovegrove (2000, 2003) has examined biogeographical patterns in mammalian resting metabolism, and demonstrated clear differences between habitats and zoogeographical zones. These differences were, however, fairly small and confined to some groups.

The vast majority of organisms, of course, are not endotherms, and for these such anthropocentric judgments are entirely misplaced. There is as yet no compelling evidence that a polar ectotherm is any more physiologically stressed or disadvantaged than a tropical one, although evolutionary adaptation to a particular temperature does have powerful ecological consequences (Clarke, 2003). In particular Clarke and Johnston (1999) showed that at higher temperatures there were a larger range of metabolic niches available, with more active lifestyles possible in warmer waters. Interestingly, Anderson and Jetz (2005) have recently shown something similar for endotherms, although here it is lifestyles involving lower field metabolic rates that appear in warmer environments.

What is not clear is precisely how temperature might regulate diversity directly. Clearly particular habitats might set specific physiological challenges that only certain groups of organisms could meet. Examples might be polar regions with shallow permafrost, cold temperate regions with regular winter frosts, or tropical areas with low rainfall. It might also seem intuitive that as one moves from tropics to poles, habitats somehow become tougher with increasingly fewer organisms able to tolerate the conditions. We must, however, be wary of anthropocentric judgments of perceived stress. This was recognized by Hutchinson (1959) who posed the question "if we can have one or two species of a large family adapted to the rigors of Arctic existence, why can we not have more?"

Despite these theoretical concerns ecologists have long documented strong correlations between diversity and temperature. In most areas of the world endotherms show strong clines in diversity with environmental temperature, despite a physiology which renders activity significantly independent of temperature (Fig. 11.1a). Although most traditional examples come from the terrestrial environment, similar correlations are also observed in the sea (Fig. 11.1b). These two examples emphasize that any theory linking macroecological patterns in diversity to temperature or climate must apply to both endotherms and ectotherms, despite their very different thermal ecologies.

A recent hypothesis that links biological diversity directly to temperature is that of Allen, Brown and Gillooly (2002), who argue that diversity is linked mechanistically to temperature through "the generally faster biological rates observed at higher temperatures" (Brown, Allen & Gillooly, 2003). Allen and colleagues base their argument on the energy equivalence rule of Damuth (1987), namely that the total energy flux of a population per unit area is invariant with respect to body size. This is based on the widely (but not universally) observed inverse relationship between abundance and body size. Allen et al. (2002) extend the assumption of energy equivalence by incorporating the biochemical kinetics developed within the metabolic theory of ecology (Brown et al., 2004), and predict a relationship between diversity and temperature which they test with data for a range of terrestrial, freshwater and marine taxa. This prediction is matched fairly well by the data, but Currie (this volume) has shown that the slope of the relationship is far from universal.

Several studies have suggested that the energy-equivalence rule does not apply to all communities (for example Marquet, Navarrete & Castilla, 1995; Ackerman, Bellwood & Brown, 2004), and Storch (2003) has questioned the conceptual basis of the model. Nevertheless we are left with the observation of strong correlations between diversity and temperature (Fig. 11.1), correlations which require mechanistic explanation. Allen et al. (this volume) have recently recast their hypothesis and in doing so make a distinction between the different roles played by thermal and chemical energy in influencing diversity. This revised hypothesis abandons the dependence on energy equivalence, and provides a conceptual model linking the more individuals mechanism with theories relating evolutionary rate to temperature.

(a)

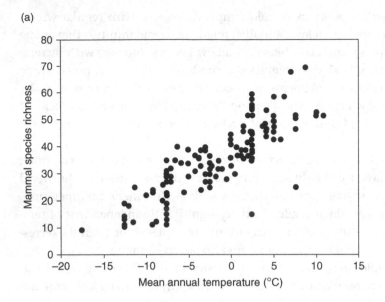

(b)

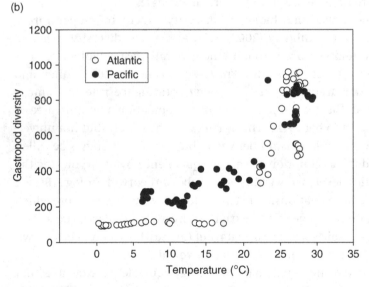

**Figure 11.1** Correlations between animal diversity and environmental temperature. (a) Mammal diversity and temperature in Canadian mammals (redrawn from data in Kerr & Parker, 1997). (b) Gastropod mollusc diversity and seawater temperature for North American continental shelves (redrawn from data in Roy *et al.*, 1998).

## Temperature, speciation and extinction: the evolutionary timescale

Many hypotheses postulating a direct influence of temperature on diversity carry the implicit assumption that we live in an equilibrium world: temperature sets limits to maximum diversity through its absolute value (or perhaps its seasonal variability), and organisms have diversified until those limits are reached and the habitats saturated. This explanation is not convincing theoretically in the simple form described, and its predictions are not matched by observation.

An alternative explanation which has long attracted attention is that climate, or more specifically temperature, influences the rates of speciation and extinction. In a nonequilibrium world, where the process of diversification in colder regions is slower and has not proceeded as far as it has in tropical regions, this would result in a latitudinal diversity cline. Equilibrium explanations are, however, also possible. Rosenzweig (1995) has proposed a simple model whereby absolute speciation and extinction rates are dependent on standing diversity but also vary with area, such that in the larger tropics speciation is more rapid and extinction slower than in the less widespread subtropics. This is proposed as a species–area effect, which results in a higher standing diversity in the warmer tropics (because these are more extensive). Anyway, species richness reaches a steady-state value when speciation and extinction rates are equal, and the resultant steady-state diversity is correlated with temperature if speciation rate is correlated with it. The neutral model of Hubbell (2001) also provides a mechanism by which speciation and extinction dynamics can lead to differences in standing diversity.

These explanations beg the question of why speciation rates might be faster at higher temperatures. Two possible mechanisms that have attracted considerable attention are temperature-related variations in mutation rate, and generation time. Martin (1995) suggested that the increased metabolic rate in ectotherms at higher temperatures might lead to an enhanced rate of mutation through increased free radical damage. Data to test this are hard to acquire and Held (2001) could find no evidence for a reduced rate of molecular substitutions in polar marine ectotherms. Gillooly et al. (2005) have recently proposed that a significant proportion of the variation in the rate of nucleotide substitution in organisms can be explained by the joint influence of body size and temperature on metabolic rate. The predictions of this model are well matched by data for the mitochondrial genome but data from the nuclear genome were more equivocal. Allen et al. (this volume) have formalized the assumption of a temperature-related generation of molecular evolution into a quantitative model of the generation of diversity. When integrated with neutral biodiversity theory, and simplifying assumptions concerning energy flow through food webs, this model predicts variation in diversity with temperature that broadly matches observation.

Considerable attention has also been directed at the possibility that generation time might influence diversification rate (Marzluff & Dial, 1991). Since generation time tends to be shorter in small organisms and among ectotherms at higher temperatures, this hypothesis leads to very specific predictions. Careful tests of these two predictions have, however, yielded mixed results to date (Cardillo, 1999; Bromham, 2002; Bromham & Cardillo, 2003).

Diversification rates are difficult to estimate, though Willis and Yule (1922) pioneered the idea that taxonomic structure might provide a guide to diversification rate. Working principally with plants, they examined the frequency distribution of subtaxa per taxon (species per genus, genera per family and so on) and concluded that these tended to exhibit a pattern Willis (1922) called a "hollow curve". Furthermore the shape of this curve would be different in slowly diversifying and rapidly diversifying clades. Such a conclusion, of course, relies on the assumption that the taxonomy in question reflects the phylogenetic history of the clade accurately, and some workers (e.g. Walters, 1986) regard taxonomy as an entirely artificial construct with no meaningful evolutionary content at all. Nee (2004) has placed Willis' arguments on a more formal mathematical footing, though as yet the technique has not been able to indicate significant differences in diversification rates with latitude. More recently Goldberg et al. (2005) have developed a dynamical model involving speciation, extinction and dispersal to allow direct testing of historical hypotheses.

Recent molecular studies of plants (e.g. that of Wright, Gray & Gardner, 2003 on *Mearnsia*) have suggested that greater "biological energy" (by which in this context is meant a higher mean annual temperature) available at low latitudes drives more rapid diversification. Other explanations are, however, possible (Pawar, 2005; Brown & Pauly, 2005) and the labile nature of diversification rates among the major lineages of flowering plants likely reflects a highly complex relationship with environmental factors (Davies et al., 2004).

An alternative approach to test for any relationship between diversification rate and latitude is to use the fossil record. Crame and Clarke (1997) used the exponential lineage diversification model discussed by Nee and could find no significant difference in the diversification rate of tropical and polar families of gastropods. In contrast, Flessa and Jablonski (1996) examined the rate of turnover of whole bivalve faunas and showed that tropical faunas turned over more rapidly. Variation between different clades is, however, high and this suggests a range of factors at work in determining speciation rate. Recently Buzas, Collins and Culver (2002) reported higher diversification rates in tropical than temperate foraminifera in the Cenozoic, though these data are not directly comparable with other studies because the authors used a different measure of diversification from the more traditional paleoecological studies (namely proportional increase in diversity through time as measured by Fisher's alpha for the entire fossil community at a given location, rather than absolute or *per species* diversification rate).

Speciation is, however, only one aspect of diversity. Diversity is the net product of speciation and extinction, and the balance between these two processes is integral to many of the theoretical approaches to equilibrium diversity. Unfortunately extinction rates are difficult to estimate, and we currently lack a complete theory of extinction in ecological or evolutionary terms. Paleobiological studies can demonstrate correlations between extinction

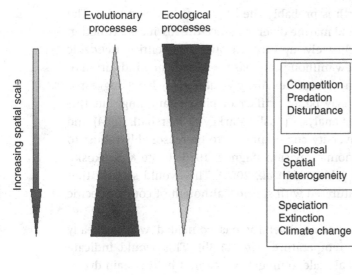

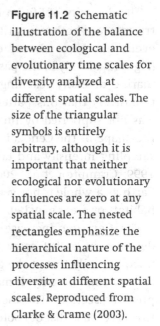

Evolutionary processes    Ecological processes

Increasing spatial scale

Competition
Predation
Disturbance

Dispersal
Spatial
heterogeneity

Speciation
Extinction
Climate change

**Figure 11.2** Schematic illustration of the balance between ecological and evolutionary time scales for diversity analyzed at different spatial scales. The size of the triangular symbols is entirely arbitrary, although it is important that neither ecological nor evolutionary influences are zero at any spatial scale. The nested rectangles emphasize the hierarchical nature of the processes influencing diversity at different spatial scales. Reproduced from Clarke & Crame (2003).

intensity in particular taxa and factors such as geographical range, larval type or feeding mode. Very few studies, however, have been able to demonstrate any clear latitudinal signals (for one example see Smith & Jeffrey, 1998). Furthermore many of these studies have been carried out using data from mass extinction events, which may represent different processes from normal or background extinction. However, the spectacular increase in the diversity of marine invertebrates during the Cenozoic does provide a powerful insight into those factors influencing diversification, and brings into sharp focus the importance of historical processes in shaping the global patterns of diversity we see today.

## The role of history

It has long been recognized that spatial and temporal scales of variability are closely linked in physical environmental processes (Stommel, 1963; Steele, 1985). This is also true for biological and ecological processes, although here there are important differences between the marine and terrestrial environments (Myers, 1994; Clarke & Crame, 2003). The importance of these relationships is in the shift in the balance between ecological and evolutionary processes with increasing spatial scale (Fig. 11.2). To understand patterns on a global scale we therefore cannot ignore the role of evolutionary processes operating over long timescales: history is important.

The diversity of life on Earth is probably the highest it has ever been. The trajectory of both terrestrial and marine diversity since the K/T mass extinction event has been almost exclusively upward through the entire Cenozoic (Fig. 11.3a). Only in the past few million years has there been any indication of marine diversity reaching an asymptote. Alroy *et al.* (2001) have suggested tentatively that this pattern may be an artifact of biased sampling, but this was not supported by further analysis (Bush, Markey & Marshall, 2004) and the shape of the Cenozoic diversity curve appears to be reasonably robust to sampling intensity and taxonomic revision (Signor, 1985; Foote & Sepkoski, 1999; Crampton *et al.*, 2003; Jablonski *et al.*, 2003). This would suggest that Earth as a whole is not yet saturated with species (although of course specific habitats or areas may be).

The Cenozoic increase in marine diversity has coincided with a steady decrease in global seawater temperature (Fig. 11.3b). This would indicate unequivocally that at the global scale, temperature cannot be the main driver for standing diversity. It may, however, drive the process of diversification (see previous section). The most thorough study of rates of diversification in the fossil record is that of Foote (2005). Data for the Cenozoic show that there was a peak of net diversification immediately following the K/T extinction event (Fig. 11.3c). This pulse was associated with a period of history when the global ocean temperature was warmer than today, and has been followed by a slowing of diversification and a global ocean cooling. There is, however, no significant correlation between *per species* net diversification rate and mean global seawater temperature, averaged per stratigraphic interval, for the period since the Lower Eocene (the period for which suitable paleotemperature data are available) (Pearson $r = 0.479$, $P > 0.2$, $n = 9$). The *per species* rate of origination of new taxa is, however, significantly correlated with mean temperature (Pearson $r = 0.753$, $P < 0.05$), whereas *per species* extinction rate is not (Pearson $r = 0.551$, $P > 0.1$). The shape of the time-course of post-K/T origination (Fig. 11.3c) makes it difficult to be sure the relationship with temperature is causal rather than being related primarily to the internal dynamics of diversification following a mass extinction event. The fossil record thus shows clearly that there is no simple relationship between temperature and diversity, but this is an important area for further testing of ideas relating diversification to environmental temperature.

From the viewpoint of what paleontologists call deep time, we live in an unusual world. Latitudinal clines in climate as extreme as those we see today are not typical of the Phanerozoic as a whole. Taking just the Cenozoic, diversity has risen significantly since the K/T extinction (Fig. 11.3a), and detailed work with molluscan faunas has shown that the present strong latitudinal diversity cline is a relatively recent feature (Crame & Clarke, 1997; Crame, 2001). Bambach (1977) showed that the Cenozoic increase in marine diversity involves marked diversification within provinces, and Crame (2001) has shown that in

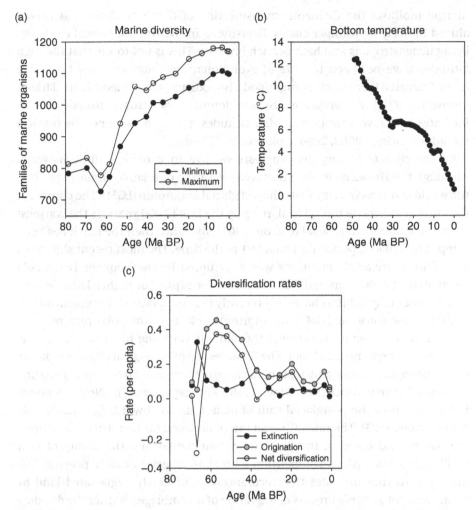

**Figure 11.3** Marine diversity and temperature during the Cenozoic. (a) Marine diversity during the Cenozoic: data from the Fossil II database (courtesy Mike Benton). Data are plotted at family level and both maximum and minimum estimates of family diversity are plotted. (b) Cenozoic paleotemperatures for the Southern Ocean determined from Mg/Ca ratios in the skeletons of foraminifera (Lear, Elderfield & Wilson, 2000). This paleotemperature proxy avoids the difficulties associated with glaciation which beset the more widely used oxygen isotope proxy. Comparison with the diversity curve (a) reveals the inverse relationship through time of marine diversity and global seawater temperature. (c) Origination and extinction rates for marine taxa since the Late Eocene (the period for which Mg/Ca paleotemperature data are available) (Foote, 2005). Data are calculated as *per species* rates averaged over stratigraphic intervals, and plotted as a function of the mean absolute date for that interval.

marine molluscs the Cenozoic intensification of diversity clines was driven almost entirely by younger clades diversifying in the tropics, typical examples being neogastropods and heteroconch bivalves. This is not to say that the high latitudes have not been the site of evolutionary novelty, as many taxa have indeed radiated there, such as amphipods, isopods and some teleost fish (Clarke & Johnston, 2003). Nevertheless the development of strong diversity clines indicates that diversification at high latitudes has been swamped by tropical radiations (Briggs, 2003, 2004; Goldberg *et al.*, 2005).

Recent climate history also suggests we live in a nonequilibrium world. Although the Holocene is often portrayed as a time of relative climate stability, the world is still recovering from the last glacial maximum (LGM). The climate of the current Holocene interglacial, roughly the last 12 000 years, is the warmest since the Eemian interglacial of about 130 ka BP. Since then the Earth has been gripped by a glacial period for about 90% of the time. The most recent shift from glacial to interglacial conditions was interrupted by the Younger Dryas cold event about 11 000 years ago, but was otherwise rapid. For higher latitudes this means that many habitats have only recently become available for colonization, with the time since the LGM being shorter the closer to the polar regions.

The retreat of the ice sheets and the climatic warming had dramatic consequences for the terrestrial biota. The fossil record of ecological change is particularly good for plants and insects, although there are also detailed marine records of faunal shifts (Valentine, 1966). Extensive work in North America has documented the postglacial shift of plant taxa northwards in considerable detail (Gates, 1993). The rate of spread varied between taxa, and depended upon the nature and speed of the dispersal of propagules and the ability of new seedlings to establish in competition with those species already present. The fossil record thus indicates that recolonization of newly deglaciated land by plants was not a simple process of migration of assemblages. Rather the development of new assemblages is stochastic, being dependent on the availability of suitable habitat, dispersal dynamics and establishment ecology (Verheyen & Hermy, 2001). Rates of postglacial range movement were typically slower than the shift of climatic conditions, although some plant taxa have recolonized at rates markedly greater than their dispersal mechanism would suggest, a feature sometimes known as Reid's paradox (Clark, 1998). Taken together these results would suggest that the vegetation of North America has not been in equilibrium with climate since the LGM (see discussion in Gates, 1993).

The important question in understanding current patterns of diversity is whether equilibrium has now been achieved. Existing plant assemblages have sufficiently well defined environmental correlates that they can be classified into clearly defined biomes, and Currie (1991) has argued that sufficient time has elapsed since the LGM for Arctic plant assemblages to have achieved equilibrium. However, a powerful role for history is indicated by the existence of diversity anomalies at a global scale (Qian & Ricklefs, 1999, 2000; Xiang *et al.*, 2004).

Patterns of marine diversity also suggest a strong role for history and a non-equilibrium world. The marine biota of the Arctic was eliminated during the last glacial event; the current fauna is thus relatively young (Dunton, 1992) and recolonization of the Arctic basin and northern North Atlantic is continuing, principally from the North Pacific (Vermeij, 1991). In contrast the shallow water fauna of the Antarctic continental shelf appears to have survived the last glacial maximum, either in refugia or by moving into deeper water (Clarke & Crame, 1989, 1992), and diversity is higher than in the younger Arctic fauna (Clarke & Johnston, 2003). The asymmetry in patterns of diversity between the northern and southern hemisphere is clear indication of an important role for history in shaping large-scale patterns of diversity (Clarke & Crame, 1997, 2003; Chown *et al.*, 2004). At northern high latitudes recolonization is continuing, and global patterns of diversity thus reflect the powerful role of glacial history. As with plants, the process of recolonization was not always related directly to dispersal potential and the existence of local refugia is strongly suggested in some cases (e.g. Marko, 2004).

Although most attention has been directed at biotic response to the most recent glacial cycle, it has long been recognized that climatic and glacial cycles driven by Milankovitch orbital variability have been a powerful mechanism driving speciation and extinction dynamics throughout much of the Cenozoic (Clarke & Crame, 1989, 1997, 2003; Crame, 2001). In the marine realm this influence is mediated principally through changes in sea level (Wallace, 1876; Palumbi, 1996, 1997), driven by variability in the size of the polar ice caps, and can thus drive evolutionary dynamics in the tropics (Crame, 2001; Clarke & Crame, 2003). On land, the principal response has been shifts in range, and the mechanism has recently been termed "orbitally forced species' range dynamics" (Dynesius & Jansson, 2000; Jansson & Dynesius, 2002). The much later development of northern hemisphere ice has also meant that range dynamics on land have tended to be a more recent feature than in the sea.

## The relative importance of climate and history in global patterns of diversity

The impact of history thus has a major confounding effect on interpretation of climate/diversity patterns, as shown diagrammatically in Fig. 11.4. Two extreme possibilities are that diversity is controlled directly by climate such that the influence of history is minimal (Fig. 11.4, left), or that diversity is independent of climatic factors and the global diversity cline is dictated purely by historical factors such as the time since glaciation (Fig. 11.4, centre). The first possibility represents an equilibrium world: no matter how long we wait, global patterns of diversity remain the same. The second possibility represents a highly

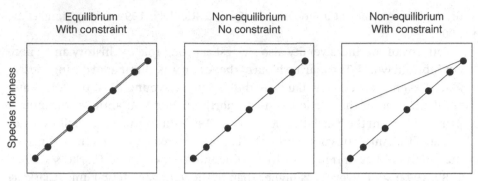

Figure 11.4 A conceptual illustration of possible relationships between climatic constraints and historical processes in determining the present relationships between diversity and climate. The line shows the maximum diversity possible in an equilibrium world, and hence describes fundamental constraints of climate on diversity. The filled circles show a hypothetical distribution of diversity across a spatial gradient, such as a latitudinal cline. Left: The pattern is dictated entirely by climatic constraints on diversity, and diversity is at equilibrium. Processes driving diversity can be deduced directly from the observed patterns. Center: The pattern is dictated entirely by historical processes. There are no constraints on diversity from climate, and global patterns reflect spatial variations in the time since glaciation or other historical factors. Right: Global patterns of diversity are influenced by both climatic constraints and historical processes. The nonequilibrium nature of the geographical distribution of diversity means that the observed patterns cannot be used to deduce the nature of environmental constraints on diversity.

nonequilibrium world. The most likely position is a combination of climatic and historical control: climate sets an upper bound on diversity (through a mechanism that is not yet entirely clear) but the short time since the last glacial maximum means that diversity has yet to reach this boundary (Fig. 11.4, right). This intermediate position would mean that the observed relationship between diversity and climate cannot give direct insight into the underlying mechanistic relationship unless the effect of history can somehow be factored out.

## Acknowledgments

I thank David Storch and Pablo Marquet for the invitation to attend the SFI/CTS Symposium in Prague, and Kevin Gaston for stimulating discussion on the possible links between climate and diversity. Several colleagues very kindly provided data for figures in this chapter: Mike Benton provided the marine diversity data for plotting Fig. 3(a), Carrie Lear the Mg/Ca paleotemperature data for plotting Fig. 3(b), and Mike Foote the diversification data plotted in Fig. 3(c). Finally it is a pleasure to thank David Storch for his careful reading of the text and for his sensitive editorial work.

# References

Ackerman, J. L., Bellwood, D. R. & Brown, J. H. (2004). The contribution of small individuals to density-body size relationships: examination of energetic equivalence in reef fishes. *Oecologia*, **139**, 568–571.

Allen, A. P., Brown, J. H. & Gilooly, J. F. (2002). Global biodiversity, biochemical kinetics, and the energy-equivalence rule. *Science*, **297**, 1545–1548.

Alroy, J., Marshall, C. R., Bambach, R. K., *et al.* (2001). Effects of sampling standardisation on estimates of Phanerozoic marine diversification. *Proceedings of the National Academy of Sciences of the United States of America*, **98**, 6261–6266.

Anderson, K. J. & Jetz, W. (2005). The broad-scale ecology of energy expenditure of endotherms. *Ecology Letters*, **8**, 310–318.

Angel, M. V. (1994). Spatial distribution of marine organisms: patterns and processes. In *Large Scale Ecology and Conservation Biology*, ed. P. J. Edwards, R. M. May & N. R. Webb, pp. 59–109. Oxford: Blackwell Scientific Publications.

Angel, M. V. (1997). Pelagic biodiversity. In *Marine Biodiversity: Causes and Consequences*, ed. R. F. G. Ormond, J. D. Gage & M. V. Angel, pp. 35–68. Cambridge: Cambridge University Press.

Bambach, R. K. (1977). Species richness in marine habitats through the Phanerozoic. *Paleobiology*, **3**, 152–167.

Barthlott, W., Lauer, W. & Placke, A. (1996). Global distribution of species diversity in vascular plants: towards a world map of phytodiversity. *Erdkunde*, **50**, 317–327.

Briggs, J. C. (2003). Marine centres of origin as evolutionary engines. *Journal of Biogeography*, **30**, 1–18.

Briggs, J. C. (2004). Older species: a rejuvenation on coral reefs. *Journal of Biogeography*, **31**, 525–530.

Bromham, L. (2002). Molecular clocks in reptiles: life history influences rate of molecular evolution. *Molecular Biology and Evolution*, **19**, 302–309.

Bromham, L. & Cardillo, M. (2003). Testing the link between the latitudinal gradient in species richness and rates of molecular evolution. *Journal of Evolutionary Biology*, **16**, 200–207.

Brown, J. H., Allen, A. P. & Gilooly, J. F. (2003). Response to heat and biodiversity (Huston). *Science*, **299**, 512–513.

Brown, J. H., Gilooly, J. F., Allen, A. P., Savage, V. M. & West, G. B. (2004). Toward a metabolic theory of ecology. *Ecology*, **85**, 1771–1789.

Brown, J. M. & Pauly, G. B. (2005). Increased rates of molecular evolution in an equatorial plant clade: an effect of environment or phylogenetic nonindependence. *Evolution*, **59**, 238–242.

Bush, A. M., Markey, M. J. & Marshall, C. R. (2004). Removing bias from diversity curves: the effects of spatially organized biodiversity on sampling-standardization. *Paleobiology*, **30**, 666–686.

Buzas, M. A., Collins, L. S. & Culver, S. J. (2002). Latitudinal difference in biodiversity caused by higher tropical rate of diversification. *Proceedings of the National Academy of Sciences of the United States of America*, **99**, 7841–7843.

Cardillo, M. (1999). Latitude and rates of diversification in birds and butterflies. *Proceedings of the Zoological Society of London, Series B*, **266**, 1221–1225.

Chown, S. L. & Gaston, K. J. (2000). Areas, cradles and museums: the latitudinal gradient in species richness. *Trends in Ecology and Evolution*, **15**, 311–315.

Chown, S. L., Sinclair, B. J., Leinas, H. P. & Gaston, K. J. (2004). Hemispheric asymmetries in biodiversity – a serious matter for ecology. *PLoS Biology*, **2**, 1701–1707.

Clark, J. S. (1998). Why trees migrate so fast: confronting theory with dispersal biology and the paleorecord. *American Naturalist*, **152**, 204–224.

Clarke, A. (2003). Costs and consequences of evolutionary temperature adaptation. *Trends in Ecology and Evolution*, **18**, 573–581.

Clarke, A. & Crame, J. A. (1989). The origin of the Southern Ocean marine fauna. In *Origins and Evolution of the Antarctic Biota*, ed. J. A. Crame, pp. 253–268. London: The Geological Society.

Clarke, A. & Crame, J. A. (1992). The Southern Ocean benthic fauna and climate change: a historical perspective. *Philosophical Transactions of the Royal Society of London, Series B*, **338**, 299–309.

Clarke, A. & Crame, J. A. (1997). Diversity, latitude and time: patterns in the shallow sea. In *Marine Biodiversity: Causes and Consequences*, ed. R. F. G. Ormond, J. D. Gage & M. V. Angel, pp. 122–147. Cambridge: Cambridge University Press.

Clarke, A. & Crame, J. A. (2003). The importance of historical processes in global patterns of diversity. In *Macroecology: Concepts and Consequences*, ed. T. M. Blackburn & K. J. Gaston, Vol. 43, pp. 130–151. Oxford: Blackwell.

Clarke, A. & Gaston, K. J. (2006). Climate, energy and diversity. *Proceedings of the Royal Society of London, Series B*, **273**, 2257–2266.

Clarke, A. & Johnston, N. M. (1999). Scaling of metabolic rate with body mass and temperature in teleost fish? *Journal of Animal Ecology*, **68**, 893–905.

Clarke, A. & Johnston, N. M. (2003). Antarctic marine benthic diversity. *Oceanography and Marine Biology: an Annual Review*, **41**, 47–114.

Crame, J. A. (2001). Taxonomic diversity gradients through geological time. *Diversity and Distributions*, **7**, 175–189.

Crame, J. A. & Clarke, A. (1997). The historical component of taxonomic diversity gradients. In *Marine Biodiversity: Causes and Consequences*, ed. R. F. G. Ormond,

J. D. Gage & M. V. Angel, pp. 258–273. Cambridge: Cambridge University Press.

Crampton, J. S., Beu, A. G., Cooper, R. A., Jones, C. M., Marshall, B. & Maxwell, P. A. (2003). Estimating the rock volume bias in paleo-biodiversity studies. *Science*, **301**, 358–360.

Currie, D. J. (1991). Energy and large-scale patterns of animal and plant species richness. *American Naturalist*, **137**, 27–49.

Damuth, J. (1987). Interspecific allometry of population density in mammals and other animals: the independence of body mass and population energy use. *Biological Journal of the Linnean Society*, **31**, 193–246.

Darwin, C. (1859). *On the Origin of Species by Means of Natural Selection*. London: John Murray.

Davies, T. J., Barraclough, T. G., Savolainen, V. & Chase, M. W. (2004). Environmental causes for plant biodiversity gradients. *Philosophical Transactions of the Royal Society of London, Series B*, **359**, 1645–1656.

Dunton, K. (1992). Arctic biogeography: the paradox of the marine benthic fauna and flora. *Trends in Ecology and Evolution*, **7**, 183–189.

Dynesius, M. & Jansson, R. (2000). Evolutionary consequences of changes in species' geographical distributions driven by Milankovitch climate oscillations. *Proceedings of the National Academy of Sciences of the United States of America*, **97**, 9115–9120.

Evans, K. L., Warren, P. H. & Gaston, K. J. (2004). Species-energy relationships at the macroecological scale: a review of the mechanisms. *Biological Reviews*, **79**, 1–25.

Flessa, K. W. & Jablonski, D. (1996). The geography of evolutionary turnover: a global analysis of extant bivalves. In *Evolutionary Paleobiology*, ed. D. Jablonski, D. H. Erwin & J. H. Lipps, pp. 376–397. Chicago: University of Chicago Press.

Foote, M. (2005). Pulsed origination and extinction in the marine realm. *Paleobiology*, **31**, 6–20.

Foote, M. & Sepkoski, J. J. (1999). Absolute measures of the completeness of the fossil record. *Nature*, **398**, 415–417.

Francis, A. P. & Currie, D. J. (2003). A globally consistent richness-climate relationship for angiosperms. *American Naturalist*, **161**, 523–536.

Gaston, K. J. (2000). Global patterns in biodiversity. *Nature*, **405**, 220–227.

Gates, D. M. (1993). *Climate Change and its Biological Consequences*. Sunderland, MA: Sinauer Associates.

Gillooly, J. F., Allen, A. P., West, G. B. & Brown, J. H. (2005). The rate of DNA evolution: effects of body size and temperature on the molecular clock. *Proceedings of the National Academy of Sciences of the United States of America*, **102**, 140–145.

Goldberg, E. E., Roy, K., Lande, R. & Jablonski, D. (2005). Diversity, endemism, and age distributions in macroevolutionary sources and sinks. *American Naturalist*, **165**, 623–633.

Gulick, J. T. (1872). On the variation of species as related to their geographical distribution, illustrated by the Achatinellinae. *Nature*, **6**, 222–224.

Hawkins, B. A., Field, R., Cornell, H. V., *et al.* (2003). Energy, water, and broad-scale geographic patterns of species richness. *Ecology*, **84**, 3105–3117.

Held, C. (2001). No evidence for slow-down of molecular substitution rates at subzero temperatures in Antarctic serolid isopods (Crustacea, Isopoda, Serolidae). *Polar Biology*, **24**, 497–501.

Hubbell, S. P. (2001). *The Unified Neutral Theory of Biodiversity and Biogeography*. Princeton: Princeton University Press.

Hutchinson, G. E. (1959). Homage to Santa Rosalia, or why are there so many kinds of animals? *American Naturalist*, **93**, 145–159.

Irigoien, X., Huisman, J. & Harris, R. P. (2004). Global biodiversity patterns of marine phytoplankton and zooplankton. *Nature*, **429**, 863–867.

Jablonski, D., Roy, K., Valentine, J. W., Price, R. M. & Anderson, P. S. (2003). The impact of the pull of the recent on the history of marine diversity. *Science*, **300**, 1133–1135.

Jansson, R. & Dynesius, M. (2002). The fate of clades in a world of recurrent climatic change: Milankovitch oscillations and evolution. *Annual Review of Ecology and Systematics*, **33**, 741–777.

Kerr, J. T. & Packer, L. (1997). Habitat heterogeneity as a determinant of mammal species richness in high-energy regions. *Nature*, **385**, 252–254.

Kier, G., Mutke, J., Dinerstein, E., *et al.* (2005). Global patterns of plant diversity and floristic knowledge. *Journal of Biogeography*, **32**, 1107–1116.

Lear, C. H., Elderfield, H. & Wilson, P. H. (2000). Cenozoic deep-sea temperatures and global ice volumes from Mg/Ca in benthic foraminiferal calcite. *Science*, **287**, 269–272.

Lovegrove, B. G. (2000). The zoogeography of mammalian basal metabolic rate. *American Naturalist*, **156**, 201–219.

Lovegrove, B. G. (2003). The influence of climate on the basal metabolic rate of small mammals: a slow-fast metabolic continuum. *Journal of Comparative Physiology B*, **173**, 87–112.

MacArthur, R. H. (1964). Environmental factors affecting bird species diversity. *American Naturalist*, **98**, 387–397.

Marko, P. B. (2004). "What's larvae got to do with it?" Disparate patterns of post-glacial population structure in two benthic marine gastropods with identical dispersal potential. *Molecular Ecology*, **13**, 597–611.

Marquet, P. A., Navarrete, S. A. & Castilla, J. C. (1995). Body size, population density and the energy-equivalence rule. *Journal of Animal Ecology*, **64**, 325–332.

Martin, A. P. (1995). Metabolic rate and directional nucleotide substitution in animal mitochondrial DNA. *Molecular Biology and Evolution*, **12**, 1124–1131.

Marzluff, J. M. & Dial, K. P. (1991). Life history correlates of taxonomic diversity. *Ecology*, **72**, 428–439.

Myers, A. A. (1994). Biogeographic patterns in shallow-water marine systems and the controlling processes at different scales. In *Aquatic Ecology: Scale, Pattern and Process*, ed. P. S. Giller, A. G. Hildrew & D. G. Raffaelli, pp. 547–574. Oxford: Blackwell Scientific Publications.

Nee, S. (2004). Extinct meets extant: simple models in palaeontology and molecular phylogenetics. *Paleobiology*, **30**, 172–178.

Öpik, H. & Rolfe, S. A. (2005). *The Physiology of Flowering Plants*. 4th edn. Cambridge: Cambridge University Press.

Palumbi, S. R. (1996). What can molecular genetics contribute to marine biogeography? An urchin's tale. *Journal of Experimental Marine Biology and Ecology*, **203**, 75–92.

Palumbi, S. R. (1997). Molecular biogeography of the Pacific. *Coral Reefs*, **16**, S47–S52.

Pawar, S. S. (2005). Geographical variation in the rate of evolution: effect of available energy or fluctuating environment. *Evolution*, **59**, 234–237.

Peters, R. H. (1983). *The Ecological Implications of Body Size*. Cambridge: Cambridge University Press.

Peters, R. H. (1991). *A Critique for Ecology*. Cambridge: Cambridge University Press.

Pianka, E. R. (1967). On lizard species diversity: North American flatland deserts. *Ecology*, **48**, 333–350.

Qian, H. & Ricklefs, R. E. (1999). A comparison of the taxonomic richness of vascular plants in China and the United States. *American Naturalist*, **154**, 160–181.

Qian, H. & Ricklefs, R. E. (2000). Large-scale processes and the Asian bias in species diversity of temperate plants. *Nature*, **407**, 180–182.

Quigg, A., Finkel, Z. V., Irwin, A. J., *et al.* (2003). The evolutionary inheritance of elemental stoichiometry in marine phytoplankton. *Nature*, **425**, 291–294.

Recher, H. F. (1969). Bird species diversity and habitat diversity in Australiia and North America. *American Naturalist*, **103**, 75–80.

Rosenzweig, M. L. (1995). *Species Diversity in Space and Time*. Cambridge: Cambridge University Press.

Roy, K., Jablonski, D., Valentine, J. W. & Rosenberg, G. (1998). Marine latitudinal diversity gradients: tests of causal hypotheses. *Proceedings of the National Academy of Sciences of the United States of America*, **95**, 3699–3702.

Signor, P. W. (1985). Real and apparent trends in species richness through time. In *Phanerozoic Diversity Patterns: Profiles in Macroevolution*, ed. J. W. Valentine, pp. 129–150. Princeton: Princeton University Press.

Smith, A. B. & Jeffrey, C. H. (1998). Selectivity of extinction among sea urchins at the end of the Cretaceous period. *Nature*, **392**, 69–71.

Steele, J. H. (1985). A comparison of terrestrial and marine ecological systems. *Nature*, **313**, 355–358.

Stommel, H. (1963). Varieties of oceanographic experience. *Science*, **139**, 572–576.

Storch, D. (2003). Comment on "global biodiversity, biochemical kinetics, and the energy-equivalence rule". *Science*, **299**, 346b.

Valentine, J. W. (1966). Numerical analysis of marine molluscan ranges on the extratropical northeastern Pacific shelf. *Limnology and Oceanography*, **11**, 198–211.

Verheyen, K. & Hermy, M. (2001). The relative importance of dispersal limitation of vascular plants in secondary forest succession in Muizen Forest, Belgium. *Journal of Ecology*, **89**, 829–840.

Vermeij, G. J. (1991). Anatomy of an invasion: the trans-Arctic interchange. *Paleobiology*, **17**, 281–307.

von Humboldt, A. (1808). *Ansichten der Natur mit wissenschaftlichen Erlauterungen*. Tübingen: J. G. Cotta.

Wallace, A. R. (1876). *The Geographical Distribution of Animals: With a Study of the Relations of Living and Extinct Faunas as Elucidating the Past Changes of the Earth's Surface*. New York: Harper.

Walters, S. M. (1986). The name of the rose: a review of ideas on the European bias in angiosperm classification. *New Phytologist*, **104**, 527–546.

Whittaker, R. H. (1972). Evolution of measurements of species diversity. *Taxon*, **21**, 213–251.

Willis, J. C. (1922). *Age and Area: A Study in Geographical Distribution and Origin of Species*. Cambridge: Cambridge University Press.

Willis, J. C. & Yule, G. U. (1922). Some statistics of evolution and geographical distribution in plants and animals, and their significance. *Nature*, **109**, 177–179.

Wright, D. H., Currie, D. J. & Maurer, B. A. (1993). Energy supply and patterns of species richness on local and regional scales. In *Species Diversity in Ecological Communities: Historical and Geographical Perspectives*, ed. R. E. Ricklefs & D. Schluter, pp. 66–74. Chicago and London: University of Chicago Press.

Wright, S. D., Gray, R. D. & Gardner, R. C. (2003). Energy and the rate of evolution: inferences from plant rDNA substitution rates in the western Pacific. *Evolution*, **57**, 2893–2898.

Xiang, Q.-Y., Zhang, W. H., Ricklefs, R. E., *et al.* (2004). Regional differences in rates of plant speciation and molecular evolution: a comparison between eastern Asia and eastern North America. *Evolution*, **58**, 2175–2184.

# CHAPTER TWELVE

# Inverse latitudinal gradients in species diversity

PAVEL KINDLMANN

*Institute of Systems Biology and Ecology,*
*Academy of Sciences of the Czech Republic, University of South Bohemia,*
*Agrocampus Rennes*

IVA SCHÖDELBAUEROVÁ

*Institute of Systems Biology and Ecology,*
*Academy of Sciences of the Czech Republic, University of South Bohemia*

ANTHONY F. G. DIXON

*University of East Anglia*

## Introduction

No single pattern of biodiversity has attracted ecologists more than the observed increase in species richness from the poles to the tropics (Pianka, 1966; Rohde, 1992; Rosenzweig & Sandlin, 1997; Gaston & Blackburn, 2000; Willig, Kaufman & Stevens, 2003; Hillebrand, 2004). An obstacle in the search for the primary cause of this latitudinal gradient is the ever-increasing number of hypotheses (Pianka, 1966; Rohde, 1992; Clarke, this volume), their interdependence (Currie, 1991; Gaston & Blackburn, 2000) and lack of rigorous falsification (Currie, Francis & Kerr, 1999; Currie, this volume). However, a general decline in species richness with latitude is commonly observed (Pielou, 1977; Colwell & Hurtt, 1994; Willig & Lyons, 1998; Colwell & Lees, 2000; Zapata, Gaston & Chown, 2003; Colwell, Rahbek & Gotelli, 2004).

Some groups of organisms, however, show an opposite trend: a strong latitudinal decline in species diversity towards the tropics. These trends have been almost neglected in the literature and little is known about their underlying ecological and evolutionary causes. Therefore, the ecological explanations proffered are usually specific to the group in question. Here an account of the most important cases of inverse latitudinal gradients is given. The existing hypotheses explaining this phenomenon are summarized and the evidence that tends to favor one of these is presented.

## Groups showing inverse latitudinal gradients
### North American breeding birds

Cook (1969) in his detailed study of gamma diversity in North American breeding birds revealed that a transect through central and eastern North

*Scaling Biodiversity*, ed. David Storch, Pablo A. Marquet and James H. Brown. Published by Cambridge University Press. © Cambridge University Press 2007.

America showed an unambiguous decrease in regional diversity with decreasing latitude within the boundaries of the United States. This decrease was most marked in deciduous forests of the eastern United States, in which regional diversity declined sharply from New England toward the southeastern United States.

### The pitcher plant mosquito

Buckley *et al.* (2003) studied geographical variation in species richness of the entire food web of invertebrates, protozoa and bacteria that inhabit the water-filled leaves (pitchers) of the purple pitcher plant, *Sarracenia purpurea* L. Species richness at the site scale (data collected from 39 undisturbed populations, randomly distributed throughout the range of *S. purpurea*, across North America) increased linearly with latitude; more species were recorded at the northern sites. Pitcher richness was *c.* 30% of the site richness and also increased linearly with latitude. A separate analysis of each taxonomic group (invertebrates, protozoa and bacteria) at the site scale showed that the increase in species richness with latitude was because of an increase in protozoan and bacterial richness; invertebrate richness exhibited no significant relationship with latitude. At the pitcher scale, the relationships between richness and latitude were slightly different: richness of all three components of the community increased with latitude and the abundance of the top predator in the system, the pitcher plant mosquito (*Wyeomyia smithii*), decreased significantly with latitude.

### Shallow-water molluscs

Molluscs are the most diverse group of ocean-shelf macrobenthos, for which good comparative taxonomic data are available. Valdovinos, Navarrete and Marquet (2003) quantified latitudinal diversity gradients of Prosobranchia, Bivalvia and Placophora, from northern Peru (10° S) to Cape Horn (55° S), in particular their relationship to temperature and shelf area, and compared their results with the trends documented for both the northwestern Atlantic and northeastern Pacific Oceans. They analyzed the diversity and distribution of 629 species of shelled molluscs, including only those known to live in waters shallower than 200 m. Strong latitudinal changes in mollusc species diversity were evident along the Peru–Chilean shelf, for all major mollusc taxa studied, especially for Prosobranchia, the most diverse group within molluscs. However, the change in species diversity was not monotonous across latitudes. Diversity of prosobranch species remained relatively low and constant around a value of 100 species/latitudinal band between 10 and 40° S, and then sharply increased to the south, reaching *c.* 300 species/band around Cape Horn. This general pattern was similar for all taxonomic groups, but stronger for shelled species inhabiting mostly hard substrates (Prosobranchia and Placophora), than for Bivalvia, which inhabit mostly soft substrates. Unlike temperature, shelf area explained a significant portion of the variance (59%) in species diversity south of the equator.

## Marine benthic algae

On the Atlantic coast of Europe, the seaweed flora shows the classical pattern, with species richness increasing towards the equator (van den Hoek, 1975). However, in temperate Pacific South America, the number of species increases between 10° S to 55° S (Santelices, 1980).

## Ichneumonids

The next unexpected decline in diversity towards the tropics is that observed in Ichneumonidae (first published by Owen & Owen, 1974), which belong to the largest insect families (Townes, 1969). The anomalous latitudinal gradient in ichneumonid diversity is a composite of separate trends in distinct lineages, some of which are more, and some less, species-rich in tropical than in temperate latitudes (Janzen, 1981; Gauld, 1986). Ichneumonid subfamilies with increasing diversity towards the tropics are usually generalists, with low potential growth rates (measured in terms of the number of eggs laid), or – if they are specialists – they attack exposed hosts. Ichneumonid subfamilies scarcer in the tropics are usually specialists, often attacking concealed hosts, and have high growth rates (Janzen, 1981; Gauld, 1986; Noyes, 1989; Askew, 1990; Gaston, 1991; Stork, 1991; Gauld, Gaston & Janzen, 1992; Hawkins, 1994).

## Aphids

Dixon *et al.* (1987) analyzed data on the area-adjusted regional species numbers of plants and aphids from 23 countries. They found a strong exponential decline in the ratio of the number of aphid to plant species, if plotted against the number of plant species. The regional species diversity of aphids was maximal at some intermediate latitudes, and declined in areas of high vegetation complexity – in the tropics. The paucity of aphids in the tropics and subtropics has been attributed to the aphids' adaptation to temperate conditions, which results in a reduced incidence of sexual reproduction in the tropics, causing reduced genetic recombination and therefore reduced speciation rate (Bodenheimer & Swirski, 1957). However, within the family Aphididae, the Aphidinae and Drepanosiphinae, which comprise 70% of modern aphids, are not restricted to a particular region, and the Greenideinae and Hormaphidinae, which comprise 7%, are restricted mostly to southern Asia and Australia (Eastop, 1977). Thus, some species from the major aphid subfamilies are endemic to the tropics and subtropics and are well adapted to the climatic conditions that prevail there (Hales, 1976;

Agarwala & Dixon, 1986). Although continuous parthenogenesis is more common in species living in the tropics and subtropics than in many temperate regions, sexual forms have been described for many of the endemic species in the tropical regions. In addition, the distribution of aphids does not appear to be restricted by the association with particular groups of plants, since most groups of vascular plants serve as hosts for aphids (Eastop, 1978); that is, at least 97% of the vascular flora of the world could potentially host aphids. Thus, because some species of aphids are able to survive and thrive in the tropics and subtropics and because their speciation is unlikely to have been limited by a lack of genetic recombination or of suitable host plants, it is difficult to understand why aphids as a group have not flourished on the rich tropical and subtropical floras.

## General explanations of the inverse latitudinal trends in species diversity

In some cases species diversity of the group in question depends more strongly on some biotic or abiotic factor (for example, energy available, abundance of a "keystone" predator) than on latitude:

1.  Southern parts of North America, for example, are considerably drier and have accordingly lower plant productivity, measured, for example, by the Normalized Difference Vegetation Index, NDVI, than more northern areas (see Hurlbert & Haskell, 2003). It is therefore not surprising that the species richness of North American breeding birds also declines towards the south, as – according to the species–energy relationship (Storch, Evans & Gaston, 2005) – there is a positive correlation between species richness and plant productivity.

2.  One possible explanation for why species richness of invertebrates, protozoa and bacteria that inhabit the pitchers of S. purpurea generally increases with latitude, is that predation plays an important "keystone" role in structuring this community (Power et al., 1996). As the abundance of the top predator, a filter-feeding mosquito, decreases, a greater number of taxa in lower trophic levels (protozoa and bacteria) were able to persist. This is supported by experimental studies on this system, which have shown that the pitcher-plant mosquito is a keystone predator regulating the species richness of protozoa and bacteria (Addicott, 1974; Cochran-Stafira & von Ende, 1998; Kneitel & Miller, 2002; Buckley et al., 2003).

3.  The inverted latitudinal pattern shown by seaweeds (Santelices, 1980) is the result of the coexistence along the coastlines of Peru and Chile of species with different geographic origins (Santelices, 1980). This region is characterized by high endemism (32.3% of the flora) and a very unequal contribution of tropical (3.4%) and sub-Antarctic (34.4%) species. The number of

tropical species decreases towards the South Pole, while the sub-Antarctic elements increase. The abundance of endemic species is relatively similar along most of the coastline, as is the abundance of the other two algal groups found there, namely the widely distributed (22.8% of the flora) and bipolar (7.1%) species.

However, sometimes the situation is more complicated and requires a more comprehensive explanation. This is especially the case for ichneumonids and aphids. Three hypotheses have been proposed:

The *"resource fragmentation hypothesis"* (RFH; Janzen & Pond, 1975; Janzen, 1981) has been used to explain the inverse latitudinal trends in species richness of Ichneumonidae. It assumes that as species richness becomes very high, the increasing number of potential host species does not support an increasing richness of parasitoid species because each of the additional potential host species is too rare to be exploited by specialist parasitoids. Below some threshold host density, parasitoids cannot find specific hosts, or cannot maintain viable population sizes over ecological time. The effect may be promoted by aspects of the lowland tropical climate: prey "bloom" of hosts that could support specialists, producing temporal fragmentation of resources (Janzen & Pond, 1975). To overcome resource fragmentation, tropical ichneumonids must be more polyphagous, or better at finding rare hosts (Janzen, 1981; Gauld & Gaston, 1994). Shaw (1994) proposed a related idea that fragmentation of hosts in the tropics affects speciation rates, so that radiations of parasitoids, particularly specialists, have not occurred in the tropics as extensively as in the temperate regions. When hosts are abundant and populations large, specialists can radiate by colonizing new hosts; smaller and more dispersed tropical populations present fewer opportunities for parasitoids to speciate in this manner. Further, predation may be more intense in tropical than in temperate ecosystems (Paine, 1966; Elton, 1973). Adult ichneumonids also suffer predation and, in the tropics, important predators such as birds, asiliid flies and dragonflies are abundant. If specialists spend more time searching for hosts, they will be more exposed to predators and thus would be more constrained than generalists in the tropics (Gauld, 1987).

The *"nasty host hypothesis"* (NHH) is based on the observations that toxicity is more common in tropical than in temperate plant communities (Levin, 1976; Coley & Aide, 1991; Basset, 1994) and that plant allelochemicals in host tissue can injure immature parasitoids (for example Duffey, Bloem & Campbell, 1986). Thus Gauld *et al.* (1992) proposed that increased toxicity, accompanied by great variety in the types of toxins, may make hosts in the tropics on average less accessible to parasitoids, leading to the observed decline in species richness. To overcome host toxicity, a parasitoid lineage will have to become more specialized. As evidence, Gauld *et al.* (1992) noted that diversity is not lower among tropical parasitoids attacking life-stages of their hosts that are not chemically well-defended, such as eggs or pupae (except of the pupae of insects that sequester plant chemicals into adulthood), or attacking insects that feed on plant tissues containing few allelochemicals, such as sap or wood. Sime and Brower (1998) suggest that for parasitoids associated with the Papilionoidea, the NHH is the most and the RFH the least likely to explain their diversity patterns. Predation hypotheses may apply to parasitoid lineages whose hosts vary in concealment from predators. However, these mechanisms do not explain why this should have a disproportionately adverse effect on parasitoid diversity relative to host diversity.

*The "common host hypothesis"* (CHH). From Dixon *et al.* (1987) and Kindlmann (1988) it follows that inverse latitudinal trends in species richness should be found in groups, in which species are characterized by five main attributes: (1) host specificity, (2) necessity to look for the host periodically, (3) random host search, (4) short time available to find the host, and (5) the species richness of the group, to which their host belongs, increases towards the tropics. Host is understood here in the commonest sense, i.e. host for a parasite, plant for an herbivore etc. Actually, because of (1) and (2), the survival of the species is vitally dependent on periodical looking for the specific host. However, because of (3) and (4), the host of such species must be "relatively common" (that is, its abundance must exceed a certain critical value) – otherwise the individuals are not able to find it, as they have only a limited time for random search (Fig. 12.1). In the tropics, only a small proportion of the host species is "relatively common", as – because of (5) – there are many potential host species in the tropics, only few of them can therefore be "relatively common" (Fig. 12.1). In a sense, the CHH is a generalization and refinement of the RFH.

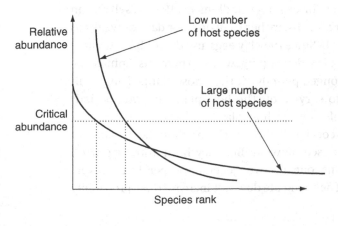

Figure 12.1 Illustration of the "common host hypothesis". Regionally present species from the host group are ranked here according to their relative cover. In communities where the total regional number of host species is large, the proportion of species whose relative cover (or abundance) exceeds the critical abundance is low.

## Testing the common host hypothesis

Aphids are an ideal group, as they satisfy five main attributes. Most aphids feed on only one or a few species of plants, or commute between two plant species, a winter host and a summer host (host-alternating aphids) – (1). Because of their enormous population growth rates, they frequently overexploit their host plants and then it is advantageous for individuals to fly off and seek hosts elsewhere – (2). Because of their small size, they have little control of the direction of their flight, and therefore they look for their host plant at random – (3). It is advantageous for aphids to have high growth rates and short generation times. This is nicely illustrated by the parthenogenesis and telescoping of generations (a female has her own granddaughter developing in her gonads), characteristic of aphids. Thus migrant aphids have only a short time to search for a host plant – (4). The species richness of plants, the group they feed on, increases towards the tropics – (5).

The subfamilies of ichneumonids scarcer in the tropics are usually specialists – (1), they are parasitoids and have to search for hosts – (2), they often attack concealed hosts, which introduces a random element into their host search – (3), they lay many eggs and therefore they do not have much time for laying each egg – (4) and the diversity of their hosts increases towards the tropics – (5). Therefore it is not surprising that the diversity of these ichneumonids declines towards the tropics.

Janzen and Pond (1975) and Janzen (1981) suggest that low host population density acts as a barrier to ichneumonid species-richness by rendering certain species too scarce to serve as a specialist's host. The common host hypothesis (CHH) suggests that besides the absolute host density the relative one could also play a role.

Psyllids can serve as a counterexample. They are similar to aphids in terms of their host specificity (Hodkinson, 1974) and ability to find their host plants (Moran, 1968; Moran & Brown, 1973). Nevertheless they are most numerous in terms of species in the tropics (see for example Hodkinson, 1986). Psyllids can live for a long time as adults – for months, rather than only for days or weeks as do aphids – so they do not satisfy (4). Since they lay eggs and do not have to meet the high food demands of embryos developing within them, as aphids do, psyllids possibly survive for prolonged periods off their host plants. Long adult life combined with the ability to survive off the host plant for long periods greatly increase the probability of finding a host plant.

A similar situation occurs in coccids. They search for their host plants at random – they are passively dispersed by wind. But they have a lower growth rate than aphids, only completing one or two generations per year (Dixon, Hemptinne & Kindlmann, 1987). Their long life does not increase their probability

**Table 12.1** *Reproductive success of orchids, measured as the percentage of flowers pollinated per plant, in various parts of the world*

| Geographic area | Nectar bearing Rewarding | | Nectarless Deceptive | |
|---|---|---|---|---|
| | % RS | (N) | % RS | (N) |
| North America | 49.3 | (11) | 19.5 | (9) |
| Europe | 63.1 | (8) | 27.7 | (29) |
| Temperate zones, southern hemisphere | 74.4 | (3) | 41.4 | (8) |
| Temperate zones of Asia | 43.0 | (3) | – | – |
| **Temperate zones** | **56.0** | **(25)** | **28.5** | **(46)** |
| **Tropics** | **24.9** | **(5)** | **11.5** | **(27)** |

Numbers of species considered are in brackets.
*Source:* Neiland & Wilcock (1998)

of finding a host plant, as is the case for psyllids. However, due to their low growth rate they are less likely to overexploit their hosts. Consequently, for coccids there is less urgency to find another host plant of the same species – so they do not satisfy (2). That is, there is not such a great advantage in regularly dispersing and searching for more suitable hosts, and dispersal is less important for their survival. They can exploit even uncommon plants and therefore their species diversity may increase towards the tropics.

The CHH is supported indirectly by the following: if the CHH is correct, then the host plants of aphids should be common. Dixon *et al.* (1987) checked the percentage of plants of three plant families (Asteraceae, Ranunculaceae and Daucaceae) in Czechoslovakia that host aphids. This revealed that the common species of plants (as indicated by the Flora of Czechoslovakia, where each plant species is characterized as "common", "scattered" or "rare" by the authors) are five times more likely to have aphids associated with them than are scattered or rare species. Similarly, the most abundant species of the families Euphorbiaceae, Lamiaceae and Viciaceae are more likely to host aphids than the rarer species. Most of the plant species that host aphids, but are indicated as rare in the Flora of Czechoslovakia, are more abundant in adjacent countries (Dixon *et al.*, 1987).

Beyond the scope of species richness patterns is another application of the CHH: the reproductive success of orchids, measured as the percentage of flowers pollinated per plant, consistently declines towards the tropics (Table 12.1, Neiland & Wilcock, 1998). With respect to the assumptions of the CHH, for successful pollination, the insect pollinators have to transfer pollen from one species to the same plant species – (1), they have to do it every flowering season – (2), they visit the plants at random – (3), the visitation sequence has to be short – otherwise they lose the pollinia they are carrying – (4), and the species richness in Orchidaceae increases towards the tropics – (5). Thus the CHH predicts the pattern observed in Table 12.1.

## Conclusion

Certain taxonomic groups do not follow the usual trend of increasing species richness from the poles to the tropics. One explanation for this is that it is a consequence of the constraints imposed by the way of life of the group. In groups where dispersal from one host patch to another occurs frequently and the individuals look for hosts at random, the common host hypothesis suggests that their species diversity should be inversely related to the species diversity of their hosts. Any deviation from the above-mentioned assumptions results in the usual trend in the latitudinal gradient in species richness.

The empirical data for several groups indicate that the CHH can explain several inverse latitudinal gradients. Nevertheless, the very diversity of nature makes it likely that this is not the only explanation.

## References

Addicott, J. F. (1974). Predation and prey community structure: an experimental study of the effect of mosquito larvae on the protozoan communities of pitcher plants. *Ecology*, **55**, 475–492.

Agarwala, B. K. & Dixon, A. F. G. (1986). Population trends of *Cervaphis schouteniae* v.d. Goot on *Microcos paniculata* and its relevance to the paucity of aphid species in India. *Indian Biologist*, **18**, 37–39.

Askew, R. R. (1990). Species diversities of hymenopteran taxa in Sulawesi. In *Insect and the Rain Forests of South East Asia (Wallacea)*, ed. W. J. Knight & J. D. Holloway, pp. 255–260. London: Royal Entomological Society.

Basset, Y. (1994). Palatability of tree foliage to chewing insects: a comparison between a temperate and a tropical site. *Acta Oecologica*, **15**, 181–191.

Bodenheimer, F. S. & Swirski, E. (1957). *The Aphidoidea of the Middle East.* Jerusalem: Weizmann Science Press.

Buckley, H. L., Miller, T. E., Ellison, A. M. & Gotelli, N. J. (2003). Reverse latitudinal trends in species richness of pitcher-plant food webs. *Ecology Letters*, **6**, 825–829.

Cochran-Stafira, D. L. & von Ende, C. N. (1998). Integrating bacteria into food webs: studies with *Sarracenia purpurea* inquilines. *Ecology*, **79**, 880–898.

Coley, P. D. & Aide, T. M. (1991). Comparison of herbivory and plant defences in temperate and tropical broad-leaved forests. In *Plant-Animal Interactions: Evolutionary Ecology in Tropical and Temperate Regions*, ed. P. W. Price, T. M. Lewinsohn, G. W. Fernandes & W. W. Benson, pp. 25–50. New York: John Wiley.

Colwell, R. K. & Hurtt, G. C. (1994). Nonbiological gradients in species richness and a spurious Rapoport effect. *American Naturalist*, **144**, 570–595.

Colwell, R. K. & Lees, D. C. (2000). The mid-domain effect: geometric constraints on the geography of species richness. *Trends in Ecology and Evolution*, **15**, 70–76.

Colwell, R. K., Rahbek, C. & Gotelli, N. J. (2004). The mid-domain effect and species richness patterns: what have we learned so far? *American Naturalist*, **163**, E1–E23.

Cook, R. E. (1969). Variation in species density in North American birds. *Systematic Zoology*, **18**, 63–84.

Currie, D. J. (1991). Energy and large-scale patterns of animal- and plant-species richness. *American Naturalist*, **137**, 27–49.

Currie, D. J., Francis, A. P. & Kerr, J. T. (1999). Some general propositions about the study of spatial patterns of species richness. *Écoscience*, **6**, 392–399.

Dixon, A. F. G., Kindlmann, P., Lepš, J. & Holman, J. (1987). Why are there so few species of aphids, especially in the tropics? *American Naturalist*, **129**, 580–592.

Dixon, A. F. G., Hemptinne, J.-L. & Kindlmann, P. (1997). Effectiveness of ladybirds as biological control agents: patterns and processes. *Entomophaga*, **42**, 71–83.

Duffey, S. S., Bloem, K. A. & Campbell, B. C. (1986). Consequences of sequestration of plant natural products in plant-insect-parasitoid interactions. In *Interactions of Plant Resistance and Parasitoids and Predators of Insects*, ed. D. J. Boethel & R. D. Eikenbary, pp. 31–60. New York: John Wiley.

Eastop, V. F. (1977). Worldwide importance of aphids as virus vectors. In *Aphids as Virus Vectors*, ed. K. F. Harris & K. Maramorosch, pp. 3–62. London: Academic Press.

Eastop, V. F. (1978). Diversity of the Stenorrhyncha within major climatic zones. *Symposia of the Royal Entomological Society of London*, **9**, 71–88.

Elton, C. S. (1973). The structure of invertebrate populations inside neotropical rain forest. *Journal of Animal Ecology*, **42**, 55–104.

Gaston, K. J. (1991). The magnitude of global insect species richness. *Conservation Biology*, **5**, 283–296.

Gaston, K. J. & Blackburn, T. M. (2000). *Pattern and Process in Macroecology*. Oxford: Blackwell Scientific.

Gauld, I. D. (1986). Latitudinal gradients in ichneumonid species-richness in Australia. *Ecological Entomology*, **11**, 155–161.

Gauld, I. D. (1987). Some factors affecting the composition of tropical ichneumonid faunas. *Biological Journal of the Linnean Society*, **30**, 299–312.

Gauld, I. D. & Gaston, K. J. (1994). The taste of enemy-free space: parasitoids and nasty hosts. In *Parasitoid Community Ecology*, ed. B. A. Hawkins & W. Sheehan, pp. 279–299. Oxford: Oxford University Press.

Gauld, I. D., Gaston, K. J. & Janzen, D. H. (1992). Plant allelochemicals, tritrophic interactions and the anomalous diversity of tropical parasitoids: the "nasty" host hypothesis. *Oikos*, **65**, 353–357.

Hales, D. F. (1976). Biology of *Neophyllaphis brimlbecombei* Carver (Homoptera: Aphididae) in the Sydney region. *Australian Zoologist*, **19**, 77–83.

Hawkins, B. A. (1994). *Pattern and Process in Host-Parasitoid Interactions*. Cambridge: Cambridge University Press.

Hillebrand, H. (2004). On the generality of the latitudinal diversity gradient. *American Naturalist*, **163**, 192–211.

Hodkinson, I. D. (1974). The biology of the Psylloidea (Homoptera): a review. *Bulletin of Entomological Research*, **64**, 325–338.

Hodkinson, I. D. (1986). The psyllids (Homoptera: Psylloidea) of the oriental zoogeographical region: an annotated check-list. *Journal of Natural History*, **20**, 299–357.

Hurlbert, A. H. & Haskell, J. P. (2003). The effect of energy and seasonality on avian species richness and community composition. *American Naturalist*, **161**, 83–97.

Janzen, D. H. (1981). The peak in North American ichneumonid species richness lies between 38° and 42° N. *Ecology*, **62**, 532–537.

Janzen, D. H. & Pond, C. M. (1975). A comparison by sweep sampling of the arthropod fauna of secondary vegetation in Michigan, England and Costa Rica. *Transactions of the Royal Entomological Society of London*, **127**, 33–50.

Kindlmann, P. (1988). Extraordinary latitudinal gradients in species richness – one explanation. In *Mathematical Ecology*, ed. T. G. Hallam, L. J. Gross & S. A. Levin, pp. 149–157. Berlin: Springer.

Kneitel, J. M. & Miller, T. E. (2002). Resource and top-predator regulation in the pitcher plant (*Sarracenia purpurea*) inquiline community. *Ecology*, **83**, 680–688.

Levin, D. A. (1976). Alkaloid-bearing plants: an ecogeographic perspective. *American Naturalist*, **110**, 261–284.

Moran, V. C. (1968). Preliminary observations on the choice of host plants by adults of the citrus psylla, *Trioza erytreae* (Del Guercio) (Homoptera: Psyllidae). *Journal of the Entomological Society of South Africa*, **31**, 403–409.

Moran, V. C. & Brown, R. P. (1973). The antennae, host plant chemoreception and probing activity of the citrus psylla, *Trioza erytreae* (Del Guercio) (Homoptera: Psyllidae), *Journal of the Entomological Society of South Africa*, **36**, 191–202.

Neiland, M. R. M. & Wilcock, C. C. (1998). Fruit set, nectar reward, and rarity in the Orchidaceae. *American Journal of Botany*, **85**, 1657–1671.

Noyes, J. S. (1989). The diversity of Hymenoptera in the tropics with special reference to Parasitica in Sulawesi. *Ecological Entomology*, **14**, 197–207.

Owen, D. F. & Owen, J. (1974). Species diversity in temperate and tropical Ichneumonidae. *Nature*, **249**, 583–584.

Paine, R. T. (1966). Food web complexity and species diversity. *American Naturalist*, **100**, 65–75.

Pianka, E. R. (1966). Latitudinal gradients in species diversity: a review of concepts. *American Naturalist*, **100**, 33–46.

Pielou, E. C. (1977). The latitudinal spans of seaweed species and their patterns of overlap. *Journal of Biogeography*, **4**, 299–311.

Power, M. E., Tilman, D., Estes, J. A., Menge, B. A., Bond, W. J. & Mills, L. S. (1996). Challenges in the quest for keystones. *BioScience*, **46**, 609–620.

Rohde, K. (1992). Latitudinal gradients in species diversity: the search for the primary cause. *Oikos*, **65**, 514–527.

Rosenzweig, M. L. & Sandlin, E. A. (1997). Species diversity and latitudes: listening to area's signal. *Oikos*, **80**, 172–176.

Santelices, B. (1980). Phytogeographic characterization of the temperate coast of Pacific South America. *Phycologia*, **19**, 1–12.

Shaw, M. R. (1994). Parasitoid host ranges. In *Parasitoid Community Ecology*, ed. B. A. Hawkins & W. Sheehan, pp. 111–144. Oxford: Oxford University Press.

Sime, K. R. & Brower, A. V. Z. (1998). Explaining the latitudinal gradient anomaly in ichneumonid species richness: evidence from butterflies. *Journal of Animal Ecology*, **67**, 387–399.

Storch, D., Evans, K. L. & Gaston, K. J. (2005). The species–area–energy relationship. *Ecology Letters*, **8**, 487–492.

Stork, N. E. (1991). The composition of the arthropod fauna of Bornean lowland rain forest trees. *Journal of Tropical Ecology*, **7**, 161–180.

Townes, H. (1969). The genera of Ichneumonidae, Part 1. *Memoirs of the American Entomological Institute*, **11**, 1–300.

Valdovinos, C., Navarrete, S. A. & Marquet, P. A. (2003). Mollusk species diversity in the southeastern Pacific: why are there more species towards the pole? *Ecography*, **26**, 139–144.

van den Hoek, C. (1975). Phytogeographic provinces along the coast of the northern Atlantic Ocean. *Phycologia*, **14**, 317–330.

Willig, M. R. & Lyons, S. K. (1998). An analytical model of latitudinal gradients of species richness with an empirical test for marsupials and bats in the New World. *Oikos*, **81**, 93–98.

Willig, M. R., Kaufman, D. M. & Stevens, R. D. (2003). Latitudinal gradients in biodiversity: pattern, process, scale, and synthesis. *Annual Review of Ecology, Evolution and Systematics*, **34**, 273–309.

Zapata, F. A., Gaston, K. J., Chown, S. L. (2003). Mid-domain models of species richness gradients: assumptions, methods and evidence. *Journal of Animal Ecology*, **72**, 677–690.

CHAPTER THIRTEEN

# Regional-to-global patterns of biodiversity, and what they have to say about mechanisms

DAVID J. CURRIE

*University of Ottawa*

## Introduction

One of the most striking patterns in ecology is broad-scale variation of species richness (e.g. Fig. 13.1). Ecologists have noted these patterns for at least two centuries (von Humboldt & Bonpland, 1807; Wallace, 1878). Since then, geographical patterns of diversity have been extensively documented (see references in Table 1 in Hawkins *et al.*, 2003a) and numerous reviews and textbooks have discussed factors hypothesized to have generated them (Huston, 1994; Rosenzweig, 1995; Chesson, 2000).

Two distinct points of view have characterized this discussion. The first, I would characterize as the *multiple substituting influences* family of hypotheses. According to this view, a wide variety of factors influence richness in very context-specific manners. The second view, I will call the *strong constraint* family of hypotheses. These hypotheses propose that, as in physical systems, a small number of general principles exert strong constraints on the behavior of ecological systems. Thus, the propensity (*sensu* Popper, 1990) of ecological systems to behave in particular ways can be related to one, or a small number of variables, while the rest of the world's complexity adds a bit of noise.

To reveal my own prejudice, I believe that the goal of science is to develop predictive models of the behavior of natural systems (Peters, 1991; Rigler & Peters, 1995). A search for strong propensities, perhaps reflecting strong constraints, is a logical way to begin to approach this goal.

## Multiple substituting influences

Textbooks of ecology and reviews of this subject typically present lists of processes that can potentially affect richness. For example, diversity has been observed to vary in ways that suggest effects of disturbance, competition, predation, mutualism, habitat complexity, evolutionary factors, dispersal limitation, etc. It is typically postulated that these factors vary strongly among regions. For example, Qian and Ricklefs (1999) propose that richness of

*Scaling Biodiversity*, ed. David Storch, Pablo A. Marquet and James H. Brown. Published by Cambridge University Press. © Cambridge University Press 2007.

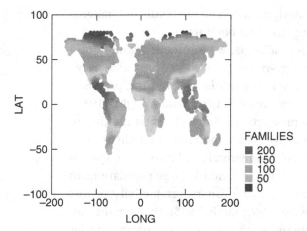

FAMILIES
■ 200
□ 150
■ 100
■ 50
□ 0

**Figure 13.1** The global variation in angiosperm family richness, adapted from Francis and Currie (2003). (For color version see Plate 9.)

flowering plants is higher in temperate forests of eastern Asia than in North America because angiosperms' evolutionary origin was in Southeast Asia. Starnes and Etnier (1986) suggest that fish species richness in the Cumberland Plateau in the southeastern USA is high because of vicariance events during the Pleistocene. Sax (2001) proposes that richness reflects abiotic stresses at high latitudes, and biotic stresses at low latitudes. Kerr and Packer (1997) propose that mammal species richness in North America depends upon climate (annual potential evapotranspiration, specifically) in cold parts of the continent, and habitat heterogeneity in warm areas. Diversity may spatially vary because of the geography of glacial refugia (Adams & Woodward, 1989; Petit *et al.*, 2003), disturbances (Connell, 1978), community assembly (Fukami & Morin, 2003), or many other factors. Variation of diversity has been related to all of these factors, under at least some circumstances and at some spatial scales.

## Strong constraint

In contrast, richness may be constrained under all circumstances by a small number of factors (or perhaps only one), while other factors may further influence diversity locally. Global constraints should be globally reflected in statistical relationships in any data set in which the constraint varies (e.g. Lawton's, 1999, generalizations). These constraints may or may not be easily expressible in terms of particular mechanisms. For example, virtually every aspect of the ecology of individual organisms scales with body size, e.g. metabolic rates, reproductive rates, home range size, population dynamics, life expectancy, etc. (Peters, 1983). A characteristic such as life expectancy is presumably influenced by myriad mechanisms ranging from apoptosis to susceptibility to predation and exposure to environmental extremes, all of which scale with body size. To predict life expectancy from underlying mechanisms would be challenging indeed, but it is possible to get close based on body size.

Regarding spatial variation in species richness, a prominent example of a strong-constraint hypothesis is the *energy–richness hypothesis* (or *species–energy hypothesis*, sometimes also called the *more individuals hypothesis*), first proposed by Hutchinson (1959) and developed by Brown (1981) and Wright (1983). According to this hypothesis, primary productivity limits the total number of individual organisms that can exist in a given area. Individuals are distributed among species. Areas where there are more individuals will have more species because a greater number of species will have sufficiently large populations to avoid extinction. Since geographic variation in primary productivity results mainly from varying climate (Rosenzweig, 1968; Lieth, 1975), the climatic variables that constrain primary productivity should also constrain species richness.

A more recent strong-constraint hypothesis is the *metabolic theory of ecology* (Allen, Brown & Gillooly, 2002; Brown *et al.*, 2004; Allen, Gillooly & Brown, this volume). This hypothesis proposes that patterns of richness derive from two considerations. The first is the "energy equivalence rule". This "rule" is based on the empirical observations that the metabolic rate of individual animals scales in proportion to mass (M) to the power 0.75, and the number of individuals per unit area scales as mass to the power $-0.75$. Consequently, total metabolic rate per unit area, which is the product of metabolism per individual times the number of individuals, is independent of mass. Thus, populations of different species (among endotherms or among ectotherms) should use approximately equivalent amounts of energy. The second consideration is the temperature dependence of enzyme kinetics. Most metabolic processes, including energy acquisition, rates of cellular division, accumulation of mutations, etc. are temperature dependent. To a first approximation, the body temperature of ectothermic organisms (including plants) depends on ambient temperature. Therefore, these processes are universally constrained by temperature. If a population uses a fixed amount of energy, and if energy use by individuals increases with temperature, then individual population densities of ectotherms must vary inversely with temperature. Assuming that the total number of individuals of all species is independent of temperature, Allen *et al.* (2002) predict that species richness should vary positively with temperature. Endotherms, by maintaining a constant body temperature, escape the temperature constraint. Their population densities and species richness should therefore be independent of temperature. Allen *et al.* (2002) show a number of data sets that are consistent with this hypothesis.

There are other strong-constraint hypotheses. For example, Kleidon and Mooney (2000) noted that many aspects of plant physiology are strongly constrained by temperature and water availability. They hypothesize that the

number of possible combinations of physiological parameters that yield a positive energy balance (net primary productivity greater than zero) covaries with
climate. In essence, richness is higher in warm, wet places because there are
more possible physiologies that survive under those conditions. This hypothesis
predicts patterns of species richness that are at least qualitatively consistent
with the global variation in species density observed by Barthlott, Lauer and
Placke (1996).

Most strong-constraint hypotheses about species richness hypothesize that
climate – some aspect of temperature, solar radiation, and/or water availability –
is the main constraint on richness. Even though the proposed mechanisms
differ, this family of hypotheses makes a set of predictions in common.
(a) Richness should relate to its climatic drivers in a consistent manner in any
region of the globe, despite regional differences in evolutionary history, sub-
strate, disturbance, etc. (b) Richness–climate relationships should be independent of spatial extent. The parameters of the relationship, and the residual mean
squared error, should both be independent of spatial extent. In contrast, the
proportion of variance that is statistically related to climate (i.e. $R^2$) should
depend upon the range of climate within the area considered, which will
depend upon spatial extent. (c) Spatial grain should affect the parameters of
any richness–climate relationship because richness covaries with area (Holt
et al., 1999; Venevsky & Veneskaia, 2003). Moreover, large-grain studies should
be relatively insensitive to local variation in nonclimatic factors that might
affect local richness (e.g. edaphic conditions), because they integrate over
large areas. Fine-grained studies, in contrast, might be expected to reflect local
influences (e.g. Smith, 2001).

Individual strong-constraint hypotheses make additional predictions. The
energy–richness hypothesis predicts relationships between climate and the
numbers of individuals, between numbers of individuals and numbers of species, as well as relationships as these factors change temporally (Currie et al.,
2004). Metabolic theory makes the same prediction for endotherms (Allen et al.,
2002, this volume).

Metabolic theory (Allen et al., 2002) makes an additional prediction that is
astoundingly strong: that the geographic variation in the natural logarithm of
richness of ectotherms should scale as a linear function of the reciprocal of
temperature (kelvin) with a slope of $-0.78$. Allen et al. (2002) test this prediction
using the variation of richness across North America using data from (among
other sources) Currie (1991).

### Extant evidence

A vast body of evidence is consistent with the hypothesis that broad-scale
variation in species richness of most taxa is constrained by climate. Richness
within higher taxa (orders and up) and functional groups are strongly correlated

with climatic variables (Wright, Currie & Maurer, 1993). Among 85 studies of broad-scale patterns of richness reviewed by Hawkins *et al.* (2003a), 82 reported that richness was more strongly related to climate (measures of heat and water availability) than to any other environmental characteristic. In a study of the global variation in angiosperm family and species richness among quadrats $10^4 \, \mathrm{km}^2$ in area, Francis and Currie (2003) found that richness could be statistically related to a variety of variables involving heat and water. The following regression model made good predictions of richness ($R^2 = 0.83$, $n = 4224$):

$$FR = 8.78 + 0.220 * PET + 6.79 \times 10^{-5} * PET^2 - 0.0641 * WD, \tag{13.1}$$

where FR is angiosperm family richness, PET is annual potential evapotranspiration (in mm/year), and WD is annual water deficit (mm/year). Further, Francis and Currie (2003) argued that the climate–richness relationship is globally consistent, since richness in any one part of the world could be accurately predicted from the richness–climate relationship derived for the rest of the world (their Fig. 5).

In contrast, other studies appear to support multiple substituting influences determining global variation in richness. For example, Schall and Pianka (1978) observed that mammal richness is positively correlated with insolation in North America, whereas it is negatively correlated in Australia. Similarly, Kerr and Packer (1997) observed that mammal richness in North America correlates with potential evapotranspiration (or temperature) only in cold regions; richness is more strongly correlated with habitat heterogeneity in warm areas. Francis and Currie (2003) showed that these regional discrepancies disappear when richness is modeled as a function of both heat and water. However, in many cases, significant differences in richness among biogeographic regions of the world remain after controlling for climate (Latham & Ricklefs, 1993a,b; Qian & Ricklefs, 2004). Further, within some biogeographic areas, the richness–climate relationship is weak (Qian & Ricklefs, 2004). These differences may indicate that regional processes such as evolutionary history have left a signature on contemporary richness patterns (Latham & Ricklefs, 1993a,b; Ricklefs, Latham & Qian, 1999).

The present study addresses three questions. First, to what extent do climate–richness relationships differ among regions? Second, if there is a single, global richness–climate relationship, could subsamples differing in spatial extent or spatial grain also appear to differ in the ways (described above) that have led some researchers to conclude that different variables control richness in different localities? Third, is extant evidence consistent with either of the two most prominent strong-constraint hypotheses: the species–energy hypothesis, and metabolic theory?

## Methods

In this study, we compare richness–climate relationships at several spatial scales. To do this, I have used the following extant data sets.

To examine regional effects on richness, I re-examined the global angiosperm data of Francis and Currie (2003). Francis and Currie used the range maps of angiosperm families presented by Heywood (1993). We overlayed distributions on a global equal-area grid with 4224 quadrats, each $10\,500\,km^2$ ($2°$ latitude $\times$ $2°$ longitude at $45°$ N or S). This grain size corresponded to the apparent resolution of Heywood's maps: the smallest patches of distribution recorded, and the smallest holes in otherwise continuous distributions, were this size. We then tallied the number of families occurring in each grid. All parts of the globe in which angiosperms are present were included, except small oceanic islands, since Heywood's maps excluded these.

Using the same grid, Francis and Currie (2003) sampled the vascular plant species richness map of Barthlott *et al.* (1996). These authors had estimated vascular plant species richness in $10^4\,km^2$ areas, based on local and regional floras. In some parts of the world with few data (notably, tropical Africa), Barthlott *et al.* (1996) interpolated their richness surface using climatic and topographic information.

To study the effect of changing spatial extent, I estimated richness–climate relationships both globally, and within the biogeographic regions first described by R. Wallace: Nearctic, Neotropical, Palearctic, Ethiopian (sub-Saharan Africa), Oriental (Asia south of the Himalayas) and Australian (Brown & Lomolino, 1998, p. 26). Each region is further divided into four subregions. I also compared relationships within 23 subregions. The available data excluded the Neotropical subregion comprised entirely of Caribbean islands.

To study the effect of spatial grain, I compared coarse- and fine-grained data of continental to global spatial extent. Francis and Currie (2003) provided coarse-grained, global vascular plant species richness. Coarse-grained North American tree species richness was taken from Currie and Paquin (1987). In that study, we had superimposed distribution maps of the native North American tree species (Little, 1971) on a quadrat system that was $2.5°$ latitude $\times$ $2.5°$ longitude south of $50°$ N, and $2.5°$ latitude $\times$ $5.0°$ longitude north of $50°$ N. Quadrat area therefore varied by approximately a factor of 2, but it averaged $50\,500\,km^2$. Quadrats covered Canada and the continental United States, excluding offshore islands.

Fine-grained, broad-extent data were taken from Alwyn Gentry's set of 0.1 ha transects through forests in many parts of the world (Phillips & Miller, 2002). The spatial extent is nominally global, although the Neotropics are overrepresented in Gentry's samples, and high latitudes are undersampled. Gentry recorded tree species and some other species in his transects; we have used only the tree data. The data are available in raw form on the web at www.mobot.org/MOBOT/Research/gentry/transect.shtml. Gentry's transects that were smaller than 0.1 ha were excluded from the present analysis.

I also compared coarse- and fine-grained bird species richness. Coarse-grained data were taken from Currie (1991), using the same grid as Currie and Paquin

(1987). In that study, I had resampled the bird species richness map of Cook (1969) and recorded the highest richness occurring in each quadrat. Fine-grained data are available from the North American Breeding Bird Survey (Bystrak, 1981; Sauer, Hines & Fallon, 2004). This program samples routes across the continental United States (including Alaska) and the parts of Canada that are accessible by road (this excludes most northern areas outside the Yukon). Three-minute point counts are done at 0.8 km intervals along 40 km routes following secondary roads. Using point counts, birds are detectable over a radius of approximately 400 m. Consequently, the area nominally sampled along a route is 25 km². The data can be downloaded from www.mbr-pwrc.usgs.gov/bbs/bbs.html.

Climate data were taken from published maps, as cited in the publications listed above. Precipitation data were transformed to the power 0.3 to make the frequency distribution of the data approximately symmetrically distributed. Temperature data were transformed as suggested by Allen *et al.* (2002): $1/kT$ where $k$ is Boltzmann's constant ($8.62 \times 10^{-5}$ eV K$^{-1}$) and $T$ is temperature in kelvins. The frequency distribution of the quantity $1/kT$, which I shall call Boltzmann temperature, is strongly positively skewed. To be consistent with Allen *et al.* (2002), I did not transform this variable. The frequency distribution of potential evapotranspiration, measured in mm/year, was not improved by trans-formation and was therefore left untransformed. Water deficit, calculated as annual potential evapotranspiration minus annual actual evapotranspiration, was also left untransformed. Species richness was fifth-root transformed to improve normality. Family richness required no transformation. Richness was log-transformed in cases where comparison with earlier theory so required.

## Results

### Regional effects on richness

Climatic variation can account for most, but not all, of the broad-scale variation in richness. Richness differs dramatically among biogeographic regions (as Darwin and Wallace noted). However, interregional differences are almost entirely collinear with climate (Fig. 13.2). Francis and Currie's (2003) global climatic model (Eq. 13.1) statistically accounts for 83.7% of the variance in angiosperm family richness. One can add biogeographic subregion as a covariate:

$$FR = (c_0 + c_1 D) + (c_2 \, PET + c_3 \, D \, PET) + \left(c_4 \, PET^2 + c_5 \, D \, PET^2\right) \\ + (c_6 \, WD + c_7 \, D \, WD),$$

(13.2)

where $D$ is a categorical dummy variable distinguishing among regions or subregions and $c_1$ to $c_7$ are empirical constants. Additional variance explained by region after accounting for climate is small, but significant (Fig. 13.2; $R^2$ increases to 0.906).

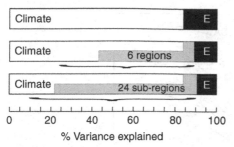

**Figure 13.2** The variance in the global variation in angiosperm family richness statistically explained in multiple regressions by climate (potential evapotranspiration and water deficit) alone, or in combination with a categorical variable distinguishing among Wallace's biogeographic regions (6) or subregions (23). The length of the white bar is the proportion of the variance in richness that can be related to climate. Similarly, the length of gray-shaded part of the bar represents the proportion of variance that can be related to (sub)region. The overlap of white and gray bars is the proportion of the variance in richness that is related to the collinearity of climate and region. The black areas labeled E represent unexplained residual variance (error). The braces under the bars represent the strength of the collinearity between region and potential evapotranspiration. Climate differs very strongly among regions. After accounting for climate, relatively little variance in angiosperm richness can be related to region or subregion, whereas there is considerable variation in richness that is related to climate, after accounting for region.

Most climate–richness relationships within biogeographic regions fall close to the global relationship (Fig. 13.3). The global richness–climate relationship predicts richness in most biogeographic regions and subregions as precisely as it predicts richness in a random selection of global points (Fig. 13.4). Richness in some regions, however, is predicted more precisely by local relationships than by the global relationship (the points significantly above the confidence interval in Fig. 13.4).

The tropics do not depart in a consistent manner from the global relationship, in contrast to the suggestion that richness depends upon climatic constraints in cold places, and biotic constraints in the tropics (cf. Sax, 2001). In some tropical areas (e.g. the southern Sahara and the Congo basin) the richness–climate relationship flattens out and leads to high residuals (Fig. 13.5), whereas in others (e.g. Southeast Asia, western equatorial Africa), richness follows the global relationship quite closely. Similarly, richness varies less closely with climate in certain temperate areas (e.g. southern Africa, New Zealand) than in others (e.g. northern Eurasia and North America).

Areas with the most striking residuals seem to be associated with specific climatic or physiographic features (Fig. 13.3 and top panel of Fig. 13.5). The Sahara, the Australian Outback, New Zealand, the North American Great Plains, and the African tropical forests all have fewer angiosperm families than climate

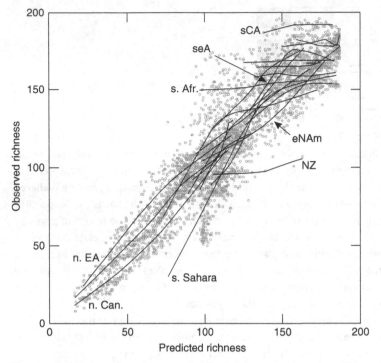

**Figure 13.3** Observed angiosperm family richness, as a function of the predictions of a global model relating richness to potential evapotranspiration, water deficit, and their interaction. The lines represent LOWESS fits within each of 23 Wallace biogeographic subregions. Selected regions are labeled: eNAm – eastern North America, n. Can. – northern Canada, n. EA – northern Eurasia, NZ – New Zealand, s. Sahara – southern Sahara, s. Afr. – southern Africa, sCA – southern Central America, seA – Southeast Asia.

alone predicts. Other areas – the Atacama Desert and the west slope of the Andes, the Namib Desert and the western Kalahari, desert areas of northern Mexico, and northern Queensland in Australia – all have higher richness than climate alone would predict. Within-quadrat elevation range statistically accounts for some of the difference in richness among ecoregions after controlling for climate ($R^2$ increases to 0.845) but most of the variation remains.

It is not clear what accounts for differences in richness among biogeographic subregions after controlling for climate and elevation. It is possible that the residual differences reflect contemporary climatic differences not captured by Currie and Francis's model. For example, Venevsky and Veneskaia (2003) found that a model that includes the seasonal timing of precipitation makes significantly better predictions of vegetation richness than the annual mean climatic variables that we used. Alternatively, Qian and Ricklefs (2004) suggested that angiosperm richness is higher in East Asia, where angiosperms first evolved. However, the spatial pattern of residuals shows no evidence of this. The most

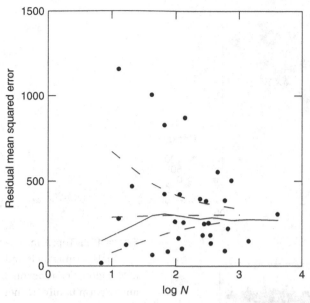

**Figure 13.4** Residual mean squared errors from the global richness–climate relationship, tallied within Wallace's biogeographic regions (6) and subregions (23). The dashed lines represent the mean and 95% confidence interval around errors on 1000 samples randomly drawn from the global set. The solid line is a LOWESS fit to the data. The global relationship predicts richness in most biogeographic regions and subregions at least as well as it predicts richness in points randomly selecting from anywhere on the globe. This indicates that there is no reason to postulate special regional influences on richness in these areas. The exceptions, the points falling above the top dashed line, are areas where there are plausibly regional, nonclimatic influences on richness. These are shown in the lower panel of Fig. 13.5.

intriguing pattern in the residuals (Fig. 13.5) is that certain desert areas have significantly lower than expected richness (southern Sahara, western Australia, Arabia), whereas others have high richness (northern Chile, northern Mexico, Namibia). Whatever accounts for these regional differences (I would hypothesize seasonality), it represents a relatively small influence, accounting for only about 8% as much variance as annual climate.

**Do richness–climate relationships depend upon spatial extent?**
The strength of richness–climate relationships as measured by $R^2$ increases with increasing spatial extent for angiosperm families (Fig. 13.6a) and species (not shown; similar to Fig. 13.6a). Climate typically accounts for a smaller proportion of the variance within regions than it does in an equal number of quadrats selected randomly from the global set. This is not surprising; the variability of both physical variables and richness is smaller in small regions (Fig. 13.7a,b). Thus, the strength of richness–climate relationships is largely a function of the

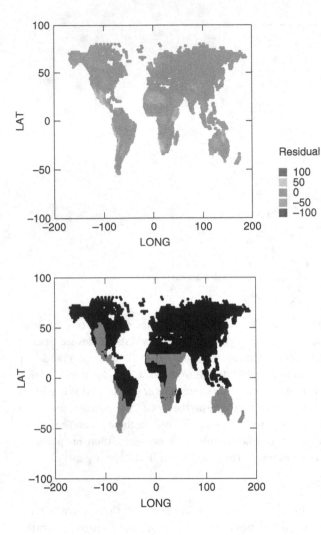

**Figure 13.5** Top: A map of the residuals from Francis and Currie's (2003) global relationship between angiosperm family richness and climate. Bottom: Wallace biogeographic subregions in which the mean squared residual is significantly ($P \leq 0.05$) greater than would be expected in comparison with an equal number of quadrats randomly selected from the global set (gray areas; other areas are shown in black). Thus, regional, nonclimatic influences on richness might be hypothesized in those regions. (For color version see Plate 10.)

variability of richness and climate within the study area (second degree polynomial $R^2 = 0.61$; Fig. 13.7c).

Even though the correlation $R$ between richness and climate within regions is typically lower than that of the global relationship, residual error is significantly *smaller* in regional relationships (Fig. 13.6b). This is also not surprising. Richness–climate relationships within a region can be more closely tuned to local sets of conditions. Note, however, that although richness–climate relationships derived within regions may not account for a large portion of the within-region variability in richness, their predictions are closer to observed richness than are the predictions from the global relationship. The only exceptions globally are Wallace's Ethiopian biogeographic region, and the subregion encompassing the Sahel and eastern Africa.

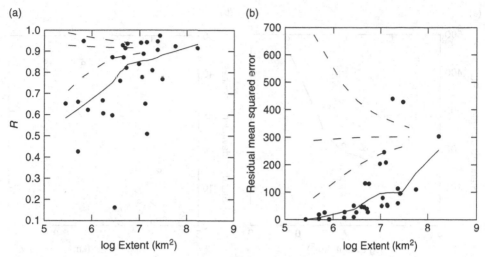

**Figure 13.6** Richness–climate relationships within biogeographic regions compared with random subsets of the global relationship. (a) The multiple correlation coefficients (R) of relationships relating angiosperm family richness to PET (potential evapotranspiration), $PET^2$ and water deficit. Each point represents a regression using the $10\,500\ km^2$ quadrats entirely within one of Wallace's biogeographic regions ($n = 6$) or subregions ($n = 23$). Extent refers to the area (in $km^2$) of the region. The dashed lines represent the expected correlations (upper 95% confidence limit, mean, and lower 95% confidence limit), based on points selected randomly from the global set, rather than from a single contiguous region. The solid line represents the LOWESS trend in the data: the explained variance (i.e. the $R^2$) of richness–climate relationships increases with spatial extent. (b) The residual mean squared error (RMSE) of the same regressions. Local relationships typically make significantly more accurate predictions of richness than does the global relationship. The two exceptions are sub-Saharan Africa generally (Wallace's Ethiopian region), and the Sahel and East Africa specifically. Thus, regional relationships are actually stronger than the global relationship (they have lower residual variance) even though their $R^2$ values are typically weaker.

In sum, richness–climate relationships are largely consistent worldwide, within and among regions. Residual differences in richness after controlling for climate are small. Apparently weak relationships within regions reflect the fact that the ranges of variation of richness and of climate are small in small areas.

## Do broad-extent richness–climate relationships depend upon grain size?

Ideally, to test for grain-size effects, one would compare richness–climate relationships in nested sampling units over a range of grain sizes. This is possible over small spatial extents (e.g. Palmer & White, 1994; Stohlgren et al., 1999), but it would be logistically very difficult over continental to global spatial extents.

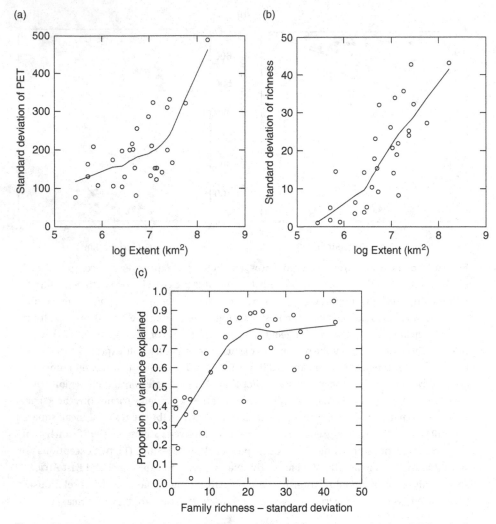

**Figure 13.7** The standard deviation of (a) annual potential evapotranspiration (PET) and of (b) angiosperm family richness within Wallace biogeographic regions and subregions, as functions of the spatial extent (area) of the (sub)region in km$^2$. The solid lines represent LOWESS trend lines. The variability of physical variables and of richness increase with increasing spatial extent. Not surprisingly, in areas where climate (PET and water deficit) varies little, the richness–climate relationship is weak (c).

As a compromise, we compared tree species richness (fifth root transformed) in 50 500 km$^2$ quadrats (Currie & Paquin, 1987), species richness of angiosperms in 10 000 km$^2$ areas (Barthlott *et al.*, 1996) and species richness of trees in 0.1 ha transects.

The first difference among grain sizes is that the distributions of underlying data differ (Fig. 13.8d). Fine-grained data include more extreme conditions

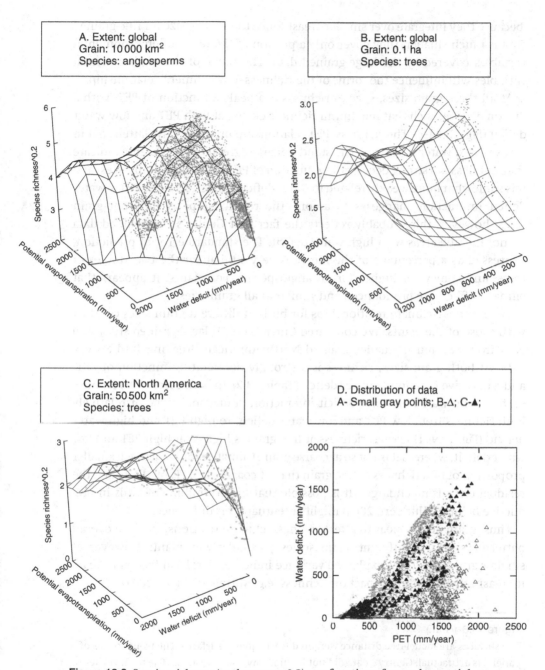

**Figure 13.8** Species richness (to the power 0.2) as a function of annual potential evapotranspiration and water deficit. (A) Species density of angiosperms based on species densities estimated in 10 000 km² quadrats by Barthlott *et al*. (1996). (B) Species richness of trees only in 0.1 ha transects studied by Alwyn Gentry (Phillips & Miller, 2002). (C) Species richness of trees in Currie and Paquin's (1987) North American data. Note that the water deficit scale is reversed; thus, from left to right, it represents a gradient from dry to wet.

(because they integrate over smaller areas). Since the sample size for fine-grained data is much smaller, they cover only a portion of the range of environmental variables covered by the large-grained data. The range of the environmental variables will influence the forms of the richness–environment relationships.

At all three grain sizes, species richness is a peaked function of PET, with a diagonal ridge, such that maximum richness occurs at high PET and low water deficit (Fig. 13.8a–c). The richness–PET relationship progressively flattens out in areas where water is scarcer. The standardized regression coefficients indicate that richness is a strong decelerating function of PET at all three grain sizes, and it is somewhat more weakly related to water deficit (Table 13.1). The PET × water deficit interaction changes sign among the relationships at different grain sizes; however, this probably reflects the fact that Gentry's fine-grained data do not include areas with high water deficit. The standard error of prediction, expressed as a percentage of the mean, is very similar for the two studies of trees, and somewhat higher for all angiosperms. For plants, it appears that climatic effects are pronounced and similar at all grain sizes.

The richness–climate relationships for birds at different grain sizes contrast with those of the plants. We compared Currie's (1991) large-grained study and data from the much smaller grained North American Breeding Bird Survey data. At both grain sizes, richness is a strongly decelerating function of PET, and a negative function of water deficit (Table 13.2). In both cases, the response surfaces show a PET × water deficit interaction (a diagonal ridge of relatively high richness from low PET and low water deficit, to high PET and high water deficit) (Fig. 13.9). However, richness at fine grain is highest at high PET and low water deficit, whereas it is not so at coarse grain. Climate explains a much smaller proportion of bird richness at fine grain than at coarse grain (Table 13.2), and the residual error is much larger. It is possible that undersampling of birds in productive habitats (Hurlbert, 2004) might accentuate this difference.

Thus, grain does appear to affect richness–climate relationships. The overall pattern is similar at different spatial scales, particularly for plants. However, at smaller grain, the lower explained variance indicates that local factors have an increasingly important impact on richness (e.g. Mittelbach et al., 2001).

---

**Figure 13.8** (cont.)

The surfaces are model-free distance-weighted least squares surfaces. The front corner of panel B is artifactual; Gentry's data did not include any cold, dry areas. The front corner of panel C has been removed for the same reason. The general shapes of the patterns at the three scales are similar. Panels B and C are bumpier than panel A largely because their sample sizes are much smaller (A: $n = 4224$; B; $n = 198$, C: $n = 337$). Note that the coverage of the potential evapotranspiration × water deficit surface (panel D) is less complete in the Currie and Paquin and the Gentry studies. Differences in the smoothed surfaces reflect, in part, differences in data coverage.

**Table 13.1** *Richness–climate relationships in plants*

The data are based upon Currie and Paquin's (1987) coarse-grained tally of tree richness, Barthlott *et al.*'s (1996) coarse-grained estimates of angiosperm species richness, and Gentry's (Phillips & Miller, 2002) fine-grained (0.1 ha) censuses of trees and shrubs. Despite different grains and very different methods, the models are quite similar. PET (potential evapotranspiration, mm/year); WD (water deficit, mm/year).

| Model characteristics | | Independent variables | Coefficient | Standardized coefficient |
|---|---|---|---|---|
| Taxon | Trees | PET | $3.59 \times 10^{-3}$ | 3.49 |
| Grain | $5 \times 10^4 \, km^2$ | $PET^2$ | $-1.42 \times 10^{-6}$ | −2.60 |
| Extent | Canada and USA | WD | $-1.87 \times 10^{-3}$ | −1.47 |
| Data | Currie & Paquin (1987) | PET × WD | $9.37 \times 10^{-7}$ | 1.24 |
| Model $R^2$ | 0.852 | | | |
| $n$ | 337 | | | |
| s.e./mean | 9.59% | | | |
| Taxon | Angiosperms | PET | $3.84 \times 10^{-3}$ | 2.40 |
| Grain | $10^4 \, km^2$ | $PET^2$ | $-1.25 \times 10^{-6}$ | −1.48 |
| Extent | Global | WD | $-1.61 \times 10^{-3}$ | −0.82 |
| Data | Barthlott *et al.* (1996); Francis & Currie (2003) | PET × WD | $1.70 \times 10^{-7}$ | 0.12 |
| Model $R^2$ | 0.577 | | | |
| $n$ | 4224 | | | |
| s.e./mean | 18.2% | | | |
| Taxon | Trees | PET | $1.42 \times 10^{-3}$ | 1.42 |
| Grain | 0.1 ha | $PET^2$ | $-2.54 \times 10^{-7}$ | −0.62 |
| Extent | Global | WD | $-1.01 \times 10^{-4}$ | −0.074 |
| Data | Phillips & Miller (2002) – Alwyn Gentry | PET × WD | $-2.86 \times 10^{-7}$ | −0.35 |
| Model $R^2$ | 0.710 | | | |
| $n$ | 198 | | | |
| s.e./mean | 11.7% | | | |

## Energy–richness hypothesis

The energy–richness hypothesis predicts that richness should be correlated to the total number of individuals, which is correlated with primary productivity, which in turn is correlated with climate. Correlations closer in the causal chain should be stronger than distal correlations because additional variance enters at every link. Currie *et al.* (2004) examined the evidence for these, and other, predictions. They concluded that extant evidence is largely inconsistent with the energy–richness hypothesis. Correlations other than richness–climate

**Table 13.2** *Richness–climate relationships in birds*
Except for water deficit and its interaction with PET, the models are similar.

| Model characteristics | | Independent variables | Coefficient | Standardized coefficient |
|---|---|---|---|---|
| Taxon | Birds | PET | 0.441 | 4.32 |
| Grain | $5 \times 10^4\,\text{km}^2$ | $PET^2$ | $-2.61 \times 10^{-4}$ | $-4.81$ |
| Extent | USA and Canada | WD | $1.96 \times 10^{-2}$ | $-0.87$ |
| Data | Currie (1991) | PET × WD | $1.54 \times 10^{-4}$ | 2.07 |
| Model $R^2$ | 0.852 | | | |
| s.e./mean | 13.7% | | | |
| Taxon | Birds | PET | 0.157 | 2.01 |
| Grain | $14\,\text{km}^2$ | $PET^2$ | $-7.24 \times 10^{-5}$ | $-2.03$ |
| Extent | USA and southern Canada | WD | $-1.40 \times 10^{-1}$ | $-1.82$ |
| Data | Breeding Bird Survey | PET × WD | $6.94 \times 10^{-5}$ | 1.52 |
| Model $R^2$ | 0.285 | | | |
| s.e./mean | 24.3% | | | |

were weak or inconsistent. We tentatively rejected the energy–richness hypothesis.

**Metabolic theory of species richness**
Like the energy–richness hypothesis, the hypothesis that broad-scale patterns of richness reflect the temperature dependence of metabolism (Allen *et al.*, 2002; Venevsky & Veneskaia, 2003) predicts that richness will be correlated with climatic variables. However, the metabolic theory proposed by Allen *et al.* (2002, this volume) makes some additional, remarkably strong, predictions. Among these is the prediction that the natural logarithm of richness should scale as a linear function of $1/(kT)$, where $k$ is Boltzmann's constant ($8.62 \times 10^{-5}$ $eVK^{-1}$). The slope is predicted to be the activation energy of metabolism, $-0.78\,eV$ (Allen *et al.*, 2002).

I examined this prediction for angiosperm species using the data of Barthlott *et al.* (1996), as sampled by Francis and Currie (2003), and the tree species richness data of Currie and Paquin (1987). Water deficit (which I used in the figures above) depends upon both temperature and water availability. Therefore, to

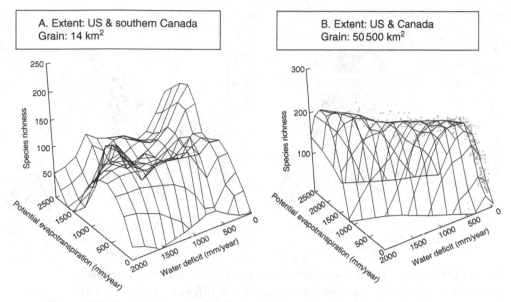

**Figure 13.9** Species richness of birds as a function of mean annual potential evapotranspiration and water deficit. (A) Point count data from the North America Breeding Bird Survey (Sauer *et al.*, 2004). (B) Data from superimposed range maps (Currie, 1991). Both data sets cover similar extents (except for the far North); therefore the distributions of the climate data are similar. Note that, in both data sets, the front and back corners of the fitted surfaces are extrapolations beyond the limits of the data. It is therefore unwise to draw inferences from those parts of the graph.

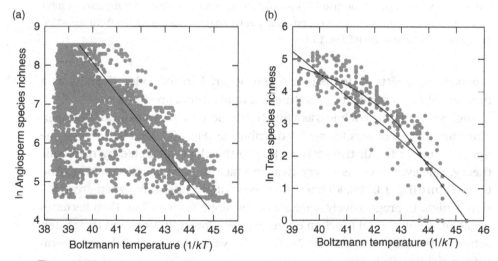

**Figure 13.10** (a) Lognormal angiosperm species richness as a function of temperature (expressed as $1/kT$, where $k$ is Boltzmann's constant and $T$ is temperature in K). The solid line is the slope of the relationship predicted by the hypothesis of metabolic control of richness (Allen *et al.*, 2002; Brown *et al.*, 2004). (b) The same relationship using Currie and Paquin's (1987) tree species richness data. The straight line is a linear fit to the data, the slope of which ($-0.74 \pm 0.05$) is very close to the predicted slope ($-0.78$), whereas the curved line is a LOWESS fit.

(a)

(b)

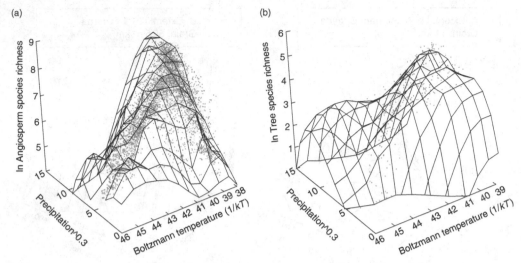

**Figure 13.11** The logarithm of angiosperm richness and as functions of total annual precipitation and mean annual temperature, expressed as $1/kT$, where $k$ is Boltzmann's constant ($8.62 \times 10^{-5}$ eV K$^{-1}$) and $T$ is temperature in kelvins (Allen *et al.*, 2002). The Boltzmann temperature scale is reversed to present a better perspective of the response surface. In this projection, temperature increases from left to right. In both panels, the front and the right corners of the graph (i.e. the extremes of precipitation at $1/kT = 46$) are extrapolations beyond the range of the data (shown as gray points). (a) Global angiosperm species richness. (b) Tree species richness in North America (Currie & Paquin, 1987). In the global angiosperm data set, the slope of the richness–Boltzmann temperature relationship (indicated by the slopes of the grid lines parallel to the temperature axis) is negative at high precipitation, and positive at low precipitation. The tree data set lacks samples from areas that are extremely hot and dry (cf. Fig. 13.12).

separate the effects of temperature and water, I instead plot richness as a function of mean annual temperature and total annual precipitation.

Angiosperm species richness as a function of Boltzmann-transformed temperature has a more or less triangular distribution (Fig. 13.10a). The slope of the upper bound of the distribution is close to the slope predicted by metabolic theory. However, there is a very clear interaction between precipitation and temperature (Fig. 13.11a). Richness increases with temperature when precipitation is high. In progressively drier areas, the slope flattens, and then becomes negative. A polynomial function of temperature, precipitation, and their interaction statistically accounts for 74.9% of the variability in global angiosperm species richness ($SR$):

$$\ln SR = -216.1 + 1.024\,B - 0.118\,B^2 + 5.45\,P - 0.0266\,P^2 - 0.121\,B \times P, \quad (13.3)$$

where $B$ is Boltzmann temperature, and $P$ is total annual precipitation (to the power 0.3).

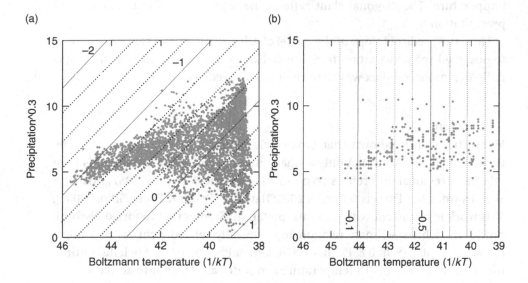

**Figure 13.12** The slope of the log species richness – Boltzmann $T$ relationship (i.e. the partial derivative of ln richness as a function of temperature and precipitation), as it varies with Boltzmann $T$ and total annual precipitation. Metabolic theory predicts a slope of $-0.78$. (a) Vascular plant species richness, from Barthlott *et al.* (1996) and Francis and Currie (2003) global data set. The points represent the range of observed conditions. (b) Tree species richness from Currie and Paquin (1987). In both cases, the predicted slope falls within the data, but observed slope varies a great deal from the predicted slope because richness is a nonlinear function of Boltzmann temperature. In the case of angiosperm richness, there is also a significant interaction with precipitation.

In Currie and Paquin's tree data (Fig. 13.10b), the slope of a linear relationship between tree richness and Boltzman-transformed temperature ($-0.74 \pm 0.05$, 95% c.i.) falls remarkably close to the predicted slope ($-0.78$), as Allen *et al.* (2002), who also analyzed these data, noted. However, closer examination shows that richness is again a significantly nonlinear function of Boltzmann temperature. The interaction term is not statistically significant in the tree data set:

$$\ln SR = -145.4 + 7.15\,B - 0.0962\,B^2 + 1.43\,P - 0.0863\,P^2$$

$$(R^2 = 0.786,\ n = 337,\ P < 10^{-9}).$$

(13.4)

Figure 13.12 shows $\partial(\ln SR)/\partial B$, the log-normal richness–Boltzmann temperature slope (holding precipitation constant) over the range of $B$ and $P$ observed in our data. Metabolic theory predicts to be a constant $-0.78$ eV. The observed slope varies from roughly $-1$ to $+1$ in the global angiosperm data, and from $-1.3$ to $-0.1$ in the North American tree data (Fig. 13.12). The variation of slope with temperature reflects the quadratic dependence of richness on temperature. The diagonal slant reflects the interaction of temperature and precipitation.

Thus, the predicted slope of the model of Allen *et al.* (2002) is remarkably close to observed spatial variation in richness. However, richness clearly varies spatially in a more complex way than their model predicts.

## Discussion

Many studies have shown that broad-scale patterns of richness are strongly related to climate, and that only a small amount of residual variability is then related to regional differences (Wright, 1983; Currie & Paquin, 1987; Adams & Woodward, 1989; Francis & Currie, 2003; Hawkins, Porter & Diniz-Filho, 2003b). This work is consistent with that interpretation. Studies that reported discontinuities in richness–climate relationships typically related richness to a single climatic variable (Schall & Pianka, 1978; Kerr & Packer, 1997). Such discontinuities disappear when both temperature and water are taken into account.

Weak richness–climate relationships within regions are exactly what one would expect when the within-region range of the variables in question is small. Thus, low $R^2$ values noted in some regional studies (Hawkins *et al.*, 2003a; Qian & Ricklefs, 2004) do not argue against the generality of a global richness–climate relationship. Rather, they indicate that, at scales at which climate varies little, climatic variation is not responsible for variation in richness.

It is sometimes argued that interregional differences (without controlling for climate) reflect regional processes such as evolutionary history (Latham & Ricklefs, 1993a,b; Ricklefs *et al.*, 1999). This argument suffers from several problems. First, different regions of the globe differ so strongly in climate (Francis & Currie, 1998) that it is difficult to distinguish between hypothesized regional effects on diversity, versus those of climate. The variance in richness that is collinear with both climate and region might be due to either. However, climate typically explains a large amount of residual variance after controlling for region, whereas regional differences after controlling for climate are generally small (e.g. Fig. 13.5).

Richness–climate relationships within regions around the world generally fall within a single, general relationship. New Zealand is a clear outlier with low richness, perhaps due to isolation. In contrast to the suggestion of Sax (2001), richness does not seem to depend upon abiotic factors (climate) in polar to temperate regions and biotic variables in the tropics. There are areas in the tropics (e.g. the Amazon and Southeast Asia) where richness follows climate very closely, and other areas where it does not. The same can be said regarding temperate regions. Rather, the striking residuals from the global relationship seem often to be found in very dry areas of the globe, some of which have higher than expected richness, and others lower. This might be due to evolutionary factors; however, a more obvious possibility is differences in the seasonality of precipitation (cf. Venevsky & Veneskaia, 2003).

This begs the question of what mechanism acts as the general constraint? The species–energy (a.k.a. climate–richness) hypothesis, first proposed by Hutchinson (1959), has received a great deal of interest in recent years. Correlations between richness and climate are consistent with this hypothesis (Hawkins et al., 2003a). However, the hypothesis makes many other predictions, hardly any of which appear to be consistent with extant data (Currie et al., 2004). This is apparently not the mechanism underlying global patterns of species richness.

Metabolic theory (Allen et al., 2002; Brown et al., 2004) made a highly orginal attempt to relate broad-scale patterns of richness to temperature gradients. Its most remarkable aspect was its very specific prediction of the slope of the relationship between log richness and Boltzmann-transformed temperature. We find that the upper bound of angiosperm richness as a function of temperature is very close to this predicted slope. However, much of the variation in richness is clearly related to water availability for trees, angiosperms, and most animal groups (A. Algar, J. T. Kerr & D. J. Currie, in prep.).

The original work of Allen et al. (2002) related richness solely to temperature (using some of these same data). More recent work (Allen et al., this volume) argues that broad-scale richness gradients reflect both temperature dependence of metabolism (and rate of evolution), as well as productivity-controlled gradients of abundance of individuals. Many studies (see Wright et al., 1993; Hawkins et al., 2003a) have observed that richness varies as a function of temperature, water and their interaction. This is consistent with an effect of productivity. However, the evidence does not suggest that productivity influences richness through increased numbers of individuals. Numbers of individuals do not vary markedly over climatic gradients, in contrast to richness (e.g. Currie et al., 2004; Fig. 13.1, Fig. 13.2; cf. Pautasso & Gaston, 2005, and look closely at their correlation coefficients). This is obvious walking through wet tropical forests versus boreal forests: diversity is strikingly greater in the tropics, but not the density of trees. Further, richness–climate relationships are typically much stronger than either richness–individuals, or individuals–climate relationships.

I suspect that Allen et al. (this volume) are correct in postulating that productivity influences richness (albeit through some mechanism other than numbers of individuals). Unfortunately, the current version of metabolic theory (Allen et al., this volume) no longer makes an explicit prediction about the expected relationship between richness and climatic variables. Rather, it predicts simply a correlation between richness, temperature and production, as do many other hypotheses.

Other strong-constraint hypotheses include the hypothesis that the number of possible ways to survive physiologically varies with climate. This hypothesis can make explicit, interesting predictions (Kleidon & Mooney, 2000; Anderson & Jetz, 2005), although it has not been tested adequately (Currie et al., 2004).

Similarly, the hypothesis that evolutionary rates vary with climate is also still relatively poorly tested (Currie *et al.*, 2004).

## Conclusion

I believe that this evidence is consistent with the view that one, or a small number, of factors act as general constraints on variation in richness on the regional to global scale. I see no reason to postulate that regional factors contribute more than relatively small amounts of variance to richness–climate relationships. There are no obvious differences in the richness–climate relationship between continents (as evolutionary hypotheses postulate) or between the tropics and colder regions. Changing extent may make richness–climate relationships appear to be weak, but their residual variability is, in fact, generally lower than the global relationship predicts. At fine grains, factors other than climate may also have strong effects on richness.

This suggests that textbooks should begin with the climatic constraint on richness, and discuss other factors as minor influences, much as textbooks present phosphorus concentration as the principal factor determining the abundance of aquatic organisms, with other factors such as predation, mixing depth, etc., as minor contributors.

## Acknowledgments

Thanks to Anthony Francis, Tania Sendel and Bryan Wilson for allowing me to use their data. David Storch, Andrew Allen, and Andrew Clarke offered very constructive feedback on earlier drafts. This work was supported by a grant from the Natural Sciences and Engineering Research Council of Canada, and by travel funds from the Santa Fe Institute.

## References

Adams, J. M. & Woodward, F. I. (1989). Patterns in tree species richness as a test of the glacial extinction hypothesis. *Nature*, **339**, 699–701.

Allen, A. P., Brown, J. H. & Gillooly, J. F. (2002). Global biodiversity, biochemical kinetics, and the energetic-equivalence rule. *Science*, **297**, 1545–1548.

Anderson, K. J. & Jetz, W. (2005). The broad-scale ecology of energy expenditure of endotherms. *Ecology Letters*, **8**, 310–318.

Barthlott, W., Lauer, W. P. A. & Placke, A. (1996). Global distribution of species diversity in vascular plants: toward a world map of phytodiversity. *Erkunde*, **50**, 317–327.

Brown, J. H. (1981). Two decades of homage to Santa Rosalia: toward a general theory of diversity. *American Zoologist*, **21**, 877–888.

Brown, J. H. & Lomolino, M. V. (1998). *Biogeography*. Sunderland, MA: Sinauer Associates.

Brown, J. H., Gillooly, J. F., Allen, A. P., Savage, V. M. & West, G. B. (2004). Toward a metabolic theory of ecology. *Ecology*, **85**, 1771–1789.

Bystrak, D. (1981). The North American Breeding Bird Survey. *Studies in Avian Biology*, **6**, 34–41.

Chesson, P. (2000). Mechanisms of maintenance of species diversity. *Annual Reviews of Ecology and Systematics*, **31**, 343–366.

Connell, J. H. (1978). Diversity in tropical rain forests and coral reefs. *Science*, **199**, 1302–1310.

Cook, R. E. (1969). Variation in species density of North American birds. *Systematic Zoology*, **18**, 63–84.

Currie, D. J. (1991). Energy and large scale patterns of animal and plant species richness. *American Naturalist*, **137**, 27–49.

Currie, D. J. & Paquin, V. (1987). Large-scale bio-geographical patterns of species richness in trees. *Nature*, **329**, 326–327.

Currie, D. J., Mittelbach, G. G., Cornell, H. V., *et al.* (2004). Predictions and tests of climate-based hypotheses of broad-scale variation in taxonomic richness. *Ecology Letters*, **7**, 1121–1134.

Francis, A. & Currie, D. J. (1998). Global patterns of tree species richness in moist forests: another look. *Oikos*, **81**, 598–602.

Francis, A. P. & Currie, D. J. (2003). A globally-consistent richness-climate relationship for angiosperms. *American Naturalist*, **161**, 523–536.

Fukami, T. & Morin, P. J. (2003). Productivity-diversity relationships depend upon the history of the community assembly. *Nature*, **424**, 423–426.

Hawkins, B. A., Field, R., Cornell, H. V., *et al.* (2003a). Energy, water, and broad-scale patterns of species richness. *Ecology*, **84**, 3105–3117.

Hawkins, B. A., Porter, E. E. & Diniz-Filho, J. A. F. (2003b). Productivity and history as predictors of the latitudinal diversity gradient of terrestrial birds. *Ecology*, **84**, 1608–1623.

Heywood, V. H. (1993). *Flowering Plants of the World*. New York: Oxford University Press.

Holt, R. D., Lawton, J. H., Polis, G. A. & Martinez, N. D. (1999). Trophic rank and the species-area relationship. *Ecology*, **80**(5), 1495–1504.

Hurlbert, A. H. (2004). Species-energy relationships and habitat complexity in bird communities. *Ecology Letters*, **7**, 714–720.

Huston, M. (1994). *Biological Diversity: The Coexistence of Species on a Changing Landscape*. Cambridge: Cambridge University Press.

Hutchinson, G. E. (1959). Homage to Santa Rosalia, or why are there so many kinds of animals? *American Naturalist*, **93**, 145–159.

Kerr, J. T. & Packer, L. (1997). Habitat hetero-geneity as a determinant of mammal species richness in high-energy regions. *Nature*, **385**, 252–254.

Kleidon, A. & Mooney, H. A. (2000). A global distribution of biodiversity inferred from climatic constraints: results from a process-based modelling study. *Global Change Biology*, **6**, 507–523.

Latham, R. E. & Ricklefs, R. E. (1993a). Continental comparisons of temperate-zone tree species diversity. In *Species Diversity in Ecological Communities: Historical and Geographical Perspectives*, ed. R. E. Ricklefs & D. Schluter, pp. 294–314. Chicago: University of Chicago Press.

Latham, R. E. & Ricklefs, R. E. (1993b). Global patterns of tree species richness in moist forests – energy-diversity theory does not account for variation in species richness. *Oikos*, **67**, 325–333.

Lawton, J. H. (1999). Are there general laws in ecology? *Oikos*, **84**, 177–192.

Lieth, H. (1975). Modeling the primary productivity of the world. In *Primary Productivity of the Biosphere*, ed. H. Lieth & R. H. Whittaker, pp. 237–263. New York: Springer-Verlag.

Little Jr., E. J. (1971). *Atlas of United States Trees*. Vols. 1–5. Washington, DC: U.S. Government Printing Office.

Mittelbach, G., Steiner, C., Scheiner, S. M., *et al.* (2001). What is the observed relationship between species richness and productivity? *Ecology*, **82**, 2381–2396.

Palmer, M. W. & White, P. S. (1994). Scale dependence and the species-area relationship. *American Naturalist*, **144**, 717–740.

Pautasso, M. G. & Gaston, K. J. (2005). Resources and global avian assemblage structure in forests. *Ecology Letters*, **8**, 282–289.

Peters, R. H. (1983). *The Ecological Implications of Body Size*. Cambridge: Cambridge University Press.

Peters, R. H. (1991). *A Critique for Ecology*. Cambridge: Cambridge University Press.

Petit, R. J., Aguinagalde, I., de Beaulieu, J.-L., *et al.* (2003). Glacial refugia: hotspots but not melting pots of genetic diversity. *Science*, **300**, 1563.

Phillips, O. & Miller, J. S. (2002). *Global Patterns of Plant Diversity: Alwyn H. Gentry's Forest Transect Data Set*. St. Louis, MO: Missouri Botanical Garden Press.

Popper, K. R. (1990). *A World of Propensities*. Bristol: Thoemmes.

Qian, H. & Ricklefs, R. E. (1999). A comparison of the taxonomic richness of vascular plants in China and the United States. *American Naturalist*, **154**, 160–181.

Qian, H. & Ricklefs, R. E. (2004). Taxon richness and climate in angiosperms: is there a globally consistent relationship that precludes region effects? *American Naturalist*, **163**, 773–779.

Ricklefs, R. E., Latham, R. E. & Qian, H. (1999). Global patterns of tree species richness in moist forests: distinguishing ecological influences and historical contingency. *Oikos*, **86**, 369–373.

Rigler, F. H. & Peters, R. H. (1995). *Science and Limnology*. Oldendorf/Luhe: Ecology Institute.

Rosenzweig, M. L. (1968). Net primary productivity of terrestrial communities: predictions from climatological data. *American Naturalist*, **102**, 67–74.

Rosenzweig, M. L. (1995). *Species Diversity in Time and Space*. Cambridge: Cambridge University Press.

Sauer, J. R., Hines, J. E. & Fallon, J. (2004). *The North American Breeding Brid Survey, Results and Analysis 1966–2003. Version 2004.1*. Laurel, MD: USES Patuxent Wildlife Research Center.

Sax, D. F. (2001). Latitudinal gradients and geographic ranges of exotic species: implications for biogeography. *Journal of Biogeography*, **28**, 139–150.

Schall, J. J. & Pianka, E. R. (1978). Geographical trends in the numbers of species. *Science*, **201**, 679–686.

Smith, F. (2001). Historical regulation of local species richness across a geographic region. *Ecology*, **82**, 792–801.

Starnes, W. C. & Etnier, D. A. (1986). Drainage evolution and fish biogeography of the Tennessee and Cumberlan Rivers drainage realm. In *The Zoogeography of North American Fishes*, ed. C. H. Hocutt & E. O. Wiley, pp. 325–362. New York: Wiley.

Stohlgren, T. J., Binkley, D., Chong, G. W., *et al.* (1999). Exotic plant species invade hot spots of native plant diversity. *Ecological Monographs*, **69**, 25–46.

Venevsky, S. & Veneskaia, I. (2003). Large-scale energetic and landscape factors of vegetation diversity. *Ecology Letters*, **6**, 1004–1016.

von Humboldt, A. & Bonpland, A. (1807). *Essai sur la géographie des plantes accompagné d'un tableau physique des régions équinoxales*. Paris: Shoell, reprinted by Arno Press, New York.

Wallace, A. R. (1878). *Tropical Nature and Other Essays*. New York: Macmillan.

Wright, D. H. (1983). Species-energy theory: an extension of species-area theory. *Oikos*, **41**, 496–506.

Wright, D. H., Currie, D. J. & Maurer, B. A. (1993). Energy supply and patterns of species richness on local and regional scales. In *Species Diversity in Ecological Communities: Historical and Geographical Perspectives*, ed. R. E. Ricklefs & D. Schluter, pp. 66–74. Chicago: University of Chicago Press.

CHAPTER FOURTEEN

# Recasting the species–energy hypothesis: the different roles of kinetic and potential energy in regulating biodiversity

ANDREW P. ALLEN
*National Center for Ecological Analysis and Synthesis*
JAMES F. GILLOOLY
*University of Florida*
JAMES H. BROWN
*University of New Mexico, Albuquerque and The Santa Fe Institute*

## Introduction

Understanding the causes and consequences of variation in biodiversity has long been a central focus of research in ecology and biogeography (von Humboldt, 1808; Hutchinson, 1959; MacArthur, 1969; Brown, 1981; Tilman, 1999; Hubbell, 2001; Clarke, this volume). Ecologists have been particularly fascinated by the latitudinal gradient of increasing biodiversity from the poles to the equator since at least the time of Darwin (1859) and Wallace (1878). Contemporary data indicate that this gradient holds for nearly all major groups of terrestrial, aquatic, and marine ectotherms, both plant and animal, and for endothermic birds and mammals (Rohde, 1992; Gaston, 2000; Allen, Brown & Gillooly, 2002; Willig, Kaufman & Stevens, 2003; Currie *et al.*, 2004; Pautasso & Gaston, 2005; Clarke, this volume; Currie, this volume). Furthermore, fossil data indicate that this gradient has been maintained for over 200 million years (Stehli, Douglas & Newell, 1969). Despite more than 150 years of inquiry, the mechanisms responsible for the gradient are still not well understood (Allen, Brown & Gillooly, 2003; Hawkins *et al.*, 2003; Huston *et al.*, 2003; Storch, 2003; Currie *et al.*, 2004; Clarke, this volume; Currie, this volume), but a large and growing list of hypotheses has been proposed to explain it (Rohde, 1992; Gaston, 2000; Hawkins *et al.*, 2003; Currie *et al.*, 2004).

In recent years, particular attention has focused on what we will refer to as the *species–energy hypothesis*, which proposes that the latitudinal biodiversity gradient has somehow been generated and maintained as a direct consequence of greater energy availability towards the equator. The species–energy hypothesis is consistent with extensive empirical work showing strong positive correlations between geographic gradients in biodiversity and climatic measures that

*Scaling Biodiversity*, ed. David Storch, Pablo A. Marquet and James H. Brown. Published by Cambridge University Press. © Cambridge University Press 2007.

directly or indirectly reflect energy availability in the environment (Currie, 1991; Wright, Currie & Maurer, 1993; Hawkins *et al.*, 2003; Currie *et al.*, 2004, Clarke, this volume; Currie, this volume). These climatic measures can be classified into one of two distinct classes: (1) those that directly reflect fluxes of solar radiation, such as temperature and potential evapotranspiration; and (2) those that are directly or indirectly related to the rate of conversion of solar radiation to reduced carbon compounds through photosynthesis, such as precipitation, net primary production, and actual evapotranspiration.

Several mechanisms have been proposed to account for species–energy relationships; these include the effects of temperature on biochemical reaction rates (Rohde, 1992; Allen *et al.*, 2002), the effects of temperature on the ability of organisms to maintain homeostasis (Currie, 1991; Hawkins *et al.*, 2003; Currie *et al.*, 2004), and the effects of ecosystem productivity on total community abundance (Hutchinson, 1959; Brown, 1981; Wright, 1983; Allen *et al.*, 2002; Clarke, this volume). Despite the strength and ubiquity of species–energy correlations, no consensus has yet emerged about the mechanisms that generate them (Hawkins *et al.*, 2003; Currie *et al.*, 2004).

Here we suggest that our present gap in knowledge about the origins of species–energy relationships stems from three interrelated issues. First, "energy" comes in not one, but two basic forms – kinetic and potential – that affect biota in different ways. Second, as a consequence, while both forms of energy may influence biodiversity, they necessarily do so through different mechanisms. And third, while we recognize that biodiversity is ultimately an integrated measure of speciation–extinction dynamics, we still have only limited understanding of how speciation rates, extinction rates, and the standing stock of species are dynamically linked to each other (Hubbell, 2001), and to the availability of kinetic and potential forms of energy in the environment (Allen *et al.*, 2003; Huston *et al.*, 2003; Storch, 2003). Together, these three issues highlight the need to recast the species–energy hypothesis in terms of the two basic forms of energy in nature – kinetic and potential – and the different ways they affect biota. (See also Clarke, this volume.)

In this chapter, we address these three key issues from the perspective of recent advances toward a metabolic theory of ecology (MTE) (Brown *et al.*, 2004). This recent work indicates that the availability of both forms of energy, kinetic and potential, influences biodiversity, but through different mechanisms. The first mechanism is related to the constraint of thermal kinetic energy, characterized by environmental temperature, on cellular- and individual-level metabolic processes. It is consistent with the *evolutionary speed hypothesis* (Rohde, 1992; Allen *et al.*, 2002). The second mechanism is related to the constraint of chemical potential energy, characterized by net primary production, on total community abundance. It is consistent with the *more individuals hypothesis* (Hutchinson, 1959; Brown, 1981; Wright, 1983; Allen *et al.*, 2002). We argue that these mechanisms do not operate in isolation, but rather in concert, to help regulate biodiversity gradients. Furthermore, despite fundamental differences between these two mechanisms, we propose that they both influence biodiversity through their effects on speciation rates in biological communities.

We develop these ideas as follows in the remaining sections of this chapter. In the second section, we define kinetic and potential energy, and discuss their relationships to rates of biological metabolism for individuals, communities, and ecosystems. In the third section, we discuss mechanisms that may link biodiversity to energy availability in the environment through their effects on speciation rates in biological communities. Then, in the following section, we present empirical evidence that kinetic and potential energy each play important, but fundamentally different roles in regulating biodiversity. In the final section, we discuss theoretical and empirical challenges that will need to be addressed in order to rigorously test the hypothesis that energy availability regulates biodiversity through its effects on speciation rates.

## Relationships of kinetic and potential energy to biological metabolism

We propose that a more mechanistic understanding of species–energy relationships can be achieved by explicitly focusing on the two fundamental forms of energy in nature – kinetic and potential – and their different roles in sustaining life. We therefore begin this section by briefly reviewing basic energy concepts from physics. We then discuss biological metabolism in light of these concepts. We conclude this section by discussing how the availability of kinetic and potential forms of energy constrains the biological metabolism of individuals, communities, and ecosystems.

Energy is defined as the capacity of a system to do work. For a simple mechanical system, work involves moving a mass (kg) over a distance (m) by applying a force ($m\,s^{-2}$). Regardless of the type of work being performed, its magnitude can be expressed in energy units of joules ($1\,J = 1\,kg\,m^2\,s^{-2}$). From physics, we know that all energy comes in one of two basic forms, kinetic and potential. Kinetic energy is the energy of motion. Thermal kinetic energy is essential to life because, without it, biochemical reactions cannot proceed. Thermal kinetic energy is indexed by absolute temperature, $T$ in kelvins (K), which is proportional to the average kinetic energy of randomly moving atoms and molecules in a system. At higher temperatures, atoms and molecules move at higher velocities, $v$, and therefore have more thermal kinetic energy ($T \propto v^2$). Solar radiation, another type of kinetic energy, is also essential because it is used by plants to photosynthesize reduced carbon compounds. Once formed, these compounds represent the second basic form of energy, potential energy, which is defined as energy stored in an object. The chemical potential energy stored in reduced carbon compounds fuels virtually all biochemical reactions in the biosphere.

Metabolism is the process of transforming kinetic energy to potential forms (and vice versa) through biochemical reactions. The metabolic rate of an organism is equal to its total rate of energy transformation for fitness-enhancing processes of survival, growth, and reproduction (Brown *et al.*, 2004). This rate can be expressed in units of watts ($1\,W = 1\,J\,s^{-1}$). As a point of reference, a human being has a resting metabolic rate about equal to the energy flux of a standard 100 W light bulb. Following the definition of biological metabolism, the metabolic rate of an autotroph is its total rate of photosynthesis, $P_i$:

$$CO_2 + H_2O \xrightarrow{P_i} CH_2O + O_2 \tag{14.1}$$

and the metabolic rate of a heterotroph is its total rate of respiration, $R_i$:

$$CH_2O + O_2 \xrightarrow{R_i} CO_2 + H_2O. \tag{14.2}$$

Autotrophic metabolism is thus governed by the photosynthesis of chemical potential energy in the form of reduced carbon compounds ($CH_2O$), whereas heterotrophic metabolism is governed by the utilization of chemical potential energy in respiration. Due to mass and energy balance, the gross rate of photosynthesis by a plant, $P_i$, can be expressed as the sum of two other individual-level rates, respiration plus growth. Thus, for autotrophic individuals, the metabolic rate *exceeds* the respiration rate. By contrast, for heterotrophic individuals, the metabolic rate *equals* the respiration rate, $R_i$. This is because heterotrophs take in materials that have already been "prepackaged" by plants through photosynthesis, and because respiration fuels any additional energy transformations that are required to convert these prepackaged materials to heterotrophic biomass.

For a heterotroph, the process of consuming chemical potential energy in respiration is primarily constrained by two variables: individual body size, $M_i$ (g), and temperature, $T$ (K) (Gillooly *et al.*, 2001). The combined effects of these two variables on individual respiration, $R_i$ (W), can be described by the following equation (Gillooly *et al.*, 2001):

$$R_i = r_0 M_i^{3/4} e^{-E/kT}, \tag{14.3}$$

where $r_0$ is a normalization constant, independent of body size and temperature ($W\,g^{-3/4}$), that varies about 10-fold between multicellular animals and microbes (Gillooly *et al.*, 2001). The 3/4-power scaling exponent on the body size term reflects geometric and biophysical constraints on the delivery of energy and materials to cells through biological distribution networks (West, Brown & Enquist, 1997). Based on this size dependence, Eq. (14.3) predicts a $10^{15}$-fold increase in metabolic rate over the body size range $10^{-12}\,g$ to $10^8\,g$ from microbes to whales ($[10^8/10^{-12}]^{3/4} = 10^{15}$-fold). The Boltzmann–Arrhenius factor, $e^{-E/kT}$, characterizes the exponential effects of temperature on individual metabolic rate, where $E$ is the average activation energy of the respiratory complex ($\sim$0.65 eV), and $k$ is Boltzmann's constant ($8.62 \times 10^{-5}\,eV\,K^{-1}$) (Gillooly *et al.*, 2001). This Boltzmann–Arrhenius factor quantifies the relationship of temperature to the proportion of molecules in a system that have kinetic energies exceeding the activation energy, $E$, required to react. Based on this temperature dependence, Eq. (14.3) predicts a 34-fold increase in metabolic rate over the biological temperature range 0–40 °C from an Antarctic fish to an endothermic bird or mammal ($e^{-E/k313}/e^{-E/k273} = 34$-fold from 273–313 K).

By extending these basic energy concepts, we can quantify the relationship of the individual respiration rate, $R_i$ (Eq. 14.3), to the respiratory flux of the entire heterotrophic community. Due to mass and energy balance, the total respiration rate per unit area for a heterotrophic community comprised of $J$ individuals in an area of size $A$, $R_{Tot}$ ($W\,m^{-2}$), is equal to the sum of the individual respiration rates, $R_i$, from Eq. (14.3).

$$R_{Tot} = \frac{1}{A}\sum_{i=1}^{J} R_i = (J/A)\langle R_i \rangle_J = (J/A) r_0 \langle M^{3/4} \rangle_J e^{-E/kT}, \tag{14.4}$$

where $J/A$ is the abundance of individuals per unit area ($m^{-2}$), $\langle R_i \rangle_J$ is the average metabolic rate of an individual ($= (1/J) \sum_{i=1}^{J} R_i = r_0 \langle M^{3/4} \rangle_J e^{-E/kT}$), and $\langle M^{3/4} \rangle_J$ is an average for body size ($= (1/J) \sum_{i=1}^{J} M_i^{3/4}$) (Enquist et al., 2003; Allen, Gillooly & Brown, 2005).

Four issues arise in using Eq. (14.4) to derive and test predictions. First, while $R_{Tot}$ exactly equals the sum of the individual respiration rates, $r_0$ can vary among taxa (Gillooly et al., 2001). Accuracy of predictions may therefore be improved by aggregating organisms into different functional groups. Second, Eq. (14.4) assumes that $r_0$ is independent of resource availability, $N(L_i)$, but organisms sometimes depress their metabolic rates in response to food scarcity. Equation (14.4) will be robust to such facultative responses provided that the scope for change in $r_0$ is small relative to variation in $N(L_i)$. One study supports this assumption by demonstrating that metabolic rates of a rodent species declined by only ~25% over a more than 10-fold decline in ecosystem net primary production (Mueller & Diamond, 2001). Third, the average for body size in Eq. (14.4), $\langle M_i^{3/4} \rangle_J$, does not equal the arithmetic mean of body size raised to the 3/4-power, i.e. $\langle M_i^{3/4} \rangle_J \neq \langle M \rangle_J^{3/4}$, where $\langle M \rangle_J = (1/J) \sum_{i=1}^{J} M_i$. This point is relevant because frequency distributions of body size are often highly skewed in biological communities, resulting in pronounced differences between $\langle M_i^{3/4} \rangle_J$ and $\langle M \rangle_J^{3/4}$ (Savage, 2004). Finally, fourth, Eq. (14.4) does not apply to long-term respiration rates of autotrophic communities. This is because plant metabolism is governed by photosynthesis (Eq. 14.1), which has a non-exponential temperature dependence (Allen et al., 2005). Furthermore, photosynthesis may be limited or colimited by other variables in addition to temperature (Farquhar, von Caemmerer & Berry, 1980; Allen et al., 2005); these variables include water (Lieth, 1973; Huxman et al., 2004), light (Monteith, 1972; Field et al., 1998), nutrients (Vitousek, 1984; Chapin, Matson & Mooney, 2002), and space (Enquist & Niklas, 2001). (See also Clarke, this volume.) For what follows, we will collectively denote those resources limiting photosynthesis by $L_i$, and we will denote the rate of net primary production of reduced carbon compounds by the function $N(L_i)$ $(\text{W m}^{-2})$ to reflect resource limitation on photosynthesis in ecosystems.

By imposing mass and energy balance on the production and consumption of chemical potential energy in ecosystems, we can extend Eq. (14.4) to predict the relationship of ecosystem net primary production to the total abundance and metabolism of heterotrophic individuals. If the total rate of respiration by all of the heterotrophs comprising a community, $R_{\text{Tot}}$, is limited by the availability of reduced carbon compounds, $N(L_i)$, as indicated by recent work (Allen et al., 2005), then

$$R_{\text{Tot}} = (J/A)r_0\left\langle M_i^{3/4}\right\rangle_J e^{-E/kT} \approx N(L_i). \tag{14.5}$$

Rearranging the terms in Eq. (14.5) shows how the total abundance of heterotrophs is limited by net primary production:

$$(J/A) \approx N(L_i)e^{E/kT}/r_0\left\langle M_i^{3/4}\right\rangle_J \approx N(L_i)/\langle R_i\rangle_J. \tag{14.6}$$

Equation (14.6) yields different predictions for endotherms and ectotherms. For endotherms, body temperatures, and hence average metabolic rates $\langle R_i\rangle_J$, are relatively high and constant across global temperature gradients (Anderson & Jetz, 2005). Thus, after controlling for body size, $\left\langle M_i^{3/4}\right\rangle_J$, community abundance is predicted to increase approximately linearly with the rate of consumption of net primary production, $N(L_i)$, in agreement with recent work (Pautasso & Gaston, 2005). By contrast, for ectotherms, abundance is predicted to decline exponentially with increasing temperature $(\propto e^{E/kT})$ if $N(L_i)$ and $\left\langle M_i^{3/4}\right\rangle_J$ are both held constant in Eq. (14.6) (Savage et al., 2004; Allen et al., 2005) because of increases in per-individual metabolic demands, $\langle R_i\rangle_J$ (Eq. 14.3). Thus, for the community abundance of ectotherms to even remain constant across global temperature gradients, the total rate of consumption of net primary production, $N(L_i)$, must increase with increasing temperature. Ecosystem net primary production does in fact increase with temperature (Lieth, 1973), but the response is not exponential (Allen et al., 2005). Modeling the overall global relationship between abundance and net primary production for heterotrophic ectotherms therefore requires explicit consideration of temperature and its differential effects on heterotrophic respiration versus autotrophic photosynthesis (Allen et al., 2005).

The issues discussed above arise as direct consequences of differences in the controls on metabolism for plants, heterotrophic ectotherms, and endotherms, and can be quantified using Eqs. (14.3) to (14.6). More generally, these equations demonstrate that the availability of thermal kinetic energy in the environment, indexed by $T$, fundamentally constrains the consumption of chemical potential energy by heterotrophs at the individual level, $\langle R_i \rangle_J$, and that the net rate of production of chemical potential energy by autotrophs, $N(L_i)$, fundamentally constrains the consumption of chemical potential energy by heterotrophs at the community level, $R_{Tot}$. These ecosystem-level rates of energy transformation, $N(L_i)$ and $R_{Tot}$, are, in turn, both constrained by the availability of resources, $L_i$, required for photosynthesis to proceed.

## Linking kinetic and potential energy to biodiversity through speciation

In this section, we discuss processes and mechanisms that may link kinetic and potential energy to biodiversity through their effects on speciation rates. There is now significant theoretical and empirical support for the idea that comprehensive understanding of biodiversity gradients will require a synthesis of new approaches that explicitly link short-term species coexistence to long-term speciation–extinction dynamics (Allen & Gillooly, 2006). In particular, the recently proposed Neutral Theory of Biodiversity (NTB) demonstrates that increasing the overall rate of speciation in biological communities can result in higher steady-state levels of biodiversity (Hubbell, 2001). Furthermore, there exists fossil evidence indicating that biodiversity peaks in the tropics as a direct consequence of elevated speciation rates (Stehli *et al.*, 1969; Crane & Lidgard, 1989; Jablonski, 1993; Flessa & Jablonski, 1996; Crame, 2002), although this remains an important topic of debate (Chown & Gaston, 2000; Currie *et al.*, 2004; Allen & Gillooly, 2006).

We hypothesize that kinetic and potential forms of energy both help regulate biodiversity through their effects on speciation rates, but via different mechanisms (arrows 1–3, Fig. 14.1). The process of speciation involves the evolution of genetic differences among species populations, which accumulate to induce reproductive isolation and influence ecological roles (Coyne & Orr, 2004). The overall speciation rate in a community can therefore be increased in one of two ways (Fig. 14.1): (arrow 4) by increasing the rates of genetic divergence among species populations, or (arrow 5) by increasing the total number of species populations. This reasoning implies that the overall rate of speciation in a community should be expressed as the product of a per capita rate (species individual$^{-1}$ time$^{-1}$) and total community abundance (Allen *et al.*, 2006). Characterizing speciation on a per capita basis runs counter to the long-standing tradition among evolutionists and paleontologists of expressing speciation on a per species basis (species species$^{-1}$ time$^{-1}$) (Yule, 1925; Coyne & Orr, 2004). Nevertheless, it is consistent with evolutionary theory because speciation occurs at the level of populations, not species (Coyne & Orr, 2004). It is also consistent with the NTB, which predicts that the overall speciation rate

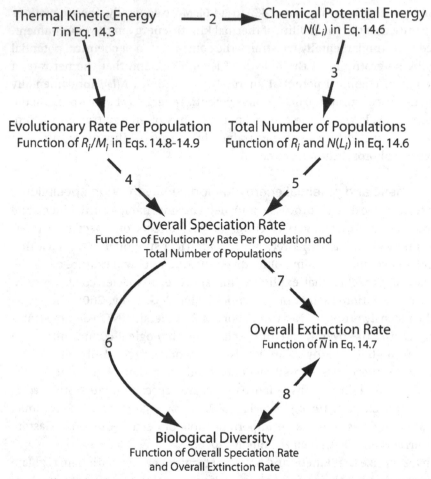

**Figure 14.1** Framework proposed in this chapter for the relationship of biological diversity to the availability of kinetic and potential forms of energy in the environment. The arrows are numbered to facilitate discussion in the text. See Allen *et al*. (2005) for theory and data on how thermal kinetic energy, *T*, influences net primary production, $N(L_i)$, in terrestrial ecosystems (denoted by arrow 2).

determines the number of species maintained in a community of fixed total abundance, and not vice versa (Hubbell, 2001).

Biodiversity is an integrated measure of speciation–extinction dynamics because the number of species in existence at any given time equals the total number of speciation events minus the total number of extinction events (arrows 6, 8; Fig. 14.1). Recent work indicates that global biodiversity is at or near steady state, and has been for hundreds of millions of years (Alroy *et al.*, 2001). This implies that overall rates of speciation and extinction are approximately equal for many taxa. Following the early work of Rozenzweig (1975) and

Sepkoski (1978), among others, and the more recent work of Hubbell (2001) and Alroy et al. (2001), we assume here that biodiversity is at or near steady state. We also assume that this steady state arises because increasing the overall rate of speciation in a community of fixed size reduces the average abundance per species per unit area, $\overline{N}$, resulting in higher rates of stochastic extinction (Hubbell, 2001). Given that the stochastic extinction rate is expected to increase with decreasing $\overline{N}$ (Lande, Engen & Saether, 2003) (arrow 7), and that

$$\overline{N} = (J/AS),\tag{14.7}$$

where $S$ is species richness in a plot of area $A$ (Allen et al., 2002), the extinction rate is directly related to species richness (arrow 8). This line of reasoning (Fig. 14.1) yields the hypothesis that the speciation rate is an important driving variable of speciation–extinction dynamics, and therefore of geographic gradients in biodiversity (Allen & Gillooly, 2006). For the remainder of this section, we will therefore speculate on how the availability of kinetic and potential forms of energy may help regulate biodiversity (arrows 1–3) through their effects on speciation rates (arrows 4–5), and the dynamic interplay between speciation, extinction, and the standing stock of species (arrows 6–8).

Based on the MTE results presented in the previous section, and other MTE results discussed below, we propose that thermal kinetic energy influences speciation rates through its effects on rates of genetic divergence among species populations (arrow 1, Fig. 14.1), and that chemical potential energy influences speciation rates through its effects on the total numbers of individuals and populations that are maintained in an ecosystem (arrow 3, Fig. 14.1).

We hypothesize that the availability of thermal kinetic energy is linked to speciation rates through the constraints of environmental temperature, $T$, on rate processes controlled by mass-specific metabolic rate, $R_i/M_i$ (following Eq. 14.3; arrow 1, Fig. 14.1). The rate at which a population evolves is constrained by two individual-level variables, the generation time and mutation rate (Fisher, 1930; Kimura, 1983). Recent work has shown that the rate of turnover of individuals, $g$ (generations $s^{-1}$), increases directly with mass-specific metabolic rate, $R_i/M_i$ (Gillooly et al., 2002; Savage et al., 2004):

$$g = g_0(R_i/M_i) = g_0 r_0 M_i^{-1/4} e^{-E/kT},\tag{14.8}$$

where $g_0$ is a normalization constant that characterizes the number of generations per joule of energy flux through a gram of tissue ($J^{-1}g$ generations) (Fig. 14.2a). More recently, we have shown that rates of mutation in nuclear and mitochondrial genomes, $\alpha$ (mutations nucleotide$^{-1}$ $s^{-1}$), also increase directly with mass-specific metabolic rate (Gillooly et al., 2005):

$$\alpha = \alpha_0(R_i/M_i) = \alpha_0 b_0 M_i^{-1/4} e^{-E/kT},\tag{14.9}$$

where $\alpha_0$ is a normalization constant that characterizes the number of joules of metabolic energy required to induce one mutation per site in a genome

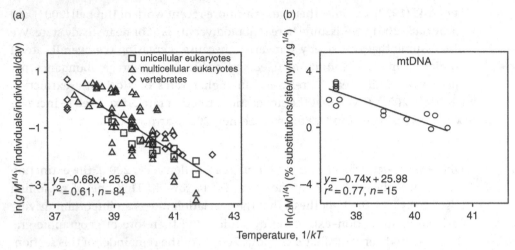

**Figure 14.2** Effects of temperature, expressed as $1/kT$, on the natural logarithm of (a) individual turnover of unicellular and multicellular eukaryotes, and (b) molecular evolution in mitochondria of multicellular eukaryotes. Rates were body size-corrected as described in Brown *et al.* (2004) prior to logarithmic transformation. Negative linear relationships between the variables, with slopes close to $-E \approx -0.65$ eV, indicate that rates increase exponentially with temperature according to the Boltzmann–Arrhenius relationship for respiration ($\propto e^{-E/kT}$, Eq. 14.3). Turnover data are from Savage *et al.* (2004), and mitochondrial RFLP data are from Gillooly *et al.* (2005).

($J^{-1}$ g mutations nucleotide$^{-1}$) (Fig. 14.2b). There are also population-level variables that influence how quickly populations evolve; these variables include effective population size, the migration rate among populations, and the intensity of natural selection (Fisher, 1930; Kimura, 1983). Furthermore, speciation requires not only evolution within populations, but also an ecological mechanism that facilitates genetic divergence among populations, e.g. a geographic barrier to dispersal in the allopatric mode of speciation (Mayr, 1942). Speciation is thus an inherently ecological as well as evolutionary process. Nevertheless, using Eqs. (14.7) and (14.8), it can be shown that if the population-level variables affecting genetic divergence rates are held constant, rates of genetic divergence will increase exponentially with temperature in the same way as individual metabolic rate (Allen *et al.*, 2006).

We hypothesize that the availability of chemical potential energy is linked to the speciation rate through the constraints of ecosystem net primary production, $N(L_i)$, on total community abundance (following Eq. 14.6; arrow 3, Fig. 14.1). Our reasoning is that if the total abundance of individuals in a community is increased through enhancement of net primary production (Eq. 14.6), total rates of population subdivision via allopatric, parapatric, sympatric mechanisms should also increase, resulting in higher speciation rates. We note one important complication with this argument. Equation (14.6) assumes that hete-rotrophs make use of all of the chemical potential energy made available by plants through net primary production. While this assumption is reasonable for the entire heterotrophic communities (Allen *et al.*, 2005), only a small fraction of total net primary production in the ecosystem, $N(L_i)$, is consumed by any of the more restricted heterotrophic "communities" that ecologists typically study (e.g. amphibians, birds, reptiles). Abundance for a restricted taxon is a function not only of ecosystem net primary production, but also of biotic and abiotic variables that interact with attributes of the taxon to uniquely determine its environmental niche (Kaspari, 2001). As a consequence, we expect the relation-ship between $N(L_i)$ and community abundance to be idiosyncratic for restricted taxa (Kaspari, 2005).

## The different roles of kinetic and potential energy in regulating biodiversity

In the preceding sections, we proposed that kinetic and potential energy each play important, but fundamentally different, roles in regulating biodiversity. Specifically, we proposed that the availability of thermal kinetic energy, char-acterized by environmental temperature $T$, helps regulate biodiversity through its effects on cellular- and individual-level processes (Eq. 14.3; arrow 1, Fig. 14.1), and that the availability of chemical potential energy, characterized by $N(L_i)$, helps regulate biodiversity through its effects on community abundance (Eq. 14.6; arrow 3, Fig. 14.1). Furthermore, we speculated that both mechanisms contribute to the maintenance of biodiversity through their effects on specia-tion rates (arrows 4–5, Fig. 14.1).

Building on our proposed framework, it is possible to decompose energetic determinants of biodiversity into those that operate through their effects on individual metabolic rate, $R_i$, and those that operate through their effects on community abundance, $J/A$ (Allen *et al.*, in preparation). However, it is important to note that these two sets of determinants are rarely if ever independent. For example, in terrestrial ecosystems, increasing the environmental temperature, $T$, not only enhances the metabolic rates of heterotrophic ectotherms ($R_i$, Eq. 14.3), it also enhances net primary production, $N(L_i)$ (Allen *et al.*, 2005) (arrow 2, Fig. 14.1), which in turn interacts with $R_i$ to influence community abundance (Eq. 14.6). Marine ecosystems perhaps offer the greatest opportunity for disentangling the effects of kinetic and potential energy on biodiversity because broad-scale gradients in the net primary production of the world's oceans are largely decoupled from temperature by nutrient limitation (Field *et al.*, 1998).

The analysis of Currie (this volume) illustrates the complexities involved in disentangling the determinants of biodiversity. In particular, Currie shows in Fig. 13.10(a) of his chapter that there exists an upper bound on tree diversity that is well fitted by the exponential Boltzmann temperature relationship predicted by Allen et al. (2002), but that there exists significant residual variation below this upper bound. Allen et al. (2002) were careful to point out in their derivation that the Boltzmann relationship is only predicted if total community abundance is held constant across temperature gradients. Thus, according to Allen et al. (2002), and to the framework proposed here (Fig. 14.1), this variation is largely attributable to variation in total plant abundance. Specifically, we hypothesize that the upper bound in Fig. 13.10(a) of Currie (this volume) is comprised predominantly of well-watered sites where plant abundance is high, relatively constant, and largely independent of latitudinal gradients in temperature (Enquist & Niklas, 2001). Because plant abundance is held constant along this upper bound, the predicted exponential effects of temperature on plant diversity are manifested. By contrast, we hypothesize that points below this upper bound are predominantly water-limited sites that have lower total plant abundance, and thus diversity. Furthermore, because precipitation and temperature interact to determine water deficit, and hence total plant abundance, we would also expect temperature and precipitation to strongly interact in determining the plant diversity of water-limited ecosystems. This is consistent with Eq. (14.3) and Fig. 13.8 of Currie (this volume), the theoretical derivation of Allen et al. (2002), and the framework proposed here (Fig. 14.1). Thus, we strongly disagree with Currie (this volume) that "plant richness does not vary with temperature in the manner predicted by metabolic theory." Indeed, we feel that the analysis of Currie provides strong support for our arguments.

In spite of these issues, our framework predicts that the energetic determinants of biodiversity should fundamentally differ for ectotherms and endotherms. In general, for ectotherms, biodiversity should increase with increases in environmental temperature and total community abundance through the combined effects of these variables on speciation rates (Fig. 14.1). Importantly, even if community abundance is held constant across latitudes, and the "more individuals hypothesis" (Hutchinson, 1959; Brown, 1981; Wright, 1983; Allen et al., 2002) therefore does not apply, ectotherm diversity is predicted to increase exponentially with latitudinal gradients of increasing temperature (Allen et al., 2002; as demonstrated by Currie et al., 2004). According to our proposed framework (Fig. 14.1), this is a direct consequence of how temperature-induced increases in the metabolic rates of individuals (Eqs. 14.3, 14.7, 14.8; arrow 2) influence the evolutionary rates of populations (arrow 4). By contrast, for endotherms, which show only modest changes in metabolic rate across latitudinal gradients in environmental temperature (Anderson & Jetz, 2005), biodiversity should be regulated primarily by the availability of chemical potential energy through its effects on total community abundance (Eq. 14.6; arrow 3) and the total numbers of populations contributing to speciation–extinction dynamics (arrow 5).

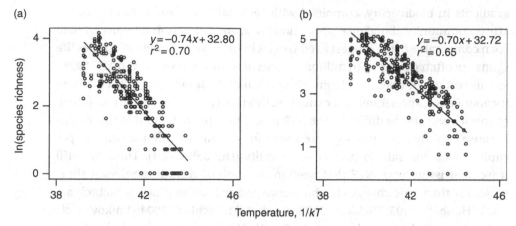

**Figure 14.3.** Effects of mean annual temperature, expressed as $1/kT$, on the natural logarithm of regional species richness for (a) amphibians and (b) trees of North America (Allen *et al.*, 2002). Negative linear relationships between the variables, with slopes close to $-E \approx -0.65$ eV, indicate that species richness increases exponentially with temperature according to the Boltzmann–Arrhenius relationship for respiration ($\propto e^{-E/kT}$, Eq. 14.3). Data from Currie (1991).

Community-level data strongly support the hypothesis that the controls on biodiversity fundamentally differ for ectotherms and endotherms. Our analysis of community-level data for ectotherms demonstrates that regional species richness increases exponentially with temperature in the same way as individual metabolic rate ($S \propto e^{-E/kT}$) when total community abundance is held constant (Allen *et al.*, 2002) (Fig. 14.3). By contrast, another analysis of community-level data for endotherms has shown that the latitudinal gradient in bird diversity is driven largely by geographic variation in total community abundance (Pautasso & Gaston, 2005). Environmental temperature thus has little or no independent effect on biodiversity of the world's avifaunas. Finally, our analysis of population-level data for ectotherms and endotherms supports this hypothesis (Allen *et al.*, 2002). In that analysis, we showed that, after correcting for body size, average abundance per species per unit area, $\bar{N}$, was independent of environmental temperature for endothermic mammal populations, but declined exponentially with increasing temperature for ectotherms. These population- and community-level data thus support the hypothesis that kinetic and potential forms of energy regulate biodiversity through fundamentally different mechanisms.

## Conclusions and caveats

Much remains to be done in order to establish the proposed chain of causality linking species diversity to energy availability (Fig. 14.1). Testing this proposed framework poses significant empirical and theoretical challenges. Empirical testing will require the analysis of regionally resolved data on contemporary gradients in biodiversity, combined with regionally resolved data on temperature, community abundance, speciation rates, and extinction rates over a time span comparable to the longest lived species in the taxon of interest. Species life spans are often measured in millions to tens of millions of years (Stanley, 1998), so this will not be easy. Developing theoretical understanding of how community abundance, speciation, and extinction interact to control the standing stock of species will also be difficult. The NTB model may prove helpful in this regard because NTB incorporates separate terms for community abundance and per capita speciation rate to predict biodiversity (Hubbell, 2001). There are still important issues with NTB that need to be resolved regarding relevant time-scales for stochastic changes in abundance and speciation (Clark & McLachlan, 2003; Hubbell, 2003; Ricklefs, 2003; Clark & McLachlan, 2004; Volkov et al., 2004). Nevertheless, synthesizing NTB with MTE appears to hold significant progress for the road ahead. Through such a synthesis, it is our hope that it will be possible to develop a more comprehensive understanding of biodiversity gradients that encompasses processes operating at the individual, population, and community levels of biological organization while remaining firmly grounded in rates of evolutionary change at the molecular level.

## References

Allen, A. P., Brown, J. H. & Gillooly, J. F. (2002). Global biodiversity, biochemical kinetics, and the energetic-equivalence rule. *Science*, **297**, 1545–1548.

Allen, A. P., Brown, J. H. & Gillooly, J. F. (2003). Response to comment on "Global biodiversity, biochemical kinetics, and the energetic-equivalence rule". *Science*, **299**, 346c.

Allen, A. P. & Gillooly, J. F. (2006). Assessing latitudinal gradients in speciation rates and biodiversity at the global scale. *Ecology Letters*, **9**, 947–954.

Allen, A. P., Gillooly, J. F. & Brown, J. H. (2005). Linking the global carbon cycle to individual metabolism. *Functional Ecology*, **19**, 202–213.

Allen, A. P., Gillooly, J. F., Savage, V. M. & Brown, J. H. (2006). Kinetic effects of temperature on rates of genetic divergence and speciation. *Proceedings of the National Academy of Sciences of the United States of America*, **103**, 9130–9135.

Alroy, J., Marshall, C. R., Bambach, R. K., et al. (2001). Effects of sampling standardization on estimates of phanerozoic marine diversification. *Proceedings of the National Academy of Sciences of the United States of America*, **98**, 6261–6266.

Anderson, K. J. & Jetz, W. (2005). The broad-scale ecology of energy expenditure of endotherms. *Ecology Letters*, **8**, 310.

Brown, J. H. (1981). Two decades of homage to Santa Rosalia: toward a general theory of diversity. *American Zoologist*, **21**, 877–888.

Brown, J. H., Gillooly, J. F., Allen, A. P., Savage, V. M. & West, G. B. (2004). Toward a metabolic theory of ecology. *Ecology*, **85**, 1771–1789.

Chapin, F. S. I., Matson, P. A. & Mooney, H. A. (2002). *Principles of Terrestrial Ecosystem Ecology*. New York: Springer-Verlag.

Chown, S. L. & Gaston, K. J. (2000). Areas, cradles and museums: the latitudinal gradient in species richness. *Trends in Ecology and Evolution*, **15**, 311–315.

Clark, J. S. & McLachlan, J. S. (2003). Stability of forest biodiversity. *Nature*, **423**, 635–638.

Clark, J. S. & McLachlan, J. S. (2004). Neutral theory (communication arising): the stability of forest biodiversity. *Nature*, **427**, 696–697.

Coyne, J. A. & Orr, H. A. (2004). *Speciation*. Sunderland, MA: Sinaur Associates.

Crame, J. A. (2002). Evolution of taxonomic diversity gradients in the marine realm: a comparison of late Jurassic and recent bivalve faunas. *Paleobiology*, **28**, 184–207.

Crane, P. R. & Lidgard, S. (1989). Angiosperm diversification and paleolatitudinal gradients in Cretaceous floristic diversity. *Science*, **246**, 675–678.

Currie, D. J. (1991). Energy and large-scale patterns of animal- and plant-species richness. *American Naturalist*, **137**, 27–49.

Currie, D. J., Mittelbach, G. G., Cornell, H. V., et al. (2004). Predictions and tests of climate-based hypotheses of broad-scale variation in taxonomic richness. *Ecology Letters*, **7**, 1121–1134.

Darwin, C. (1859). *On the Origin of Species*. London: John Murray.

Enquist, B. J. & Niklas, K. J. (2001). Invariant scaling relations across tree-dominated communities. *Nature*, **410**, 655–660.

Enquist, B. J., Economo, E. P., Huxman, T. E., Allen, A. P., Ignace, D. D. & Gillooly, J. F. (2003). Scaling metabolism from organisms to ecosystems. *Nature*, **423**, 639–642.

Farquhar, G. D., von Caemmerer, S. & Berry, J. A. (1980). A biochemical model of photosynthetic $CO_2$ assimilation in leaves of C3 plants. *Planta*, **149**, 78–90.

Field, C. B., Behrenfeld, M. J., Randerson, J. T. & Falkowski, P. (1998). Primary production of the biosphere: integrating terrestrial and oceanic components. *Science*, **281**, 237–240.

Fisher, R. A. (1930). *The Genetical Theory of Natural Selection*. Oxford: Clarendon Press.

Flessa, K. W. & Jablonski, D. (1996). The geography of evolutionary turnover: a global analysis of extant bivalves. In *Evolutionary Paleobiology*, ed. D. Jablonski, D. H. Erwin, and J. H. Lipps, pp. 376–397, Chicago: University of Chicago Press.

Gaston, K. J. (2000). Global patterns in biodiversity. *Nature*, **405**, 220–227.

Gillooly, J. F., Brown, J. H., West, G. B., Savage, V. M. & Charnov, E. L. (2001). Effects of size and temperature on metabolic rate. *Science*, **293**, 2248–2251.

Gillooly, J. F., Charnov, E. L., West, G. B., Savage, V. M. & Brown, J. H. (2002). Effects of size and temperature on developmental time. *Nature*, **417**, 70–73.

Gillooly, J. F., Allen, A. P., West, G. B. & Brown, J. H. (2005). The rate of DNA evolution: effects of body size and temperature on the molecular clock. *Proceedings of the National Academy of Sciences of the United States of America*, **102**, 140–145.

Hawkins, B. A., Field, R., Cornell, H. V., et al. (2003). Energy, water, and broad-scale geographic patterns of species richness. *Ecology*, **84**, 3105–3117.

Hubbell, S. P. (2001). *A Unified Neutral Theory of Biodiversity and Biogeography*. Princeton, NJ: Princeton University Press.

Hubbell, S. P. (2003). Modes of speciation and the lifespans of species under neutrality: a response to the comment of Robert E. Ricklefs. *Oikos*, **100**, 193–199.

Huston, M. A., Brown, J. H., Allen, A. P. & Gillooly, J. F. (2003). Heat and biodiversity. *Science*, **299**, 512–513.

Hutchinson, G. E. (1959). Homage to Santa Rosalia or why are there so many kinds of animals. *American Naturalist*, **93**, 145–159.

Huxman, T. E., Smith, M. D., Fay, P. A., et al. (2004). Convergence across biomes to a common rain-use efficiency. *Nature*, **429**, 651–654.

Jablonski, D. (1993). The tropics as a source of evolutionary novelty through geological time. *Nature*, **364**, 142–144.

Kaspari, M. (2001). Taxonomic level, trophic biology and the regulation of local abundance. *Global Ecology and Biogeography*, **10**, 229–244.

Kaspari, M. (2005). Global energy gradients and size in colonial organisms: worker mass and worker number in ant colonies. *Proceedings of the National Academy of Sciences of the United States of America*, **102**, 5079–5083.

Kimura, M. (1983). *The Neutral Theory of Molecular Evolution*. Cambridge: Cambridge University Press.

Lande, R., Engen, S. & Saether, B. E. (2003). *Stochastic Population Dynamics in Ecology and Conservation*. Oxford: Oxford University Press.

Lieth, H. (1973). Primary production: terrestrial ecosystems. *Human Ecology*, **1**, 303–332.

MacArthur, R. H. (1969). Patterns of communities in the tropics. *Biological Journal of the Linnean Society*, **1**, 19–31.

Mayr, E. (1942). *Systematics and the Origin of Species from the Viewpoint of a Zoologist*. New York: Columbia University Press.

Monteith, J. L. (1972). Solar radiation and productivity in tropical ecosystems. *Journal of Applied Ecology*, **9**, 747–766.

Mueller, P. & Diamond, J. (2001). Metabolic rate and environmental productivity: well-provisioned animals evolved to run and idle fast. *Proceedings of the National Academy of Sciences of the United States of America*, **98**, 12550–12554.

Pautasso, M. & Gaston, K. J. (2005). Resources and global avian assemblage structure in forests. *Ecology Letters*, **8**, 282–289.

Ricklefs, R. E. (2003). A comment on Hubbell's zero-sum ecological drift model. *Oikos*, **100**, 185–192.

Rohde, K. (1992). Latitudinal gradients in species diversity: the search for the primary cause. *Oikos*, **65**, 514–527.

Rosenzweig, M. L. (1975). On continental steady states of biodiversity. In *Ecology and Evolution of Communities*, ed. M. L. Cody and

J. M. Diamond, pp. 121–140, Cambridge: MA: Belnap Press.

Savage, V. M. (2004). Improved approximations to scaling relationships for species, populations, and ecosystems across latitudinal and elevational gradients. *Journal of Theoretical Biology*, **227**, 525–534.

Savage, V. M., Gillooly, J. F., Brown, J. H., West, G. B. & Charnov, E. L. (2004). Effects of body size and temperature on population growth. *American Naturalist*, **163**, E429–E441.

Sepkoski, J. J., Jr. (1978). A kinetic model of phanerozoic taxonomic diversity I. Analysis of marine orders. *Paleobiology*, **4**, 223–251.

Stanley, H. E. (1998). *Macroevolution, Pattern and Process*. Baltimore, MD: Johns Hopkins University Press.

Stehli, F. G., Douglas, D. G. & Newell, N. D. (1969). Generation and maintenance of gradients in taxonomic diversity. *Science*, **164**, 947–949.

Storch, D. (2003). Comment on "Global biodiversity, biochemical kinetics, and the energetic-equivalence rule". *Science*, **299**, 346b.

Tilman, D. (1999). The ecological consequences of changes in biodiversity: a search for general principles. *Ecology*, **80**, 1455–1474.

Vitousek, P. M. (1984). Litterfall, nutrient cycling, and nutrient limitation in tropical forests. *Ecology*, **65**, 285–298.

Volkov, I., Banavar, J. R., Maritan, A. & Hubbell, S. P. (2004). Neutral theory (communication arising): the stability of forest biodiversity. *Nature*, **427**, 696.

von Humboldt, A. (1808). *Ansichten der Natur mit wissenschaftlichen Erlauterungen*. Tubingen: J. G. Cotta.

Wallace, A. R. (1878). *Tropical Nature and Other Essays*. London: Macmillan.

West, G. B., Brown, J. H. & Enquist, B. J. (1997). A general model for the origin of allometric scaling laws in biology. *Science*, **276**, 122–126.

Willig, M. R., Kaufman, D. M. & Stevens, R. D. (2003). Latitudinal gradients of biodiversity:

pattern, process, scale, and synthesis. *Annual Review of Ecology, Evolution, and Systematics*, **34**, 273–309.

Wright, D. H. (1983). Species-energy theory: an extension of species-area theory. *Oikos*, **41**, 496–506.

Wright, D. H., Currie, D. J. & Maurer, B. A. (1993). Energy supply and patterns of species richness on local and regional scales. In *Species*

*Diversity in Ecological Communities*, ed. R. E. Ricklefs and D. Schluter, pp. 66–74, Chicago: University of Chicago Press.

Yule, G. U. (1925). A mathematical theory of evolution, based on the conclusions of Dr. J. C. Willis, F.R.S. *Philosophical Transactions of the Royal Society of London, Series B*, **213**, 21–87.

# CHAPTER FIFTEEN

# Scaling species richness and distribution: uniting the species–area and species–energy relationships

DAVID STORCH
*Charles University, Prague, The Santa Fe Institute*
ARNOŠT L. ŠIZLING
*Charles University, Prague*
KEVIN J. GASTON
*University of Sheffield*

## Introduction

Two macroecological patterns of species richness are sufficiently common and occur across such a wide range of taxa and geographic realms that they can be regarded as universal. The first is an increase in the number of species with the area sampled, the species–area relationship (hereafter SAR). The other is the relationship between species richness and the availability of energy that can be turned into biomass – the species–energy relationship (hereafter SER). Both patterns have a long history of exploration (e.g. Arrhenius, 1921; Gleason, 1922; Preston, 1960; Wright, 1983; Williamson, 1988; Currie, 1991; Rosenzweig, 1995; Waide *et al.*, 1999; Gaston, 2000; Hawkins *et al.*, 2003). However, attempts to interpret them within one unifying framework, or at least to relate them to each other, have been surprisingly rare. The most notable exception has been Wright's (1983) attempt to derive both patterns from the assumed relationship between total energy availability (defined as the product of available area and energy input per unit area) and population size. According to this theory, both area and energy positively affect species' population abundances, which decreases probabilities of population extinction, and thus increases the total number of species that can coexist on a site. Then, species richness should increase with increasing area or increasing energy in the same way.

Although this theory can be valid in island situations where the total number of species is determined by the rate of extinctions which are not balanced by immigration events (MacArthur & Wilson, 1967), the situation on the mainland is more complicated. The local occurrence of a species is given not only by the viability of this population itself, but by the broader spatial context (Rosenzweig,

*Scaling Biodiversity*, ed. David Storch, Pablo A. Marquet and James H. Brown. Published by Cambridge University Press. © Cambridge University Press 2007.

1995; Gaston & Blackburn, 2000). The shape and slope of the SAR measured on a continuous landscape is thus related to the spatial distribution of species (He & Legendre, 2002), which is affected by total population sizes, habitat heterogeneity (Rosenzweig, 1995), and spatial population or metapopulation dynamics (Hanski & Gyllenberg, 1997; Storch, Šizling & Gaston, 2003a). Consequently, the exact properties of the SER can change with scale (Waide et al., 1999; Mittelbach et al., 2001; Chase & Leibold, 2002), habitat structure (Hurlbert, 2004) and the taxa involved (Allen, Brown & Gillooly, 2002). Moreover, it has been reported that although species richness does increase with environmental productivity, this may often not be the case with population sizes (Currie et al., 2004). This violates the "more individuals hypothesis" of the SER (Gaston, 2000) which states that species richness is higher in more productive areas because they enable persistence of larger populations that are less vulnerable to extinction, in accord with Wright's (1983) proposition.

Given this situation, a simple unified framework for both the SAR and SER seems unlikely to exist. However, the fact that both patterns are inevitably related to patterns in the spatial distributions of species can provide a clue to understanding both of them, as well as their relationship. Every species richness pattern is proximately driven by patterns of occurrence of individual species (both in space and along environmental gradients), and therefore the challenge is to relate species richness patterns to regularities in the spatial distribution of individual species (Storch & Gaston, 2004), and to explore whether similar regularities can be responsible for both the SAR and SER. Our goal is to reveal these connections between the spatial distributions of species and the two biodiversity patterns, and to explore the interrelationships between the SAR and the SER in the light of these connections.

## The species–area relationship and spatial species distribution

Traditionally, the increase of species numbers with area within a contiguous mainland has been attributed to three factors (Storch et al., 2003a). The first is a pure sampling effect: larger areas may contain species that are too rare to occur in smaller areas. Second, larger areas contain more habitat types, enabling coexistence of species with different habitat requirements (i.e. habitat heterogeneity is responsible for the increase of species numbers with area). Third, spatial population dynamics leads to an aggregated pattern of species occurrence, such that the probability of finding a species within smaller areas is substantially lower than in larger areas. All these factors apparently contribute to observed SARs, although their relative importance has seldom been tested (but see Storch et al., 2003a). Importantly, although all three inevitably lead to an increase of species richness with area, it is unclear how they contribute to the quantitative properties of the SAR (i.e. its exact slope and shape). These properties seem to be relatively invariant, SARs being well approximated as power laws (but see Tjørve, 2003 for a review of alternative expressions) with relatively predictable slopes (Connor & McCoy, 1979; Rosenzweig, 1995).

A promising way of deriving the slope and shape of the SAR is by studying its proximate cause, the geometry of spatial distribution of individual species. Indeed, all three factors thought to generate an increase of species numbers with area can be seen as ultimate causes of the primary driver of the pattern, the spatial aggregation of species, because of which not all species occur within every possible area (Plotkin *et al.*, 2000; He & Legendre, 2002). Analyzing which types of species spatial distribution lead to which types of observed SARs can be relatively easily done if we define the SAR as the relationship between area and *mean* species number averaged across all plots of a given area. Then the SAR can be obtained by superimposition of functions relating the *probability of occurrence* of an individual of a given species to area. Mean species number (hereafter $\bar{S}$) is exactly equal to the sum of the probabilities of finding every species within a plot of a particular area,

$$\bar{S}_{(A)} \equiv \sum_{i=1}^{S_{tot}} p_{occ\ i(A)}, \tag{15.1}$$

where $S_{tot}$ is the total number of species considered and $p_{occ\ i}$ is the probability of occurrence of species $i$ within plots whose area is $A$ (Coleman, 1981; Williams, 1995; Ney-Nifle & Mangel, 1999; He & Legendre, 2002). It is thus possible to analyze the relationships between $A$ and $p_{occ}$ for different types of species' spatial distributions, and to study how these functions can be assembled to produce the resulting SARs.

The first models of the SAR attempted to derive it on the basis of an assumed random spatial distribution of individuals – this was the case in the widely cited paper of Arrhenius (1921), first describing the SAR as an approximate power law, as well as many of its descendants (e.g. Preston, 1960; Coleman, 1981; Williams, 1995). This assumption can give the power-law SAR, but only for very unrealistic distributions of species abundances (Fig. 15.1; see Williamson & Lawton, 1991). For more realistic species-abundance distributions it predicts a much more rapid increase of species richness for relatively small areas, and relatively quick saturation (Rosenzweig, 1995; Storch *et al.*, 2003a), i.e. rather a logarithmic function than a power law. Moreover, the assumption of a random spatial distribution is plainly unrealistic, except perhaps at very local spatial scales. Therefore, other models were derived which made exactly the opposite assumption of an ideally clumped distribution. That is, they assumed that a better approximation of a species' spatial distribution is a contiguous and spatially restricted geographic range, within which the species occurs everywhere (Maurer, 1999; Ney-Nifle & Mangel, 1999). Again, the model is

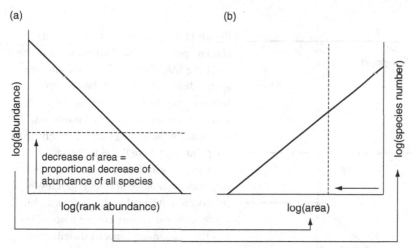

**Figure 15.1** Graphical model deriving the power-law SAR from the assumption of the power-law distribution of species abundances and random spatial distribution of individuals. (a) Assume that the rank–abundance curve of an assemblage in the total area is in this case represented by a power law, i.e. log abundance decreases linearly with logarithmized rank. Then the decrease of area to some proportion of the original area is followed by the proportional decrease of abundance of all species, which can be modeled by a shift along the abundance axis (arrow). This leads also to the decrease of number of species, as the abundances of some of them decrease below one. (b) This means that the abundance axis can be understood as equivalent to the area axis, and the rank axis is equivalent to the species number axis. If the slope of the log(rank)–log(abundance) curve is $t$, then the slope of the SAR $z = 1/t$. Modified from Williamson and Lawton (1991).

unrealistic in its assumption of a homogeneous distribution of individuals within the species' range, and thus fails to predict realistic SARs across all spatial scales, although it seems to be quite appropriate at some scales. Generally, the predicted relationship in this case is a rapid increase of species richness at the beginning, then approximate linearity on a log-log scale (i.e. close to the power law), and then a steep increase again as the spatial scale exceeds the extent of most range sizes (Allen & White, 2003).

Recently, models assuming that species distribution is aggregated on many scales of resolution have been proposed. Harte, Kinzig and Green (1999) were the first fully to acknowledge that the power law indicates scale invariance (or self-similarity), providing a model that explicitly related the power-law SAR to self-similarity at the community level. This model is based on the assumption that if a species is present within an area, the probability of its occurrence within a constant portion of that area remains the same, regardless of the absolute size of the area (see also Harte, this volume). However, using a numerical model, Lennon, Kunin and Hartley (2002) claimed that self-similarity at the level of the distribution of individual species would lead to the power-law SAR

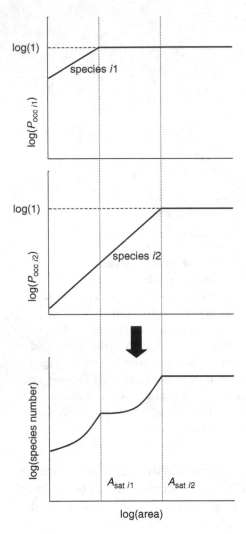

**Figure 15.2** Relationship between self-similar species' spatial distribution and the resulting SAR. If species have self-similar spatial distributions, the relationship between their probability of occupancy $P_{occ}$ and area $A$ is approximately a power law (i.e. a line on the log-log scale), but only up to the point $A_{sat}$ where $P_{occ} = 1$. This point represents the area which contains at least one individual of the species regardless of the position of the plot of this area, and its existence is a necessary consequence of the fact that we measure species distributions within finite areas. If species' distributions were self-similar with different fractal dimensions, the increasing part of their relationships between $P_{occ}$ and area $A$ would have a different slope in log-log space (as is the case here), and the SAR obtained by summing these linear functions using Eq. (15.1) would be upward accelerating on the log-log scale (Lennon *et al.*, 2002). But the fact that these functions are linear and increasing only up to the point $A_{sat}$ (and then they are constant) leads to a more complicated shape, because summing the functions for individual species leads to the upward-accelerating curve only between subsequent $A_{sat}$. This leads to the SAR which is not exactly linear on a log-log scale, but which mostly does not reveal any apparent upward or downward curvature (according to Šizling & Storch, 2004).

only if all species' spatial distributions had identical fractal dimensions, which seems to be very unrealistic (in fact, it would occur only if all species occupied the same proportions of the total area). Nevertheless, Šizling and Storch (2004) have shown that even if species differ in their fractal dimensions and occupancies, the resulting SAR can be very close to the power law (Fig. 15.2), and that this is indeed the case for central European birds which have a spatial distribution that is indistinguishable from self-similar. That is, if we replace the complex individual species' spatial distributions by exactly self-similar patterns with

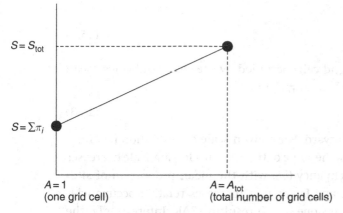

**Figure 15.3.** Estimating the slope of the SAR from the extremes of the function. As the coordinates of both minimum and maximum of the SAR measured on a grid are given, the slope on the log-log scale can be calculated as $Z = (\ln S_{tot} - \ln \sum \pi_i)/(\ln A_{tot} - n(1))$. This directly gives Eq. (15.2).

fractal dimensions extracted from those observed patterns we get accurate predictions of the shape and slope of the SAR.

This finding has some interesting implications. It suggests that a fractal spatial distribution is a better approximation of a real spatial distribution than is a random distribution or a distribution aggregated on only one spatial level (i.e. a nonstructured geographic range). Although there is no reason that individual species distributions should be fractal in a strict sense (even the abiotic environment is only rarely self-similar, and there is no reason to expect that biological processes should produce preferentially fractal structures; see Palmer, this volume), it seems that this assumption captures quite well the fact that spatial distributions are aggregated on many scales of resolution (Šizling & Storch, this volume). It is even possible that the function relating probability of species occurrence to area is not a bounded power law (which it would be in the case of an approximately self-similar distribution, see Fig. 15.2), but a different function with a similar shape (see He & Condit, and Lennon *et al.*, this volume), that is, an increasing function which becomes saturated for larger areas.

Regardless of the exact nature of species' spatial distributions, the slope of the SAR on a log-log scale for distributions measured on a grid can be calculated on the basis of species' occupancies, i.e. numbers of grid cells where species occur (Šizling & Storch, 2004). The reason is that if the SAR is approximately linear on a log-log scale, we can estimate its slope from its maximum and minimum (Fig. 15.3). The maximum is given by the total area within which we determine species distributions, measured as the total number of grid cells considered, and the total number of species considered ($A = A_{tot}$; $S = S_{tot}$). The minimum is given by the area of the basic grid cell ($A = 1$) and mean species richness within the basic grid cell, which is equal to the sum of the probabilities of occupancy of one grid cell ($\bar{S} = \sum \pi_i$). The slope of the line defined by these two extreme points in log-log space is then

$$Z = \frac{\ln\left(\frac{S_{tot}}{\sum \pi_i}\right)}{\ln(A_{tot})},$$

(15.2)

where $\pi_i$ is the proportion of grid cells occupied by species $i$. And since mean relative species occupancy $\bar{\pi} = \sum \pi_i / S_{tot}$, then

$$z = -\ln(\bar{\pi})/\ln(A_{tot}).$$

(15.3)

The implications are straightforward. For a given scale of resolution (i.e. for a given number of basic grid cells) the slope of the SAR on a log-log scale decreases with mean species relative occupancy (i.e. with the mean proportion of sites occupied by each species) and any factor that increases relative occupancies must consequently decrease the slope of the resulting SAR. Interestingly, the most often reported slope of mainland SARs is about 0.15 (0.1–0.2), which corresponds to a mean relative occupancy of about 0.5 for most reasonable grid sizes (Fig. 15.4). The reason why species on average occupy about half of grid cells remains unclear. Nevertheless, there is an explicit relationship between species' occupancy patterns, and the properties of the resulting species–area relationship, which is independent of the exact properties of species distributions and the exact shape of the SAR.

## The species–energy relationship and the distribution of species along an energy gradient

The relationship between energy availability (or environmental productivity) and species richness has largely not been considered by studying the distributions of species along the gradient of increasing productivity. This is quite surprising, considering that species distributions are a major proximate driver of any bio-diversity pattern. There has probably been an implicit assumption that the increase of species richness with productivity must trivially be accompanied by an increase in species' probability of occurrence. However, there are actually several ways in which species can be distributed along the productivity gradient, and each of them suggests different processes that could be acting (Fig. 15.5).

One extreme is where all species respond to the gradient of energy availability in a similar way, such that they all have a higher probability of occurrence in more productive areas. If this is the case, most species should occupy more localities in more productive areas (there should be fewer gaps in their extent of occurrence) and they should differ only in total range size and/or the range of levels of energy availability under which they occur: whereas common species would occur within the majority of productivity levels (albeit with higher occupancy in more productive areas), rare species would occupy only high productivity levels. The opposite extreme is represented by a "niche division" of species along the pro-ductivity gradient: every species occupies only a part of the gradient (sometimes

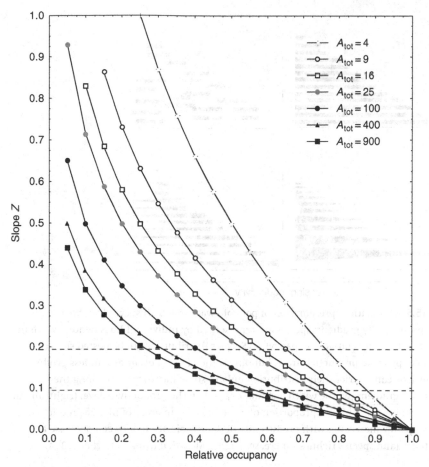

**Figure 15.4** Relationship between mean species relative occupancy and the slope of the SAR on a log-log scale. For a reasonable range of $A_{tot}$ (from c. 25 to 900 grid cells) the slope falls between 0.1 and 0.2 (dashed lines) when mean relative occupancy is about 0.5 (dotted line). For higher numbers of grid cells relative occupancy should have been lower to fall into that interval; however, grids of more than 30 × 30 cells are rarely considered, and occupancy patterns within such fine grids would probably reflect different processes from those considered here.

narrower, sometimes broader) and the SER is caused simply by the fact that more species are adapted to higher levels of productivity than to lower levels (Kleidon & Mooney, 2000). Whereas the first extreme suggests rather a simple ecological factor (resource abundance etc.) affecting the occurrence of each species independently of every other species, the other extreme indicates that evolutionary forces, such as adaptation, niche division, and species pool evolution, contribute to the increase of species richness with energy availability. Moreover, if every species occupies only a portion of the entire energy gradient (Fig. 15.5a, right), the resulting SER need not necessarily be monotonically increasing. Indeed, the

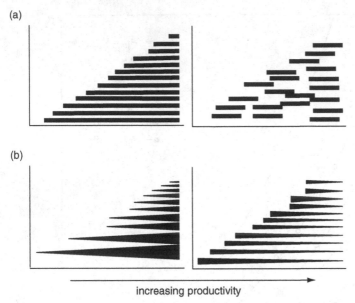

**Figure 15.5** Schematic representation of possible ways in which species can be distributed along a productivity gradient; species are represented by individual lines (whose width in row b refers to their relative occupancy). (a) Species distribution can be nested such that all species occupy more productive areas, but only some of them occur also in less productive areas (left), or can restrict their distribution only to some narrow region along the productivity gradient, whose width does not depend on the productivity level (right). (b) All species can occur in a higher proportion of available sites in areas of higher productivity, their occupancy increasing with productivity (left) or their occupancy can decrease as productivity (and species richness) increases (right). Modified from Bonn *et al.* (2004).

reported decrease of species richness within the highest energy levels (Rosenzweig, 1995; Waide *et al.*, 1999; Mittelbach *et al.*, 2001) can be related simply to the fact that species pools for different levels of productivity are different and for high productivity levels are somehow depauperate (e.g. for historical reasons).

It is very probable that both extremes, and anything in between, occur in nature, and that this contributes to the variability of reported SERs. However, it is useful to take a well-resolved data set and explore the real relationship between the SER and the distribution of species along the productivity gradient. For this purpose we took data on bird distributions in South Africa (Harrison *et al.*, 1997), for which species richness increases linearly with productivity (van Rensburg, Chown & Gaston, 2002; Chown *et al.*, 2003), and analyzed the distribution of individual species along the productivity gradient (Bonn, Storch & Gaston, 2004). For all the following considerations we assume that productivity can be measured by the normalized difference vegetation index (NDVI), which has been shown to be closely correlated with net primary productivity (Woodward, Lomas & Lee, 2001; Kerr & Ostrovsky, 2003). The results show that most species conform to the first model, with rare species occurring more frequently within areas of high productivity, whereas common species are those that live in areas of both high and low productivity, as indicated by a substantially lower mean range size of species occuring at high productivity levels (Fig. 15.6c). Moreover, even species occurring in both high and low productivity areas occupy on average more localities in more productive areas, and species turnover between neighboring cells consequently decreases with productivity (Bonn et al., 2004).

The increase of species richness with productivity seems therefore to be related directly to the increase in the probability of occurrence of most species along this gradient. This does not imply, however, that this increase is causally *responsible* for the observed SER. We can ask whether the assumption of increasing probability of species occurrence with productivity is sufficient to explain observed patterns of species richness and distribution – i.e. whether they can be predicted just on the basis of this assumption. To answer this, we have built a simple simulation model of the dynamics of species' geographic ranges across South Africa, based on a few very simple rules (Storch et al., unpublished manuscript). For each species, first, an initial grid cell is chosen for occupancy with a probability that is directly proportional to productivity (i.e. grid cells with double the productivity have double the probability of being selected). Second, each species spreads from this point of origin so that any cell adjacent to any already occupied can be occupied in the next step, but again with a probability proportional to productivity (probability that cell $i$ will be occupied in the next step $P_i = NDVI_i/NDVI_{adj.tot}$, where $NDVI_{adj.tot}$ is the sum of NDVI values for all empty cells adjacent to those already occupied). Third, the process stops when the observed number of occupied grid cells is reached (i.e. the observed distribution of species' range sizes is maintained). In the final model (model 4 in Table 15.1), we have also made an additional assumption that the ranges of species are not perfectly contiguous, by adding some random distributional gaps. This was done by enlarging the original range size of each species by a random number of cells between zero and the total number actually occupied, and simulating the dynamics using these new ranges. After each simulation the additional number of occupied cells was randomly set as unoccupied, yielding the observed range size distribution.

The results of this model are quite striking (Fig. 15.6). It predicts accurately the slope of the observed SER (the observed and predicted slopes are statistically indistinguishable), as well as the observed increase of mean species' occupancies along the productivity gradient. Moreover, the mean range size of species occurring within each productivity class (i.e. a set of grid cells sharing approximately the same productivity level) decreases with productivity almost exactly in the same way as observed. Importantly, other models with some of the assumptions relaxed did not produce accurate quantitative predictions (Table 15.1). For example, a model (model 1) that assumed a proportional increase of probability of occurrence with productivity but not spatially

310 DAVID STORCH, ARNOŠT L. ŠIZLING & KEVIN J. GASTON

(a)

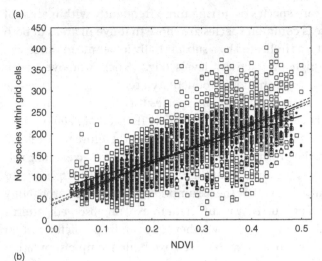

(b)

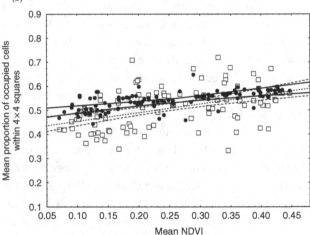

(c)

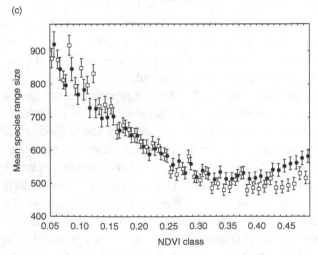

**Figure 15.6** Comparison between observed patterns of species richness and distribution along the productivity gradient (white squares) and those predicted by the simulation model (black circles). (a) Relationship between NDVI and species richness for every grid cell; thin dotted line refers to the observed regression line, dashed lines to observed confidence intervals of this line, and bold solid lines refer to nonparametric confidence intervals of the predicted regression lines obtained from 500 simulation runs. Black circles refer to one randomly selected model run. (b) Relationship between mean NDVI and mean relative species occupancy within nonoverlapping squares of $4 \times 4$ grid cells, the same marking as in the previous case. Mean relative occupancy was calculated as $\frac{1}{S}\sum_{i=1}^{S}\frac{N_{occi}}{16}$, where $S$ is the number of species present within the respective $4 \times 4$ square, and $N_{occ}$ is the number of occupied grid cells for species $i$. Note that mean relative species occupancy is not equivalent to the probability of occurrence assumed in the model, because whereas occupancy refers to the realized spatial distribution of species within defined spatial units, probability of occurrence always refers to the set of grid cells that can be occupied only in a particular step of range dynamics, i.e. to the potential occupancy of empty available cells at the respective simulation step. (c) Relationship between NDVI and mean range size measured as total number of cells occupied within South Africa, calculated for all species occurring within each NDVI class. The whiskers represent standard errors of means.

**Table 15.1** *Comparison of quantitative properties of predicted and observed relationships for four models simulating range dynamics across South Africa, and differing in their assumptions*

Model 1 assumed that species distribute according to productivity without assuming range contiguity, i.e. in each step, one unoccupied cell was set as occupied with $P_i = NDVI_i/NDVI_{tot}$, where $NDVI_i$ is the value for the particular cell, and $NDVI_{tot}$ is the sum for all unoccupied cells at a particular step. Model 2 assumed random spreading of contiguous species ranges without accounting for productivity. Model 3 assumed both range contiguity and the proportional increase of probability of occurrence with increasing productivity (see the text). Model 4 added the assumption that species ranges are not perfectly contiguous but contain some (random) amount of gaps. The first two columns give the slope of regression lines for the observation (95% confidence intervals, CIs, of these coefficients in parentheses) and 95% nonparametric CIs of these slopes obtained from 500 model simulations. Underlined are those intervals that overlap with the 95% CIs of observed slopes. Note that these measures of CIs are very conservative, as individual grid cells are not independent of each other due to spatial autocorrelation, and accounting for the autocorrelation would broaden them. The third column gives the proportion of NDVI classes with overlapping standard errors of means of species range sizes for each NDVI class (i.e. total numbers of occupied grid cells across South Africa, calculated for species present in respective NDVI level) between the models and the observation.

|  | Species-NDVI | Occupancy-NDVI | Range size-NDVI |
|---|---|---|---|
| *Observed slope* | 457.1 | 0.351 | |
| | (435.6–478.7) | (0.215–0.486) | |
| Prediction of model 1 | 425.4–451.2 | 0.647–0.677 | 47.7% |
| Prediction of model 2 | −172.0–32.7 | −0.001–0.002 | 11.4% |
| Prediction of model 3 | 485.1–638.6 | 0.381–0.686 | 59.1% |
| Prediction of model 4 | 343.8–452.1 | 0.155–0.348 | 76.7% |

contiguous ranges (i.e. species could occupy any unoccupied cells at each step of the simulation, not only those adjacent) predicted the slope of the observed SER quite well, but at the same time predicted too high a slope of the productivity–occupancy relationship, and too rapid a decrease of mean range size with productivity level (because even species with small ranges finally fell into most productivity classes). By contrast, a model (model 2) relaxing the assumption of the relationship between productivity and probability of being occupied (and keeping the range contiguity assumption) did not predict any SER at all.

The fit of model 4 does not mean that it captures all the processes that contribute to the observed SER. In fact, it is quite simplistic, and in some respects unrealistic. For example, all models of stochastic spreading of contiguous ranges necessarily produce the mid-domain effect, i.e. an increase of species richness in the center of a geographic domain due to the inevitable co-occurrence there of species with large ranges (Colwell & Lees, 2000; Jetz & Rahbek, 2001). Our model treated the northern border of South Africa as a hard boundary, not allowing species to spread across it, and consequently artificially strenghtened the mid-domain effect in a north–south direction. Fortunately, this did not affect our results, because the productivity gradient is almost exactly perpendicular to this direction (productivity increases from west to east), and the range dynamics along the productivity gradient (i.e. the spreading of species in the west–east direction) which were responsible for the observed patterns were affected by western and eastern boundaries that are genuinely hard. This has been confirmed by confining all the analyses to the southern part of South Africa, which does not substantially change the results. Nevertheless, the mid-domain effect is an inevitable outcome of simulated dynamics of ranges whose size is comparable to the area of the geographic realm considered, and thus the model would be more appropriate for regions with well-defined hard boundaries.

The findings concerning species distribution along the productivity gradient and the fit of the model have two implications that are relatively general. First, it seems that it is at least sometimes useful to consider the SER as emerging from mutually independent patterns of distribution of individual species along the gradient. Second, the SER has a geographic dimension, which is revealed by the fact that only the model assuming contiguity of species' ranges gave good results. The SER should therefore be viewed from a geographic perspective, as a product of spatial population processes modulated by available energy.

The increase of species' probabilities of occurrence with productivity can have several causes, and does not directly confirm or reject any theory comprising biological mechanisms proposed as explanations of the positive SER (Evans, Warren & Gaston, 2005). One possibility is that it is associated with higher population abundances in more productive areas, and thus is directly linked to the more individuals hypothesis (see above). This is supported by the common observation that abundances and occupancies (and/or range sizes) are positively correlated (Brown, 1984; Gaston, Blackburn & Lawton, 1997; Gaston et al., 2000; He & Gaston, 2000, 2003). However, Bonn et al. (2004) have shown for the South African bird data that species' reporting rates – proportions of checklists with presence records for a given species from all checklists submitted for a given grid cell – are lower in more productive areas. And since they are assumed to be correlated with local population abundances, this would not support the simple link between local abundance, occupancy and species richness. The other option would be that small-scale habitat heterogeneity could increase the chance that a species finds a suitable habitat. Heterogeneity may be positively related to productivity (Kerr, Southwood & Cihlar, 2001; Hurlbert, 2004), although the causes and universality of the relationship are unclear, and this option would therefore deserve much more detailed study. Regardless, for now we can rely on the finding that productivity increases the chance of a site to be occupied, irrespective of the biological reason for it.

## The species–area–energy relationship

So far, we know that the slope of the SAR on a log-log scale decreases with increasing species' mean relative occupancy, and that species' occupancies increase along a productivity gradient. Therefore, the SAR should have a lower slope in more productive regions, and consequently the SER should be more pronounced for smaller areas. In other words, we should expect a negative interaction between logarithmically transformed area and productivity in their effects on species richness.

We have tested this theory using two of the most comprehensive sets of quadrat-based distributional data, those for bird distributions in South Africa and Britain (Storch, Evans & Gaston, 2005). The results confirmed our expectations: both logarithmically transformed area and available energy were positively related to species richness, with a negative interaction between them even after controlling for spatial autocorrelation (Fig. 15.7). The pattern remained even when using another measure of productivity than NDVI (temperature; following Turner, Lennon & Lawrenson, 1988; Lennon, Greenwood & Turner, 2000), and regardless of whether the productivity measure was logarithmically transformed or not (area and species richness were always logarithmically transformed to obtain comparable slopes of the SAR). Since the slope $z$ of the SAR is one of the possible measures of species turnover (Lennon et al., 2001; Koleff, Gaston & Lennon, 2003), this finding is in accord with that of Bonn et al. (2004) that species turnover is lower in more productive areas. In a sense – and quite contrary to common intuition – more productive areas are more homogeneous in terms of geographical differences in the species composition of local assemblages.

Some previous findings seem at odds with the observed patterns. The latitudinal gradient of species richness, for example, has been reported to be more pronounced for large sample areas (Stevens & Willig, 2002; Hillebrand, 2004). If productivity systematically decreased with latitude, as is generally believed (Rosenzweig, 1995), this would challenge our results that the SER is more pronounced in smaller areas. However, latitudinal gradients of species richness are not that simple, and other factors including topography and habitat diversity contribute to them (Rahbek & Graves, 2001; Hawkins & Diniz-Filho, 2004). On some continents, the lower latitudes are even less productive than the higher latitudes: southern parts of North America are considerably drier and less productive than more northern areas (see Hurlbert & Haskell, 2003), and the finding that low latitudes here are associated with SARs of higher slope (Rodríguez & Arita, 2004) is thus in accord with our theory. Indeed, when similar analyses have been performed including humid Central and South America, the pattern predicted by our theory was found, $z$ decreasing toward the tropics (Lyons & Willig, 2002).

(a)

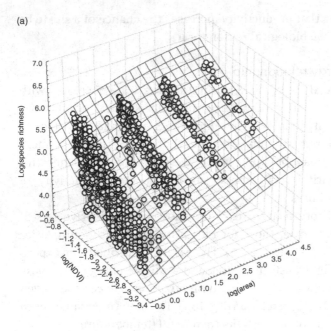

(b)

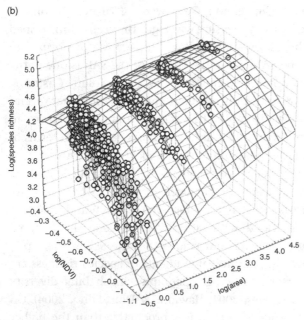

**Figure 15.7** Relationship between log(area), log(productivity) and log(species richness) for birds in (a) South Africa and (b) Great Britain. The surface is fitted by spline. Modified from Storch *et al.* (2005).

Our theory thus seems to be rather universal, at least as long as environmental productivity is associated with higher species' occupancies. Note that the theory relating the SAR and SER, as well as their interactions, to patterns of species occupancy (or rather probability of occupancy) treats all species as mutually independent, deriving the patterns without considering any interspecific interactions. This does not mean that interspecific interactions do not exist at the

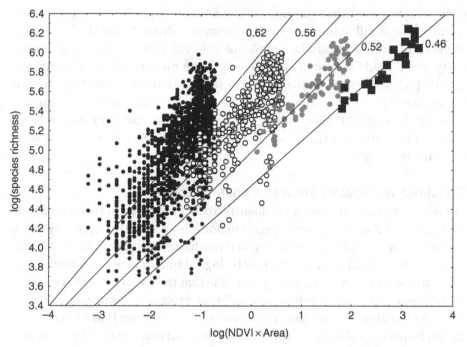

**Figure 15.8** Relationship between species richness and the product area × productivity in South Africa, with the relationship for each area marked separately: black dots, basic grid cells; white circles, squares of 2 × 2 (4) grid cells; gray circles, squares of 4 × 4 (16) grid cells; black squares, squares of 16 × 16 (64) grid cells. Regression lines for the relationships (numbers refer to regression coefficients, i.e. slopes of the relationships between species number and productivity in the log-log scale) for different areas indicate that the data points do not fall onto one universal relationship, indicating that the SAR and SER are driven by different factors.

macroecological scale – it is, for example, possible that they determine some species' properties which enter the models as input parameters, especially the distribution of species' range sizes (number of grid cells occupied by each species). However, whenever the species-range-size distribution is given, the species–area–energy relationship with predictable properties emerges, with no necessity to consider species interdependence.

Wright's (1983) notion that the SAR and SER must be closely interrelated has proven to be correct. However, area and available energy do not affect species richness in the same way. According to Wright (1983), the important variable affecting species richness is not area or energy per se, but the product of the two. In that case, the slopes of the SAR and SER on a logarithmic scale should be the same, with no interaction between productivity and area, because an increase in species richness with energy would necessarily be identical for small and large areas. But this is not the case. Moreover, from the plot of species richness against the product of area and energy (Fig. 15.8) we can see that the slope of the SER is

considerably higher than the slope of the SAR, and individual samples consequently do not fall onto one general relationship. Note, however, that even if
Wright's hypothesis was right, samples of different areas and different productivity levels would fall along one line only if the measure of productivity was
exactly proportional to abundance (in the same way as area), which is doubtful
in the case of NDVI. Therefore, our data are not too appropriate for a strong test
of Wright's original theory, although the negative interaction between NDVI
and area indicates that the emergence of the SER and SAR is not as simple as
expected by Wright.

## Conclusions – what we know and what we don't

We do not provide a definitive mechanistic theory of scaling of species richness
with area and available energy. Species richness is apparently affected by many
factors acting on different scales of spatial resolution (Whittaker, Willis & Field,
2001; Rahbek, 2005), differing in their biological importance as we move from
finer to coarser scales. It is also very probable that the species richness patterns
in different taxa emerge due to very different processes; some evidence indicates, for instance, that whereas the richness of endotherms is to a large extent
driven by resource abundance constraining the total number of individuals that
can be maintained in an area, for ectotherms evolutionary forces such as
diversification rate are more important (Allen *et al.*, 2002; Allen, Brown &
Gillooly, this volume). This seems quite reasonable, as there is indeed evidence
that total abundances and total energy consumption of species assemblages are
higher in more productive areas in endotherms (Pautasso & Gaston, 2005),
whereas this does not hold for ectotherms (Allen *et al.*, 2002; Currie *et al.*,
2004). However, we show that scaling patterns of species richness are intrinsically linked to patterns of species distribution, regardless of the exact biological
mechanisms.

Let us summarize what is actually known, and what is still unknown. First,
mainland SARs are proximately driven by aggregated patterns of spatial distribution of individual species, and their slope on a log-log scale can be calculated
from mean relative species occupancy (i.e. from knowledge of what portion of
the studied area individual species occupy). Moreover, self-similarity is a very
good approximation of observed species' spatial aggregation on several scales,
but the estimate of the slope of the SAR does not depend on the exact relationship between area and probability of occupancy (which is a power law in the
case of self-similarity). We do not know, however, to what extent species' spatial
distributions are truly self-similar, and which factors or processes should lead to
the apparent self-similarity. One candidate is fractal structure of the environment. Some indications of self-similarity in environmental variables have been
found (e.g. Storch, Gaston & Cepák, 2002), although spatial structuring of
habitat is quite variable (Palmer, this volume). But habitat is not the only

determinant of species distribution, and often cannot sufficiently explain its patterns, spatial population processes being of great importance even in such mobile groups as birds (Storch & Šizling, 2002; Storch et al., 2003a,b). Some random processes of aggregation on several spatial scales (Šizling & Storch, this volume) could provide a clue to understanding scaling of species distributions, but their biological significance (i.e. relationships to habitat structure and population/metapopulation processes) remains unexplored.

Second, we do know that when productivity is positively associated with species richness, it is often associated with a higher probability of occurrence for most species. Moreover, the SER can in some cases be derived directly from the assumption of higher probability of species occurrence in more productive areas, together with some assumptions concerning species' range dynamics. But this pattern may not be universal, and even in the case where it has been documented we do not know its biological causes. The more individuals explanation is probably the simplest and most popular, but the evidence against (Bonn et al., 2004; Currie et al., 2004) indicates that small-scale habitat heterogeneity increasing the chance that a species finds a suitable habitat could be more important (see also Hurlbert, 2004).

Third, we have shown that whenever higher productivity is associated with higher probability of occurrence of individual species, the slope of the SAR on a log-log scale must be lower in more productive areas. But we do not know how universal is the increase of species' occupancies with productivity. If the species richness of ectotherms increases with temperature without an increase in the population densities of individual species (Allen et al., 2002), it is possible that their occupancies also would not increase with productivity – assuming that there is a positive correlation between abundance and occupancy, and between temperature and productivity. Unfortunately, most tests of the relationships between productivity, population sizes, occupancies, and species richness have been performed using data on endothermic animals (particularly birds), for which these data exist at an appropriate resolution (Bonn et al., 2004; Hurlbert, 2004; Pautasso & Gaston, 2005; Storch et al., 2005; but see Kaspari, Zuan & Alonso, 2003 as an exception from this trend).

Finally, we know that scaling of species richness with energy and area can be understood in terms of patterns occurring at the level of individual species, and can be modeled assuming total species independence and no interspecific interactions. This is quite surprising, because most models and theories concerning the SER have assumed that energy availability limits total abundances or biomasses, and that this constraint on the total numbers of species that can coexist at a site is the driving force of species richness differences. But it may not be true if the increase of species richness with productivity is mediated by habitat heterogeneity (see Hurlbert, 2004). However, we do not know to what extent species independence is real, and to what extent it is just a useful property of the models which capture the relationship between several different patterns – which themselves can be affected by interspecific interactions and external constraints limiting the number of individuals and/ or species within an area (i.e. any sort of "biotic saturation"). The models we have presented assume that the distribution of species' range sizes is given, and this distribution may in fact reflect the mentioned constraints. Similarly, the increase of species' occupancies with productivity may or may not be related to limits which energy places on species abundance and occurrence. But the lesson is: so far no macroecological species richness pattern itself provides evidence for interspecific interactions or biotic saturation as a major driving force behind it. These effects can be important, but macroecological patterns themselves are not sufficient – as far as we know – for their demonstration.

## Acknowledgments

We thank the thousands of volunteers who collected the ornithological data on which the empirical results summarized in this chapter were based. The British data were kindly supplied by J.J.D. Greenwood and the British Trust for Ornithology, and the South African data by L. Underhill and the Avian Demography Unit, University of Cape Town. The study was supported by the Grant Agency of the Czech Republic (GACR 206/03/D124) the Grant Agency of the Academy of Sciences of the CR (KJB6197401), and the Czech Ministry of Education (grants LC06073 and MSM0021620845).

## References

Allen, A. P., Brown, J. H. & Gillooly, J. F. (2002). Global biodiversity, biochemical kinetics, and the energetic-equivalence rule. *Science*, **297**, 1545–1548.

Allen, A. P. & White, E. P. (2003). Effects of range size on species-area relationships. *Evolutionary Ecology Research*, **5**, 493–499.

Arrhenius, O. (1921). Species and area. *Journal of Ecology*, **9**, 95–99.

Bonn, A., Storch, D. & Gaston, K. J. (2004). Structure of the species-energy relationship. *Proceedings of the Royal Society of London, Series B*, **271**, 1685–1691.

Brown, J. H. (1984). On the relationship between abundance and distribution of species. *American Naturalist*, **124**, 255–279.

Chase, J. M. & Leibold, M. A. (2002). Spatial scale dictates the productivity-biodiversity relationship. *Nature*, **416**, 427–429.

Chown, S. L., van Rensburg, B. J., Gaston, K. J., Rodrigues, A. S. L. & van Jaarsveld, A. S. (2003). Species richness, human population size and energy: conservation implications at a national scale. *Ecological Application*, **13**, 1233–1241.

Coleman, D. B. (1981). On random placement and species-area relations. *Mathematical Biosciences*, **54**, 191–215.

Colwell, R. K. & Lees, D. C. (2000). The mid-domain effect: geometric constraints on the geography of species richness. *Trends in Ecology and Evolution*, **15**, 70–76.

Connor, E. F. & McCoy, E. D. (1979). The statistics and biology of the species-area relationship. *American Naturalist*, **113**, 791–833.

Currie, D. (1991). Energy and large-scale patterns of animal- and plant-species richness. *American Naturalist*, **137**, 27–49.

Currie, D. J., Mittelbach, G. G., Cornell, H. V., *et al.* (2004). Predictions and tests of climate-based hypotheses of broad-scale variation in taxonomic richness. *Ecology Letters*, **7**, 1121–1134.

Evans, K. L., Warren, P. H. & Gaston, K. J. (2005). Species-energy relationships at the macro-ecological scale: a review of the mechanisms. *Biology Review*, **80**, 1–25.

Gaston, K. J. (2000). Global patterns in biodiversity. *Nature*, **405**, 220–227.

Gaston, K. J. & Blackburn, T. M. (2000). *Pattern and Process in Macroecology*. Oxford: Blackwell Science.

Gaston, K. J., Blackburn, T. M. & Lawton, J. H. (1997). Interspecific abundance-range size relationships: an appraisal of mechanisms. *Journal of Animal Ecology*, **66**, 579–601.

Gaston, K. J., Blackburn, T. M., Greenwood, J. J. D., Gregory, R. D., Quinn, R. M. & Lawton, J. H. (2000). Abundance-occupancy relationships. *Journal of Applied Ecology*, **37** (Suppl. 1), 39–59.

Gleason, H. A. (1922). On the relation between species and area. *Ecology*, **3**, 158–162.

Hanski, I. & Gyllenberg, M. (1997). Uniting two general patterns in the distribution of species. *Science*, **275**, 397–400.

Harrison, J. A., Allan, D. G., Underhill, L. G., *et al.* (1997). *The Atlas of Southern African Birds.* Vols. I & II. Johannesburg: Bird Life South Africa.

Harte, J., Kinzig, A. & Green, J. (1999). Self-similarity in the distribution and abundance of species. *Science*, **284**, 334–336.

Hawkins, B. A. & Diniz-Filho, J. A. F. (2004). "Latitude" and geographic patterns in species richness. *Ecography*, **27**, 268–272.

Hawkins, B. A., Field, R., Cornell, H. V., *et al.* (2003). Energy, water, and broad-scale geographic patterns of species richness. *Ecology*, **84**, 3105–3117.

He, F. L. & Gaston, K. J. (2000). Estimating species abundance from occurrence. *American Naturalist*, **156**, 553–559.

He, F. L. & Gaston, K. J. (2003). Occupancy, spatial variance, and the abundance of species. *American Naturalist*, **162**, 366–375.

He, F. L. & Legendre, P. (2002). Species diversity patterns derived from species-area models. *Ecology*, **85**, 1185–1198.

Hillebrand, H. (2004). On the generality of the latitudinal diversity gradient. *American Naturalist*, **163**, 192–211.

Hurlbert, A. H. (2004). Species-energy relationships and habitat complexity in bird communities. *Ecology Letters*, **7**, 714–720.

Hurlbert, A. H. & Haskell, J. P. (2003). The effect of energy and seasonality on avian species richness and community composition. *American Naturalist*, **161**, 83–97.

Jetz, W. & Rahbek, C. (2001). Geometric constraints explain much of the species richness pattern in African birds. *Proceedings of the National Academy of Sciences of the United States of America*, **98**, 5661–5666.

Kaspari, M., Zuan, M. & Alonso, L. (2003). Spatial grain and the causes of regional diversity gradients in ants. *American Naturalist*, **161**, 459–477.

Kerr, J. T. & Ostrovsky, M. (2003). From space to species: ecological applications for remote sensing. *Trends in Ecology and Evolution*, **18**, 299–305.

Kerr, J. T., Southwood, T. R. E. & Cihlar, J. (2001). Remotely sensed habitat diversity predicts butterfly species richness and community similarity in Canada. *Proceedings of the National Academy of Sciences of the United States of America*, **98**, 11365–11370.

Kleidon, A. & Mooney, H. A. (2000). A global distribution of biodiversity inferred from climatic constraints: results from a process-based modelling study. *Global Change Biology*, **6**, 507–523.

Koleff, P., Gaston K. J. & Lennon, J. J. (2003). Measuring beta diversity for presence-absence data. *Journal of Animal Ecology*, **72**, 367–382.

Lennon, J. J., Greenwood, J. J. D. & Turner, J. R. G. (2000). Bird diversity and environmental gradients in Britain: a test of species energy hypothesis. *Journal of Animal Ecology*, **96**, 581–598.

Lennon, J. J., Koleff, P., Greenwood, J. J. D. & Gaston, K. J. (2001). The geographical structure of British bird distributions: diversity, spatial turnover and scale. *Journal of Animal Ecology*, **70**, 966–979.

Lennon, J. J., Kunin, W. E. & Hartley, S. (2002). Fractal species distributions do not produce power-law species area distribution. *Oikos*, **97**, 378–386.

Lyons, S. K. & Willig, M. R. (2002). Species richness, latitude, and scale-sensitivity. *Ecology*, **83**, 47–58.

MacArthur, R. H. & Wilson, E. O. (1967). *The Theory of Island Biogeography*. Princeton: Princeton University Press.

Maurer, B. A. (1999). *Untangling Ecological Complexity? The Macroscopic Perspective.* Chicago: University of Chicago Press.

Mittelbach, G. G., Steiner, C. F., Scheiner, S. M., et al. (2001). What is the observed relationship between species richness and productivity? *Ecology*, **82**, 2381–2396.

Ney-Nifle, M. & Mangel, M. (1999). Species-area curves based on geographic range and occupancy. *Trends in Ecology and Evolution*, **196**, 327–342.

Pautasso, M. & Gaston, K. J. (2005). Resources and global avian assemblage structure in forests. *Ecology Letters*, **8**, 282–289.

Plotkin, J. B., Potts, M. D., Leslie, N., Manokaran, N., LaFrankie, J. & Ashton, P. S. (2000). Species-area curves, spatial aggregation, and habitat specialization in tropical forests. *Journal of Theoretical Biology*, **207**, 81–89.

Preston, F. W. (1960). Time and space and the variation of species. *Ecology*, **29**, 254–283.

Rahbek, C. (2005). The role of spatial scale and the perception of large-scale species-richness patterns. *Ecology Letters*, **8**, 224–239.

Rahbek, C. & Graves, G. R. (2001). Multiscale assessment of patterns of avian species richness. *Proceedings of the National Academy of Sciences of the United States of America*, **98**, 4534–4539.

Rodríguez, P. & Arita, H. T. (2004). Beta diversity and latitude in North American mammals: testing the hypothesis of covariation. *Ecography*, **27**, 547–556.

Rosenzweig, M. L. (1995). *Species Diversity in Space and Time*. Cambridge: Cambridge University Press.

Šizling, A. L. & Storch, D. (2004). Power-law species-area relationships and self-similar species distributions within finite areas. *Ecology Letters*, **7**, 60–68.

Stevens, R. D. & Willig, M. R. (2002). Geographical ecology at the community level: Perspectives on the diversity of new world bats. *Ecology*, **83**, 545–560.

Storch, D. & Šizling, A. L. (2002). Patterns in commonness and rarity in central European birds: reliability of the core-satellite hypothesis. *Ecography*, **25**, 405–416.

Storch, D. & Gaston, K. J. (2004). Untangling ecological complexity on different scales of space and time. *Basic and Applied Ecology*, **5**, 389–400.

Storch, D., Gaston, K. J. & Cepák, J. (2002). Pink landscapes: 1/f spectra of spatial environmental variability and bird community composition. *Proceedings of the Royal Society of London, Series B*, **269**, 1791–1796.

Storch, D., Šizling, A. L. & Gaston, K. J. (2003a). Geometry of the species-area relationship in central European birds: testing the mechanism. *Journal of Animal Ecology*, **72**, 509–519.

Storch, D., Konvicka, M., Benes, J., Martinková, J. & Gaston, K. J. (2003b). Distributions patterns in butterflies and birds of the Czech Republic: separating effects of habitat and geographical position. *Journal of Biogeography*, **30**, 1195–1205.

Storch, D., Evans, K. L. & Gaston, K. J. (2005). The species-area-energy relationship. *Ecology Letters*, **8**, 487–492.

Tjørve, E. (2003). Shapes and functions of species-area curves: a review of possible models. *Journal of Biogeography*, **30**, 827–835.

Turner, J. R. G., Lennon, J. J. & Lawrenson, J. A. (1988). British bird species distributions and the energy theory. *Nature*, **335**, 539–541.

van Rensburg, B. J., Chown, S. L. & Gaston, K. J. (2002). Species richness, environmental correlates, and spatial scale: a test using South African birds. *American Naturalist*, **159**, 566–577.

Waide, R. B., Willig, M. R., Steiner, C. F., *et al.* (1999). The relationship between productivity and species richness. *Annual Review of Ecology and Systematics*, **30**, 257–300.

Whittaker, R. J., Willis, K. J. & Field, R. (2001). Scale and species richness: towards a general, hierarchical theory of species diversity. *Journal of Biogeography*, **28**, 453–470.

Williams, M. R. (1995). An extreme-value function model of the species incidence and species-area relationship. *Ecology*, **76**, 2607–2616.

Williamson, M. H. (1988). Relationship of species number to area, distance and other variables. In *Analytical Biogeography*, ed. A. A. Myers & P. S. Giller, pp. 91–115. London: Chapman & Hall.

Williamson, M. H. & Lawton, J. H. (1991). Fractal geometry of ecological habitats. In *Habitat Structure: The physical Arrangement of Objects in Space*, ed. S. S. Bell, E. D. McCoy & H. R. Mushinsky, pp. 69–86. London: Chapman & Hall.

Woodward, F. I., Lomas, M. R. & Lee, S. E. (2001). Predicting the future production and distribution of global terrestrial vegetation. In *Terrestrial Global Productivity*, ed. J. Roy, B. Saugier & H. Mooney, pp. 519–539. San Diego: Academic Press.

Wright, D. H. (1983). Species-energy theory: an extension of species-area theory. *Oikos*, **41**, 496–506.

PART IV

# Processes, perspectives, and syntheses

CHAPTER SIXTEEN

# Spatiotemporal scaling of species richness: patterns, processes, and implications

ETHAN P. WHITE

*Utah State University, University of Arizona, University of New Mexico*

The resemblance between time and space, in its simplest form, may be seen by driving a stake into the open water of a lake and then taking a transect toward the shore. We pass first through planktonic vegetation, then perhaps water lilies, then marsh, then grassland, then a succession of forest stages to climax forest. But we can pass through the same succession in the same order without moving at all. We may just sit by the stake for a few years or centuries and the seral stages will come to us one after the other as the lake fills in or drains.

Frank W. Preston (1960)

## Introduction

Understanding observed patterns of species diversity is a major focus of ecological research (e.g. Hutchinson, 1959; Brown, 1981; Gaston, 2000). However, it is increasingly well established that observed patterns and correlates of species richness are strongly dependent on the spatial scale of analysis (e.g. Levin, 1992; Wright, Currie & Maurer, 1993; Mittelbach *et al.*, 2001; Rahbek & Graves, 2001). This dependence results from differences in how species richness changes with the area sampled (Scheiner *et al.*, 2000; Chase & Leibold, 2002; Lyons & Willig, 2002).

There are literally hundreds of studies on the effects of spatial scale on species richness (the species–area relationship), and numerous additional studies on spatial species turnover (e.g. Connor & McCoy, 1979; Rosenzweig, 1995; Koleff, Gaston & Lennon, 2003). In fact, a number of chapters in this book represent important contributions to this field (e.g. Palmer, this volume; Gaston *et al.*, this volume; Storch, Šizling & Gaston, this volume). However, less attention has been paid to the equivalent patterns in time. Ecological systems are inherently dynamic, a fact often ignored in studies of species diversity. While spatial patterns of species richness and composition tell us much about community ecology, failing to consider temporal variability, and the ways in which it manifests itself, would be to miss half of the interesting behavior of

*Scaling Biodiversity*, ed. David Storch, Pablo A. Marquet and James H. Brown. Published by Cambridge University Press. © Cambridge University Press 2007.

ecological systems. In addition, by combining spatial and temporal patterns we can gain more information than by using either of them alone. While there are many different statistical and modeling approaches that can replicate observed spatial or temporal patterns alone, far fewer will be able to produce realistic static and dynamic patterns simultaneously (McGill, 2003; Adler, 2004; Maurer & McGill, 2004). Here I attempt to synthesize the rapidly expanding literature quantifying temporal patterns of diversity using traditionally spatial analyses, and attempt to demonstrate that these patterns are just as general and important to ecology as their spatial counterparts.

## The species–time relationship

In general, the average species richness at a site remains relatively constant from year to year[1] (Williamson, 1987; Ernest & Brown, 2001; Parody, Cuthbert & Decker, 2001; Lekve et al., 2002), but species both colonize and go locally extinct resulting in an increase in the total number of species detected as the site is monitored for increasingly long periods of time (Rosenzweig, 1995; Brown et al., 2001). This increase in the length of the species list with the period of observation was noted by Grinnell (1922) over 80 years ago. This general idea was also discussed by Williams, who noted an approximately constant increase in the number of species of insects observed in light traps at Rothamsted, England, with each doubling of the time span sampled (Fisher, Corbet & Williams, 1943; Williams, 1964). This doubling rule received empirical support from Preston (1948), though he believed this pattern to be driven by simple sampling processes (see below). Revisiting the pattern, Preston argued that because the processes generating this species–time relationship (STR) should be the same as those generating the species–area relationship (SAR) the two patterns should have the same functional form – likely that of a power function (Preston, 1960). The STR then disappeared into obscurity until Rosenzweig (1995) discussed it in his influential book.

### Processes underlying the species–time relationship

While the specific processes generating the STR and the manner in which they combine to produce the observed pattern are not fully understood, it seems clear that these processes should fall into three major categories: sampling, ecological, and evolutionary (Preston, 1960). In addition, these three groups should tend to dominate the observed patterns at different timescales, potentially creating three separate phases for the STR similar to those suggested to exist for the SAR (Williams, 1943; Preston, 1960; Allen & White, 2003).

---

[1] In cases where the environment does not undergo substantial transitions such as those during succession.

*Sampling*

For a static community (or regional pool) as more individuals are sampled the number of species observed will tend to increase (Fisher *et al.*, 1943; Bunge & Fitzpatrick, 1993; Gotelli & Colwell, 2001). Because most species–time relationships (STR) are constructed by accumulating successive samples, longer time spans also contain a greater number of individuals and therefore a greater number of species (Rosenzweig, 1995; White, 2004). There are two discrete components of sampling present in STRs. First, due to the fact that most ecological studies do not census completely all of the individuals occurring at a site at a given time, some individuals that are actually present will be missed. Some species will be so rare that by chance no individuals will be recorded during a survey even though the species was actually present at the time of the survey. As the site is then sampled repeatedly through time the chances of observing a particular species will increase solely because of the increasing number of individuals sampled. Second, even in the case of a complete census of the individuals at a site in any given year, random dynamics linking the local community to the species pool can result in random sampling patterns. This would result if individuals present in the local community were a random sample of the regional pool. For most communities both of these sampling components will be operating simultaneously. However, both individually and in combination they should produce similar patterns.[2]

*Ecological*

At intermediate timescales species turnover will result from local colonization and extinction events driven by processes such as temporal environmental variability, succession, and dispersal limitation. The expected functional outcome of the combination of these various ecological processes is unclear. Because many processes could be operating simultaneously with different strengths and outcomes in different taxa and environments, we might expect a certain amount of idiosyncrasy to occur in this phase. However, generality could emerge if there is regularity in environmental fluctuations or dispersal limitation. The potential for regularity in both environmental variability (Storch, Gaston & Cepak, 2002) and dispersal (Bell, 2001; Hubbell, 2001) to generate regular patterns for the SAR has received some support. However,

---

[2] This assumes that there are no differences in detection probability among species, which is likely a poor assumption (Nichols *et al.*, 2000). However, until some type of general model for, or complete classification of, detection probabilities for different species in different environments is available, it will be difficult to address this limitation in macroecological studies. This problem is not alleviated by attempts to determine detection probabilities from observed presence–absence data (Cam *et al.*, 2002) because both real absences and missed presences occur in the data. This results in the underestimation of detection probabilities and the overestimation of the contribution of sampling to observed patterns of turnover/ accumulation.

while STRs appear to display somewhat regular patterns at ecological time-scales, it is not clear how they are related to the underlying environment and taxon-specific ecological attributes.

*Evolutionary*

At long enough timescales speciation and extinction events will begin to dominate the observed cumulative increase in species richness (Preston, 1960; Rosenzweig, 1995). This should cause the STR to converge to a linear relationship (Preston, 1960; Rosenzweig, 1998). That is, at sufficiently long timescales doubling the timescale of analysis will add a completely new suite of species.

It is worth noting that while these different processes may be dominant at particular scales, they will not necessarily be confined entirely to those scales. The result, at least in some cases, is likely to be gradual transitions and multiple classes of processes combining to influence the functional form of the STR.

## Construction of species–time relationships

Species–time relationships are typically constructed using a sliding window approach equivalent to that used to construct fully nested SARs (e.g. Plotkin *et al.*, 2000). A window of time span, $T$, is passed over a time series of species lists, one for each time step, and all species occurring within the window are counted. This results in a linear decrease in the number of windows with increasing time span (e.g. a 20 year time series will have 20 1-year windows, 19 2-year windows, etc.). Typically, the richness values for each time span are then averaged to provide a single estimate of mean species richness for a particular time span and the means are plotted as a function of time span (e.g. Fig. 16.1). Arithmetic and geometric means appear to provide equivalent results (White, 2004) and the logical choice depends on the distribution of richness values within a time span and whether nonlinear or ordinary least squares (OLS) techniques (on log-transformed data) are to be applied to the data. An alternative approach would be to use weighted regression, weighting each time span by one over the number of windows (J. L. Green, personal communication). This will produce identical parameter estimates to arithmetic means if the data within each time span are normally distributed, and to geometric means if the data are log-normally distributed.

Nested STRs, like nested SARs, suffer from a variety of statistical issues. First and foremost is the lack of independence between data points. The only way to avoid this problem would be to use only unique portions of the time series for each time span (e.g. year 1 for the 1 year time span, years 2–6 for the 5 year time span, etc.). However, this is impractical because we do not have time series long enough to generate STRs of more than a few years using this technique, and it also risks confounding the effects of time span with those of environmental variables that may change over the course of the time series. Another problem is

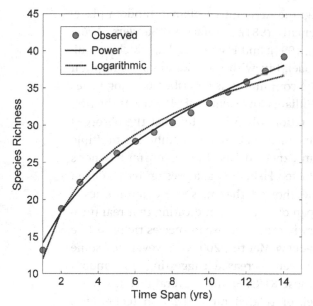

**Figure 16.1** An example of a species–time relationship constructed using data from the summer annual plant community at Portal Arizona (for details on methodology at the site see Brown, 1998). Circles represent the average observed species richness across control plots for each possible time span. As the site is observed for increasingly long periods of time, the number of species increases monotonically. Both a power function (solid line) and a logarithmic function (dotted line) provide reasonably good fits to the observed data, though in this case the power function appears to perform somewhat better.

that sample size is initially exaggerated by using sliding windows that can share substantial numbers of actual samples. This problem is reduced by averaging the values within a time span, but this ignores real variability in the data. An alternative approach would be to only use nonoverlapping windows for each time span (while still allowing longer time span windows to include windows of shorter time spans), but this results in either ignoring time spans that do not divide evenly into the length of the total time series or excluding data at one end of the time series for some time spans but not others. Given these statistical limitations, the statistics of STRs should be interpreted with caution. In general, parameter estimates for fitting of statistical functions to these types of data should be unbiased, but the estimated error in those parameters will not be valid.

There are also examples of nonnested STRs equivalent to island SARs (Rosenzweig, 1995; Rosenzweig, 1998; Hadly & Maurer, 2001). These relationships come from fossil data and are constructed by counting the total number of species occurring in a single stratum and approximating the time span of sampling by assuming it to be proportional to the depth of that strata. Perhaps surprisingly, the exponents of these long timescale, nonnested STRs are well within the range of nested, ecological timescale STRs.

## Sampling and the species–time relationship

The simplest model for the STR would be one in which the observed increases in species richness with time span are driven entirely by the associated increase in the number of individuals sampled. There are a number of approaches to quantifying how species richness should change as a function of the increased

sampling from a static pool including: the Arrhenius–Coleman random placement model (Arrhenius, 1921; Coleman, 1981); rarefaction (Sanders, 1968;
Hurlbert, 1971; Brewer & Williamson, 1994); and Fisher's alpha, which is equivalent to the Arrhenius–Coleman model, but with the additional assumption
that the abundance distribution of the community is described by a log series
(Fisher et al., 1943; Coleman, 1981). Williams (in Fisher et al., 1943) was the first
to compare a STR to a random expectation when he noted that the observed
increase in species richness with abundance generated by combining multiple
years of sampling was different from expected based on a constant Fisher's
alpha. Rosenzweig (1995, 1998) conducted Fisher's $\alpha$ analyses on half a dozen
communities with mixed results. He showed that in some communities $\alpha$
increased as a function of the time span of sampling, indicating that real turnover, not simply sampling, was generating the increase in species richness (see
also McKinney & Frederick, 1999; Hadly & Maurer, 2001). However, for some
communities $\alpha$ remained constant, or even decreased, suggesting that random
sampling alone was responsible for those STRs. Finally, several recent studies
using the Arrhenius–Coleman model, or related randomization techniques,
have demonstrated that for almost 1000 species–time relationships the
observed STR is never generated entirely by random sampling (Adler &
Lauenroth, 2003; White, 2004; White et al., 2006).[3]

While it appears that random sampling does not completely explain observed
STRs, it must have some influence on the pattern, particularly over short
periods of time where relatively few individuals are identified (Preston, 1960).
Using data on Lepidoptera, Rosenzweig (1998) noted that at short timescales
Fisher's $\alpha$ remained constant, but started to increase at longer timescales,
suggesting (as had Preston, 1960) that the STR could be divided into phases:
one dominated by sampling and the other dominated by other factors. In an
attempt to quantify the timescales of the transition between these two phases,
White (2004) fit random placement models to short timescales and power/
logarithmic functions to longer timescales, with the transition between the
two functions determined by minimizing the overall residual variation around
the two-phase model. These results suggest that, on average, ecological communities transition from sampling to ecological phases within 1–4 years (White,
2004; White et al., 2006). But, if sampling processes alone cannot describe the
observed form of the STR, then we are left with the questions: what is the shape
of the relationship and what generates it?

---

[3] These approaches should all give good estimates of sampling-based STRs in most systems, but
they all ignore the fact that in STRs (unlike SARs) an individual can occur in more than one
time period. This persistence of individuals through time complicates the construction of
sampling models of the STR and more work incorporating persistence into these methods is
clearly necessary. This complexity should have little effect on results for communities
composed of mostly short-lived individuals (like those discussed in the next paragraph), but
may prove more important in analyses of long-lived taxonomic groups.

**Functional form**

There is a long history of debate in the spatial literature over the appropriate statistical model for the SAR (e.g. Arrhenius, 1921; Gleason, 1922; Connor & McCoy, 1979; Lomolino, 2000; Williamson, Gaston & Lonsdale, 2001). The two most common are the power law and the logarithmic function (Connor & McCoy, 1979; Rosenzweig, 1995; Lennon et al., 2001). These two models are also the ones most commonly fit to the STR. Williams (in Fisher et al., 1943) originally suggested the logarithmic form, $S = c + w \log T$, based on empirical data on insects at Rothamsted, England. Preston (1948) found additional empirical support for this function in two moth communities, but also suggested that the power function, $S = cT^w$, might be appropriate (Preston, 1960). In both of these equations $S$ is species richness, $T$ is time span of sampling, and $c$ and $w$ are fitted constants. Rosenzweig (1995) revisited these early data sets (including more extensive Rothamsted data from Williams, 1964) and based on visual comparisons concluded that it was impossible to tell which form better described the pattern. He called for more extensive analyses.[4] The next several STR studies offered no comparison of models, but showed that their data were well fit by simple power functions (McKinney & Frederick, 1999; Hadly & Maurer, 2001).

Adler & Lauenroth (2003) provided the first quantitative comparison of the power and logarithmic models for the STR. Using 15 permanent grassland plant quadrats they compared power and logarithmic functions using $r^2$ values from OLS fits to appropriately log-transformed data. In all 15 quadrats the power function provided a better fit to the observed data. However, this was followed by a study of 521 breeding bird communities that showed that the logarithmic function actually provided a better fit in 60% of the communities (White, 2004; reanalyzed by White et al., 2006).

In an attempt to resolve the question of whether power or logarithmic functions better describe the observed STR, White et al. (2006) gathered together a total of 984 community time series (including the plant and breeding bird data discussed above), and generated STRs for all of the communities. A comparison of power and logarithmic functions for these communities showed that while in particular combinations of ecosystems and taxonomic groups there was some

[4] Rosenzweig also proposed a novel functional form for the pattern by adding a constant to the power function ($S = k + cT^w$; Rosenzweig, 1998). This form has the advantage of allowing nonzero species richness when time span is equal to zero. However, this new form of the STR is still an arbitrary statistical model and as such its value for describing the STR should be based on the quality of fit to the observed data. The new model provided very little improvement over a simple power function (Rosenzweig, 1998), and as such the use of the additional parameter ($k$) will likely not be supported using appropriate model comparison techniques. While this model has generally been ignored, if the model were to hold up under model comparison then its use would be warranted. However, the temptation to compare the exponent in this model to the exponent from simple power function fitting (as done by Rosenzweig) should be avoided unless $k$ is not significantly different from zero.

bias towards one functional form or the other, overall there was no difference in the fits of the different statistical functions.

One of the major goals of the extensive curve fitting that has been conducted on both species–time and species–area relationships is the hope that regular behavior of particular statistical functions will provide clues about where to focus our search for the predominant processes underlying the observed patterns (e.g. Brown *et al.*, 2002). One of the challenges for using curve fitting to isolate regular patterns in the STR is that the STR is likely composed of three phases each dominated by different sets of processes (Preston, 1960; see section on Processes above). Therefore some lack of consensus in curve fitting could result from the inclusion of multiple phases of the STR. However, White's (2004) two-phase analysis resulted in power and logarithmic functions each providing the best fit to the ecological portion of the STR about half the time, and the fits of the two models were not distinguishable from one another across the communities. This approach of describing the form of the STR using multiple phases is an improvement over simply fitting statistical functions to the entire relationship, because it allows the interpretation of the parameters from the statistical models to focus on the ecological portion of the relationship. However, it still fails to give consistent discrimination between the power and logarithmic functions.

Collectively these studies suggest that the STR may not necessarily be described by either a power law or a logarithmic function, but simply be well approximated by both. This would be quite different from some of the other well-established scale-free relationships in biology such as the allometries relating organismal characteristics to their body size, which are clearly best described by power functions (e.g. Peters, 1983; Calder, 1984; Schmidt-Nielsen, 1984). However, it may also mean that these functions are simply indistinguishable from one another over the observed scales of variation in time span and species richness (see McGill, 2003). In either case, it seems desirable to take a more bottom-up, process-based modeling approach to understand how observed STRs result from a combination of ecological factors.

The good news is that both functions do provide a good quantification of the relationship, and even extrapolating the two functions beyond the scale of the observed data provides very similar results (White *et al.*, 2006). Therefore, either function is a reasonable choice for empirical description. That said, for comparative work it makes sense to focus on the power-law exponent for the STR, $w$, because this form provides a measure of relative turnover. Most measures of temporal turnover are relative measures, because most ecologists consider a change (or addition) of 5 species in a 10 species community to be much different from a change of 5 species in a 100 species community (e.g. Diamond, 1969; Russell *et al.*, 1995; Russell, 1998). The exponent of the power function gives the proportional increase in species richness for each doubling of the timescale of observation,[5] whereas the slope of the logarithmic function describes the absolute rate of increase. Therefore, the discussion that follows will be based largely on the power function exponent.

Before leaving this section it is worth noting that while published analyses have focused on power and logarithmic functions, there may well be other models – both statistical and mechanistic – that do an equally good job of describing the observed patterns. One possibility is that the pattern will show an asymptote at long timescales, justifying the use of asymptotic statistical models such as those proposed for the SAR (Lomolino, 2000; but see Williamson *et al.*, 2001). This asymptote might occur because eventually all of the species in the regional pool may have occurred at the sampling site, so no additional species would be available to colonize. However, I suspect that by the time all species from the original pool would have been recorded at the site, the pool itself would have changed in composition. This reorganization of the regional pool would potentially allow the STR to continue to increase until evolutionary processes become the predominant influence. Residual plots for STRs present some evidence for this possibility. After fitting nonasymptotic statistical models to the data, there is no indication of negative residuals at the longest time spans, which is contrary to expectation if the STR is actually asymptotic (White, 2004). Another possible model for the STR is one proposed by He and Legendre (1996) for the SAR, which behaves like a logarithmic function at short timescales, a power law at intermediate timescales, and a logistic curve at long timescales. This could explain the better fits of the logarithmic function at short timescales and the power function at long timescales seen in breeding bird STRs prior to accounting for sampling (F. He, personal communication; residual plots in White, 2004). In addition, SAR models that produce results that are similar to power functions (e.g. Šizling & Storch, 2004; Harte *et al.*, 2005) should also provide reasonable fits to STRs.

## Generality

One reason for the wide interest in the SAR is that the pattern appears to be general, taking similar shapes and exhibiting similar parameter estimates across a wide variety of taxonomic groups and locations (e.g. Williamson, 1988; Rosenzweig, 1995). Preston (1960) argued that like the SAR, the STR should exhibit a consistent pattern across taxa and habitats. But until recently there was not enough temporal data to evaluate whether this was true.

Preston (1960) not only proposed that the STR should be a fairly general pattern, but that it should behave similarly to the SAR. If so, parameters of the statistical functions describing the two relationships should be similar. He

---

[5] The proportional increase in species richness per doubling of time span is actually equal to $2^w - 1$, not simply $w$, but $w$ is still a measure of relative turnover. Since they are simply different transformations of the same fitted constant either would be a reasonable choice for comparative work.

supported his argument using comparisons of logarithmic function slopes for the SAR and STR in several bird communities that appeared to be approximately equivalent. Focusing on the power law treatments, the nested STRs are logically most similar to SARs constructed from spatially nested subsets of intracontinental floras and faunas, which tend to yield SAR exponents on the order of 0.1 to 0.2 (Williamson, 1988; Rosenzweig, 1995). Early estimates of STR exponents appeared to suggest that they might on average be higher than those observed for intracontinental SARs (Rosenzweig, 1995), although some of these relationships were for fossil data and might be expected to have larger exponents as a result of the influence of evolutionary processes (Preston, 1960; Rosenzweig, 1995; Rosenzweig, 1998; McKinney & Frederick, 1999). In the first study to compare power law species–area and species–time relationships for the same region and taxon, Hadly and Maurer (2001) showed that the STR for a montane mammal community had an identical scaling exponent (0.27) to that of the SAR. This study was conducted on an island-type SAR (each point represented the area of appropriate habitat on a single mountain and the accompanying species richness) and an island-type STR (each point was a fossil stratum and its associated richness), and only a single STR was available. Analyses of additional data sets with multiple STRs produced conflicting results with average exponents both similar to (White, 2004) and much higher than (Adler & Lauenroth, 2003) standard SAR exponents. The most comprehensive study of STRs to date found that most sites and taxonomic groups had average exponents between 0.2 and 0.4 (White et al., 2006). Compiling data on all known published power-law STR exponents suggests a tendency for STRs to have exponents averaging around 0.3 (Fig. 16.2), a central tendency that appears to be at least as strong as that exhibited by SARs.

While there does appear to be some central tendency in observed STR exponents, there is significant variability between different sites and taxonomic groups. Understanding this observed variability offers a potential avenue for understanding the processes that generate species–time relationships as a whole. There are currently two major factors known to influence the STR exponent: spatial scale (discussed separately later in the chapter), and mean annual species richness. Both positive (Clarke & Lidgard, 2000; Stevens & Willig, 2002) and negative (Lennon et al., 2001; Lyons & Willig, 2002; Koleff et al., 2003) correlations between turnover and local species richness have been reported for studies of spatial turnover, and either sign of correlation is theoretically possible (Gaston et al., this volume). However, all 20 correlations between temporal turnover and mean annual species richness that have been conducted are either negative (9/20) or nonsignificant (11/20 with 8/11 showing a negative tendency, White, 2004; White et al., 2006). In addition, there appears to be a relationship between richness and turnover that holds across different habitats and taxonomic groups (Fig. 16.3, White et al., 2006). This suggests that a negative correlation between richness and turnover may be a general feature of temporal

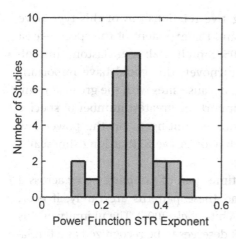

**Figure 16.2** Histogram of power-law species–time relationship (STR) exponents from all studies that published them (data from Rosenzweig, 1995; McKinney & Frederick, 1999; Hadly & Maurer, 2001; Adler & Lauenroth, 2003; White *et al.*, 2006). For studies which presented a single STR that exponent was used. For studies presenting exponents for multiple STRs for a single taxonomic group in a single region the average of these was included. For studies presenting STR exponents from multiple sites and or multiple taxonomic groups the values were averaged within unique site–taxonomic group combinations. This averaging allowed the inclusion of studies with widely varying numbers of STRs and the points generating the resulting distribution should be independent of one another.

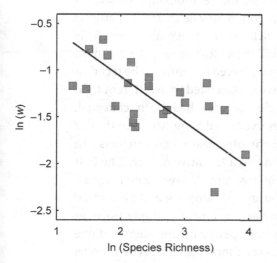

**Figure 16.3** Cross-site relationship between mean annual species richness and the power function exponent of the STR (*w*). Each point represents the average values for a unique site–taxon combination (data from White *et al.*, 2006). The data was natural log transformed and then fit using reduced major axis (RMA) regression. The regression line is $\ln(w) = -0.1 - 0.48 \ln(richness)$. The difference in slope between this analysis and that already published ($-0.3$, White *et al.*, 2006) is the result of using RMA regression on log-transformed data as opposed to nonlinear regression on untransformed data. There is no obviously correct choice for regression approaches for this data, and as such the two values represent likely bounds on the real relationship.

variability in species composition. It also suggests that variables that are positively correlated with richness such as productivity (e.g. Wright, 1983; Hawkins *et al.*, 2003), temperature (e.g. Rohde, 1992; Allen, Brown & Gillooly, 2002), and habitat heterogeneity (e.g. MacArthur, 1964; Blackburn & Gaston, 1996) may be negatively correlated with turnover. Negative relationships of this type have been documented between productivity and the exponent of the species–area relationship (Storch, Evans & Gaston, 2005; Storch, Šizling & Gaston, this volume). If the same is true for temporal turnover, this could have important implications for conservation assessment, because sites with the greatest number of species in a single year may not support the greatest number of species over some longer timescale. However, this is contingent on the power law function appropriately describing the behavior of the STR at long timescales (White *et al.*, 2006).

Increases in species richness with the time span of sampling occur across a wide variety of taxa and ecosystems, and these patterns are rarely, if ever, generated entirely by random sampling (White *et al.*, 2006). The ubiquity of this nonrandom increase suggests that the STR deserves to be recognized as a fundamental ecological pattern (White *et al.*, 2006). In addition, the fact that the STR shows regular behavior in functional form, and regular patterns in its parameters (Figs. 16.2 and 16.3), suggests that it has the potential to provide valuable insights into the potentially general nature of the dynamics of species composition.

## The species–time–area relationship

It appears that both species–area and species–time relationships behave in similar and regular ways. The question then becomes how do these two patterns combine to govern the scaling of species richness in space and time. This question, as far as I can tell, was first hinted at by Rosenzweig (1998). In an attempt to generate a fossil STR, Rosenzweig was forced to confront the fact that different periods of time in the fossil record were associated with different total areas of preserved rock from which species records had been collected. Therefore both space (the area of rock preserved) and time (the duration of each period in the fossil record) influenced the observed species richness. In order to control for this Rosenzweig proposed two alternative models. The first was a simple multiplicative combination of two power laws producing an equation of the form $S = cA^z T^w$, where $A$ is the area of sampling and $z$ is a fitted constant. This model (hereafter the "no interaction model") simply assumes that species–area and species–time relationships operate independently of one another and can both be characterized by power functions. The second model was conceptually similar, but included an extra constant to describe the time dependence. While this assumption of independent effects of space and time may seem reasonable, as discussed below it turns out that this form of the combined species–time–area relationship (STAR) is too simple to describe the observed behavior of ecological data.

The next step in the statistical modeling of the combined scaling of species richness with time and area was proposed by Adler and Lauenroth (2003). They suggested that the rate of species accumulation in time should depend on the

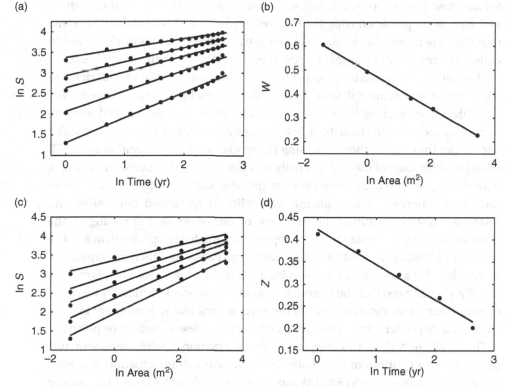

**Figure 16.4** An example species–time–area relationship using data from the summer annual plant community at Portal, AZ (for details on the site see Brown, 1998; for details on spatial aggregation of data see Adler *et al.*, 2005). For all panels points represent observed data and lines represent OLS fits to transformed data. (a) The species–time relationship (STR) as a function of temporal scale. Data from bottom to top are the STRs for spatial scales of 0.25, 1, 4, 8, and 32 m$^2$. (b) Change in the fitted exponent of the STR as a function of spatial scale. (c) The species–area relationship (SAR) as a function of time scale. Data from bottom to top are the SARs for temporal scales of 1, 2, 4, 8, and 14 years. (d) Change in the fitted exponent of the SAR as a function of timescale. The negative relationship between the opposing scale and the exponent of the accumulation relationship in (b) and (d) indicate the need for an interaction term to describe the observed species–time–area relationship.

spatial scale of observation, and that the rate of species accumulation in space should depend on the timescale of observation[6] (Fig. 16.4). This interaction between scales makes intuitive sense. For example, consider a list of all plant species occurring in a large geographic area (such as a country in Europe) during a single year. The number of new species seen in this large region by observing it

---

[6] The authors attributed this general concept to Preston (1960), but careful rereading of Preston's paper by Dr. P. B. Adler (personal communication) and myself revealed that this attribution, while generous, was in fact incorrect.

for a second year will be small, because most of the species that can occur there will have been present during the first year. However, if we conduct the same thought experiment for a much smaller area (someone's backyard) we would expect to see a greater number of new species occurring in the second year.[7]

This interaction would be expected to occur if the increases in species richness with spatial and temporal scale were being driven by similar processes. For example, if the observed increases in species richness were determined predominantly by increases in the habitat heterogeneity sampled at larger spatial scales and longer time spans, then increasing the spatial scale of observation for a STR would capture some of the heterogeneity that would drive the increase in richness with time span. The interaction between the SAR and STR would then be determined by patterns of environmental variability in space and time. Adler and Lauenroth (2003) quantified the influence of one scale on the scaling of the other by taking the simple statistical approach of modeling species richness as a function of log-transformed time, log-transformed area, and their multiplicative interaction, $\log S = \log c + z \log A + w \log T + u \log A \times \log T$. For one plant community, they showed that the interaction parameter, $u$, was significantly negative, demonstrating that the exponents of the species–area and species–time relationships were dependent on the temporal and spatial scales of analysis respectively.

This "full model" and Rosenzweig's "no interaction model" represent two points along a continuum of hypotheses for how much information is needed to describe the observed STAR. The most basic, or null, model would, as for the SAR and STR, be that the observed increase in species richness is simply that expected to result as an increasing number of individuals is sampled from a static abundance distribution (Adler *et al.*, 2005). The Arrhenius–Coleman random placement model can be easily modified for this task. The other three models are power law based models of increasing complexity. The simplest possibility is that species richness is not related uniquely to either space or time per se, but to the total space–time volume (hereafter the "volume model", Adler *et al.*, 2005). For example, observing a $10\,\mathrm{m}^2$ plot for 5 years would yield a species list of the same length as observing a $50\,\mathrm{m}^2$ plot for 1 year and a $1\,\mathrm{m}^2$ plot for 50 years. Slightly more complex is the possibility that species richness increases with time and area in different ways, but the scaling with time and area are independent of each another – the "no interaction model" (Rosenzweig, 1998). The most complex description of the STAR to date is the "full model", which not only allows the scaling of richness with space and time to be different, but it also allows these scalings to depend on the scale of the other variable (Adler & Lauenroth, 2003). The three nonsampling models all represent special cases of the full model proposed by Adler and Lauenroth (2003), which can be rewritten as

---

[7] To be precise, because we are discussing relative turnover it is really that a smaller percentage of new species occurs in the larger area, not necessarily a smaller absolute number.

$$S = cA^{z_1 + \frac{u}{2} \ln T} T^{w_1 + \frac{u}{2} \ln A},$$  (16.1)

where $A$ is the area sampled, $T$ is the time sampled, $z_1$ is the fitted exponent of the SAR at the unit timescale, $w_1$ is the fitted exponent of the STR at the unit spatial scale, $c$ is a fitted constant describing the expected richness at a single unit area and a single unit time, and $u$ is a fitted parameter quantifying the interaction between time and area (Adler et al., 2005). The "no interaction" model is the special case where $u = 0$ and the "volume" model occurs when $u = 0$ and $z_1 = w_1$.

While there is no theoretical justification for any of these models, comparing the models with different levels of complexity should at least point us towards an understanding of how much information is needed to understand combined spatiotemporal scaling. In addition, if the models do a good job of describing the observed data they will provide a valuable method for translating across scales and quantifying the relative importance of spatial and temporal turnover at different scales. A recent comparison of these four models, for eight different STARs with data ranging from zooplankton in lakes to desert rodents, supported Adler and Lauenroth's hypothesis that interaction between scales is important. For all eight STARs the full model performed better than all other models, even after correcting for differences in the number of parameters,[8] and all interaction terms were negative (Adler et al., 2005).

Because there is an interaction between spatial and temporal scaling this means that there will be combinations of spatial and temporal scale at which the exponents of STRs and SARs are equal (Adler & Lauenroth, 2003). Calculating these "scales of equivalence" tells us at what scales spatial and temporal turnover are the same. This should provide information about how the life histories of the taxa involved combine with environmental variability to produce the observed patterns.[9] These scales of equivalence can be determined by setting the exponents of the SAR and STR equal to one another and solving for area to give

$$A = b^{\left(\frac{z_1 - w_1}{u}\right)} T,$$  (16.2)

---

[8] Comparisons were done using Akaike's information criteria (AIC) with unknown variance (Burnham & Anderson, 1998; Venables & Ripley, 1999). However, due to the inherent lack of independence present in nested species–area and species–time relationships AIC represents only an arbitrary correction for the number of parameters.

[9] Preston (1960) attempted to calculate a scale of equivalence by determining scales at which the exponents of SAR and STR each reached unity due to the complete influence of evolutionary processes on the relationships (remember the predicted increase in the exponent at extremely long timescales). This assumed that SARs and STRs were independent of one another (which they are not) and that the scales at which evolutionary processes dominated the observed relationships provided information about the patterns at ecological timescales (which seems unlikely to be the case). While Preston's approach to calculating a scale of equivalence was simplistic, his estimate of ~1000 acres/year for birds may not have been too far off.

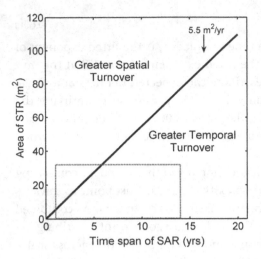

Figure 16.5 Plot indicating the scales at which the observed species–time and species–area relationship exponents will be equal to one another for the summer annual plant community at Portal, AZ (for details on the site see Brown, 1998; for details on spatial aggregation of data see Adler *et al.*, 2005). The line indicates combinations of scales where spatial and temporal scale are equal. For combinations of scale above and below the line, greater spatial turnover and greater temporal turnover, respectively, will occur. The gray dashed box encompasses the scales sampled at the site.

where $b$ is the base of the logarithm chosen for transformation (Adler *et al.*, 2005). Adler and Lauenroth's (2003) original scale of equivalence calculation determined the spatial scale at which the STR exponent was the same as the SAR exponent calculated during a single year (i.e. they set $T = 1$ yr). At combinations of scales that produce constant ratios greater than the one in the solution above, spatial turnover will be greater than temporal turnover. At scale combinations with ratios smaller than this constant, temporal turnover will be greater (Fig. 16.5, Adler *et al.*, 2005). These ratios of equivalence (the constant in the above equation) are of interest because they tell us something about how natural communities perceive and respond to the environment. For example, small mammals have much larger ratios of equivalence than annual plants, suggesting that much larger spatial scales are necessary to generate equivalent spatial and temporal turnover in rodents (Adler *et al.*, 2005). This makes sense because animals operate at much larger spatial scales than plants, effectively smoothing out, or decreasing the perception of, spatial heterogeneity in the environment (e.g. Morse *et al.*, 1985). The ability to quantify the relative importance of space and time to turnover should prove valuable when considering alternative experimental and observational designs for collecting species composition data.

## Species richness, spatial scale, and temporal turnover

Applying the species–time–area relationships discussed above to our understanding of the STR leaves us with some difficult, still unanswered questions about cause and effect. We now know that the exponent of the STR is negatively correlated with both species richness and spatial scale. However, species richness and spatial scale are positively correlated with one another (i.e. the SAR exists) making it difficult to determine the relative contributions of these processes to the observed correlations with temporal turnover (White *et al.*, 2006). The fact that temporal turnover is correlated with species richness within studies that sample at the same spatial scale (i.e. turnover and richness are negatively correlated even in the absence of any variability in spatial scale) suggests that species richness is an appropriate proximate correlate in some cases, but more extensive analyses attempting to understand and quantify the mechanisms underlying temporal turnover are needed. It is likely that environmental processes are largely responsible for these correlations, and that they have opposite influences on species richness and turnover, thereby generating the observed negative correlations. Phenomenologically, this may result from the fact that increasing the average probability of occurrence for a species will both increase mean annual richness and decrease turnover (Plotkin *et al.*, 2000; He & Legendre, 2002; Šizling & Storch, 2004). This type of causality has recently been demonstrated in spatial studies (Storch *et al.*, 2005; Storch, Šizling & Gaston, this volume). Understanding the processes causing observed increases in the average probability of occurrence represents a promising area for continuing research into these patterns.

## Concluding remarks

The influence of temporal scale on species richness, both on its own and through its impact on the spatial scaling of species richness, has several implications for the study of ecological systems. The first is that comparative studies of species richness must use data collected at the same timescales. Or, if only different timescale data are available, they should be "corrected" to the same timescale using STRs (Adler & Lauenroth, 2003; White *et al.*, 2006) in much the same way as is often done for differences in spatial scale using SARs (Inouye, 1998; Gross *et al.*, 2000; Scheiner *et al.*, 2000). Second, especially given the observed negative relationship between richness and temporal turnover, it is possible that patterns and determinants of species richness may vary with temporal scale, much as they do for spatial scale (White *et al.*, 2006). However, in the one case in which this actually has been tested, the temporal scale was found not to influence the observed patterns (Chalcraft *et al.*, 2004). Third, dynamic models of species richness patterns should be tested to see if they generate patterns describing their dynamic behavior (such as the STR) as well as their static behavior (such as the SAR). For example, Adler (2004) tested a neutral community model (Bell, 2001) to see if it could reproduce realistic species–area and species–time relationships for a Kansas grassland. While the neutral model could generate reasonable SAR and STR exponents, it required different parameterizations to produce the observed spatial and temporal patterns, thus calling into question its validity for this particular system.

There remains one important area of species–area research that has been basically untouched by those working on the temporal pattern and that is the quantification of aggregation of individuals. The SAR literature is full of studies examining the spatial aggregation of individuals and its influence on the observed spatial scaling of species richness (Plotkin et al., 2000; He & Legendre, 2002; Lennon, Kunin & Hartley, 2002; Šizling & Storch, 2004; Harte et al., 2005). Similar work on temporal aggregation should prove equally valuable (E. P. White and M. A. Gilchrist, unpublished manuscript).

The species–area and species–time relationships were on nearly equal footing in ecology when Preston wrote his seminal paper almost 50 years ago. Since then the SAR has become one of the most studied patterns in ecology, while the STR lay relatively dormant. Thanks to a spurt of recent activity on the STR, I believe that we are again coming close to having similar levels of knowledge about the two patterns.

As we compare spatial and temporal patterns it is important to remember that space and time are in fact different. One fundamental difference between time and space is that time is directional and one-dimensional whereas space is nondirectional and two-dimensional. However, these differences have barely been addressed in comparisons of the species–area and species–time relationships. Logically it seems possible that the STR is more similar to a SAR that is expanded along a linear transect of increasing length as opposed to one expanding relatively evenly in two dimensions. There may also be important differences between space and time in the variability of the environment, and in how species respond to this variability (Adler & Lauenroth, 2003). For example, it is likely that there are fewer temporal barriers to dispersal than spatial ones. These and other questions exploring the similarity and differences between space and time in ecological systems should prove a fruitful area for basic research.

In general, the STR reminds us that ecological systems are inherently dynamic. While this observation is neither novel nor surprising, it is often forgotten in diversity studies where spatial data are easier to obtain and have been extensively analyzed. The temporal scaling patterns presented here suggest that we need to consider the time dimension in order to fully quantify the patterns, and to better understand the processes of the distribution and turnover of species.

## Acknowledgments
I thank first and foremost James H. Brown, who first pointed me toward the species–time relationship as an interesting and understudied pattern. He has had a substantial influence on how I think about the STR through a number of conversations over the past eight years. Thanks to David Storch and Pablo Marquet for organizing a truly excellent workshop and inviting me to attend.

Michael Palmer and Bruce Milue pointed out the issue of persistence in sampling models to me. S. K. Morgan Ernest, James H. Brown, Peter B. Adler, Bruce Milne, David Storch and an anonymous reviewer provided valuable comments on previous versions of this manuscript. Data collection for the Portal Project was supported by NSF (most recently by DEB-0348896). During the writing of this chapter I was supported by an NSF Graduate Research Fellowship and an NSF Postdoctoral Fellowship in Biological Informatics (DBI-0532847).

## References

Adler, P. B. (2004). Neutral models fail to reproduce observed species-time and species-area relationships in Kansas grasslands. *Ecology*, **85**, 1265–1272.

Adler, P. B. & Lauenroth, W. K. (2003). The power of time: spatiotemporal scaling of species diversity. *Ecology Letters*, **6**, 749–756.

Adler, P. B., White, E. P., Lauenroth, W. K., Kaufman, D. M., Rassweiler, A. & Rusak, J. A. (2005). Evidence for a general species-time-area relationship. *Ecology*, **86**, 2032–2039.

Allen, A. P. & White, E. P. (2003). Interactive effects of range size and plot area on species-area relationships. *Evolutionary Ecology Research*, **5**, 493–499.

Allen, A. P., Brown, J. H. & Gillooly, J. F. (2002). Global biodiversity, biochemical kinetics, and the energetic-equivalence rule. *Science*, **297**, 1545–1548.

Arrhenius, O. (1921). Species and area. *Journal of Ecology*, **9**, 95–99.

Bell, G. (2001). Ecology: neutral macroecology. *Science*, **293**, 2413–2418.

Blackburn, T. M. & Gaston, K. J. (1996). Spatial patterns in the species richness of birds in the New World. *Ecography*, **19**, 369–376.

Brewer, A. & Williamson, M. (1994). A new relationship for rarefaction. *Biodiversity and Conservation*, **3**, 373–379.

Brown, J. H. (1981). Two decades of homage to Santa-Rosalia: toward a general theory of diversity. *American Zoologist*, **21**, 877–888.

Brown, J. H. (1998). The desert granivory experiments at Portal. In *Experimental Ecology*, ed.

W. J. J. Resetarits & J. Bernardo, pp. 71–95. New York: Oxford University Press.

Brown, J. H., Ernest, S. K. M., Parody, J. M. & Haskell, J. P. (2001). Regulation of diversity: maintenance of species richness in changing environments. *Oecologia*, **126**, 321–332.

Brown, J. H., Gupta, V. K., Li, B. L., Milne, B. T., Restrepo, C. & West, G. B. (2002). The fractal nature of nature: power laws, ecological complexity and biodiversity. *Philosophical Transactions of the Royal Society of London, Series B*, **357**, 619–626.

Bunge, J. & Fitzpatrick, M. (1993). Estimating the number of species: a review. *Journal of the American Statistical Association*, **88**, 364–373.

Burnham, K. P. & Anderson, D. R. (1998). *Model Selection and Inference: a Practical Information-theoretic Approach*. New York: Springer.

Calder, W. A. (1984). *Size, Function, and Life History*. Mineola, NY: Dover.

Cam, E., Nichols, J. D., Hines, J. E., Sauer, J. R., Alpizar-Jara, R. & Flather, C. H. (2002). Disentangling sampling and ecological explanations underlying species-area relationships. *Ecology*, **83**, 1118–1130.

Chalcraft, D. R., Williams, J. W., Smith, M. D. & Willig, M. R. (2004). Scale dependence in the relationship between species richness and productivity: the role of spatial and temporal turnover. *Ecology*, **85**, 2701–2708.

Chase, J. M. & Leibold, M. A. (2002). Spatial scale dictates the productivity-biodiversity relationship. *Nature*, **416**, 427–430.

Clarke, A. & Lidgard, S. (2000). Spatial patterns of diversity in the sea: bryozoan species richness in the North Atlantic. *Journal of Animal Ecology*, **69**, 799–814.

Coleman, B. D. (1981). On random placement and species-area relations. *Mathematical Biosciences*, **54**, 191–215.

Connor, E. F. & McCoy, E. D. (1979). Statistics and biology of the species-area relationship. *American Naturalist*, **113**, 791–833.

Diamond, J. M. (1969). Avifaunal equilibria and species turnover rates on the channel islands of California. *Proceedings of the National Academy of Sciences of the United States of America*, **64**, 57–63.

Ernest, S. K. M. & Brown, J. H. (2001). Homeostasis and compensation: the role of species and resources in ecosystem stability. *Ecology*, **82**, 2118–2132.

Fisher, R. A., Corbet, A. S. & Williams, C. B. (1943). The relation between the number of species and the number of individuals in a random sample of an animal population. *Journal of Animal Ecology*, **12**, 42–58.

Gaston, K. J. (2000). Global patterns in biodiversity. *Nature*, **405**, 220–227.

Gleason, H. A. (1922). On the relation between species and area. *Ecology*, **3**, 158–162.

Gotelli, N. J. & Colwell, R. K. (2001). Quantifying biodiversity: procedures and pitfalls in the measurement and comparison of species richness. *Ecology Letters*, **4**, 379–391.

Grinnell, J. (1922). The role of the "accidental". *Auk*, **39**, 373–380.

Gross, K. L., Willig, M. R., Gough, L., Inouye, R. & Cox, S. B. (2000). Patterns of species density and productivity at different spatial scales in herbaceous plant communities. *Oikos*, **89**, 417–427.

Hadly, E. A. & Maurer, B. A. (2001). Spatial and temporal patterns of species diversity in montane mammal communities of western North America. *Evolutionary Ecology Research*, **3**, 477–486.

Harte, J., Conlisk, E., Ostling, A., Green, J. L. & Smith, A. B. (2005). A theory of spatial-abundance and species-abundance distributions in ecological communities at multiple scales. *Ecological Monographs*, **75**, 179–197.

Hawkins, B., Field, R., Cornell, H., *et al.* (2003). Energy, water, and broad-scale geographic patterns of species richness. *Ecology*, **84**, 3105–3117.

He, F. L. & Legendre, P. (1996). On species-area relations. *American Naturalist*, **148**, 719–737.

He, F. L. & Legendre, P. (2002). Species diversity patterns derived from species-area models. *Ecology*, **83**, 1185–1198.

Hubbell, S. P. (2001). *The Unified Neutral Theory of Biodiversity and Biogeography*. Princeton, NJ: Princeton University Press.

Hurlbert, S. H. (1971). The nonconcept of species diversity: a critique and alternative parameters. *Ecology*, **52**, 577–586.

Hutchinson, G. E. (1959). Homage to Santa Rosalia: or, Why are there so many animals? *American Naturalist*, **93**, 145–159.

Inouye, R. S. (1998). Species-area curves and estimates of total species richness in an old-field chronosequence. *Plant Ecology*, **137**, 31–40.

Koleff, P., Gaston, K. J. & Lennon, J. J. (2003). Measuring beta diversity for presence-absence data. *Journal of Animal Ecology*, **72**, 367–382.

Lekve, K., Boulinier, T., Stenseth, N. C., *et al.* (2002). Spatio-temporal dynamics of species richness in coastal fish communities. *Proceedings of the Royal Society of London, Series B*, **269**, 1781–1789.

Lennon, J. J., Koleff, P., Greenwood, J. J. D. & Gaston, K. J. (2001). The geographical structure of British bird distributions: diversity, spatial turnover and scale. *Journal of Animal Ecology*, **70**, 966–979.

Lennon, J. J., Kunin, W. E. & Hartley, S. (2002). Fractal species distributions do not produce power-law species-area relationships. *Oikos*, **97**, 378–386.

Levin, S. A. (1992). The problem of pattern and scale in ecology. *Ecology*, **73**, 1943–1967.

Lomolino, M. V. (2000). Ecology's most general, yet protean pattern: the species-area relationship. *Journal of Biogeography*, **27**, 17–26.

Lyons, S. K. & Willig, M. R. (2002). Species richness, latitude, and scale-sensitivity. *Ecology*, **83**, 47–58.

MacArthur, R. H. (1964). Environmental factors affecting bird species diversity. *American Naturalist*, **98**, 387–396.

Maurer, B. A. & McGill, B. J. (2004). Neutral and non-neutral macroecology. *Basic and Applied Ecology*, **5**, 413–422.

McGill, B. (2003). Strong and weak tests of macroecological theory. *Oikos*, **102**, 679–685.

McKinney, M. L. & Frederick, D. L. (1999). Species-time curves and population extremes: ecological patterns in the fossil record. *Evolutionary Ecology Research*, **1**, 641–650.

Mittelbach, G. G., Steiner, C. F., Scheiner, S. M., *et al.* (2001). What is the observed relationship between species richness and productivity? *Ecology*, **82**, 2381–2396.

Morse, D. R., Lawton, J. H., Dodson, M. M. & Williamson, M. H. (1985). Fractal dimension of vegetation and the distribution of arthropod body lengths. *Nature*, **314**, 731–733.

Nichols, J. D., Hines, J. E., Sauer, J. R., Fallon, F. W., Fallon, J. E. & Heglund, P. J. (2000). A double-observer approach for estimating detection probability and abundance from point counts. *Auk*, **117**, 393–408.

Parody, J. M., Cuthbert, F. J. & Decker, E. H. (2001). The effect of 50 years of landscape change on species richness and community composition. *Global Ecology and Biogeography*, **10**, 305–313.

Peters, R. H. (1983). *The Ecological Implications of Body Size*. New York: Cambridge University Press.

Plotkin, J. B., Potts, M. D., Leslie, N., Manokaran, N., LaFrankie, J. & Ashton, P. S. (2000). Species-area curves, spatial aggregation, and habitat specialization in tropical forests. *Journal of Theoretical Biology*, **207**, 81–99.

Preston, F. W. (1948). The commonness, and rarity, of species. *Ecology*, **29**, 254–283.

Preston, F. W. (1960). Time and space and the variation of species. *Ecology*, **41**, 611–627.

Rahbek, C. & Graves, G. R. (2001). Multiscale assessment of patterns of avian species richness. *Proceedings of the National Academy of Sciences of the United States of America*, **98**, 4534–4539.

Rohde, K. (1992). Latitudinal gradients in species-diversity: the search for the primary cause. *Oikos*, **65**, 514–527.

Rosenzweig, M. L. (1995). *Species Diversity in Space and Time*. New York: Cambridge University Press.

Rosenzweig, M. L. (1998). Preston's ergodic conjecture: the accumulation of species in space and time. In *Biodiversity Dynamics*, ed. M. L. Mckinney & J. A. Drake, pp. 311–348. New York: Columbia University Press.

Russell, G. J. (1998). Turnover dynamics across ecological and geological scales. In *Biodiversity Dynamics*, ed. M. L. Mckinney & J. A. Drake, pp. 377–404. New York: Columbia University Press.

Russell, G. J., Diamond, J. M., Pimm, S. L. & Reed, T. M. (1995). A century of turnover: community dynamics at 3 timescales. *Journal of Animal Ecology*, **64**, 628–641.

Sanders, H. L. (1968). Marine benthic diversity: a comparative study. *American Naturalist*, **102**, 243–282.

Scheiner, S. M., Cox, S. B., Willig, M., Mittelbach, G. G., Osenberg, C. & Kaspari, M. (2000). Species richness: species-area curves and Simpson's Paradox. *Evolutionary Ecology Research*, **2**, 791–802.

Schmidt-Nielsen, K. (1984). *Scaling: Why is Animal Size So Important*. Cambridge: Cambridge University Press.

Šizling, A. & Storch, D. (2004). Power-law species-area relationships and self-similar species distributions within finite areas. *Ecology Letters*, **7**, 60–68.

Stevens, R. & Willig, M. (2002). Geographical ecology at the community level: perspectives on the diversity of new world bats. *Ecology*, **83**, 545–560.

Storch, D., Gaston, K. J. & Cepak, J. (2002). Pink landscapes: 1/*f* spectra of spatial environmental variability and bird community composition. *Proceedings of the Royal Society of London, Series B*, **269**, 1791–1796.

Storch, D., Evans, K. L. & Gaston, K. J. (2005). The species-area-energy relationship. *Ecology Letters*, **8**, 487–492.

Venables, W. N. & Ripley, B. D. (1999). *Modern Applied Statistics with S-PLUS*. New York: Springer.

White, E. P. (2004). Two-phase species-time relationships in North American land birds. *Ecology Letters*, **7**, 329–336.

White, E. P., Adler, P. B., Lauenroth, W. K., *et al.* (2006). A comparison of the species-time relationship across ecosystems and taxonomic groups. *Oikos*, **112**, 185–195.

Williams, C. B. (1943). Area and number of species. *Nature*, **152**, 264–267.

Williams, C. B. (1964). *Patterns in the Balance of Nature*. London: Academic Press.

Williamson, M. (1987). Are communities ever stable? In *Colonization, Succession, and Stability*, ed. A. J. Gray, M. J. Crawley & P. J. Edwards, pp. 353–371. Oxford: Blackwell Scientific Publications.

Williamson, M. (1988). Relationship of species number to area, distance and other variables. In *Analytical Biogeography*, ed. A. A. Myers & P. S. Giller, pp. 91–115. New York: Chapman and Hall.

Williamson, M., Gaston, K. J. & Lonsdale, W. M. (2001). The species-area relationship does not have an asymptote! *Journal of Biogeography*, **28**, 827–830.

Wright, D. H. (1983). Species-energy theory: an extension of species-area theory. *Oikos*, **41**, 496–506.

Wright, D. H., Currie, D. J. & Maurer, B. A. (1993). Energy supply and patterns of species richness on local and regional scales. In *Species Diversity in Ecological Communities*, ed. R. E. Ricklefs & D. Schluter, pp. 66–74. Chicago: University of Chicago Press.

# CHAPTER SEVENTEEN

# Scaling biodiversity under neutrality

LUÍS BORDA-DE-ÁGUA
*University of Georgia*
STEPHEN P. HUBBELL
*University of Georgia, Smithsonian Tropical Research Institute*
FANGLIANG HE
*University of Alberta*

## Introduction

To better understand biodiversity scaling, it may be useful to characterize the biodiversity scaling relationships that arise from the neutral perspective. This exercise will help in formulating quantitative null hypotheses for observed biodiversity scaling relationships. Here we use the term *biodiversity* to refer not only to species richness, but also to relative species abundance, and *biodiversity scaling* to refer to how patterns of biodiversity change on increasing sampling (spatial) scales. The study of biodiversity includes questions about the spatial dispersion and geographic range of species, relative species abundance, endemism, and beta diversity, the turnover of species across landscapes. A full discussion of all-taxa biodiversity scaling in the context of neutral theory is beyond the scope of the present theory because the theory currently applies only to communities of trophically similar species (a tree community, for example). It is also individual based rather than biomass based. Despite these limitations neutral theory is nevertheless a mechanistic, dynamical theory of community assembly based on fundamental demographic processes (birth, death, dispersal, speciation) – even though its postulated assembly rules are extremely simple. Under current neutral theory, speciation, ecological drift (demographic stochasticity in birth and deaths), and dispersal govern the presence or absence and the abundance of species in communities over local to global scales. Extinction is also critically important, but under neutrality, the extinction rate can be predicted once the other three processes are known. Neutral theory asserts that, to a first approximation, trophically similar species are identical (symmetric) in these vital rates on a per-capita basis. According to the theory, species develop differences in abundance due to demographic stochasticity and accidents of dispersal. Once species become differentiated in abundance, their expected fates diverge. Common species are expected to have longer life spans and to be more persistent members of local communities than rare species.

*Scaling Biodiversity*, ed. David Storch, Pablo A. Marquet and James H. Brown. Published by Cambridge University Press. © Cambridge University Press 2007.

Since publication of the original neutral theory (Hubbell, 1997, 2001; Bell, 2000, 2001), there have been a number of significant theoretical advances, and many of the problems that were originally studied only by simulation now have analytical solutions (Volkov et al., 2003; Vallade and Houchmandzadeh, 2003; Houchmandzadeh & Vallade, 2003; McKane, Alonso & Solé, 2004; Etienne & Olff, 2004). One of the most significant advances has been the incorporation of symmetric density- and frequency-dependence (Volkov et al. 2005). Here, as we study the implications of neutrality for biodiversity scaling, we make additional improvements to the theory by incorporating more realistic models of dispersal. The original formulation (Hubbell, 2001) was constructed on the foundation of the theory of island biogeography, which only treated space implicitly in the island–mainland problem studied by MacArthur and Wilson (1967). Hubbell (2001) studied a spatially explicit model by simulation, but these studies were limited to the classical "voter model" of dispersal (e.g. Holley & Liggett, 1975; Silvertown et al., 1992; Durrett & Levin, 1996), in which dispersal is restricted to immediately adjacent sites in a single time step. However, there is steadily accumulating evidence that dispersal in virtually all organisms is characterized not only by frequent small-distance movements, but also by occasional very large, long-distance movements (e.g. Lewis 1997; Petit et al., 1997; Clark et al., 1998). Such long-distance movements or "jump-dispersal" events, even if they occur only relatively rarely, may have potentially large effects on species distributions and on biodiversity scaling. Thus, if one wants to understand how the mechanism of dispersal affects biodiversity on local to biogeographic spatial scales, characterizing the distribution of dispersal distances (dispersal "kernels"), including long-distance events, becomes an important objective.

Several theoretical approaches have been taken to the description of dispersal kernels (for a review see Nathan & Muller-Landau, 2000). The classical approach is to assume two-dimensional Gaussian diffusion (Nagylaki, 1974), which results in a Rayleigh distribution of radially calculated dispersal distances. This approach provides a good description of spatial dispersal when the process is relatively uniform and continuous, leading to an expansion of the borders of the spatial distribution at a constant velocity. However, it was the prevalence of jump-dispersal events in natural populations that led ecologists to search for other models of dispersal that would better capture the shape of observed dispersal kernels. These kernels generally have "fat tails" relative to the Gaussian, that is, higher probability of long-distance dispersal and therefore more probability in the tails of the distribution. One such distribution is the 2Dt distribution, which has recently been fit to a large number of dispersal kernels of tree species (Clark et al., 1999; Muller-Landau et al., 2004) and used as a model for dispersal in theoretical and simulation work (Chave & Leigh, 2002; Chave, Muller-Landau & Levin, 2002).

A class of probability density functions that have not yet been widely used in ecology (Kot, Lewis & Van den Driessche, 1996; Halley & Iwasa, 1998), but that

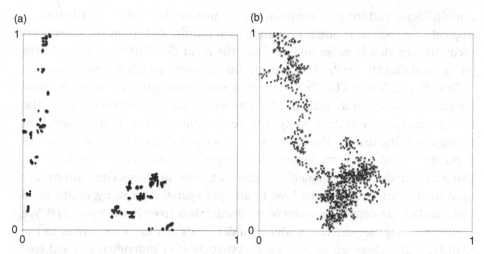

**Figure 17.1** (a) Example of Lévy flights obtained with a Cauchy distribution, and (b) a typical random walk obtained with a Gaussian distribution. Lévy flights are random walks where the position of the next point is obtained by adding to the position of the previous point distances along the $x$ and $y$ axes sampled from Lévy stable distributions. The Gaussian is a special case of the Lévy stable distributions. Because it does not have fat tails it does not give origin to a series of well-identified clusters. In both cases we used 1000 points. The scales are arbitrary.

seem highly appropriate for describing dispersal, are the probability density functions known as Lévy stable distributions (Weiss, 1994; West & Deering, 1994; Mandelbrot, 1997; Mantegna & Stanley, 2000). Although the Gaussian (normal) distribution is a member of this class, it is a special and unusual case in that it has defined moments (e.g. mean, variance, etc.). Despite the fact that they are true probability density functions whose integrals are equal to unity, most Lévy stable distributions do not have defined moments. When used to describe dispersal, the "fat tails" of Lévy stable distributions increase the probability of occasional long-distance dispersal events, resulting in a pattern of movement unlike Brownian diffusion which tends to show the steady advance of a "front". Instead, one obtains dispersal patterns aptly termed "Lévy flights", characterized by sequences of mostly local movements, terminated by occasional long jumps to the location of a new sequence of local movements. Figure 17.1 is an example, which might represent the path taken by a series of sequential parent–offspring pairs, for the simplified case of only a single offspring produced in each time step.

   An important conclusion of this work is that the population-level dispersion patterns produced by many individuals simultaneously pursuing independent Lévy flights of multiple offspring produce patterns that are characterized by multifractals. By using multifractal methods, our main purpose is to show that a multifractal pattern is a common occurrence in the spatial distribution of tropical tree species. If observed patterns are multifractal, then the onus is on theoretical models to generate them, and the point distributions obtained with our neutral simulations do show patterns that are well described by multifractals.

This chapter is about biodiversity scaling under neutrality. However, because we are introducing more realistic Lévy stable distributions for dispersal into the theory, and because of the novelty of these distributions and of multifractals in ecology, we first discuss the patterns of dispersion that arise in single species populations under neutral dynamics with non-Gaussian, Lévy stable dispersal. Using a spatially explicit model, we show that these single species patterns are multifractal, and we describe how to analyze spatial data using multifractal methods (a more detailed account on multifractals is given in the Appendix). We then show that the patterns produced under neutrality are very similar to the multifractality observed in the spatial distribution of individual tropical tree species on Barro Colorado Island (BCI), Panama. Finally, we return to our primary question, and consider how changing the parameters of the Lévy stable dispersal function affects biodiversity scaling under neutrality. In this chapter, we only consider symmetric neutrality, such that all species exhibit the average community dispersal kernel. Elsewhere we relax this assumption and allow species to have different Lévy stable dispersal kernels. We now describe the spatially explicit model of the community used in our studies.

## The model
### Modeling dispersal with Lévy stable distributions
Here we consider mainly seed dispersal by terrestrial plants, but our conclusions also apply to all species that exhibit occasional long-distance "jump" dispersal events. Empirically obtained seed dispersal distributions are often convex near the source plant and have long tails (Clark *et al.*, 1999; Jones *et al.*, 2005) that are too "fat" relative to the standard Gaussian distribution. Therefore, we seek different distribution functions that can accommodate the observed shapes both near and far from the source (Clark *et al.*, 1999). Lévy stable distributions have been rarely used in ecology but they have a venerable history in the study of fractals (e.g. Mandelbrot, 1977, 1997; West & Deering, 1994), and Gnedenko and Kolmogorov (1954) predicted the wider application of Lévy stable distributions: "All these distribution laws, called stable, ... deserve the most serious attention. It is probable that the scope of applied problems in which they play an essential role will become in due course rather wide." As mentioned, the Gaussian distribution is different from other Lévy stable distributions in two regards. First, the Gaussian distribution has moments of all orders, while, in general, Lévy stable distributions have only one moment (mean) or no moments at all. Second, the tails of the Gaussian distribution are not well described by power laws, unlike the tails of other Lévy stable distributions. From a theoretical

point of view, Lévy stable distributions result from the sum of independent, identically distributed (i.i.d.) random variables and arise from a more general form of the central limit theorem. According to the central limit theorem, the sum of i.i.d. random variables with *finite variance* converges to the Gaussian distribution. However, for distributions without finite variance (or mean), such as the Cauchy distribution, the familiar central limit theorem does not apply. It is for these other distributions that the other Lévy stable distributions are the limiting sum.

Except for a few cases, such as the Gaussian and the Cauchy, the analytical expression of the probability density function of the Lévy stable distributions is not available, but the form of their characteristic function is. For one-dimensional distributions centered at the origin and symmetrical, the characteristic function, $F(q)$, is

$$F(q) = \exp(-c\,|q|^{\alpha}), \tag{17.1}$$

where $c$ is called the scale parameter and $\alpha$ the characteristic exponent. The parameter $\alpha$ is bounded as $0 < \alpha \leq 2$. When $\alpha = 1$ we obtain the Cauchy distribution, and when $\alpha = 2$ the Gaussian distribution. Except for $\alpha = 2$, Lévy stable distributions only have moments of order lower than $\alpha$. Hence, distributions with $1 < \alpha < 2$ only have mean, and distributions with $\alpha \leq 1$ do not have moments of any order.

Although in general the form of the probability density functions is not known, it can be shown (e.g. West & Deering, 1994) that, except for the Gaussian, the tail of the probability density functions decays as a power law:

$$f(|x|) \sim |x|^{-(1+\alpha)}. \tag{17.2}$$

Figure 17.2 illustrates the probability density functions of some Lévy stable distributions for several values of $\alpha$ and $c$. The generation of Lévy stable random variables can be done easily with the algorithm suggested by Chambers, Mallows and Stuck (1976). For information on Lévy stable distributions, in addition to the references already cited, we recommend Mantegna and Stanley (2000) and Weiss (1994).

### The computer model

Our model took space explicitly into account and consisted of a hexagonal lattice with 1024 by 1024 sites, where every site is occupied with a single individual of an arbitrary species. Following common practice in the study of spatially explicit models (e.g. Chave *et al.*, 2002), we used periodic boundary conditions. However, we also checked our results with a model without periodic boundary conditions, but the results were qualitatively indistinguishable. We initialized the system by sampling individuals from a pool of 100 species in which all the species had the same probability of being chosen, or were drawn

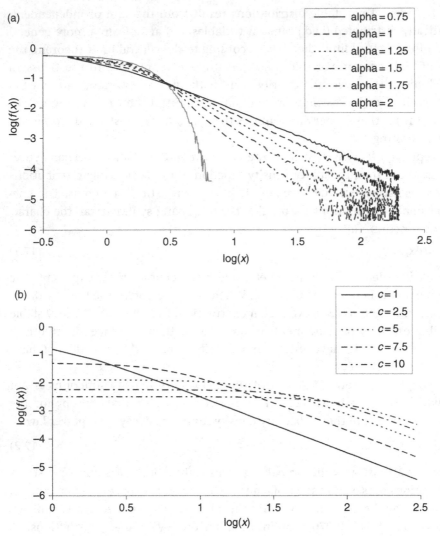

**Figure 17.2** Examples of Lévy stable distributions plotted in log-log scales. In plot (a), $c = 1$ and $\alpha = 0.75$, 1.0, 1.25, 1.5, 1,75, 2.0, and in plot (b), $\alpha = 1.0$ (Cauchy distribution) and $c = 1$, 2.5, 5, 7.5, 10. Except for $\alpha = 2.0$ (Gaussian distribution) in plot (a), the tails are approximately straight lines; the slopes are equal to $-(1 + \alpha)$.

from the relative abundance distribution expected under neutrality given the size of the community and the speciation rate (Hubbell, 2001). In each iteration we removed a percentage of the individuals (deaths), and we refilled each vacant site with a new individual (birth). This new individual might be an entirely new species (speciation), with probability $v$, or an individual of a species already present in the community, with probability $1 - v$. In our studies we varied the speciation rate from $10^{-7}$ to $10^{-4}$. When the replacement was from a species already present in the community, we chose the species by an inverse dispersal method, as follows. Centered in the site to be replaced, we randomly chose distances from a Lévy stable distribution along the $x$ and $y$ axes in positive or negative directions, and these distances determined the maternal site and therefore the species of the new individual. We performed two kinds of simulations, but the results were qualitatively similar. In one case, we preserved information on the lattice prior to imposing mortality so that there was always an individual present in the maternal site. In the second case, we choose the identity of the new individual only among the individuals that survived mortality. In this case, the selected maternal site may be vacant. When this happened, we repeated the search until we found an occupied site. Most of our simulations employed the first method, which was much faster to run. We ran each simulation until a well-established equilibrium was reached, meaning that after a transient the simulation has evolved to a regime where we observed no trend in the evolution of the number of species, and species–area curves and species-abundance distributions obtained at different time steps were qualitatively similar.

Chave et al. (2002) used a very similar model to ours. A few differences from our model to Chave et al. (2002) are: we used a hexagonal lattice and they used a square lattice, we used Lévy stable distributions and they used the 2Dt distribution, we did not allow for vacant sites (in the spirit of the zero-sum game as in Hubbell, 2001) and they allowed for vacant sites.

## Multifractal analysis of spatial dispersion of single species populations

In this section we first analyze the spatial distribution of model species obtained with different dispersal kernels under neutrality, and we use multifractals to describe these spatial distributions. We then show, using multifractals, that similar patterns are also observed in many of the tree species in the 50 ha plot of tropical forest on Barro Colorado Island (BCI), Panama, established in 1980 (Hubbell & Foster, 1983).

Figure 17.3 shows several distributions obtained with different dispersal kernels ($c = 10$ and $\alpha = 1.0$, 1.5, and 2.0). It is obvious from visual inspection that the degree of clustering depends on the dispersal kernel used. When dispersal distances decrease, which corresponds to an increase in the parameter $\alpha$ of the Lévy stable distributions, the spatial dispersion patterns become more clumped. On first inspection these results might seem to contradict our previous discussion on the spatial distributions generated by Lévy flights (Fig. 17.1). However, these point distributions are being generated by a process that is different from that of a single Lévy flight. First, in the simulations, each "parent" point may give rise to more than one "offspring" point; that is, a point can start multiple new "paths". Second, there is superimposed mortality, which removes some of the points from the landscape. Third, we are using periodic boundary

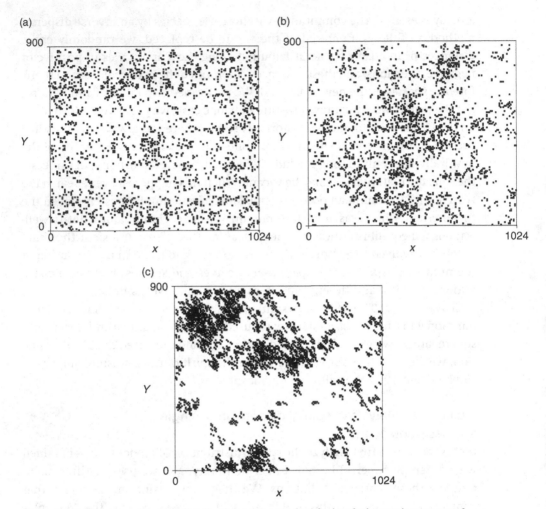

**Figure 17.3** Example of spatial distributions generated with simulations using a neutral model. Plot (a) was obtained with $\alpha = 1.0$ (Cauchy distribution), plot (b) with $\alpha = 1.5$, and plot (c) with $\alpha = 2.0$ (Gaussian distribution). Notice that an increase in the value of $\alpha$ leads to more clumped distributions.

conditions, which means that points that leave the plot from one side re-enter from the opposite side of the plot; hence, points are closer together than one would expect from a Lévy flight. This periodic boundary effect is equivalent to assuming immigration from adjacent areas of the simulated forest. Since the resulting single-species dispersion patterns are well described by multifractals, we now turn to a description of multifractal methods.

### Definition of multifractals
Most objects including point distributions that exhibit fractality are, in fact, multifractal, so multifractal methods provide a more accurate description of

such objects. The difference between fractals and multifractals lies in the detail of information used about the pattern that one is describing. In describing point distributions using fractals alone, we only use information about presence or absence. In describing point distributions using multifractals, we also use information about relative abundance. Adapting an example from Evertsz and Mandelbrot (1992), imagine a large geographical area, say, South America. If South America is divided into two regions of equal area, one region is likely to have a larger forested area than the other. If one of these regions is again subdivided into two equal areas, one of these subareas may have a larger forested area than the other. As the subdivision continues, it is likely that each of the subdivided regions will have a different proportion of forested area. Forest area is thus an "irregular" measure at all spatial scales. Now let this irregularity be self-similar, such that each time we make a subdivision, the proportions of forested area in the two halves remain the same, say $p_1$ and $p_2$. This means that in the next division of these areas, we obtain fractions $p_1p_1$, $p_1p_2$, $p_2p_1$, and $p_2p_2$. In this case, we say that the irregularity is the same ("self-similar") at all scales, and the process by which it was obtained is called a multiplicative cascade. At each scale of the construction of the multifractal we can construct histograms of values associated with the fractions in the subdivisions. The objective of the multifractal analysis is to describe the scaling properties of these histograms, which is achieved after appropriate renormalizations (Evertsz & Mandelbrot, 1992). However, dealing directly with the histograms is a very inefficient process, and, instead, we deal with the moments of the distributions and observe the scaling properties of the moments. In the next section we give a brief account of the method used in this work and give more detailed information in the Appendix.

## Estimating multifractal spectra

Whereas a fractal is described by a single number, the fractal dimension, a multifractal requires a spectrum of "dimensions"; notice the quotation marks because not all values of the spectrum can be properly interpreted as dimensions. For the purposes of this work we use the spectrum of generalized dimensions, $D_q$ (see Evertsz & Mandelbrot, 1992, for another type of multifractal spectrum). There are several methods to estimate the multifractal spectrum but not all are equally adequate for calculating all parts of the spectrum. For reasons explained in the Appendix, we use the fixed-mass method.

The fixed-mass method is based on the following relationship, valid for multifractals,

$$\langle R_i(m)^{-\tau_q}\rangle^{1/\tau_q} \sim m^{-1/D_q}, \tag{17.3}$$

where $\langle\ \rangle$ stands for average over all points, $R$ for radius, $m$ for the number of points in the vicinity of a given point $i$, and $\tau_q$ is a real number related to $D_q$ through the relationship $\tau_q = (q-1)D_q$, and $q$ is also a real number ranging

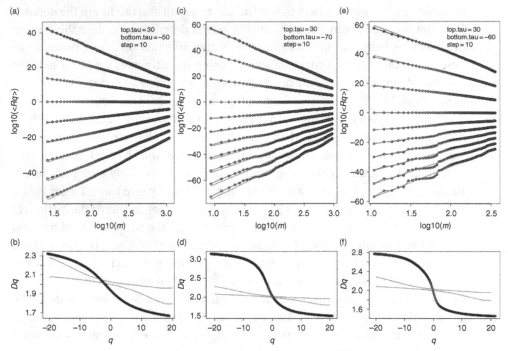

**Figure 17.4** Plot (a) shows the curves of $\log_{10}(\langle R_q \rangle) = \log_{10}(\langle R_i(m)^{-\tau_q} \rangle^{1/\tau_q})$ versus $\log_{10}(m)$ for the point distribution shown in Fig. 17.3(a) and obtained with $\alpha = 1.0$. From this plot we estimate the slope from which we obtain $q$, used for the construction of plot (b), showing the spectrum of generalized dimensions $D_q$. Notice that $D_q$ is a monotonically decreasing function of $q$. Plots (c) and (d), and (e) and (f) are the same for the distributions of Fig. 17.3(b) and Fig. 17.3(c), respectively. The red solid lines in plots (b), (d) and (f) consist of the largest and the smallest $D_q$ values obtained from 200 Poisson processes with the same number of points as the original distribution. (For color version see Plate 11.)

from $-\infty$ to $+\infty$. As we will see below, $q$ plays an important role in the characterization of a multifractal. The main idea in the fixed-mass method is to determine the minimum radius from a point $i$, $R_i$, that contains $m$ points, $R_i(m)$. The method consists of calculating $R_i(m)$ for all points in the plot and, then, the average $\langle R_i(m)^{-\tau_q} \rangle$ for several values of $\tau_q$. This process is repeated for several values of $m$, and, in order to assess and characterize the multifractality, we plot $\log\left(\langle R_i(m)^{-\tau_q} \rangle^{1/\tau_q}\right)$ as function of $\log(m)$; see Fig. 17.4(a, c, e) and Fig. 17.6(a, c, e). For a multifractal we should observe a linear relationship, or a linear relationship with oscillations superimposed (see Box 17.1). From these curves we estimate the slope, which corresponds to $-1/D_q$. We then use the relationship $\tau_q = (q-1)D_q$ to calculate $q$ and, finally, we draw $D_q$ as a function of $q$, which is the spectrum of generalized dimensions. The $D_q$ spectrum is a monotonically decreasing function, sigmoid in shape; Fig. 17.4(b, d, f) and Fig. 17.6(b, d, f) show several $D_q$ spectra.

---

**Box 17.1 Power laws, oscillations and self-similarity**

Power laws, such as $y = ax^b$, are not the only family of curves that are self-similar, although the estimation of fractal dimensions is usually performed by trying to fit a straight line in a log-log plot. A more general form that is still self-similar is

$$y = ax^b f \left( \frac{\log(x)}{\log(c)} \right), \qquad (17.4)$$

where $a$, $b$, and $c$ are constants and $f(z)$ is a function such as $f(z) = f(1+z)$ (Liebovitch, 1998). When plotted in a log-log plot, the curve obtained with this function is a straight line on which periodic oscillations are super-imposed. Hence, whenever we see such a pattern we consider it evidence of self-similarity. However, the presence of these oscillations makes the estimation of the slope associated with the power law more difficult, and may in some cases cause one to erroneously reject the hypothesis of self-similarity even when the pattern may truly be self-similar (Badii & Polity, 1984; Meneveau & Sreenivasan, 1989).

---

Changing $q$, or $\tau_q$, is somehow analogous to obtaining the moments of a probability density function. As explained in more detail in the Appendix, by choosing different $q$ values we select regions of the plane with different point densities. The part of the $D_q$ spectrum associated with positive values of $q$ gives information on dense regions of the point distribution, and the part associated with negative $q$ values gives information on sparse regions of the point distribution. In the case of a perfect fractal, all generalized "dimensions" are equal and the spectrum is a horizontal line parallel to the $q$-axis, and in the special case of a Poisson process in a plane $D_q = 2$. Deviances from a horizontal line are a measure of the heterogeneity of the point spatial distribution (see next section for examples on the estimation of multifractal spectra and the Appendix for more detailed information).

Some values of $q$ lead to well-known fractal dimensions: $q = 0$ corresponds to the box-counting dimension, and $q = 2$ corresponds to the correlation dimension. In the following sections we will pay special attention to these two fractal dimensions for two reasons. First, because we want to show that the box-counting dimension is sometimes misleading, since we obtain a value close to 2 although the distribution is not that of a Poisson process, and, second, because $D_2$ has a straightforward interpretation in terms of the degree of clustering: when $D_2$ is equal to the topological dimension, 2 in the case of a plane, the points are distributed according to a Poisson process, often called complete spatial randomness, and when $D_2$ is smaller than the topological dimension the points are clustered, and the degree of clustering increases as $D_2$ decreases.

To see this, think of a Poisson process and of a clustered distribution with the same number of points in an area of equal size and shape. For the Poisson distribution, the number of points increases as $R^2$ increases. For a clustered distribution when $R$ is small, the number of points increases faster than predicted by the Poisson distribution precisely because the points are clumped. However, after a certain value of $R$, voids start to dominate the clustered distribution, and thereafter the number of points increases more slowly than predicted by the Poisson distribution. Since for a fractal the number of points increases as $R^{D_2}$, then $D_2 < 2$.

## Spatial distributions of model species under neutrality

We now apply multifractals methods to analyze the spatial distributions of model species under neutrality with Lévy stable dispersal, and for a representative set of common tree species in BCI. In order to establish multifractality we required that a scaling region (i.e. $\log(\langle R_i(m)^{-\tau_q}\rangle^{1/\tau_q})$ versus $\log(m)$) be observed for at least one order of magnitude, and we required that the $D_q$ spectrum is a monotonically decreasing function.

We first analyze the distributions of species obtained by simulations under neutrality. As previously discussed, Fig. 17.3 shows that point distributions obtained with larger values of $\alpha$ are more clustered than those obtained with smaller $\alpha$. We now show how these characteristics are reflected in the multifractal spectrum and the steps that one always goes through in multifractal analysis. Consider the point process in Fig. 17.3(a). The estimation of the multifractal spectrum starts with the calculation of the $\log(\langle R_i(m)^{-\tau_q}\rangle^{1/\tau_q})$ curves, each obtained for a fixed value of $\tau_q$ (Fig. 17.4a). In order to avoid cluttering the figure, we show only curves for a few values of $\tau_q$, but we used more values to obtain the final estimation of the $D_q$ spectrum. We chose a large range of $\tau$ values to accommodate $q$ values in the range $-20$ to $20$, with special interest in values of $q$ close to $0$ and $2$. The next step is to assess if the curves of $\log(\langle R_i(m)^{-\tau_q}\rangle^{1/\tau_q})$ are well fit by straight lines. This is clearly true for the distribution in Fig. 17.4(a). Note that the linear relationships extend for more than one order of magnitude, $26 \le m \le 1082$. In fact, we could not identify an upper cutoff, so we speculate that the scaling region would be further extended if a larger data set had been available. We now estimate the slopes of the lines in Fig. 17.4(a), which are equal to $-1/D_q$, determine $q$ using $q = 1 + \tau_q/D_q$, and plot the multifractal spectrum (Fig. 17.4b). This figure shows that the $D_q$ spectrum is a monotonically decreasing function of $q$, as expected for a multifractal distribution. We estimate $D_0$ and $D_2$ from $\tau = -2$ and $\tau = 2$, leading, respectively, to $q = -0.03$ ($\approx 0.0$) and $q = 2.07$ ($\approx 2.0$), and from $D_q = \tau_q/(q-1)$, $D_0 = 2.004$, and $D_2 = 1.87$. The width of the spectrum, which is a measure of the difference between the scaling properties of the regions with higher and lower density of points, is $\Delta D_{-20-20} = D_{-20} - D_{20} = 0.656$ (we chose $D_{-20}$ and $D_{20}$ because it corresponds to the limits of the $q$ values used to describe the multifractal spectrum). $D_0$ is slightly larger than the maximum expected, 2. This is most likely a small error due to the fitting procedure and because we used a $q$ value slightly smaller than 0, and since $D_q$ is a monotonically decreasing function, this may lead to the value of $D_0$ being slightly larger than 2, when, in fact, its true value is 2.

Although ideally a Poisson process has $D_q = 2$ for all $q$, it is likely that for a finite collection of points this is not the case. In order to rule out the possibility that the observed $D_q$ spectrum is that of a Poisson process, we generated 200 Poisson processes and obtained the envelopes consisting of the largest and the smallest $D_q$ values, shown in Fig. 17.4(b) in red solid lines. Note that the spectrum of the distribution obtained under neutrality only falls within the two envelopes of the Poisson processes in the vicinity of $D_0$, but that for most of the region in which $q < 0$ it lies above the envelopes of the Poisson processes and for most $q > 0$, it is below. Thus we can reject the hypothesis that the distribution of the model population under neutrality with Lévy stable dispersal is a Poisson process.

For the point distribution in Fig. 17.3(b), obtained with $\alpha = 1.5$, we estimate $D_0 = 2.03$, $D_2 = 1.84$, and $\Delta D_{-20-20} = 1.64$ (Fig. 17.4c, d, colour plate), and for the distribution in Fig. 17.3(c), obtained with $\alpha = 2.0$, we estimate $D_0 = 1.95$, $D_2 = 1.69$, $\Delta D_{-20-20} = 1.31$ (Fig. 17.4c, f). We also plotted the envelopes of the spectra of 200 Poisson processes with the same number of points as the original distributions, and in both cases we observe that, except for $q$ close to 0, the spectrum is once again clearly outside the boundaries of the envelopes. Note that if we had reduced our analysis to $D_0$ (i.e. box counting), we would have concluded erroneously that the distribution was that of a Poisson process. Relative to the distribution of points obtained with $\alpha = 1.0$, we observe that $D_2$ decreases when $\alpha$ increases, in agreement with our previous finding that an increase in $\alpha$ leads to more clustered distributions.

## Single-species distributions of BCI tree species

We now turn to the analysis of the spatial distributions of common tree species in the BCI plot. For this study, we used data from the 1995 census. The 1995 census contains 300 species and 229 072 individuals. There are 75 species in the 1995 census that have more than 500 individuals. We restricted the analysis to these common species in order to have large scaling regions for the fixed-mass method. Applying our criteria for multifractality, we conclude that a multifractal model is an excellent representation for 67 (90%) of these species. We expect that this fraction will increase when data from larger areas become available. It is not possible to present the multifractal spectra here for all the species we analyzed, so we present the multifractal spectra for species that are representative of the several patterns we found. The representative species are: *Guarea guidonia* (Meliaceae) (Fig. 17.5a), *Annona acuminata* (Annonaceae) (Fig. 17.5b), and *Rinorea sylvatica* (Violaceae) (Fig. 17.5c). We summarize the

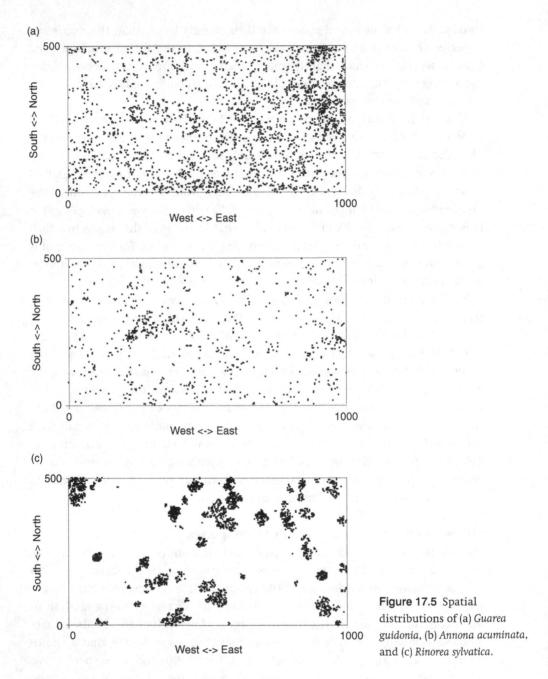

**Figure 17.5** Spatial distributions of (a) *Guarea guidonia*, (b) *Annona acuminata*, and (c) *Rinorea sylvatica*.

results in terms of $D_0$, $D_2$ and the difference $\Delta D_{-20-20}$. None of the species has a spatial distribution following a Poisson process.

The spectrum of *Guarea guidonia* (Fig. 17.6b), resembles those obtained from the neutral model species with $\alpha = 1$, but note that the width of the spectrum for *Guarea guidonia* is slightly larger, $\Delta D_{-20-20} = 0.964$, indicating a more

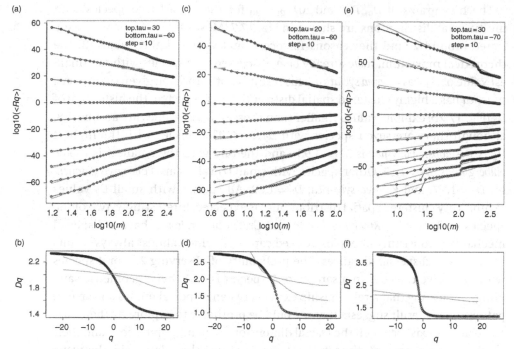

**Figure 17.6** Plot (a) shows the curves of $\log_{10}(\langle R_q \rangle) = \log_{10}(\langle R_i(m)^{-\tau_q} \rangle^{1/\tau_q})$ versus $\log_{10}(m)$, and plot (b) the spectrum of generalized dimensions for the spatial distribution of *Guarea guidonia* (Fig. 17.5a), and plots (c) and (d), and (e) and (f) are the same for *Annona acuminata* (Fig. 17.5b) and *Rinorea sylvatica* (Fig. 17.5c), respectively. The red lines in plots (b), (d) and (f) consist of the largest and the smallest $D_q$ values obtained from 200 Poisson processes with the same number of points as the original distribution. (For color version see Plate 12.)

heterogeneous distribution. The spectrum of *Annona acuminata* (Fig. 17.6d) is interesting because for negative $q$ values, i.e. sparse regions, the spectrum is undistinguishable from a Poisson process. This conclusion follows from the fact that for negative $q$ values, the spectrum lies completely within the envelopes of the simulated Poisson process. However, for positive $q$, i.e. abundant regions, it clearly lies outside the envelopes of the random simulations, and we conclude that the distribution is not that of a Poisson process. *Rinorea sylvatica* is especially intriguing because of its highly clumped distribution (see Fig. 17.5c). As expected, its multifractal spectrum (Fig. 17.6e, f), exhibits a large width ($\Delta D_{-20-20} = 2.75$). Note the oscillations in the plot of $\log(\langle R_i(m)^{-\tau_q} \rangle^{1/\tau_q})$ as a function of $\log(m)$, and that these oscillations exhibit some periodicity. According to our discussion in Box 17.1 of a more general form of self-similarity, these oscillations do not indicate an absence of self-similarity. Such oscillations often arise in cases like *Rinorea* in which there are distinct cluster sizes.

The histograms of $D_0$, $D_2$, and $\Delta D_{-20\,-20}$ for the 67 BCI tree species with multifractal distributions are shown in Fig. 17.7. Most values of $D_0$ are concentrated around 2, and the reasons for occasional values slightly above 2, the theoretical maximum, have already been discussed. The species with the smallest value of $D_0$ was *Rinorea sylvatica*. This result is not surprising given that *Rinorea sylvatica* has a highly clustered spatial distribution. As expected, the histogram of $D_2$ (Fig. 17.7b) exhibits values smaller than those of $D_0$. $D_2$ values are around 1.8, although there are seven species with $D_2 < 1.4$. The species with the highest $D_2$ is *Desmopsis panamensis* ($D_2 = 1.95$), and the one with the smallest is *Croton billbergianus*, $D_2 = 1.15$. Other species with small $D_2$ values are *Palicourea guianensis*, $D_2 = 1.17$, and *Rinorea sylvatica*, $D_2 = 1.22$. All species with small $D_2$ values exhibit very clustered spatial distributions, as expected. Interestingly, two of the species with low $D_2$, *Rinorea sylvatica* and *Croton billbergianus*, have a dispersal mechanism consisting of explosive seed capsules, which almost always results in very local dispersal distances. The probability of observing 2, 3 or 4 species with explosive capsules in a sample of 7 species is 0.05 (hypergeometric sampling), indicating that a relationship exists between dispersal modes and spatial patterns. This result suggests that it would be profitable to explore further what correlations exist between the fractal dimensions of plant populations and their mechanism or mode of dispersal. We also analyzed the relationship between regeneration guilds (9 gap species versus 58 nongap species) and found that among the 7 species with $D_2 < 1.4$, 3 were gap species, which was also significant ($P = 0.046$). Also of interest is the relationship between the average $D_2$ of the gap species, $\overline{D_2} = 1.54$, and nongap species, $\overline{D_2} = 1.77$. A randomization test (Manly, 1997) showed that the average $D_2$ of the gap species is significantly smaller (one-tail test) from the average $D_2$ of the nongap species ($P = 0.002$).

Species with highly clustered distributions show the largest differences between the most dense and most sparse regions. For this reason, it is not unexpected that two highly aggregated gap species exhibit the largest $\Delta D$ values: *Palicourea guianensis* has the largest $\Delta D_{-20-20} = 4.34$, followed by *Croton billbergianus*, $\Delta D_{-20-20} = 3.85$. The species with the smallest $\Delta D_{-20-20} = 0.708$ is *Sorocea affinis*, whose spatial distribution does not exhibit any obvious clusters. Most values of $\Delta D_{-20-20}$ occur between 0.8 and 2.2.

## Species–area relationships under neutrality

We showed in the previous sections that a neutral model with Lévy stable dispersal can lead to species distributions that are well described by multifractals. We have also shown that short distance dispersal (larger $\alpha$) leads to spatial distributions that are more aggregated than those obtained with longer distance dispersal (smaller $\alpha$).

The question for this section is what influence does long- versus short-distance dispersal have on the shape of species–area curves? Chave, *et al*. (2002)

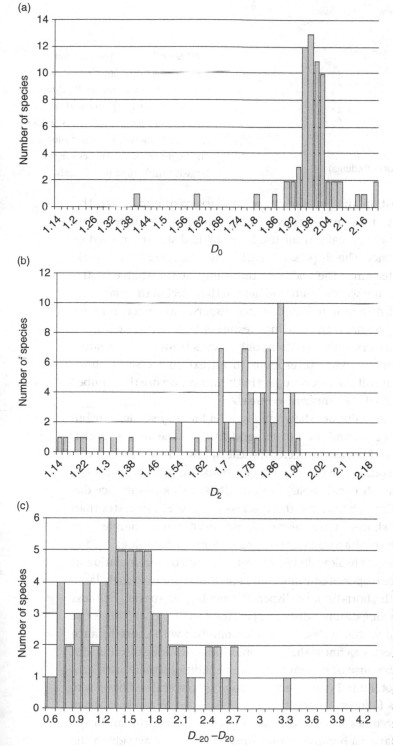

**Figure 17.7** (a) Histograms of the box-counting dimension ($D_0$), (b) the correlation dimension ($D_2$), and (c) the width of the $D_q$ spectrum ($\Delta D_{-20-20}$) for the 67 species in the 50 ha BCI plot. Only those species with more than 500 individuals and with spatial distributions well characterized by a multifractal model were included in the analysis.

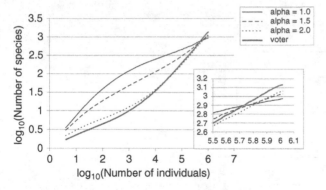

**Figure 17.8** Log of the number of species as a function of the log of the number of contiguous individuals (equivalent to area) obtained with simulations using $\alpha = 1.0$, 1.5, 2.0 and the voter's model. The inset plot is an enlargement of the curves for the largest numbers of individuals.

also addressed this question and because of the similarities of our models the results are qualitatively the same. Here we model long-distance dispersal by varying the characteristic exponent, $\alpha$, of the Lévy stable distribution used to model the dispersal kernel. The dispersal kernel is also affected by the scale parameter $c$, which determines the width of the hump at the source in the dispersal kernel, but because we are interested here in the effect of the characteristics of the tail of the distribution to long-distance dispersal we concentrate on varying $\alpha$ only. For comparison, we also include results obtained with the voter's model, assuming that dispersal (immigration) only occurs from the six nearest neighbor cells. The voter's model corresponds to an extreme case of short-distance dispersal. Because all sites are occupied in the lattice, we use the number of the contiguous individuals as a measure of area, $A$.

The species–area relationships are shown in Fig. 17.8 for Lévy stable distributions having parameters $c = 1$ and $\alpha = 1.0$, 1.5, and 2.0, and the voter's model. When dispersal distances increase ($\alpha$ decreases) the species–area relationships change from having a concave shape to a convex shape on a log-log plot. For small number of individuals (small areas), communities with long-distance dispersal have higher species richness, and the species–area curves rise faster than for communities with short-distance dispersal. However, when sample area increases further, the rate of accumulation of species of communities having long-distance dispersal starts to slow down, whereas the rate of accumulation of species for short-distance dispersal communities accelerates. For extremely large areas, communities with short-distance dispersal have higher species richness than communities with long-distance dispersal (see inset in Fig. 17.8). This is the exact opposite for small spatial scales, where communities with short-distance dispersal have lower species richness than communities with long-distance dispersal. Note, however, because of periodic boundary conditions there is an artificial reduction in the total number of species at large spatial scales. Chave *et al.* (2002) explained this as follows: "as additional area is added to a subset, eventually that added area becomes closer to the starting point because the landscape wraps around. Thus, that area becomes more similar to the area already in the sample, and fewer new species are added" (Chave *et al.*, 2002). In order to check the importance of periodic boundary conditions for species richness as a function of dispersal distances in our simulations, we also studied communities without periodic boundary conditions, but results were qualitatively similar.

Our previous studies of single species spatial patterns provide a guide to understanding the relationship between the shape of the species–area relationship and dispersal distance in terms of the degree of clustering. When dispersal distances are small (voter's model and $\alpha$ close to 2), species tend to form clusters and occupy a well delimited range. In this case, when we sample small areas, we find just a few species, or, in some extreme cases, even monodominance. When area increases, we may find just a few more species (because they are clustered), and consequently the species–area curves rise slowly. In contrast, for communities with long-distance dispersal (smaller $\alpha$), species are less clustered and more intermixed. In this case, at small spatial scales we encounter more species than in cases when species are highly clustered because of short-distance dispersal. In the most extreme case of long-distance dispersal, cluster sizes reduce to the minimum size of one individual per species. Not surprisingly, in the latter case, when area increases, the number of species rises very quickly at first. However, when we keep increasing the area, the trend reverses. Because most or all species are well mixed and encountered in relatively small areas, the rate of accumulation of species decreases.

## Scaling species abundance distributions under neutrality

In this final section, we examine the influence of dispersal on the shape of relative species-abundance distributions and, in particular, how dispersal affects the shape of species-abundance distributions as sample area increases. Bell (2000, 2001) also studied in detail the shape of species-abundance distributions under neutrality; however, Bell (2000) did not consider dispersal on space explicitly, and Bell (2001) considered the spatial location of local communities explicitly but not the spatial location of each individual in its local community. Equally, Chave *et al.* (2002) analyzed how relative abundance changes at different scales, but here we also compare species-abundance distributions obtained with different dispersal kernels at the same spatial scales.

Figure 17.9 shows species-abundance distributions (species frequencies) plotted as a function of the octaves of the number of individuals (Preston curves) for different spatial scales and for $\alpha = 1.0$, plot (a), and for $\alpha = 2.0$, plot (b). In both cases the distributions have a similar pattern of change when area increases. For the smallest number of individuals the curves resemble those of a log series, with the maximum occurring for the lowest abundance class, and then monotonically decreasing. When area increases, the curves develop a maximum (mode) in intermediate abundance classes. This is reminiscent of the "unveiling" effect of the distribution first discussed by Preston (1948) (Hubbell, 2001, chapter 2). Finally, at

(a)

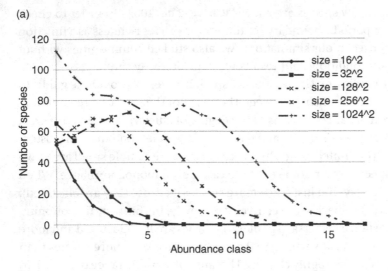

(b)

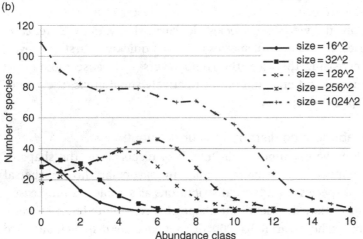

**Figure 17.9** Species–abundance distributions obtained with simulations with $c = 10$, $v = 10^{-4}$, and $\alpha = 1.0$ (a) and $\alpha = 2.0$ (b) for different number of individuals: $16^2$, $32^2$, $128^2$, $256^2$, and $1024^2$. The first abundance class corresponds to 1 individual, the second to 2 individuals, the third to 3–4 individuals, the fourth to 5–8, and so on, with the top value corresponding to a power of 2.

the largest scales the maximum tends to occur once again at the lowest abundance class, and the curves become more similar to a log series. Although both families of curves show the same changes as area increases, closer inspection reveals that there are quantitative differences between the curves. For small areas, the community obtained with longer dispersal distances ($\alpha = 1.0$) has more singleton species but fewer species in the higher abundance classes. This result is in agreement with the findings of the previous section because under long-distance dispersal species are more intermingled; therefore, for small areas we find, on average, fewer individuals per species. When area increases, the maximum for intermediate abundance classes first appears in the community with shorter dispersal distances. Again, this result is a consequence of the lower number of rare species at small spatial scales when dispersal distances are short because

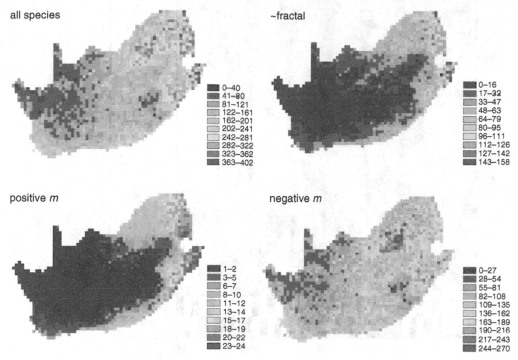

all species

| | |
|---|---|
| ■ | 0–40 |
| ■ | 41–80 |
| | 81–121 |
| | 122–161 |
| | 162–201 |
| | 202–241 |
| | 242–281 |
| | 282–322 |
| ■ | 323–362 |
| ■ | 363–402 |

~fractal

| | |
|---|---|
| ■ | 0–16 |
| ■ | 17–32 |
| | 33–47 |
| | 48–63 |
| | 64–79 |
| | 80–95 |
| | 96–111 |
| | 112–126 |
| ■ | 127–142 |
| ■ | 143–158 |

positive *m*

| | |
|---|---|
| ■ | 1–2 |
| ■ | 3–5 |
| | 6–7 |
| | 8–10 |
| | 11–12 |
| | 13–14 |
| | 15–17 |
| | 18–19 |
| ■ | 20–22 |
| ■ | 23–24 |

negative *m*

| | |
|---|---|
| ■ | 0–27 |
| ■ | 28–54 |
| | 55–81 |
| | 82–108 |
| | 109–135 |
| | 136–162 |
| | 163–189 |
| | 190–216 |
| ■ | 217–243 |
| ■ | 244–270 |

**Plate 1** Species richness maps for southern African birds.

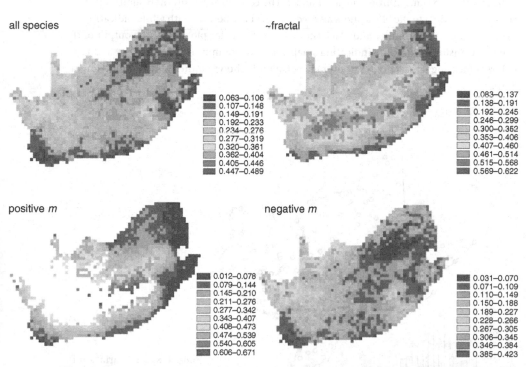

all species

| | |
|---|---|
| ■ | 0.063–0.106 |
| | 0.107–0.148 |
| | 0.149–0.191 |
| | 0.192–0.233 |
| | 0.234–0.276 |
| | 0.277–0.319 |
| | 0.320–0.361 |
| | 0.362–0.404 |
| | 0.405–0.446 |
| ■ | 0.447–0.489 |

~fractal

| | |
|---|---|
| ■ | 0.083–0.137 |
| | 0.138–0.191 |
| | 0.192–0.245 |
| | 0.246–0.299 |
| | 0.300–0.352 |
| | 0.353–0.406 |
| | 0.407–0.460 |
| | 0.461–0.514 |
| ■ | 0.515–0.568 |
| ■ | 0.569–0.622 |

positive *m*

| | |
|---|---|
| ■ | 0.012–0.078 |
| | 0.079–0.144 |
| | 0.145–0.210 |
| | 0.211–0.276 |
| | 0.277–0.342 |
| | 0.343–0.407 |
| | 0.408–0.473 |
| | 0.474–0.539 |
| ■ | 0.540–0.605 |
| ■ | 0.606–0.671 |

negative *m*

| | |
|---|---|
| ■ | 0.031–0.070 |
| | 0.071–0.109 |
| | 0.110–0.149 |
| | 0.150–0.188 |
| | 0.189–0.227 |
| | 0.228–0.266 |
| | 0.267–0.305 |
| | 0.306–0.345 |
| ■ | 0.346–0.384 |
| ■ | 0.385–0.423 |

**Plate 2** Spatial variation in *z* of the power-law species–area relationship for southern African birds. The blank (white) areas for the positive-*m* assemblage occurs where there are insufficient data to fit a SAR.

Plates 1-12 are available for download in colour from www.cambridge.org/9780521699372

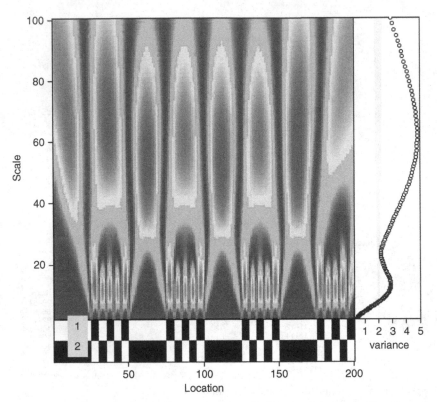

**Plate 3** Illustration of wavelet dissimilarity applied to simulated data. The 10 species were divided into two communities labeled 1 and 2. The communities alternate along a linear transect according to the black and white sequences at the bottom with white indicating the presence of that community and black the absence. The color plot shows the output of the wavelet transform with blue indicating small values of community dissimilarity and red colors indicating large values. The average behavior is shown to the right as a function of scale.

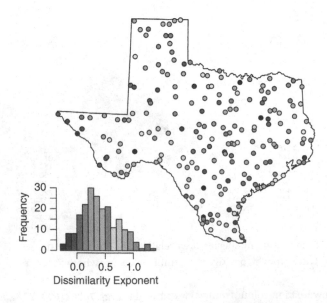

**Plate 4** Spatial variation in biodiversity scaling across the Texas BBS data set. The inset shows a frequency histogram of values.

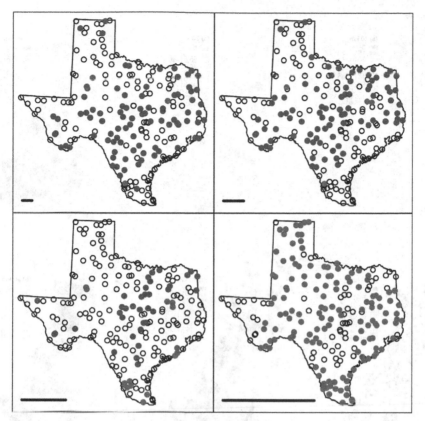

**Plate 5** Hot and cold spots for community dissimilarity plotted at four scales. Open circles correspond to BBS routes that were not significantly different from the result of 1000 bootstrap randomizations of the data. Blue-filled circles showed significantly ($\alpha = 0.05$) less turnover at that scale and red-filled circles significantly more. The horizontal bar at the lower left of each panel indicates the scale of analysis.

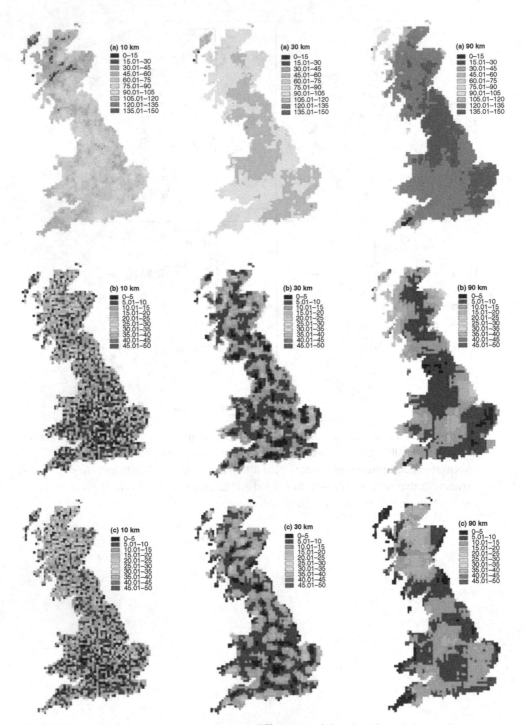

**Plate 6** Maps of the matching components at different spatial grains (from left to right, 10 km, 30 km, 90 km) for the breeding birds in Britain. Top row, species continuity; middle row, species gain; and bottom row, species loss.

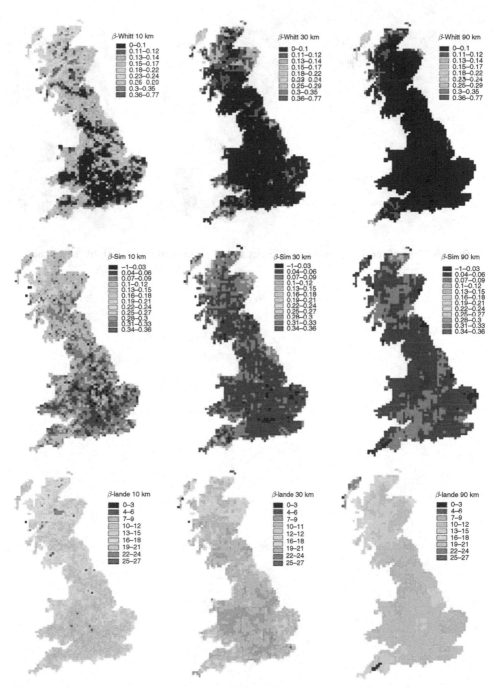

**Plate 7** Maps of beta diversity between neighbouring quadrats at different spatial grains (from left to right, 10 km, 30 km, 90 km) for the breeding birds in Britain. Top row, $\beta_w$; middle row, $\beta_{sim}$; and bottom row, $\beta_l$.

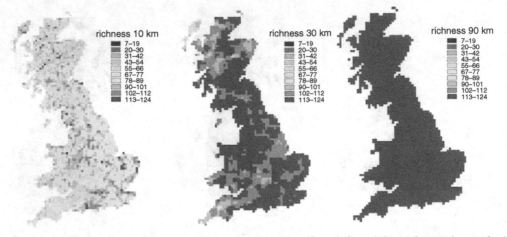

**Plate 8** Maps of species richness at different spatial grains (from left to right, 10 km, 30 km, 90 km).

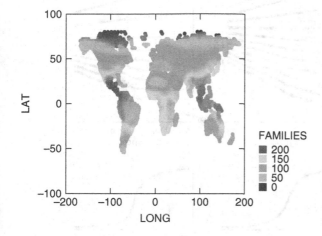

**Plate 9** The global variation in angiosperm family richness, adapted from Francis and Currie (2003).

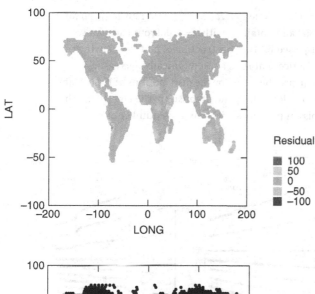

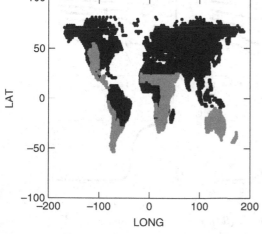

**Plate 10** Top: A map of the residuals from Francis and Currie's (2003) global relationship between angiosperm family richness and climate. Bottom: Wallace biogeographic subregions in which the mean squared residual is significantly ($P \leq 0.05$) greater than would be expected in comparison with an equal number of quadrats randomly selected from the global set (gray areas; other areas are shown in black). Thus, regional, nonclimatic influences on richness might be hypothesized in those regions.

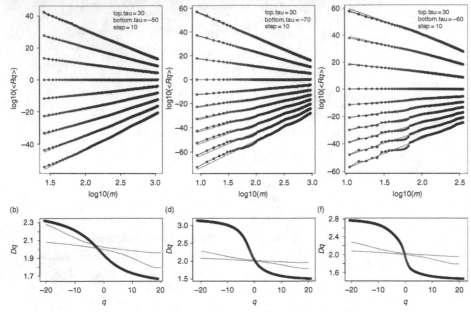

**Plate 11** Plot (a) shows the curves of $\log_{10}(\langle R_q\rangle) = \log_{10}(\langle R_i(m)^{-\tau_q}\rangle^{1/\tau_q})$ versus $\log_{10}(m)$ for the point distribution shown in Fig. 17.3(a) and obtained with $\alpha = 1.0$. From this plot we estimate the slope from which we obtain $q$, used for the construction of plot (b), showing the spectrum of generalized dimensions $D_q$. Notice that $D_q$ is a monotonically decreasing function of $q$. Plots (c) and (d), and (e) and (f) are the same for the distributions of Fig. 17.3(b) and Fig. 17.3(c), respectively. The red lines in plots (b), (d) and (f) consist of the largest and the smallest $D_q$ values obtained from 200 Poisson processes with the same number of points as the original distribution.

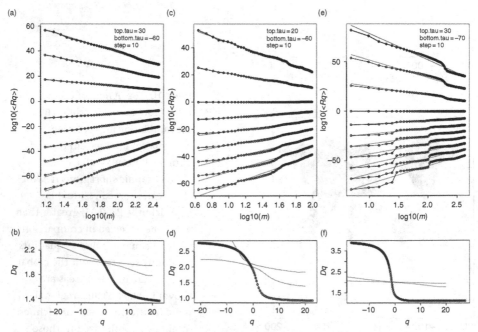

**Plate 12** Plot (a) shows the curves of $\log_{10}(\langle R_q\rangle) = \log_{10}(\langle R_i(m)^{-\tau_q}\rangle^{1/\tau_q})$ versus $\log_{10}(m)$, and plot (b) the spectrum of generalized dimensions for the spatial distribution of *Guarea guidonia* (Fig. 17.5a), and plots (c) and (d), and (e) and (f) are the same for *Annona acuminata* (Fig. 17.5b) and *Rinorea sylvatica* (Fig. 17.5c), respectively. The red lines in plots (b), (d) and (f) consist of the largest and the smallest $D_q$ values obtained from 200 Poisson processes with the same number of points as the original distribution.

species tend to occur in clusters. Above a certain area, both curves show a maximum for intermediate abundances. When the sample area increases further, the curves become progressively more similar, and the maximum for intermediate abundances is less obvious and it may disappear altogether. Interestingly, for the entire area, the species-abundance distributions for short-dispersal distances have a larger number of singleton species than the curves obtained for larger dispersal distances. The important conclusion is that the shape of the species-abundance distribution is not only a function of dispersal, but also a function of size of the sample area (see also Hubbell & Borda-de-Água, 2004).

## Discussion and conclusions

Here we have developed a neutral model that considers space explicitly and studied the effect of long- and short-distance dispersal, first, on the spatial patterns of individual species distributions and, second, on the macroecological patterns of species–area curves and species-abundance distributions. We used Lévy stable distributions to model the dispersal kernels because their power law ("fat") tails better capture long-distance dispersal events. We used multifractals to analyze the spatial distributions obtained with simulations and compared the results with the multifractal analyses of the spatial distribution of individual tree species in BCI.

Our work on the multifractal characteristics of individual species, spatial distributions is meant as a starting point. One current problem is the general inadequacy of data sets on the large-scale distribution of species. The proper study of multifractality (or fractality) requires data sets from where we can extract scaling regions that span several orders of magnitude. Data of this sort are rare in ecology. Both our simulations (because of limiting computer time and space) and the BCI data set are no exceptions to this general problem of inadequate data sets. Given these limitations, we used the most robust method we could to obtain the multifractal spectra, the fixed-mass method, and attempted to estimate the multifractal spectrum only for those species with large sample sizes, more than 500 individuals, and for species in which we observed a scaling region for at least one order of magnitude.

Given these caveats, we arrive at three important conclusions from our multifractal analyses. The first conclusion is that a large number of species, about 90% of the species in the BCI 50 ha plot with more than 500 individuals, were well described by a multifractal pattern. The second conclusion is that the distributions obtained from the neutral theory with Lévy stable dispersal were also well described by a multifractal pattern. Third, differences among BCI species in dispersal mode and in life history were significantly correlated with differences in their multifractal spectra.

Moreover, these multifractal patterns were present in the simulations regardless of the particular parameter values of the Lévy stable distribution used to model dispersal. However, the characteristics of the multifractal spectra depended on the value of the characteristic exponent, $\alpha$, of the Lévy stable distributions. When dispersal distance decreases (large $\alpha$), the spatial distributions are more heterogeneous, which is revealed in the increase of the width of the multifractal spectra, $D_q$. This observation raises the question of whether there is a quantitative relationship between the parameter $\alpha$ of the Lévy stable distributions and values of the multifractal spectrum, such as the fractal dimensions. In our limited explorations of this question, we did not find such a relationship. One reason is that there was some variability in the resulting multifractal spectra even for the same $\alpha$ value. A complicating issue is that not all species had the same number of individuals, which is likely to affect the estimation of the multifractal spectrum. Nevertheless, we did demonstrate a significant trend towards less clustering when dispersal distances increase, as revealed by an increase in the correlation dimension $D_2$, and the tendency of the multifractal spectrum to become narrower. This result was helpful in understanding the shape of the species–area curves and species-abundance distributions obtained with simulations. It has been suggested (e.g. Rosenzweig, 1995; Hubbell, 2001) that species–area relationships are triphasic. When plotted in a log-log plot they are convex near the origin, almost log-log linear on intermediate scales, i.e. scales on which they are well described by power laws, and then for very large areas they approach a slope close to 1. A slope close to 1 is usually interpreted as the result of exceeding the correlation length by sampling across regions having independent evolutionary histories and biotas. In the voter's model, a limiting slope of unity can be proven analytically (Bramson, Cox & Durrett, 1996), and Allen and White (2003) showed that a slope equal to 1 can be obtained under the assumption of restricted species ranges.

In our simulations we did not observe slopes approaching unity for large areas, but this is probably a result of the small size of the simulation lattice, and the use of periodic boundary conditions, which tend to reduce the rate of accumulation for very large areas, as mentioned. By contrast, for small and intermediate areas, we obtained curves that reproduce the shapes of those observed in real data. For intermediate scales, the species–area relationships were nearly linear in log-log plots. Note also that our simulations used the same dispersal kernel for all species, following the symmetry assumption of the neutral model. However, we know that species have different dispersal abilities. We have not yet studied what happens in this case, but the species–area relationships obtained with species having a variety of dispersal kernels may differ from the ones obtained with our simulations. We speculate that their shapes will be a mixture of the curves we obtained with the simulations and will be well described by power laws.

The region of the log-log species–area relationship in which the effect of dispersal is more visible is at small spatial scales. When dispersal distances increase, the shape of the log-log species–area relationship changes to accelerating curves at short distances and decelerating curves at long distances. The latter is the pattern most often observed in real data sets (e.g. Condit *et al.*, 1996). However, accelerating (upward bent) curves can also be observed, as shown by Palmer (this volume) for the mountainous plants in North America. Short-distance dispersal may be one explanation for such patterns, since it is easy to imagine that mountains act as barriers to plant dispersal at a variety of spatial scales. Of course, other processes, such as habitat heterogeneity and habitat specialization, may be at work as well.

An important result, in agreement with Hubbell (2001), is that short-distance dispersal may lead to lower species richness in local communities at small scales, but to greater species richness in communities at large scales (Fig. 17.8). This means that increasing dispersal distances increases local community species richness (alpha diversity) at small scales but has a complex effect on beta diversity, first increasing and then decreasing species turnover as area increases.

Concerning species abundance distributions when plotted as Preston curves, two important results were shown with the simulations. First, and in accordance with Hubbell (2001), Chave *et al.* (2002) and Hubbell and Borda-de-Água (2004), the shape of the species–abundance distribution is a function of the sampling area, and, second, for the same sampling area, the shape of the species-abundance distribution is a function of the dispersal rate. The second result is important because it shows that comparison of the evolution of the species-abundance distributions with area for two different communities may reveal the characteristic dispersal distances of their species. In conclusion, our study emphasizes the importance of defining the sampling area relative to the spatial scale of dispersal for understanding the scaling of species-abundance distributions. One caveat to our conclusions is that all of our simulations employed the "point-mutation" mode of speciation, which generates many short-lived rare species. It is known that other models of speciation, such as "random-fission" speciation (Hubbell, 2001) or "peripheral isolate" speciation (Hubbell & Lake, 2003; Hubbell, 2005), produce different steady-state distributions of relative species abundance, with fewer rare species. In particular, changing the mode of speciation may affect our conclusions regarding the shape of the relative abundance distributions, especially the relative abundance of singleton species.

It is also important to notice that there is no distinction between local communities and metacommunity in our model as there was in Hubbell (2001). Nevertheless, our results agree with the qualitative conclusions reached by Hubbell (2001). In our case, a subset of the simulation lattice is equivalent to a local community, and a reduction in the dispersal distance is equivalent to a reduction in the immigration rate, the parameter that coupled the local communities with the metacommunity in Hubbell's original model.

The results of our simulations are also in good qualitative agreement with the observations from real data sets – in particular those from tropical forest tree communities. These results of course do not prove that tropical tree communities are neutral-symmetric. However, they do suggest that symmetric neutral theory is a good first approximation, especially with the improved dispersal model and the explicit treatment of space. These results are encouraging and mean that it is profitable to ask to what extent community-level patterns are the result of species similarities rather than to their differences. The improved theory also allows us to study the spatial distribution of individual species in far greater detail. Future work will include breaking symmetry in a variety of ways, and asking to what extent species differences must be incorporated in order to explain particular aspects of biodiversity scaling relationships in different ecological communities.

## Appendix 17.I   Multifractals
This appendix describes in more detail methods to characterize multifractals.

*Characterization of multifractals by the box-counting method*
The characterization of a multifractal requires a set of numbers, some of which correspond to fractal dimensions. Hereafter we focus exclusively on describing point distributions in a plane. There are at least three methods for obtaining these numeric descriptors for point distributions: the box-counting method, familiar to many readers, the fixed-radius method and the fixed-mass method. When describing multifractals, the box-counting method is useful mainly for heuristic reasons, but is rarely used in practical situations. Consider, for example, the distributions in Fig. 17.3. Suppose we are just interested in presence-absence, i.e. the box-counting fractal dimension. In this case, we cover the points with "boxes" (squares) and count how many boxes contain at least one point. Then we repeat this process for boxes of different sizes. The theoretical definition of fractal dimension is given by

$$D = \lim_{\varepsilon \to 0} -\frac{\log(N(\varepsilon))}{\log(\varepsilon)}, \tag{17.5}$$

where $N(\varepsilon)$ is the number of occupied boxes of linear size (side length) $\varepsilon$. However, in actual situations, we estimate $D$ by plotting $\log N(\varepsilon)$ versus $\log(\varepsilon)$, and then identify a region of variation in $\varepsilon$ over which the relationship is well approximated by a straight line (this requirement should occasionally be relaxed, as explained in Box 17.1). The slope of this line segment is equal to $-D$.

In the case of multifractals, however, we also need to take into account the proportion of points, $p_i$, in each box. Now the characterization of the multifractal is done in terms of a set of generalized "dimensions", $D_q$, obtained from the equation

$$D_q = \lim_{\varepsilon \to 0} \frac{1}{q-1} \frac{\log\left(\sum_{i=1}^{N(\varepsilon)} p_i^q\right)}{\log(\varepsilon)}, \tag{17.6}$$

where $q$ is a real number ranging from $-\infty$ to $+\infty$; to avoid the division by zero, we take the limit when $q$ tends to 1, and the resulting formula is

$$D_1 = \lim_{\varepsilon \to 0} \frac{\sum_{i=1}^{N(\varepsilon)} p_i \log(p_i)}{\log(\varepsilon)}. \tag{17.7}$$

Note that Eq. (17.5) is just a special case of Eq. (17.6) when $q = 0$, and that changing $q$ is similar to obtaining the moments of the distribution of the $p_i$. The set of values of $D_q$ is called the "$D_q$ spectrum" of generalized "dimensions". In real world situations, in analogy with estimating the fractal dimension, we estimate $D_q$ by looking for straight line segments in the plots of $\log\left(\sum_{i=1}^{N(\varepsilon)} p_i^q\right)$ versus $\log(\varepsilon)$. The $D_q$ spectrum is a monotonically decreasing function of $q$ and looks like a stretched Z (see Fig. 17.4).

The utility of obtaining the $D_q$ spectrum by changing $q$ is that it reveals many different and subtle attributes of a pattern of points on a plane. For example, when $q$ is a large positive number, the sum in Eq. (17.6) is most sensitive to the largest $p_i$ values, that is, to regions of high abundance. Conversely, when $q$ is a small negative number, but large in absolute value, the sum in Eq. (17.6) is most sensitive to the smallest $p_i$ values, that is, to regions of low abundance. The width of the $D_q$ spectrum is a measure of the heterogeneity of the multifractal. Thus, for a Poisson process with no heterogeneity (complete spatial randomness) all dimensions are equal and the $D_q$ spectrum is a straight line parallel to the $q$-axis.

*Characterization of multifractals by the fixed-radius and fixed-mass methods*
Although easy to implement, the box-counting method has problems in real applications (see Cutler, 1993). For very large boxes, all boxes are likely to be occupied, and the number of boxes increases with the Euclidean dimension of the space (2, for points in the plane). For very small boxes, all boxes contain only one point, and the number of boxes remains constant. In order to overcome these problems, some authors (e.g. Grassberger & Procaccia, 1983; Badii & Broggi, 1988) have developed alternative methods based on the distance between points (for an example of a practical application see Hirabayashi, Ito & Yoshii, 1992). These methods are based on the following relationship:

$$\langle (p_i/R^{D_q})^{q-1} \rangle \sim \text{constant}, \tag{17.8}$$

where now $p_i = m/(M-1)$, $m$ is the number of points within radius $R$ of a given point, $i$, $M$ is the total number of points, and $<>$ denotes the average taken over all points. Based on Eq. (17.8), one can pursue two strategies to obtain $D_q$: the fixed-radius and the fixed-mass methods.

In the fixed-radius approach we determine how many points, $m$, lie within radius $R$ of a given point $i$, and estimate the dependency of $p_i(R)$ on $R$ according to

$$\langle p_i(R)^{q-1} \rangle \sim R^{\tau_q}, \tag{17.9}$$

where $\tau_q = (q-1)D_q$. For $q = 2$ we obtain an expression known as the "correlation sum"; hence the procedure used in calculating $D_2$ is equivalent to that for calculating Ripley's function (e.g. Diggle, 1983).

In the fixed-mass approach, we instead calculate the minimum radius from a point $i$, $R_i$, that contains $m$ points, and we write the functional dependency $R_i(m)$ on $m$ as

$$\langle R_i(m)^{-\tau_q} \rangle^{1/\tau_q} \sim m^{-1/D_q}. \tag{17.10}$$

Although the fixed-radius method is easier to implement than the fixed-mass method, it has the disadvantage of leading to very small scaling regions for $q < 1$, and, hence, it is not recommended for estimating $D_q$ for $q < 1$ (Grassberger, Badii & Politi, 1988). For this reason, we recommend the use of the fixed-mass method to obtain multifractal spectra.

The steps to determine the multifractal spectra using the fixed-mass method are: (1) for every point in the set determine the minimum value of $R$ that contains a specified number of points, $m$; (2) repeat the previous step for different values of $m$; (3) choose different values of $\tau_q$ and check if $\log(\langle R_i(m)^{-\tau_q} \rangle^{1/\tau_q})$ as a function of $\log(m)$ can be appropriately described by a linear relationship for some scaling region (but see Box 17.1); (4) if a scaling region is found, estimate the slope $(= -1/D_q)$; and (5) once $D_q$ is known, determine $q$ from $q = 1 + \tau_q/D_q$.

An important difference between the fixed-radius and the fixed-mass method is that in the former we vary $q$, while in the latter we vary $\tau$. This implies that in the fixed-mass method we do not have control over the obtained values of $q$. In some cases, however, we may like to know the exact value of a given $D_q$ ($D_2$, for example). One solution is to choose several values of $\tau$ within the range of values that we predict to lead to $q = 2$, and choose the obtained value of $q$ that is closest to 2.

In most practical situations, it is also desirable to introduce corrections for boundaries. We suggest the correction method used in the statistical analysis of spatial point processes together with Ripley's function (see Diggle, 1983).

## Acknowledgments

LBA thanks the kind hospitality provided by the Pacific Forestry Centre, Victoria BC, Canada. We thank Jayanth Banavar, Amos Maritan, and Igor Volkov for stimulating discussions. We thank David Storch, Pablo Marquet, and Jérôme

Chave for suggestions that considerably improve the content and presentation of this chapter. This work was partially carried out under a postdoctoral fellowship from Simon Fraser University and a grant from the National Science Foundation (DEB 0346488).

## References

Allen, A. P. & White, E. P. (2003). Effects of range size on species-area relationships. *Evolutionary Ecology Research*, **5**, 493–499.

Badii, R. & Broggi, G. (1988). Measurement of the dimension spectrum $f(\alpha)$: fixed mass approach. *Physics Letters A*, **131**, 339–343.

Badii, R. & Politi, A. (1984). Intrinsic oscillations in measuring the fractal dimension. *Physics Letters A*, **104**, 303–305.

Bell, G. (2000). The distribution of abundance in neutral communities. *American Naturalist*, **155**, 606–617.

Bell, G. (2001). Neutral macroecology. *Science*, **293**, 2413–2418.

Bramson, M., Cox, J. T. & Durrett, R. (1996). Spatial models for species-area curves. *Annals of Probability*, **24**, 1721–1751.

Chambers, J. M., Mallows, C. L. & Stuck, B. W. (1976). A method for simulating stable random variables. *Journal of the American Statistical Association*, **71**, 340–344.

Chave, J. & Leigh Jr., E. G. (2002). A spatially explicit neutral model of $\beta$-diversity in tropical forests. *Theoretical Population Biology*, **62**, 153–168.

Chave, J., Muller-Landau, H. C. & Levin, S. A. (2002). Comparing classical community models: theoretical consequences for patters of diversity. *American Naturalist*, **159**, 1–23.

Clark, J. S., Fastie, C., Hurtt, G., *et al.* (1998). Reid's paradox of rapid plant migration. *Bioscience*, **48**, 13–24.

Clark, J. S., Silman, M., Kern, R., Macklin, E. & HilleRisLambers, J. (1999). Seed dispersal near and far: patterns across temperate and tropical forests. *Ecology*, **80**, 1475–1494.

Condit, R., Hubbell, S. P., LaFrankie, J. V., *et al.* (1996). Species-area and species-individual relationships for tropical trees: a comparison of three 50 ha plots. *Journal of Ecology*, **84**, 549–562.

Cutler, C. D. (1993). A review of the theory and estimation of fractal dimension. In *Dimension Estimation and Models*, ed. H. Tong, pp. 1–107. Singapore: World Scientific.

Diggle, P. J. (1983). *Statistical Analysis of Spatial Point Processes*. London: Academic Press.

Durrett, R. & Levin, S. (1996). Spatial models for species-area curves. *Journal of Theoretical Biology*, **179**, 119–127.

Etienne, R. S. & Olff, H. (2004). A novel genealogical approach to neutral biodiversity theory. *Ecology Letters*, **7**, 170–175.

Evertsz, C. J. G. & Mandelbrot, B. B. (1992). Multifractal measures. In *Chaos and Fractals. New Frontiers of Science*, ed. H. O. Peitgen, H. Jürgens & D. Saupe, pp. 921–953. New York: Springer-Verlag.

Gnedenko, B. V. & Kolmogorov, A. N. (1954). *Limit Distributions for Sums of Independent Random Variables*. Cambridge, MA: Addison-Wesley.

Grassberger, P. & Procaccia I. (1983). Characterization of strange attractors. *Physical Review Letters*, **50**, 346–349.

Grassberger, P., Badii, R. & Politi, A. (1988). Scaling laws for invariant measures on hyperbolic and nonhyperbolic atractors. *Journal of Statistical Physics*, **51**, 135–178.

Halley, J. M. & Iwasa, Y. (1998). Extinction rate of a population under both demographic and environmental stochasticity. *Theoretical Population Biology*, **53**, 1–15.

Hirabayashi, T., Ito, K. & Yoshii, T. (1992). Multifractal analysis of earthquakes. *Pure and Applied Geophysics*, **138**, 591–610.

Holley, R. A. & Liggett, T. M. (1975). Ergodic theorems for weakly interacting systems and the voter model. *Annals of Probability*, **3**, 643–663.

Houchmandzadeh, B. & Vallade, M. (2003). Clustering in neutral ecology. *Physical Review E*, **68**, Art. No. 061912.

Hubbell, S. P. (1997). A unified theory of biogeography and relative species abundance and its applications to tropical rain forests and coral reefs. *Coral Reefs*, **16** (suppl.), S9–S21.

Hubbell, S. P. (2001). *The Unified Neutral Theory of Biodiversity and Biogeography*. Princeton: Princeton University Press.

Hubbell, S. P. (2005). Neutral theory of biodiversity and biogeography and Stephen Jay Gould. *Paleobiology*, **31** (suppl.), 122–132.

Hubbell, S. P. & Borda-de-Água L. (2004). The distribution of relative species abundance in local communities under neutrality: a response to the comment by Chisholm & Burgman. *Ecology*, **85**, 3175–3178.

Hubbell, S. P. & Foster, R. B. (1983). Diversity of canopy trees in a neotropical forest and implications for the conservation of tropical trees. In *Tropical Rain Forest: Ecology and Management*, ed. S. J. Sutton, T. C. Whitmore & A. C. Chadwick, pp. 25–41. Oxford: Blackwell.

Hubbell, S. P. & Lake, J. K. (2003). The neutral theory of biodiversity and biogeography, and beyond. In *Macroecology: Concepts and Consequences*, ed. T. M. Blackburn & K. J. Gaston, pp. 45–63. Oxford: Blackwell Science.

Jones, F. A., Chen, J., Weng, G. J. & Hubbell, S. P. (2005). A genetic evaluation of seed dispersal in a Neotropical tree, *Jacaranda copaia* (Bignoniaceae). *American Naturalist*, **166**, 543–555.

Kot, M., Lewis, M. A. & Van den Driessche, P. (1996). Dispersal data and the spread of invading organisms. *Ecology*, **77**, 2027–2042.

Lewis, M. A. (1997). Variability, patchiness, and jump dispersal in the spread of an invading population. In *Spatial Ecology: The Role of Space in Population Dynamics and Interspecific Interactions*, ed. D. Tilman & P. Kareiva, pp. 46–74. Princeton: Princeton University Press.

Liebovitch, L. S. (1998). *Fractals and Chaos Simplified for the Life Sciences*. Oxford: Oxford University Press.

MacArthur, R. H. & Wilson, E. O. (1967). *The Theory of Island Biogeography*, Princeton: Princeton University Press.

Mandelbrot, B. B. (1977). *Fractals: Form, Chance, and Dimension*. San Francisco: W. H. Freeman.

Mandelbrot, B. B. (1997). *Fractals and Scaling in Finance: Discontinuity, Concentration, Risk*. New York: Springer.

Manly (1997). *Randomization, Bootstrap and Monte Carlo Methods in Biology*. 2nd edn. London: Chapman & Hall/CRC.

Mantegna, R. N. & Stanley, H. E. (2000). *An Introduction to Econophysics: Correlations and Complexity in Finance*. Cambridge: Cambridge University Press.

McKane, A. J, Alonso, D. & Solé, R. V. (2004). Analytic solution of Hubbell's model of local community dynamics. *Theoretical Population Biology*, **65**, 67–73.

Meneveau, C. & Sreenivasan, K. R. (1989). Measurements of $f(\alpha)$ from scaling histograms and applications to dynamical systems and fully developed turbulence. *Physics Letters A*, **137**, 103–112.

Muller-Landau, M. C., Dalling, J. W., Harms, K. E., *et al.* (2004). Seed dispersal and density-dependent seed and seedling survival in *Trichilia turbeculata* and *Miconia argentea*. In *Tropical Forest Diversity and Dynamism: Findings From a Large-scale Plot Network*, ed. C. Losos & E. G. Leigh, Jr., pp. 340–362. Chicago: University of Chicago Press.

Nagylaki, T. (1974). The decay of genetic variability in geographically structured populations. *Proceedings of the National Academy of Sciences of the USA*, **71**, 2932–2936.

Nathan, R. & Muller-Landau, H. (2000). Spatial patterns of seed dispersal, their determinants and consequences for recruitment. *Trends in Ecology and Evolution*, **15**, 278–285.

Petit, J. R., Pineau, E., Demesure, B., Bacilieri, R., Ducousso, A. & Kremer, A. (1997). *Proceedings of the National Academy of Sciences of the USA*, **94**, 9996–10001.

Preston, F. W. (1948). The commonness, and rarity, of species. *Ecology*, **29**, 254–283.

Rosenzweig, M. L. (1995). *Species Diversity in Space and Time*. Cambridge: Cambridge University Press.

Silvertown, J., Holtier, J. S., Johnson, J. & Dale, P. (1992). Cellular automaton models of interspecific competition for space – the effect of pattern on process. *Journal of Ecology*, **80**, 527–534.

Vallade, M. & Houchmandzadeh, B. (2003). Analytical solution of a neutral model of biodiversity. *Physical Review E*, **68**, Art. No. 061902.

Volkov, I., Banavar, J. R., Hubbell, S. P. & Maritan, A. (2003). Neutral theory and relative species abundance in ecology. *Nature*, **424**, 1035–1037.

Volkov, I., Banavar, J., He, F., Hubbell, S. P. & Maritan, A. (2005). Density dependence explains tree species abundance and diversity in tropical forests. *Nature*, **438**, 658–661.

Weiss, G. H. (1994). A primer of random walkology. In *Fractals in Science*, ed. A. Bunde & S. Havlin, pp. 119–161. Berlin: Springer-Verlag.

West B. J. & Deering, W. (1994). Fractal physiology for physicists: Lévy statistics. *Physics Reports*, **246**, 1–100.

# CHAPTER EIGHTEEN

# General patterns in plant invasions: a family of quasi-neutral models

TOMÁŠ HERBEN

*Academy of Sciences of the Czech Republic, Charles University, Prague*

## Introduction

Biological invasions, i.e. cases when an alien species increases and spreads in a new region, are of enormous practical interest (Elton, 1958; Groves, 1989; Levin, 1989). Empirical studies show large differences between different community types in the number of alien species found there (Rejmánek, Richardson & Pyšek, 2005). It is therefore believed that the fact whether a community is invasible can tell us something on the "internal working" of the invaded communities; in particular, understanding why a particular species establishes in a particular community can shed light on the ecological processes structuring a community (Elton, 1958; Shea & Chesson, 2002; Moore *et al.*, 2001). Experimental studies have shown that invasion success may be affected by processes such as disturbance (Fox & Fox, 1986; Mooney & Drake, 1986; Burke & Grime, 1996), fluctuating resources (Davis, Grime & Thompson, 2000), or growth rate ranking of species (Rejmánek & Richardson, 1996).

In theoretical studies, invasibility has been routinely used as a stability measure in Lotka–Volterra or similar systems (Case, 1990; Law & Morton, 1996; Moore *et al.*, 2001; Byers & Noonburg, 2003). Nevertheless there is a certain gap between theoretical understanding of community invasibility (Shea & Chesson, 2002) and empirical studies of single invasions. The latter inevitably study events that are singular in their nature (Rejmánek *et al.*, 2005). Studies of individual invasions typically concentrate on specific biological traits of the invasive species that are essential for their invasion success. While such information is often critically needed for management of the particular invasion, these observations are often difficult to generalize. Some generalizations, such as "Invasive species have higher population growth rates" are not very useful for better understanding. Further, invasions are studied after they occur; therefore they cannot be easily compared against the background of the cases where invasion has not taken place, again making generalizations of invasion processes difficult.

This gap has been one of the driving forces behind extensive collecting of metadata in order that general patterns are identified and understood (Lonsdale, 1999; Pyšek, Richardson & Williamson, 2004). These data are typically used to address two central issues of invasion ecology: (1) are there general traits of

*Scaling Biodiversity*, ed. David Storch, Pablo A. Marquet and James H. Brown. Published by Cambridge University Press. © Cambridge University Press 2007.

invasive species, and (2) are there general parameters that determine whether a community is invasible?

While the former issue has been rather successfully approached using comparative studies (Rejmánek & Richardson, 1996), the latter remains more difficult. Part of the reason is due to the fact that the universe of possible community parameters is less easy to define than a set of possible species traits. Many community parameters have been proposed to play a role in susceptibility to invasions, such as disturbance (Fox & Fox, 1986; Burke & Grime, 1996), productivity (Tilman, 1997; Davis et al., 2000) or species richness (Lonsdale, 1999).

One of the widespread but controversial ideas in ecology says that the number of alien species establishing in a community is affected by the species richness of that community (Lonsdale, 1999). If the relationship is negative, it could be interpreted as an indication that more species-rich communities are more resistant to invasion (Lodge, 1993). This would mean that biotic resistance of a community against invasion could be assessed using its species richness. The negative relationship has been explained by how niche space is filled by native species; if there are fewer native species, it is more likely that some regions of the niche space are empty and open for an invader (Case, 1990, 1996; Law & Morton, 1996; Prieur-Richard & Lavorel, 2000; Shea & Chesson, 2002). However, in an elegant study, Moore et al. (2001) showed that invasibility of a community depends on the mechanism of diversity maintenance and both negative and positive relationships can be expected.

Currently there are plenty of field data, both observational and experimental, on the relationship between species richness and invasibility collected in the past two decades. However, one should be rather careful in the interpretation of data using richness as a community parameter. First, it should be noted that richness as a community parameter makes sense only when it is acceptable to assume that differences between species do not matter much and all species are roughly equally important. While this is never true, it is best approached by large data sets (often assembled from literature) which span a range of scales and habitat types and the patterns they show are likely to be due to rather general processes (Lonsdale, 1999; Pyšek et al., 2004). In such a case, however, functional explanations involving richness should be formulated as assuming all species to be approximately equivalent.

Second, species richness is both a community parameter and a response variable. Local species richness is often seen as a dependent variable which is a function of mechanisms operating in the community (May, 1973; Hubbell, 2001; Mouquet, Moore & Loreau, 2002). Communities differing in richness thus may differ in mechanisms that determine it and richness may serve as a proxy variable for some of these mechanisms (Moore et al., 2001; Mouquet et al., 2002). By contrast, establishing a relationship between richness and community-level parameters such as biomass production or invasibility assumes richness to be a community parameter. Using similar reasoning at a different scale, the species pool of a region is also an independent richness parameter if local species richness is studied as a response variable (Pärtel & Zobel, 1999).

Both these qualifications mean that the relationship between invasibility and richness of communities should be examined in a framework that permits treating all species as roughly equivalent and can treat richness both as a community parameter and a response variable. This can easily be done by neutral lottery models, which typically assume equivalence of all species (in size, per capita natality and mortality, immigration rates, competitive ability, etc.) and make predictions about species richness. In neutral models, community dynamics is seen as a stochastic result of these processes in communities of limited sizes and is due to processes that operate fully independently of any biological traits of species (Hubbell, 1979). They can capture well the dynamics of large species assemblages and often make good predictions of general patterns of community structure (abundance distributions) or scaling patterns (species–area relationships; Hubbell, 1979, 2001; see also Borda-de-Água et al., this volume). By virtue of assuming all species being approximately equivalent, they can be used to model processes of community invasion that involve species richness as a community parameter.

In this contribution, I will examine how specific patterns in plant invasions can be reproduced by null models with no specific assumptions about the division of the niche space or competitive structure. First, I will use a simple neutral model of community invasibility to address the scale dependence of this process. Next, I will use a generalized version of the same model to examine the effect of species pool size on invasibility of randomly assembled communities.

## Is there a relationship between the number of alien species and the richness of the local community?

Invasibility of communities has been typically studied by examination of the relationship between the number of native species and the number of aliens (slope of the native–alien relationship, further abbreviated NAR). Published data on NAR report both negative (Elton, 1958; Lodge, 1993) and positive (Pickard, 1984; Lonsdale, 1999; Pyšek, Jarošík & Kučera, 2002; Sax, 2002; Stohlgren et al., 2002) relationships. Several authors suggest that studies reporting a negative relationship are experimental, whereas a positive relationship has been shown primarily by large-scale observational studies (Levine, 2000; Naeem et al., 2000; Levine, Kennedy & Naeem, 2002; see also Fig. 18.1). More detailed analyses of published data have shown that NAR shape is typically scale dependent with negative relationships being found only at scales smaller than several meters (Levine et al., 2002; Shea & Chesson, 2002; Fridley, Brown & Bruno, 2004; Herben et al., 2004; Fig. 18.1).

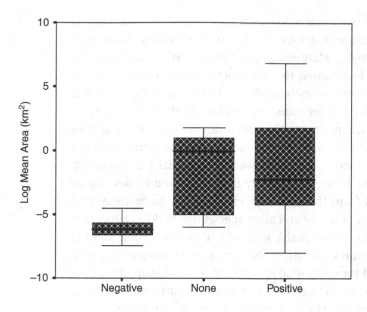

**Figure 18.1** Box-and-whisker plot of logarithm base 10 of mean study area (km$^2$) of published studies reporting significant and negative (Negative), nonsignificant (None), and significant and positive (Positive) relationships between number of aliens and number of native species (NAR). Boxes cover interquartile range, whiskers indicate total range. Based on data from Herben *et al.* (2004).

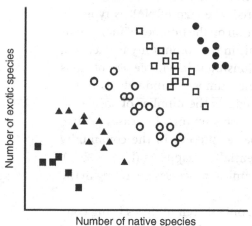

**Figure 18.2** Expected relationship between number of native and number of alien species based on competitive relationship between species at all scales. Redrawn after Shea and Chesson (2002). Identical symbols indicate communities of identical sizes.

Shea and Chesson (2002) hypothesized that a negative NAR is found at any specific (sufficiently narrow) scale because of the effects of species interactions such as competition for resources or enemy-free space (Fig. 18.2). Because the number of species depends on the size of the species assemblage, larger assemblages are bound to have higher absolute numbers of invaders simply due to the species–area relation (Shea & Chesson, 2002). Thus, any sample that spans large and small assemblages should show a positive NAR even if the relationship at each specific scale is negative.

Since the scale dependence is so universal in NAR, it should first be examined to see to what extent patterns of NAR can be due purely to neutral processes operating over different scales. For this, I am using a simple dynamic model based on drawing individuals from two pools of identical species (native and alien) and lottery processes of disturbance and local growth (the Appendix discusses a version with all species having identical population growth rates; see also Herben *et al.*, 2004). There is assumed to be a strict carrying capacity in the model such that the number of individuals in the community is fixed. Community structure is then determined by replacement probabilities of deceased individuals. Replacement probabilities are influenced by current species abundances, growth rates, and immigration rates. The only difference between native and alien species is that no aliens are allowed in the initial species composition of the community: the native community is first allowed to develop by random drawing of species from the native species pool for some time. This model thus predicts numbers of native and alien species (i.e. NAR) as a function of community size (number of individuals), sizes of both species pools and the parameters of the lottery (disturbance rate, growth rates, and immigration rates).

The analysis of the model shows that no specific interaction structure of the communities needs to be assumed to explain the observed patterns of NAR; all its major features can be generated by the neutral process. If communities with the same numbers of individuals are compared, the sign of NAR is typically negative (Fig. 18.3a). This result is due to limitation on the number of individuals in the community; if the number of individuals in the community is fixed and sufficiently small, a strong and negative relationship is inevitable. For obvious reasons, the effect is particularly strong if the number of individuals in the community is of the similar order of magnitude as the number of species in the species pool. As number of individuals in the community increases relative to the species pool, the proportion of all species present in the community increases, and NAR becomes weaker and essentially disappears (Fig. 18.3b, c). These patterns in NAR are independent of dynamical processes operating in the community (Herben *et al.*, 2004).

The neutral process predicts a positive NAR only if communities being compared are of different numbers of individuals, as also shown by Shea and Chesson (2002). Positive NAR is a result of general dependence of the number of species on the number of individuals and/or area. Variation of the number of individuals in the community is predicted by the neutral model to be the prime determinant of the sign of the NAR (Fig. 18.3). The neutral model predicts a negative NAR for small plots where there is little variation in size, while positive NAR for large plots with considerable variation in size. The strength of the positive NAR increases as differences in community size increase.

The variation in number of individuals is also a critical difference between small-scale and large-scale studies. Most biological variables have skewed distributions where variance increases with the mean (e.g. McCullagh & Nelder, 1989). The same applies to data on community richness and invasibility. In these data, this variance/mean relationship has two main sources. First, variation in

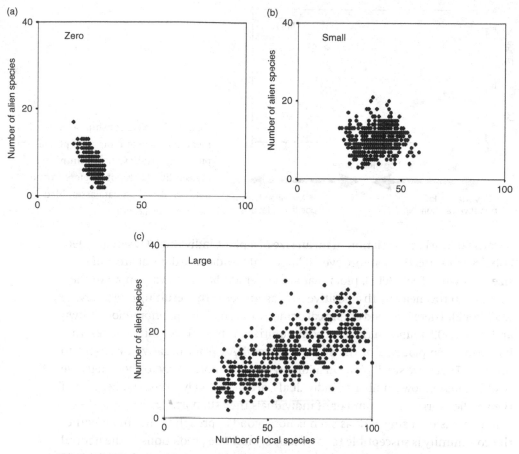

**Figure 18.3** Relationship between number of alien species and number of native species at equilibrium for communities of different size variation (500 realizations of simulated data for each community size). (a) Zero – number of individuals fixed at 50; (b) small – number of individuals sampled from the range 50–100; (c) large – number of individuals sampled from the range 50–200. Disturbance = 0.5, local replacement rate = 0.5; pool of alien species 10 000, pool of native species 500. All species are identical except immigration rates of alien species are 100 times lower than those of native species. Note the same scaling in all three plots; 500 realizations of each parameter combination. Based on data from Herben *et al.* (2004).

plot sizes is an inevitable result of the way data are collected in such studies. This has the following reason: while small-scale studies are often done on plots of deliberately fixed sizes and thus no noticeable size variation, large-scale studies rely on observational data sets often collected at physiographic or political units of variable sizes (Planty-Tabacchi *et al.*, 1996; Lonsdale, 1999; Pyšek *et al.*, 2002). Analysis of published data sets on NAR indeed shows that the range of plot sizes systematically increases with the mean plot size (Fig. 18.4). Second, plot size is not directly related to the number of individuals in the community (Zobel & Liira, 1997; Pärtel & Zobel, 1999). Their relationship is not straightforward

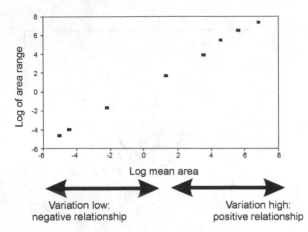

Figure 18.4 Relationship between the mean plot size and range of plot sizes in published studies on community invasibility. Each point refers to one data set. Based on data assembled by Herben *et al.* (2004).

because of the large variation in mean size of a plant individual (Oksanen, 1996; Zobel & Liira, 1997). Therefore even if large-scale studies are done at areas of fixed sizes (Brown & Peet, 2003), plots that are larger are bound to vary more in their spatial heterogeneity, with a positive NAR again being the resulting effect (Levine *et al.*, 2002). There is a good empirical demonstration of this phenomenon: Brown and Peet (2003) found, in riparian communities in the eastern United States, that increasing the plot size of the study changed NAR from negative or absent to positive. Therefore small plots, in addition to being more likely to show negative NAR because of low number of individuals, are more likely to show it because of the smaller variation in number of individuals they support.

In conclusion, using NAR as such is not a good approach to identify whether the community is susceptible to invasions or not. The predictions of the neutral model, however, can be used as a kind of null hypothesis against which the field data can be compared (Fridley *et al.*, 2004).

## Species pool and number of alien species: mass effect

Ambiguity of the concept of species richness (i.e. whether it is a response variable or a community parameter) is often treated by breaking richness down into two components: (1) local species richness, and (2) species pool. While the distinction is to some extent conventional, there is an important difference that is captured by it. Species richness is just the number of species per unit area; species pool is a set of species whose propagules can reach the community in reasonable time and therefore are the source of species that were able to prevail at the given habitat (Zobel, 1997). Local species richness is primarily determined by processes operating within a community, such as constraints of interactions between individuals and species or statistical constraints as those dealt with in the previous section. As a result, variation in species richness largely reflects the variation of factors that determine intensity of competition or other interactions within the community, intensity of disturbance, etc.; species richness itself is then better seen as a dependent variable. In contrast, species pool comprises species that do not necessarily co-occur physically in one community, but are available for immigration into that community. The size of the species pool therefore reflects primarily constraints of migration and evolution of species and is often treated as an independent variable for local species richness. If local richness is determined primarily by the species pool size, the species–area relationships for different species pool sizes are essentially parallel (Bartha & Ittzés, 2001). In contrast, if local processes of coexistence play an important role in addition to the species pool size, local richness at small scales will converge independently of the species pool size.

The distinction between local species richness and species pool should be taken into consideration wherever large differences in species pools across habitats are likely to occur. This is typically the case of oceanic islands/continents, or isolated/nonisolated islands contrasts, but is likely to be involved in many contrasts at mainland habitats as well (see e.g. Ewald, 2003). In the context of invasion ecology, the definition of the species pool of invasive plants is particularly tricky. It can be defined in two ways. It may include all potentially alien species (including those that have not yet crossed the dispersal barriers); then the alien species pool is very large, but the immigration probabilities are very low. Alternatively, one may include only species that have already crossed the dispersal barrier (i.e. alien species already occurring in the area, although not necessarily in the community itself).

Distinction between local species richness and species pool is also inherent in neutral models, no matter whether species pool is modeled as a constant (e.g. Hubbell, 1979; Bartha & Ittzés, 2001) or as a dynamic variable (e.g. Hubbell, 2001). If all species have identical immigration rates, local species richness is necessarily a function of the size of species pool (see Bartha & Ittzés, 2001, for a thorough analysis of the issue). This should have implications for NAR relationship; in particular, the size of the species pool and immigration rates should also have a strong effect on the predicted NAR relationship. First, if the species pool is small relative to the number of individuals in the community (e.g. on oceanic islands), random drawing of individuals produces communities that contain most of the species from the species pool. Therefore the constraint of the number of individuals on local community richness becomes weaker. As a result, the intensity of NAR decreases and it eventually goes to zero as the proportion of species represented in the local community approaches unity. If all species from one of the species pools are already present, NAR is bound to be exactly zero.

If species pools and immigration rates of native and alien species differ, this "saturation" begins to play a role at different community sizes for each of the species sets. In such a case, species from the species pool with larger immigration rates are more likely to establish in the community than those from the other species pool. The community then contains a larger proportion out of all species from that species pool even at rather small community sizes; further increase in community size does not add many more species from that species pool, but is still adding species from the species with lower immigration. This generates a nonlinear shape of the NAR. The degree of nonlinearity is a measure of combined difference in immigration rates and species pools of these two species groups (T. Herben, unpublished data). In the real world, the species pool of aliens is likely to be larger, because of many more species being available in geographically distant habitats in the same climatic zone than in the local species pool, but the species have on average a much lower immigration rate. The local species pool may be smaller, but its species have a much higher immigration rate. It is therefore likely that at certain community sizes most species from the native species pool are already represented, while alien species are still available for immigration. If this is the case, the nonlinear shape of NAR should result. Since the shape of NAR can be established empirically, it can be used as a means to assess relative size of these species pools and immigration probabilities.

### Invasibility of islands: sampling effects and the species pool size

Empirical examination of species pool effects has to work with communities with varying species pools (Pärtel *et al.*, 1996). However, ecologically meaningful operational definitions of species pools are difficult in most cases (Wilson & Anderson, 2001). Islands are good examples of the variation in the species pool. The low number of species on islands is typically manifested by higher average slopes of the species–area relationships if islands of different sizes are compared (Rosenzweig, 1995). This means that smaller islands are more impoverished relative to mainland plots of the same size, primarily due to restricted immigration to small and/or isolated islands (MacArthur & Wilson, 1967). Species pool differences may be thought of as reflecting the long-term difference in immigration rates to the island (which may, or need not be, at equilibrium). A steeper species–area relationship at the whole island level, however, does not necessarily mean that island communities are more species poor at a finer (within-island) scale. The effect of the smaller size of the species pool at smaller islands may be compensated, for example, by larger niche breadths of species involved ("ecological release"; Case, 1974; Kitayama & Mueller-Dombois, 1995).

Oceanic islands are typically more invasible by alien species compared with mainland (Lonsdale, 1999; Sax, 2001; Denslow, 2003). This has been extensively documented for plants (Lonsdale, 1999), birds (Case, 1996; but see Sol, 2000) as well as for other groups (Gaston *et al.*, 2003). Many functional explanations of this phenomenon (introduction of herbivores, different fire regimes) have been proposed (Courchamp, Chapuis & Pascal, 2003). While these explanations are likely to be responsible for an important part of the variation in island invasibility, they often deal with rather specific phenomena that cannot be applied universally to all island habitats.

The major difference between islands and continents does not reside in their contrasting species richness, but the fact that an island community represents a smaller sample of the set of potential species for the given set of habitat conditions. Invasibility of islands should therefore be analyzed in terms of the differences in species pools, not in differences in local species richness of the invaded community. (Local species richness is also less straightforward to address given the statistical constraints addressed in previous chapters.) Although island species pools are dynamic over a sufficiently long timescale, they may be treated as a static fixed number for the purpose of assessing invasibility, as recent immigration rates of alien species are likely to be much higher due to massive propagule input in the past few centuries (see e.g. Gaston *et al.*, 2003).

In general, species pool may have two different effects on community invasibility. First, it may be the sheer mass effect (see the previous section). The mass effect, however, will be important if immigration rates are high; if most recruitment takes place within the community (as is generally the case), its contribution will be negligible. Second, further effects may appear if the species in the species pool are not identical. If there is a variation in a certain trait among species, size of the species pool ultimately determines the range of variation in traits in these species. In a larger pool, the likelihood of finding a better adapted species or a better competitor for a given set of conditions is higher (Huston, 1997; Tilman, Lehman & Thomson, 1997). This issue has been extensively addressed in studies of the relationship between biodiversity and ecosystem functioning ("chance" or "sampling effect"; Lepš *et al.*, 2001; Hector *et al.*, 2002; Aarssen, Laird & Pither, 2003).

Such effect could also affect general patterns of invasibility due to differences in size of the native species pool (as a consistent difference between islands and continents) and can be examined by a generalized version of the model above. The important difference here is that it should permit some type of species differences in order that the sampling effect can take place. Here I use the assumption of varying population growth rates among species (see Herben, 2005; and the Appendix). This makes possible, in rather general terms, to account for species sorting by environmental conditions at a habitat and therefore for a fit between community composition and environment which is so prevalent in ecological systems. Population growth rates are used as a proxy for the ability of the species to thrive in its environment relative to other species and should be understood in relative terms within the given environment. The neutral model with growth rates identical in all species (the one used in the previous two sections) is used as a reference. Again, the only difference between native and alien species is that no aliens are allowed in the initial species composition of the community: the native community is first allowed to develop by random drawing of species from the native species pool for some time. Only then the alien species are allowed to establish together with native species. Then the model predicts invasibility of communities as a function of their species pool size and the parameters of the lottery.

The results show that the model with a nonzero variation in population growth rates consistently predicted a higher proportion of alien species and, particularly, higher proportion of individuals of alien species if local species pools were small (Fig. 18.5; Herben, 2005). The strength of the effect depended on the coefficient of variation of population growth rates (Fig. 18.5); the higher the coefficient, the higher is the sampling effect of the species pools on invasibility. The longer time the community had to sample from the native species pool, the higher was its resistance to invasion (data not shown here). Such patterns could in principle be addressed by empirical data.

This shows that if there is a variation in population growth rates, the sampling process is sufficient to explain higher invasibility of communities with smaller pools of native species. Sampling over a sufficiently long period from a sufficiently large species pool produces a community of native species with higher than average population growth rates. Such assemblage is therefore much more likely to block establishment of a randomly drawn invader, because the invader's population growth rate is on average lower than that of most species already present in the community. The invasibility thus decreases with the increasing species pool and the time period over which sampling from the local pool can take place. In reality, one may assume that an invader might have undergone a similar sampling process and therefore will have a larger potential growth rate. This would make the effect even stronger.

The species sorting according to their population growth rates tends to produce communities with higher skew in their abundance distribution as they become dominated by a few highly successful (i.e. fast growing) species (see also Bell, 2000). Nonzero variation in population growth rates changes abundance distribution curves to become more steep (median of the Simpson's index changes from 0.02 for the fully neutral model to 0.72 for the model with $CV(r) = 0.99$). Highly successful cases of massive invasions were therefore more likely when the abundance distribution of the community was rather flat, with no major dominant (Fig. 18.6).

The relationship between species pool and invasibility has rarely been explicitly addressed. In most field data sets, data are collected at only one scale and the effects of species pool thus cannot be separated from those of local species richness (see e.g. Pärtel et al., 1996; Wilson and Anderson, 2001; Grace, 2001). Data sampled at smaller scales generally provide only local richness data without any information on species pools (e.g. Davis, Grime & Thompson, 2000; Kennedy et al., 2002; Fargione, Brown & Tilman, 2003). This is clearly due to the difficulty in estimating species pools in field studies. Smith and Knapp (2001) showed that species pool does have a strong effect on invasibility; communities with larger species pools were less invasible. By contrast, large-scale data are

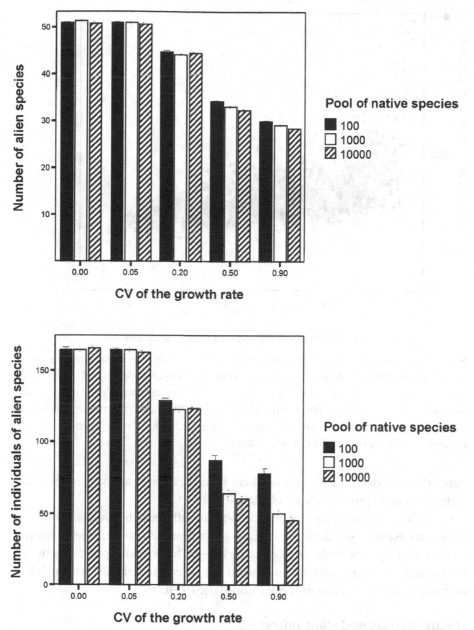

**Figure 18.5** The effect of the size of the pool of native species on the number of species and number of individuals of aliens. Other parameters: proportion of local replacement $= 0.9$, alien species pool $= 500$, number of individuals $= 500$, duration of invasion $= 10$ steps, number of steps before invasion began $= 100$. Bars indicate 1 s.e.; 500 realizations of each parameter combination. In order to separate sampling from mass effect, immigration probability is constant per total species pool. CV, coefficient of variation. Based on data from Herben (2005).

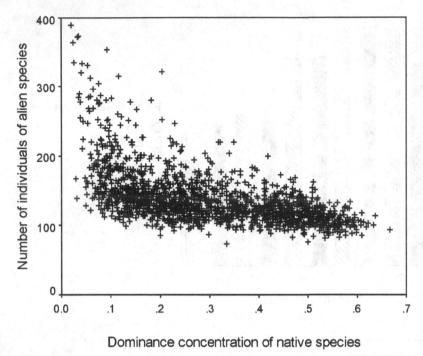

Dominance concentration of native species

**Figure 18.6** Relationship between dominance structure of native species (Simpson's index) and the number of individuals of alien species. Number of steps before species from the alien pool are allowed to establish = 100, alien species pool = 500, number of individuals = 500, duration of invasion = 100 steps, coefficient of variation of species population growth rates = 0.5, local replacement proportion = 0.7; 500 realizations of each parameter combination. Based on data from Herben (2005).

generally collected on larger plots where species richness and species pool are difficult to distinguish (see e.g. Lonsdale, 1999).

Size of species pools may also be an important difference between oceanic and terrestrial (habitat) islands; as migration is generally much easier between habitat islands, their species pools are likely to be larger. This would explain why terrestrial islands of any habitat type, in contrast to true oceanic islands, are much less affected by invasions of alien species (Lonsdale, 1999).

## Neutral models and plant individuals

If predictions of neutral models are to be compared with field patterns in a more quantitative fashion, data on numbers of individuals are necessary to assess whether the process could operate in the field (see also Oksanen, 1996). In the present case, the neutral process produces strong and negative NAR only if numbers of (independent) individuals per community are small enough (below 200, depending on the species pool size). A typical study reporting a negative NAR is done in grasslands at plots of $1\,m^2$ or smaller (Herben et al., 2004). Published data on numbers of shoots per $1\,m^2$ in grasslands range over three orders of magnitude (15–15 000; see Herben *et al.*, 2004). Assuming that an average tussock (the "independent" individual) is composed of several tens of shoots, numbers of independent sampling units in a grassland may thus range around a few hundred per $m^2$. This may already be sufficient for neutral effects to play a role.

Zobel and Liira (1997) demonstrated persuasively that the number of individuals must be known to assess diversity patterns in plants. This is often a problem in plant ecology, as numbers of individuals are rarely recorded (with a notable exception of forestry and tree research). A complicating issue for neutral and similar models is that plant individuals (shoots) are often not independent units due to ubiquitous clonal growth or short-distance dispersal and resulting intraspecific spatial aggregation; autocorrelation of species identity is typically quite high. However, a more careful analysis may help to identify "independent" individuals; the number of such individuals can be used as a model parameter and different communities can be compared based on them.

## Conclusions

The models show that many general patterns in invasion ecology can be explained by neutral or statistical processes and no specific traits of invasive species or parameters of invaded communities have to be assumed (Herben *et al.*, 2004; Fridley *et al.*, 2004). This does not necessarily mean that the patterns found are statistical artifacts that are of no relevance for ecological systems. In contrast, major mechanisms discussed here, i.e. sampling from species pools of different sizes, constraint on number of individuals and variation in growth rates among species, are present in some form in all ecological systems. Although their representation by the null model is simplistic, constraints similar to those shown by the neutral models are inevitable in any ecological system (Oksanen, 1996; Pärtel & Zobel, 1999; Zobel, 2001). This obviously does not mean that invasions as ecological process are irrelevant; cases of individual invasions will remind us painfully of the opposite. It only means that analysis of large assemblages shows patterns that are often dominated by signals produced by statistical processes. Biological explanations should then be sought only for patterns not explained by null models of these processes (Fridley *et al.*, 2004).

## Acknowledgments

This chapter greatly benefited from discussions with Kateřina Bímová, Deborah Goldberg, Bohumil Mandák, Zuzana Münzbergová, Valerio De Patta Pillar, Petr Pyšek, Marcel Rejmánek and David Storch. I also thank Pablo Marquet, Petr Pyšek, David Storch and an anonymous referee for critical comments on an earlier draft of this chapter. The research was supported by the GA ČR grant no. 206/04/0081.

## Appendix 18.I    The modeling approach

*The model*

Simulations are done by a simple simulation model of community assembly and dynamics invasion. It is based on random drawing from two distinct species pools (native and alien) into a local community and simulating disturbance, local growth and later immigration into this local community.

There is no difference between species coming from the pool of native species and those from the pool of aliens, except that alien and native species are allowed to have a different rate of immigration into the local community ($m_{alien} \neq m_{native}$) and sizes of the pools may be different ($P_{native} \neq P_{alien}$). If mass effect of species pool is not of interest (see section on "Invasibility of islands"), the immigration probability summed over all species was kept constant by changing values of immigration rates according to the size of the respective species pool ($m_{native}\, P_{native} = $ const., and $m_{alien}\, P_{alien} = $ const.).

In the version with varying population growth rates, population growth rate of each species (both native and alien) was drawn from the gamma distribution with a mean of 1 and a coefficient of variation which is one of the model parameters (for the summary of model parameters, see Table 18.1). Gamma distribution was used as a general distribution that generates skewed distributions of many biological variables (McCullagh & Nelder, 1989). Mean growth rate does not affect the model as all growth rates are relative in a null model with a fixed community size. Identical variation in growth rates was used both in native and alien species.

At the beginning of each simulation, a new local community is initialized by drawing $N$ individuals (community size) of the local community from the species pool of native species; the probability of an individual of the $i$th species being drawn is thus $1/P_{native}$, where $P_{native}$ is the size of the native species pool. Drawing is done with replacement, i.e. several individuals may be drawn from one species.

Three processes operate in the local community at each step: disturbance, local replacement, and immigration. To model disturbance, $dN$ individuals are randomly removed from the local community at each step ($0 < d < 1$); each individual has equal probability to be removed irrespective of species. Fractional numbers of individuals are rounded to the nearest integer. The individuals removed by disturbance are then replaced by local replacement (i.e. population growth of species already present) and by immigration. The local replacement, i.e. multiplication of species already present in the local community that survived the disturbance event, is simulated by drawing $l\, d\, N$ individuals from species already present in the community ($0 < l < 1$). The probability of drawing an individual from a species is a function of frequency of that species and of its population growth rate; the probability of an individual of the

**Table 18.1** *Parameters used by the simulation model; default values/values used in most simulations shown in boldface*

| Parameter | Symbol | Values used |
|---|---|---|
| Community size (number of individuals) | $N$ | **500**, 2000 |
| Number of species in the species pool of native species | $P_{native}$ | **100**, **1000**, **10 000** |
| Number of species in the species pool of aliens | $P_{alien}$ | **500**, **5000** |
| Disturbance rate (number of individuals removed from the community at each step) | $d$ | **0.1**, 0.3, 0.5, 0.7 |
| Proportion of local replacement (fraction of vacant positions filled by growth of species already present in the community) | $l$ | 0.2, **0.5**, 0.7, **0.9**, 0.99 |
| Rate of immigration of local species into the local community[a] | $m_{native}$ | **0.5**, **0.05**, **0.005** |
| Rate of immigration of alien species into the local community[a] | $m_{alien}$ | **0.1**, 0.01 |
| Coefficient of variation of species relative population growth rates | $CV(r)$ | 0, 0.05, 0.2, **0.5**, 0.7, 0.99 |
| Number of steps before alien species are allowed to arrive | | **1**, **5**, **10**, **100**, **300** |
| Number of steps after alien species are allowed to arrive | | 5, **100** |

[a] Values changed together with the species pool size in order to keep the immigration probability summed over all species in the species pool constant.

$i$th species being drawn is thus $\frac{r_i N_i}{\sum_j r_j N_j}$, where $N_i$ is the number of individuals of the $i$th species in the community after the disturbance event and $r_i$ is its (relative) population growth rate; the summation is done over all species in the local community. These individuals can be either native or alien provided they were present in the community prior to the disturbance ($N_i > 0$). Species not present in the community have zero probability to be drawn here.

The remaining individuals, i.e. $(1 - l) d N$ individuals, are replaced by immigration from outside the community, i.e. from both species pools. Initially, only species from the native species pool can immigrate; the probability of an individual of the $i$th species being drawn is then $1/P_{native}$. After a specified number of steps (which is one of the model parameters), individuals of alien species can also immigrate; the probability of an individual of the $i$th species being drawn is then $\frac{m_i}{m_{native}P_{native} + m_{alien}P_{alien}}$, where $m_{native}$ and $m_{alien}$ are relative immigration rates of native and alien species respectively, and $P_{alien}$ is the size of alien species pool; $m_i$ equals $m_{alien}$ and $m_{native}$ for alien and native species, respectively. No account is taken of whether the species to which the individual drawn belongs is already present in the community. Individuals are drawn from the species pools with replacement (i.e. several individuals may be drawn from one species); this process determines the abundance distribution of species in the community.

As a result of these processes, numbers of species present in the local community and their abundances reflect identical rules of disturbance, immigration and ecological drift (stochastic variation due to low numbers) under the constraints of varying population growth rates.

# References

Aarssen, L. W., Laird, R. A. & Pither, J. (2003). Is the productivity of vegetation plots higher or lower when there are more species? Variable predictions from interaction of the "sampling effect" and "competitive dominance effect" on the habitat templet. *Oikos*, **102**, 427–432.

Bartha, S. & Ittzés P. (2001). Local richness-species pool ratio: a consequence of the species-area relationship. *Folia Geobotanica*, **36**, 9–23.

Bell, G. (2000). The distribution of abundance in neutral communities. *American Naturalist*, **155**, 606–617.

Brown, R. L. & Peet, R. K. (2003). Diversity and invasibility of southern Appalachian plant communities. *Ecology*, **84**, 32–39.

Burke, M. J. W. & Grime, J. P. (1996). An experimental study of plant community invasibility. *Ecology*, **77**, 776–790.

Byers, J. E. & Noonburg, E. G. (2003). Scale dependent effects of biotic resistance to biological invasion. *Ecology*, **84**, 1428–1433.

Case, T. J. (1974). Interference competition and niche theory. *Proceedings of the National Academy of Sciences of the United States of America*, **71**, 3073.

Case, T. J. (1990). Invasion resistance arises in strongly interacting species-rich model competition communities. *Proceedings of the National Academy of Sciences of the United States of America*, **87**, 9610–9614.

Case, T. J. (1996). Global patterns in establishment of exotic birds. *Biological Conservation*, **78**, 69–96.

Courchamp, F., Chapuis, J. L. & Pascal, M. (2003). Mammal invaders on islands: impact, control and control impact. *Biological Reviews*, **78**, 347–383.

Davis, M. A., Grime, J. P. & Thompson, K. (2000). Fluctuating resources in plant communities: a general theory of invasibility. *Journal of Ecology*, **88**, 528–534.

Denslow, J. S. (2003). Weeds in paradise: thoughts on the invasibility of tropical islands. *Annals of Missouri Botanical Garden*, **90**, 119–127.

Elton, C. S. (1958). *The Ecology of Invasions by Animals and Plants*. London: Methuen.

Ewald, J. (2003). The calcareous riddle: Why are there so many calciphilous species in the central European flora? *Folia Geobotanica*, **38**, 357–366.

Fargione, J., Brown, C. S. & Tilman, D. (2003). Community assembly and invasion: an experimental test of neutral versus niche processes. *Proceedings of the National Academy of Sciences of the United States of America*, **100**, 8916–8920.

Fox, M. D. & Fox, B. J. (1986). The susceptibility of natural communities to invasion. In *Ecology of Biological Invasions, an Australian Perspective*, ed. R. H. Groves & J. J. Burdon, pp. 57–66. Canberra: Australian Academy of Science.

Fridley, J. D., Brown, R. L. & Bruno, J. F. (2004). Null models of exotic invasion and scale-dependent patterns of native and exotic species richness. *Ecology*, **85**, 3215–3222.

Gaston, K. J., Jones, A. G., Hanel, C. & Chown, S. L. (2003). Rates of species introduction to a remote oceanic island. *Proceedings of the Royal Society of London, Series B*, **270**, 1091–1098.

Grace, J. B. (2001). Difficulties with estimating and interpreting species pools and the implications for understanding patterns of diversity. *Folia Geobotanica*, **36**, 71–83.

Groves, R. H. (1989). Ecological control of invasive terrestrial plants. In *Biological Invasions: a Global Perspective*, ed. J. A. Drake, H. A. Mooney, F. di Castri, *et al.*, pp. 437–461. Chichester: John Wiley.

Hector, A., Bazeley-White, E., Loreau, M., Otway, S. & Schmid, B. (2002). Overyielding in grassland communities: testing the sampling effect hypothesis with replicated biodiversity experiments. *Ecology Letters*, **5**, 502–511.

Herben, T. (2005). Species pool size and invasibility of island communities: a null model of sampling effects. *Ecology Letters*, **8**, 909–917.

Herben, T., Mandák, B., Bímová, K. & Münzbergová, Z. (2004). Invasibility and species richness of a community: a neutral model and a survey of published data. *Ecology*, **85**, 3223–3233.

Hubbell, S. P. (1979). Tree dispersion, abundance, and diversity in a tropical dry forest. *Science*, **203**, 1299–1309.

Hubbell, S. P. (2001). *The Unified Neutral Theory of Biodiversity and Biogeography*. Princeton: Princeton University Press.

Huston, M. A. (1997). Hidden treatments in ecological experiments: re-evaluating the ecosystem function of biodiversity. *Oecologia*, **108**, 449–460.

Kennedy, T. A., Naeem, S., Howe, K. M., Knops, J. M. H., Tilman, D. & P. Reich. (2002). Biodiversity as a barrier to ecological invasion. *Nature*, **417**, 636–638.

Kitayama, K. & Mueller-Dombois, D. (1995). Biological invasion on an oceanic island mountain – do alien plant-species have wider ecological ranges than native species. *Journal of Vegetation Science*, **6**, 667–674.

Law, R. & Morton, R. D. (1996). Permanence and the assembly of ecological communities. *Ecology*, **77**, 762–775.

Lepš, J., Brown, V. K., Len, T. A. D., *et al.* (2001). Separating the chance effect from other diversity effects in the functioning of plant communities. *Oikos*, **92**, 123–134.

Levin, S. A. (1989). Analysis of risk for invasions and control programs. In *Biological Invasions: a Global Perspective*, ed. J. A. Drake, H. A. Mooney, F. di Castri, *et al.*, pp. 425–435. Chichester: John Wiley.

Levine, J. (2000). Species diversity and biological invasions: relating local process to community pattern. *Science*, **288**, 852–854.

Levine, J. M., Kennedy, T. & Naeem, S. (2002). Neighborhood scale effects of species diversity on biological invasions and their relationship to community patterns. In *Biodiversity and Ecosystem Functioning: Synthesis and Perspectives*, ed. M. Loreau, S. Naeema & P. Inchausti, pp. 79–91. Oxford: Oxford University Press.

Lodge, D. M. (1993). Biological invasions: lessons for ecology. *Trends in Ecology and Evolution*, **8**, 133–137.

Lonsdale, W. M. (1999). Global patterns of invasions and the concept of invasibility. *Ecology*, **80**, 1522–1536.

MacArthur, R. H. & Wilson, E. O. (1967). *The Theory of Island Biogeography*. Princeton: Princeton University Press.

May, R. M. (1973). *Stability and Complexity in Model Ecosystems*. Princeton: Princeton University Press.

McCullagh, P. & Nelder, J. A. (1989). *Generalized Linear Models*. London: Chapman & Hall.

Mooney, H. A. & Drake, J. A. (eds.) (1986). *Ecology of Biological Invasions of North America and Hawaii*. New York: Springer.

Moore, J. L., Mouquet, N., Lawton, J. H. & Loreau, M. (2001). Coexistence, saturation and invasion resistance in simulated plant assemblages. *Oikos*, **94**, 303–314.

Mouquet, N., Moore, J. L. & Loreau, M. (2002). Plant species richness and community productivity: why the mechanism that promotes coexistence matters. *Ecology Letters*, **5**, 56–65.

Naeem, S., Knops, J. M. H., Tilman, D., Howe, K. M., Kennedy, T. & Gale, S. (2000). Plant diversity increases resistance to invasion in the absence of covarying factors. *Oikos*, **91**, 97–108.

Oksanen, J. (1996). Is the humped relationship between species richness and biomass an artefact due to plot size? *Journal of Ecology*, **84**, 293–295.

Pärtel, M. & Zobel, M. (1999). Small-scale plant species richness in calcareous grasslands determined by the species pool, community age and shoot density. *Ecography*, **22**, 153–159.

Pärtel, M., Zobel, M., Zobel, K. & van der Maarel, E. (1996). The species pool and its relation to species richness: evidence from Estonian plant communities. *Oikos*, **75**, 111–117.

Pickard, J. (1984). Exotic plants on Lord Howe Island: distribution in time and space 1853–1981. *Journal of Biogeography*, **11**, 181–208.

Planty-Tabacchi, A. M., Tabacchi, E., Naiman, R. J., Deferrari, C. & Decamps, H. (1996). Invasibility of species-rich communities in riparian zones. *Conservation Biology*, **10**, 598–607.

Prieur-Richard, A. H. and Lavorel, S. (2000). Invasions: the perspective of diverse plant communities. *Australian Ecology*, **25**, 1–7.

Pyšek, P., Jarošík, V. & Kučera, T. (2002). Patterns of invasion in temperate nature reserves. *Biological Conservation*, **104**, 13–24.

Pyšek, P., Richardson, D. M. & Williamson, M. (2004). Predicting and explaining plant invasions through analysis of source area floras: some critical considerations. *Diversity and Distributions*, **10**, 179–187.

Rejmánek, M. & Richardson, D. M. (1996). What attributes make some plant species more invasive? *Ecology*, **77**, 1655–1661.

Rejmánek, M., Richardson, D. M. & Pyšek P. (2005). Plant invasions and invasibility of plant communities. In *Vegetation Ecology*, ed. E. Van Der Maarel. Oxford: Blackwell.

Rosenzweig, M. (1995). *Species Diversity in Space and Time*. Cambridge: Cambridge University Press.

Sax, D. F. (2001). Latitudinal gradients and geographic ranges of exotic species: implications for biogeography. *Journal of Biogeography*, **28**, 139–150.

Sax, D. F. (2002). Native and naturalized plant diversity are positively correlated in scrub communities of California and Chile. *Diversity and Distributions*, **8**, 193–210.

Shea, K. & Chesson, P. (2002). Community ecology theory as a framework for biological invasions. *Trends in Ecology and Evolution*, **17**, 170–176.

Smith, M. D. & Knapp, A. K. (2001). Size of the local species pool determines invasibility of a C-4-dominated grassland. *Oikos*, **92**, 55–61.

Sol, D. (2000). Are islands more susceptible to be invaded than continents? Birds say no. *Ecography*, **23**, 687–692.

Stohlgren, T. J., Chong, G. W., Schell, L. D., *et al.* (2002). Assessing vulnerability to invasion by nonnative plant species at multiple spatial scales. *Environmental Management*, **29**, 566–577.

Tilman, D. (1997). Community invasibility, recruitment limitation, and grassland biodiversity. *Ecology*, **78**, 81–92.

Tilman, D., Lehman, C. & Thomson, K. T. (1997). Plant diversity and ecosystem productivity: theoretical considerations. *Proceedings of the National Academy of Sciences of the United States of America*, **94**, 1857–1861.

Wilson, J. B. & Anderson, B. J. (2001). Species-pool relations: like a wooden light bulb? *Folia Geobotanica*, **36**, 35–44.

Zobel, M. (1997). The relative role of species pools in determining plant species richness: an alternative explanation of species coexistence? *Trends in Ecology and Evolution*, **12**, 266–269.

Zobel, K. (2001). On the species-pool hypothesis and on the quasi-neutral concept of plant community diversity. *Folia Geobotanica*, **36**, 3–8.

Zobel, K. & Liira, J. (1997). A scale-independent approach to the richness vs biomass relationship in ground-layer plant communities. *Oikos*, **80**, 325–332.

# CHAPTER NINETEEN

# Extinction and population scaling

WILLIAM E. KUNIN
*University of Leeds*

## Introduction

Arguably, the most important development in ecology in the past few decades has been the discovery of space. The spatial structure of populations and their interactions has become increasingly central to our understanding of ecological dynamics, revolutionizing many areas of both theory and application (e.g. Tilman & Kareiva, 1997). While this is true of all organisms, spatial aspects of population biology are particularly apparent in sessile organisms such as plants. Plant populations are spatially complex, with individuals typically clustered within patches that are themselves aggregated in habitats that are patchily distributed in space. Despite attempts to define the "natural" scale of patchiness (reviewed in Dale, 1999), most populations I know of appear aggregated at virtually any spatial scale. This greatly complicates the description of the abundance and distribution of species, as most of the useful measures are intrinsically scale bound. Indeed, many different aspects of abundance can be reflected by grid occupancy at some appropriate scale of resolution (Kunin, 1998). Thus the extent of a species' geographic range reflects its coarse-scale distribution, whereas population size or cover reflects fine-scale abundance, with factors such as the number of discrete subpopulations or habitat specialization being reflected at intermediate scales.

In an attempt to summarize such spatially complex patterns, the area occupied by a species may be plotted at multiple spatial scales on logarithmic axes, into a "scale area curve" that could summarize abundance scaling. These curves were renamed "range–area relationships" (or RAR) by Harte and colleagues (e.g. Ostling, Harte & Green, 2000; see also Harte, this volume) to emphasize the links to the species–area relationship (SAR), and indeed the SAR can be thought of as the sum of the RARs of all the species present (e.g. Storch, Šizling & Gaston, 2003; Šizling & Storch, 2004). For the purposes of this chapter, however, the important value of the RAR is as an efficient way to capture the spatial pattern of a population's abundance across spatial scales: the height of the RAR at any arbitrary scale reflects the amount of area occupied at that scale, whereas the slope of the curve reflects the degree of aggregation of that occupancy.

*Scaling Biodiversity*, ed. David Storch, Pablo A. Marquet and James H. Brown. Published by Cambridge University Press. © Cambridge University Press 2007.

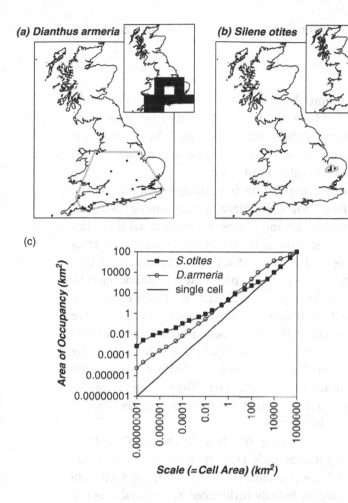

(a) Dianthus armeria   (b) Silene otites

(c)

**Figure 19.1** Spatial scaling of species abundance. The distribution of (a) the Deptford pink (*D. armeria*) in Britain is much wider but more diffuse than that of (b) the Spanish catchfly (*S. otites*). These patterns are reflected in (c) their range–area relationships (RARs), which show *D. armeria* to be far the commoner of the species at coarse scales, but much the rarer at fine scales. From Hartley and Kunin (2003).

The notion may best be demonstrated by example (Fig. 19.1). We have by now surveyed populations of quite a few British plant species over a range of scales from fractions of a meter to hundreds of kilometers, using stratified random subsampling (Hartley *et al.*, 2004). These curves differ markedly between even closely related species, reflecting different scaling patterns in their abundance. Thus, for example, two of the species we examined were the Spanish catchfly (*Silene otites*) and the Deptford pink (*Dianthus armeria*), two members of the Caryophyllaceae. The UK Red Data Book species *S. otites* is generally considered substantially rarer than the "scarce" *D. armeria* at national scales within Britain (Stewart, Pearman & Preston, 1994; Wigginton, 1999), occupying fewer than one quarter as many 10 km cells within the British national grid, and with a geographic range (measured as the size of the minimum convex polygon containing it) only 1.5% that of its more widespread counterpart. Yet the narrow distribution of *S. otites* is densely occupied, in contrast to the diffuse distribution of *D. armeria*, so that at very fine scales the "rarer" *Silene* is actually some 146 times *commoner* than *Dianthus* (Hartley & Kunin, 2003). To describe abundance, we need to take scale into account.

## Factors influencing scaling

If species distributions differ substantially in their scaling attributes, we should attempt to deduce the reasons for such differences. Too often we seem to be content to describe spatial patterns without explaining them. In the next few paragraphs, I will outline some of the processes that may be at work, before focusing on one of them for the remainder of this chapter.

The first candidate for explaining population patterning is habitat. As the physical environment is spatially complex, populations may inherit their scaling properties from the habitats they inhabit. There is a substantial literature demonstrating the scaling properties of many environmental variables, including for example geomorphology (Turcotte, 1997) and climatic variation (Pelletier, 1997). We can imagine a map of the potential population growth rate ($\lambda$) of a species across space reflecting these underlying abiotic conditions as a contour map or a fractal surface. If we slice through this map at $\lambda = 1$, we would have a map of all areas where the focal species could, in principle, maintain viable populations. For most species, such a map would be spatially complex, if not precisely fractal (indeed, if it includes finite areas of solid habitat, it cannot truly be fractal; see Halley *et al.*, 2004). The scaling properties of such maps might be strongly reflected in the distribution of the species inhabiting them (see also Palmer, this volume).

However, species are unlikely to precisely fill their "niche map". Indeed, many (especially rare) species may inhabit only a tiny fraction of the landscape potentially available to them. Where populations are far short of such constraints, their spatial patterns may be heavily influenced by dispersal, as the descendants of the initial colonists of the landscape spread out into the available terrain. Almost any realistic dispersal function produces a bias for propagules to land close to their source, resulting in some degree of aggregation, but the degree of aggregation may vary greatly; species with powerful dispersal abilities should display rather diffuse aggregations, whereas poorer dispersers may develop tightly clustered populations (see also Borda-de-Água *et al.*, this volume). If, as some ecologists believe, most natural populations are engaged in near-random walks demographically well below their full carrying capacity (e.g. Hubbell, 2001), then such dispersal-limited aggregation may not be a short-lived "transient" but may instead be important throughout a species' career.

Adopting a more deterministic ecological view, one might be tempted to think that this effect of dispersal would fade as species begin to fill up their habitat; but at this stage dispersal takes a different and perhaps equally important role. Limitations in dispersal ability mean that small, isolated patches of available habitat are likely to remain unoccupied by the species, a process that

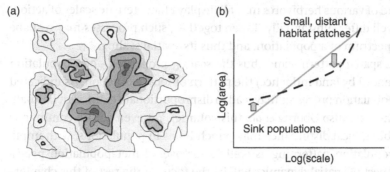

**Figure 19.2** (a) Hypothetical example of a species' niche map, with contour lines representing different values of $\lambda$, with the heavy line indicating $\lambda = 1$; the limit for population growth when rare. Shaded areas are inhabited by the species, with some isolated habitat remaining empty, whereas sink populations may be maintained in nonhabitat close to viable source areas. (b) This may be expressed in terms of RARs, with the gray line representing the RAR of the underlying habitat, and the dashed curve being that of areas actually inhabited.

has been well documented in metapopulation research (e.g. Thomas, Thomas & Warren, 1992). These small isolated patches occupy a larger share of space at coarse scale than they do at finer scales (Fig. 19.2). Conversely, "sink" populations may sometimes be maintained in areas that are not in principle suitable for occupation by the species ($\lambda < 1$) if these areas receive a substantial influx of propagules from more suitable sites. Such sinks will almost of necessity be adjacent to source populations, and so will add area to the map at fine scale, while having little or no impact at coarser scales (Fig. 19.2). Taken together, these two properties will act to make populations rather more spatially clumped than the habitats they inhabit, flattening the range–area relationship.

The population dynamics of such species may also be affected in various ways by the density of the population, but this too is scale specific. Population density is defined as the number of individuals per unit area, and so can depend critically on the size of the unit of area within which it is measured (Smallwood & Schonewald, 1996; Gaston, Blackburn & Gregory, 1999). Different individuals within a population may experience substantially different local population densities; indeed, each can be described as having its own spectrum of scale-specific densities. Various density-dependent interactions (both classical and inverse) may depend on density at different characteristic ranges of spatial scales (Roy & Hastings, 1996). In plants, for example, competition (a classical, negative density feedback) acts at very fine spatial scales, where roots or branches physically overlap. By contrast, pollination (which typically displays inverse density dependence, or Allee effects) may be most sensitive to density at the pollinator's behavioral scale (up to multiple kilometers; Steffan-Dewenter et al., 2002; Westphal, Steffan-Dewenter & Tscharntke, 2003). Similarly, the density-dependent effects of mycorrhizae, of pathogens and of various herbivores may all display characteristic scales of action, which may well differ substantially. Taken together, such processes may reshape the density spectrum of a population, and thus its spatial scaling.

Finally, the spatial pattern – and thus the scaling properties – of a population may be influenced by (and influence) the pattern of local extinction. As indicated above, metapopulation processes may lead to disproportionate extinction in small, isolated patches (see also Oborny *et al.*, this volume). Yet even within continuous swaths of habitat, local disturbance may punch holes in populations, with implications for population patterning as well as for overall metapopulation persistence. This aspect of spatial dynamics will be the focus of the rest of this chapter.

Over the next few pages, I will explore several aspects of the link between scaling and extinction. I will begin by discussing the spatial pattern of local population extinctions, and then explore the implications of such spatially structured extinctions for the persistence of metapopulations. Finally, I will examine how extinctions reshape the spatial pattern of the surviving populations, and how that pattern in turn can be used to estimate the impact of past extinctions and to gauge the risk of future losses.

## Spatial structure in extinction

Local extinctions can be the result of a wide variety of causes, ranging from demographic stochasticity, through interactions with competitors or natural enemies, to extrinsic disturbance. These processes may act on a range of spatial scales (Hartley & Kunin, 2003). This is easiest to demonstrate in the case of disturbance: while some disturbance events (e.g. a single footfall) may act at very fine scales, others (such as the plowing of a field) may occur over tens or hundreds of meters, still others (e.g. storms, plagues or fires) over tens or hundreds of kilometers, and still others (e.g. effects of a meteorite impact or shift in agricultural incentives) acting at continental or even global scales. The result of all but the finest of these disturbance components is that populations near each other in space are disproportionately likely to share the same fate: they are likely either both to be hit, or both to escape damage. The same is true when extinctions are caused by other less abrupt factors. Population fluctuations tend to be spatially correlated, for any of a variety of reasons. For one thing, weather patterns are correlated across space, so that a particularly good or bad period for one population is likely to be similarly good or bad for other populations nearby (in what has been termed the "Moran effect", Royama, 1992). Biotic interactions may also be correlated in space; for example, a pathogen or predator outbreak may spread in a contagious manner across the species' distribution. In addition, even if populations were to initially fluctuate independently, even fairly small amounts of dispersal between populations can serve to synchronize their fluctuations (e.g. Lecomte *et al.*, 2004); and if populations fluctuate synchronously in space, they are likely to wander towards extinction in lockstep. Taken together, all of these factors suggest that the fates of populations should not be independent in space.

So does it happen? Until recently, we didn't know. There has been surprisingly little research performed to date to test the spatial structure of local extinctions. There have been only a few publications purporting to test it, and even these are fraught with methodological confusion. The fact that no two published studies have used the same method makes it difficult to compare their results meaningfully. Indeed, two of the studies (Rodriguez & Delibes, 2002, 2003) come to different conclusions from the same data set! This confusion is understandable; to test for spatial correlations in extinction risk, we must first factor out the spatial structure of the population itself – after all, a population can't become extinct unless it was there in the first place. The solution is to compare the spatial autocorrelation of actual extinctions with randomized data sets with the same number of extinctions distributed at random among previously occupied populations. There are rather subtler methodological issues as well; in particular, a division between equally valid distance-based (e.g. Ripley's K) and neighbor-order based (e.g. Cuzick & Edwards, 1990) methods. These methods differ, most notably, in how they treat a pattern of disproportionate extinction in those regions with the sparsest occupancy. Such patterns are to be expected, as isolated populations may face greater inbreeding (with potential adverse consequences for individual fitness and population viability), and have lower chances of so-called "rescue" from immigration (Brown & Kodric-Brown, 1977). In a neighbor-order based measure, such patterns would be treated as positive spatial autocorrelation (as these populations tend to be each other's closest neighbors); yet a distance-based measure would regard these spatially separated extinctions as evidence of negative spatial correlations.

Recently, one of my colleagues examined the spatial distribution of extinctions in 16 species of British plants, including species chosen to have high dispersal (orchids and wind-dispersed composites) and others chosen for lower dispersal abilities (legumes and non-wind-dispersed composites). His results (McDowall, 2003) suggest that spatial autocorrelations in extinction risk are found in all the species considered, at least at some spatial scales. In general, autocorrelation was more likely to be found using neighbor-order methods than with distance-based measures, presumably because of disproportionate loss of the sparsest parts of the distribution. Moreover, significant autocorrelation was found most often at the finest spatial scales, in part because of declines in statistical power at coarser scales.

Spatial autocorrelation in extinction is observed in some very different systems as well, although it is not always described as such. Detailed observations of local extinction in prairie dog (*Cynomys ludovicianus*) colonies (Stapp, Antolin & Ball, 2004) display clear spatial autocorrelation, due to the spatial spread of disease. Similarly, the spread of invasive predatory mink across Britain has caused spatially correlated extinction of local water vole (*Arvicola terrestris*) populations (Aars *et al.*, 2001). More generally, the distributions of many species have been found to retreat over time to a narrow (and often marginal) residual range (Channell & Lomolino, 2000), implying that spatially structured extinctions apply widely.

## Modeling the implications of spatially structured extinction

If local extinctions are spatially autocorrelated, does it matter? Certainly it ought to raise alarm bells. Classical models of extinction (e.g. Levins, 1969) have generally assumed that both habitat and local extinction are distributed randomly in space. There have been some attempts to explore the implications of spatial structure in habitat (e.g. Fahrig, 1998; With & King, 1999; Flather & Bevers, 2002), but surprisingly few have explicitly explored the implications of spatially structured extinction (but see McCarthy & Lindenmayer, 2000). In this field, at least, practice has sometimes been ahead of theory; the very best applied population viability analyses (e.g. LaHaye, Gutierrez & Akçakaya, 1994; Akçakaya & Atwood, 1997) have sometimes included spatial structure in habitat quality, and thus, implicitly, in extinction risk. Nonetheless, little is known about the general implications of spatial autocorrelation in extinction processes on overall extinction risk.

It seems clear that the effects of spatially structured risk ought to depend somewhat on the spatial structure of the underlying population's habitat. As mentioned above, there is a growing body of theoretical work to suggest that aggregated habitat provides some degree of protection to populations in the face of spatially random disturbance of the sort that is generally modeled. Yet aggregating habitat in the face of spatially structured extinction processes seems a much less desirable option. Doing so puts all of one's demographic eggs in one stochastic basket: by aggregating habitat, it becomes more likely that large fractions – or indeed all – of a species' population may be lost simultaneously. Perhaps a more general formulation about extinction and habitat scaling can be inferred. If randomly scattered populations are particularly vulnerable to random disturbance, and aggregated populations seem likely to be particularly vulnerable to aggregated disturbance, one might hypothesize that, whatever the spatial pattern of a population, it should be most vulnerable to an extinction process with the same scaling properties as the population itself (Hartley & Kunin, 2003).

To test this possibility, my colleague Thanasis Kallimanis worked with me to construct a simulation model of a metapopulation occupying spatially structured habitat and subjected to spatially structured disturbance (Kallimanis *et al.*, 2005). To test the conjecture that populations were most vulnerable to a spectrum of disturbance that scales as they do, we used the same five types of spatial models for both habitat and disturbance. These models ranged from fully random at the scale of single cells, to ones having only fine-scale patchiness, to fractal models with patchiness at all scales, to models with patchiness only at coarse scales, and finally to simulations of blocks of contiguous habitat (or of disturbance).

Simulations were performed with greatly varying levels of habitat availability, ranging from >90% of the arena being habitable to <1% being suitable, and with each habitat pattern tested against all of the different disturbance regimes: some identical in spatial structure to the habitat itself and others very dissimilar to it. The simulations were, of course, fully randomized, so that even when the spatial character of habitat and disturbance were the same, the precise location of the habitat and disturbance were independent. After trying a wide range of dispersal functions, we used exponential functions in the published work (although qualitatively similar results were found for other curves), with characteristic dispersal distances (d) ranging from 1 to 256 cells; that is, from extremely local to near universal. We then monitored the rate of metapopulation extinction in each set of simulations (integrated across the full range of habitat availabilities), and the threshold amount of habitat required for a population to persist.

The results of those simulations (e.g. Fig. 19.3) both confirm established ideas about extinction, and challenge them. When disturbance was modeled as random, as it almost always is in extinction modeling, then aggregating habitat generally reduced extinction risk, as has been found by other researchers (With & King, 1999; Hill & Caswell, 1999; Flather & Bevers, 2002). However, when spatial structure was built into the disturbance process, two important changes occurred. First of all, increasing levels of autocorrelation in disturbance resulted in a substantial increase in metapopulation extinction risk: the same amount of disturbance was much more destructive if the disturbance was aggregated in space. Moreover, the ideal configuration of habitat shifted markedly as the spatial structure of disturbance shifted. As we predicted, blocks of contiguous habitat were not only not the ideal configuration when faced with blocks of disturbance, but they were instead the most vulnerable configuration. Our general prediction that each landscape would be most vulnerable to a disturbance regime that scales like the habitat itself, however, was not borne out by the simulations; fractal landscapes, for example, were relatively invulnerable to fractal disturbance processes. Indeed, fractal habitat mosaics performed fairly well in the face of most disturbance regimes – they were almost as safe as a block of habitat under random disturbance, and they were generally at least as safe as diffusely scattered habitat in the face of block disturbance. The messy, multi-scaled nature of a fractal landscape seems to fare well because it has something for everyone: blocks of contiguous habitat that survive well in the face of fine mists of random disturbance and widely scattered outposts that can escape blocks of disturbance. Perhaps we're one step closer to understanding the answer to the famous "SLOSS" (single large or several small) debate in reserve design (Diamond, 1975; Ovaskainen, 2002; McCarthy, Thompson & Possingham, 2005). Perhaps the choice given was a false dichotomy: neither clumping all the habitat together nor dispersing it all into tiny bits is optimal, but rather a mixture of many sizes ("many mixed?") may do better. The sort of messy

(a)

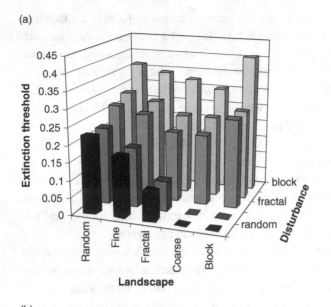

(b)

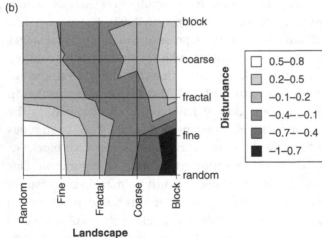

**Figure 19.3.** (a) Representative results of simulations of metapopulation persistence in a spatially structured habitat in the face of spatially structured disturbance. This example shows extinction thresholds (50% persistence for 5000 time steps, estimated by logistic regression) for populations of intermediate ($d = 16$) exponential dispersal distances. Note that the spatial aggregation of disturbance generally increases extinction risk, but does so most dramatically for populations with aggregated habitat. (b) Overall pattern of relative extinction risk in simulations, expressed relative to row means to highlight which landscape is most vulnerable to each disturbance regime. Data from Kallimanis *et al.* (2005).

multiscaled configurations we tend to find in real reserve networks may have accidentally got it right all along.

## Effects of extinction on spatial pattern

So far, I've concentrated on the impact that the spatial pattern of a population can have on its overall extinction risk, but the obverse problem is also of interest: how (local) extinction can affect population pattern. One of the recent issues that has been explored in my laboratory is the biological correlates of scaling patterns; if certain sorts of species consistently show more diffuse (or more clumped) distributions than others, it may give us a clue as to the forces responsible for shaping the distributional differences we see in the biota. We have amassed a data set covering nearly 400 species of rare and scarce British plants, and have compiled data about all manner of seemingly relevant ecological traits for these species – details of their habitat preferences, growth forms, dispersal abilities, their breeding systems, and so on. Many of these traits did in fact prove to be related to distributional pattern, as predicted (Pocock et al., 2006). Nonetheless, the single strongest association was not with any of these morphological or life-history traits, but rather with an historical one: the degree to which the population had experienced local extinctions in its recent past. In general, populations that had experienced substantial rates of recent extinction show much more sparsely dispersed spatial patterns than those that have faced few or none. Parallel work on butterflies (Wilson et al., 2004) revealed much the same pattern: species with expanding ranges tend to show relatively densely clustered distributions, whereas species that have experienced range contraction tend to show sparsely scattered patterns.

The pattern can perhaps best be understood by means of an analogy to waves washing up on a beach. Advancing waves move as a coherent front, but retreating waves leave behind scattered puddles. In the case of retreating populations, these "puddles" probably represent relictual sites where favorable conditions persist within otherwise inhospitable landscapes. Such sites may be too small or isolated to be colonized were the current landscape to be held constant, and so many of these populations are probably doomed in the medium to long term (in the absence of active management); or perhaps some may be large enough to provide long-term security of sorts. Whatever their future fate, they persist for now at least, providing a dim shadow of the species' historical distribution.

## Using spatial pattern to predict extinction risks

If recent extinction is a good predictor of spatial pattern, surely the relationship can be reversed: spatial pattern can be used as an index of recent extinction history. We have tested this idea on the UK butterfly database, mentioned above (Wilson et al., 2004). Not surprisingly, it works: butterfly species with unusually sparse distributions were generally found to be those that had declined recently. The analysis of such patterns using "box-counting" fractal dimensions ($D_B$) requires a bit of care, as in general there is a strong positive relationship between overall occupancy (that is, the fraction of all grid cells occupied by the species) and $D_B$; after all, a single point in an otherwise empty map necessarily has $D_B = 0$, and a completely occupied map must have $D_B = 2$. To factor out this trend, we examined the residuals from a regression of $D_B$ on occupancy, and thus when I refer to an "unusually sparse" distribution, I mean one with an unusually low $D_B$ for its occupancy, or more formally: one with a negative residual. Such methodological details don't matter much, as it turns out; we have also measured spatial pattern using several other well-known indices of dispersion (e.g. Condit's $D_x$ and Ripley's $L$), and the same relationship was found in each case: more diffusely scattered populations tended to be those that had declined in the recent past.

Of course, such a relationship would be of little interest if it was different in each area, so that we could only draw inferences about populations whose histories are already known. Fortunately, the relationship between spatial pattern and population history seems to be more general than that. To test the idea, we used the relationship measured for British butterflies to draw inferences about the butterflies of Flanders, in Belgium. Having already discovered the relationship between the spatial pattern of a British butterfly population and its population trajectory, we applied it directly to predict the trajectory of Flemish butterfly populations from their spatial patterns. Surprisingly, not only did the UK relationship perform well in Flanders, it actually produced better predictions there than it did in the UK, perhaps because of the higher resolution in the data set used there.

But there is one even more exciting prospect in using spatial patterning as an extinction index. Not only can inferences be drawn about past local extinctions, but future extinctions may also be predicted. We examined the spatial patterns of past butterfly surveys in the UK, and tested how well they predicted subsequent local extinction rates. They performed reasonably well, much better than would be expected by chance, although admittedly rather less well than they did in inferring past extinctions. The relationship between spatial pattern and subsequent extinction fits well with the growing body of spatial ecological theory. Small, isolated populations seem disproportionately vulnerable to extinction for a range of reasons: being isolated, they are unlikely to be "rescued" demographically (or genetically) by immigration (Brown & Kodric-Brown, 1977), and are also unlikely to be recolonized subsequently.

The fact that declining populations tend to become sparsely scattered, and that sparsely scattered populations tend to subsequently decline, together suggest a worrying future. Taken together, these two trends suggest the existence of an "extinction vortex" (Gilpin & Soulé, 1986), a positive feedback loop spiraling towards extinction. We may be able to infer and predict dynamics of such populations, but it is a far more vital matter to learn how best to intervene to prevent global extinction of such populations.

## Conclusions

Populations are spatially complex, and the patterns they display are molded by a range of ecological processes. Extinction is arguably one of the most powerful of these. Certainly, there is growing evidence that extinctions are not randomly distributed in space, and that the spatial correlation in risk may have practical consequences for conservation planning. Past extinctions leave predictable marks on the patterning of populations, and the spatial pattern of populations in turn may influence the rate of future losses. The study of extinction scaling is in its infancy, but already it is beginning to reveal intriguing patterns and to make valuable predictions.

# References

Aars, J., Lambin, X., Denny, R. & Griffin, A. C. (2001). Water vole in the Scottish uplands: distribution patterns of disturbed and pristine populations ahead and behind the American mink invasion front. *Animal Conservation*, **4**, 187–194.

Akçakaya, H. R. & Atwood, J. L. (1997). A habitat-based metapopulation model of the California gnatcatcher. *Conservation Biology*, **11**, 422–434.

Brown, J. H. & Kodric-Brown, A. (1977). Turnover rates in insular biogeography: effects of immigration on extinction. *Ecology*, **58**, 445–449.

Channell, R. & Lomolino, M. V. (2000). Dynamic biogeography and conservation of endangered species. *Nature*, **403**, 84–86.

Cuzick, J. & Edwards, R. (1990). Spatial clustering for inhomogeneous populations. *Journal of the Royal Statistical Society Series B – Methodological*, **52**, 73–104.

Dale, M. R. T. (1999). *Spatial Pattern Analysis in Plant Ecology*. Cambridge: Cambridge University Press.

Diamond, J. M. (1975). The island dilemma: lessons of modern biogeographic studies for the design of natural reserves. *Biological Conservation*, **7**, 129–146.

Fahrig, L. (1998). Relative effects of habitat loss and fragmentation on population extinction. *Journal of Wildlife Management*, **61**, 603–610.

Flather, C. H. & Bevers, M. (2002). Patchy reaction-diffusion and population abundance: the relative importance of habitat amount and arrangement. *American Naturalist*, **159**, 40–56.

Gaston, K. J., Blackburn, T. M. & Gregory, R. (1999). Does variation in census area confound density comparisons? *Journal of Applied Ecology*, **36**, 191–204.

Gilpin, M. E. & Soulé, M. E. (1986). Minimum viable populations: processes of extinction. In *Conservation Biology: Science of Scarcity and Diversity*, ed. M. E. Soulé, pp. 19–34. Sunderland, MD: Sinauer.

Halley, J. M., Hartley, S., Kallimanis, A. S., Kunin, W. E., Lennon, J. J. & Sgardelis, S. P. (2004). Uses and abuses of fractal methodology in ecology. *Ecology Letters*, **7**, 254–271.

Hartley, S. & Kunin, W. E. (2003). Scale dependency of rarity, extinction risk, and conservation priority. *Conservation Biology*, **17**, 1559–1570.

Hartley, S., Kunin, W. E., Lennon, J. J. & Pocock, M. J. O. (2004). Coherence and discontinuity in the scaling of species distribution patterns *Proceedings of the Royal Society of London, Series B*, **271**, 81–88.

Hill, M. F. & Caswell, H. (1999). Habitat fragmentation and extinction thresholds on fractal landscapes. *Ecology Letters*, **2**, 121–127.

Hubbell, S. P. (2001). *The Unified Neutral Theory of Biodiversity and Biogeography*. Princeton: Princeton University Press.

Kallimanis, A. S., Kunin, W. E., Halley, J. & Sgardelis, S. P. (2005). Metapopulation extinction risk under spatially autocorrelated disturbance. *Conservation Biology*, **19**, 534–546.

Kunin, W. E. (1998). Extrapolating species abundance across spatial scales. *Science*, **281**, 1513–1515.

LaHaye, W. S., Gutierrez, R. J. & Akçakaya, H. R. (1994). Spotted owl metapopulation dynamics in southern California. *Journal of Animal Ecology*, **63**, 775–785.

Lecomte, J., Boudjemadi, K., Sarrazin, F., Cally, K. & Clobert, J. (2004). Connectivity and homogenisation of population sizes: an experimental approach in *Lacerta vivipara*. *Journal of Animal Ecology*, **73**, 179–189.

Levins, R. (1969). Some demographic and genetic consequences of environmental heterogeneity for biological control. *Bulletin of the Entomological Society of America*, **15**, 237–240.

McCarthy, M. A. & Lindenmayer, D. B. (2000). Spatially-correlated extinction in a metapopulation model of Leadbeater's possum. *Biodiversity and Conservation*, **9**, 47–63.

McCarthy, M. A., Thompson, C. P. & Possingham, H. P. (2005). Theory for designing nature reserves for single species. *American Naturalist*, **165**, 250–257.

McDowall, W. (2003). Extinction in a spatially autocorrelated environment. MSc dissertation, University of Leeds.

Ostling, A., Harte, J. & Green, J. L., (2000). Self-similarity and clustering in the spatial distribution of species. *Science*, **290**, Supplement 671a.

Ovaskainen, O. (2002). Long term persistence of species and the SLOSS problem. *Journal of Theoretical Biology*, **218**, 419–433.

Pelletier, J. D. (1997). Analysis and modeling of the natural variability of climate. *Journal of Climate*, **10**, 1331–1342.

Pocock, M. J. O., Hartley, S., Telfer, M. G., Preston, C. D. & Kunin, W. E. (2006). Ecological correlates of range structure in rare and scarce British plants. *Journal of Applied Ecology*, **94**, 581–596.

Rodriquez, A. & Delibes, M. (2002). Internal structure and patterns of contraction in the geographic range of the Iberian lynx. *Ecography*, **25**, 314–328.

Rodriguez, A. & Delibes, M. (2003). Population fragmentation and extinction in the Iberian lynx. *Biological Conservation*, **109**, 321–331.

Roy, C. & Hastings, A. (1996). Density dependence: are we searching at the wrong scale? *Journal of Animal Ecology*, **65**, 556–566.

Royama, T. (1992). *Analytical Population Dynamics*. London: Chapman & Hall.

Šizling, A. L. & Storch, D. (2004). Power-law species-area relationships and self-similar species distributions within finite areas. *Ecology Letters*, **7**, 60–68.

Smallwood, K. S. & Schonewald, C. (1996). Scaling population density and spatial pattern for terrestrial mammalian carnivores. *Oecologia*, **105**, 329–355.

Stapp, P., Antolin, M. F. & Ball, M. (2004). Patterns of extinction in prairie dog metapopulations: plague outbreaks follow El Nino events. *Frontiers in Ecology and the Environment*, **2**, 235–240.

Steffan-Dewenter, I., Münzenberg, U., Bürger, C., Thies, C. & Tscharntke, T. (2002). Scale-dependent effects of landscape context on three pollinator guilds. *Ecology*, **83**, 1421–1432.

Stewart, A., Pearman, D. A. & Preston, C. D. (1994). *Scarce Plants in Britain*. Peterborough: JNCC.

Storch, D., Šizling, A. & Gaston, K. (2003). Geometry of the species-area relationship in central European birds: testing the mechanism. *Journal of Animal Ecology*, **72**, 509–519.

Thomas, C. D., Thomas, J. A. & Warren, M. S. (1992). Distribution of occupied and vacant butterfly habitats in fragmented landscapes. *Oecologia*, **92**, 563–567.

Tilman, D. & Kareiva, P. (eds.) (1997). *Spatial Ecology: the Role of Space in Population Dynamics and Interspecific Interactions*. Princeton: Princeton University Press.

Turcotte, D. L. (1997). *Fractals and Chaos in Geology and Geophysics*. Cambridge: Cambridge University Press.

Westphal, C., Steffan-Dewenter, I. & Tscharntke, T. (2003). Mass flowering crops enhance pollinator densities at a landscape scale. *Ecology Letters*, **6**, 961–965.

Wigginton, M. J. (1999). *British Red Data Books. 1: Vascular Plants*, 3rd edn. Peterborough: JNCC.

Wilson, R. J., Thomas, C. D., Fox, R., Roy, D. B. & Kunin, W. E. (2004). Spatial patterns in species diversity reveal biodiversity change. *Nature*, **432**, 393–396.

With, K. A. & King, A. W. (1999). Extinction thresholds for species in fractal landscapes. *Conservation Biology*, **13**, 314–326.

# CHAPTER TWENTY

# Survival of species in patchy landscapes: percolation in space and time

BEÁTA OBORNY
*Loránd Eötvös University, Budapest*
GYÖRGY SZABÓ
*Research Institute for Technical Physics and Materials Science, Budapest*
GÉZA MESZÉNA
*Loránd Eötvös University, Budapest*

## Introduction

This chapter is about some basic geometric considerations and scaling laws in the spatial structure of habitats and (meta)populations.

Conservation of a valuable species, or conversely, eradication of an invasive species can be significantly helped by mapping its potential habitats. It is not easy, however, to measure the value of a habitat patch for a population or subpopulation. Not only the quality, but also the size and shape of the patch can influence birth, death, migration or dispersal (Forman, 1995; Wiens, 1997; chapter 8 in Turner, Gardner & O'Neill, 2001). The wider context, patch-to-patch neighborhood is another matter of consideration, because it can directly influence the movement of individuals (cf. borderline penetrability; Wiens, 1997) or survival and reproduction (cf. edge effects, ecotone effects; chapter 3 in Forman, 1995; Milne *et al.*, 1996; Harrison & Bruna, 1999). Spatial patterns on larger, regional scales are not negligible either. For example, habitat fragmentation is often a serious threat to survival (Fahrig, 2003). Many species require multiple patch types for completing the life cycle, or performing different activities (e.g. feeding and breeding). In this case, the proximity of different patch types in the patchwork also matters. Finally, the patches are rarely constant: they can shrink, expand, or shift; new patches can appear and old ones disappear. The changes can seriously challenge survival (Keymer *et al.*, 2000; see also Wiens, 1997 about habitat tracking).

Some species have adapted to limitations in the availability of suitable patches in space and/or time. For example, species living on rock outcrops or in permanent lakes have been selected for tolerating habitat fragmentation. Their patches are scattered, but quite permanent over time. Those species that colonize new openings after natural disturbances (fire, landslide, etc.), typically *r*-strategists, are adapted to scattered and impermanent patches. Their habitat is *fragmented both in space and time.* A great problem about the increasing human impact on the landscape in almost every region of the Earth is that even those species are exposed to disturbance and fragmentation which lack the proper response in their life history and behavioral repertoire. For example, brown kiwi (*Apteryx australis*), a forest-inhabiting bird in New Zealand, lives nowadays in remnants of forests separated by agricultural fields. The bird is flightless, and thus it must walk across unhabitable areas in order to reach new forest patches. Observations suggest that the bird is ready to cross 80 m distance, but larger distances significantly decrease the chance of colonization. When the forest remnants are 500 m apart, then colonization is almost hopeless without "stepping stones" (Potter, 1990). Every species has its own sensitivity to a suite of characteristics of the landscape structure. To estimate the danger of extinction, it is important to relate the spatial dynamics of the landscape to the spatial dynamics of the population.

The relationship between the two dynamics is not at all trivial. The distribution of the population is continuously being matched to the distribution of suitable patches through birth and death events and movement (migration and/or dispersal), which are limited in capacity. There may be considerable mismatches between the pattern of suitable patches and the pattern of occupied patches (see more about this in Kunin, this volume). Two kinds of discrepancy may occur:

1. The population exists in unsuitable sites. For example, it is declining, but the decline is slow (cf. extinction debt; Tilman *et al.*, 1994) or it is rescued by immigrants from a source population (Hanski, 1994; Lande, Engen & Saether, 1998).
2. The population does not occur in suitable sites. This can be caused by stochastic extinction and limited dispersal/migration (Hanski, 1997). The first studies showing this effect were made in island biogeography (MacArthur & Wilson, 1967) and metapopulation ecology (Levins, 1969; Hanski & Simberloff, 1997). Early theoretical models simplified the representation of the environment: the habitable area was assumed to consist of distinct patches; the nonhabitable area was represented as a featureless medium (matrix). Later developments refined the representation of the environment (Hanski & Simberloff, 1997), especially through an interface to landscape ecology (Wiens, 1997; Keymer *et al.*, 2000).

The next section in this chapter shows some purely landscape ecological considerations. We model a landscape which consists of habitable (good) and nonhabitable (bad) sites for a hypothetical species. We describe the process whereby a gradual loss of good sites leads to a sudden breakdown in the connectivity of the good areas, and thus, *habitat fragmentation* emerges.

The following section shows the other side of the coin: the landscape structure will be neglected, by assuming that the environment is homogeneous and constant, but the dynamics of the population will be explicitly modeled in space. We use a spatially explicit analogue of the classical, Levins type of metapopulation model, the so-called contact process, to show another kind of fragmentation: *population fragmentation*, whereby gradual change in the rate of spreading of the species leads to an abrupt change in the spatial pattern and in the probability of survival.

We then connect the two models, and study a spatial population living in a patchy habitat. In addition, we let the good and bad habitat patches change over time. We investigate the relationship between habitat fragmentation and population fragmentation, summarize the external and internal reasons for extinction, and discuss the variety of *pathways to extinction*.

All the models will be very simple. They were considered as null models (neutral models) in their own field of research: *landscape ecology* (chapter 6 in Turner *et al.*, 2001) and *spatial population ecology* (including metapopulation ecology and epidemiology; Durrett & Levin, 1994; Holmes, 1997; Levin & Pacala, 1997; Snyder & Nisbet, 2000). The reason for applying these simple, minimal models is that the phenomena that we wish to show are independent of the fine-scale details of the model, and thus can be extended to more complex models too. We devote a section for discussing generalizations and applicability of these classes of models (universality classes) for real-life systems. Finally, we discuss some implications for the conservation of biodiversity.

## Habitat fragmentation: an analogy with isotropic percolation

This section is based on a null model in landscape ecology, the so-called random map (Gardner *et al.*, 1987; Gustafson & Parker, 1992; Andrén, 1994; With, Gardner & Turner, 1997; chapter 6 in Turner *et al.*, 2001). The area on which the species lives is represented by a square lattice (Fig. 20.1a). Each lattice cell can be either good (habitable) or bad (nonhabitable). The proportion of good sites[1] on the lattice is $h$. Good and bad cells are randomly distributed in the lattice (i.e. no correlation is assumed between the cells). This feature makes the model interesting as a null model, because eventual spatial structures emerge solely by neighborhood contacts (a good cell can get next to a good cell, etc.).

Neighborhood can be defined in various ways. In this chapter, we use von Neumann neighborhood, i.e. consider the four adjacent cells as neighbors. Other options would also be possible (8 cells, etc.). While the expected frequencies of the

---

[1] This is the same quantity as $h$, the proportion of nondestroyed habitat, in models of habitat destruction (Nee & May, 1992; Hanski, 1997).

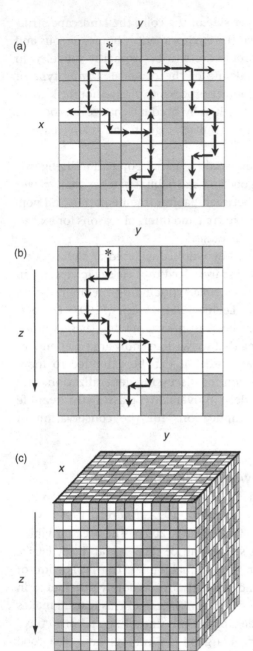

**Figure 20.1** Percolation patterns on square lattices, consisting of good (white) and bad (gray) sites. (a) An illustration for isotropic percolation. We start from a good site marked by *, and step to good sites only. One step is represented by an arrow. Any direction is permitted (up, down, left, and right). (b) Directed percolation. The rule for stepping is similar, but the upward direction is forbidden, i.e. percolation is directed vertically ($z$, shown by a gray arrow), but is isotropic horizontally ($x$). Note that one of the pathways permitted in (a) is forbidden in (b). (c) A combination of (a) and (b). The horizontal plane (coordinates $x$ and $y$) hosts isotropic percolation. The vertical axis is directed (coordinate $z$). In the present context, $x$ and $y$ are spatial coordinates, and $z$ is time. Each horizontal slice is a snapshot picture about the habitat pattern at a particular time. Any uniform column (all-gray or all-white) indicates that the quality of that particular site remains the same for a number of time steps. This panel can also be used for illustrating occupancy of a homogeneous habitat. In that case, white cells represent empty sites; gray cells represent occupied sites. Occupancy changes over time (direction $z$) by local colonization and extinction events.

configurations of good and bad cells around any focal cell can be easily calculated from $h$, the larger-scale correlations (neighbor of neighbor, etc.) become increasingly difficult to approach analytically. Therefore, Monte Carlo simulations have been used for studying the system (Stauffer & Aharony, 1992). Necessarily, numerical experimentations use finite-sized lattices ($L \times L$). To exclude finite-size effects,

(a) $h=0.5$

(b) $h=h_c=0.593$

(c) $h=0.7$

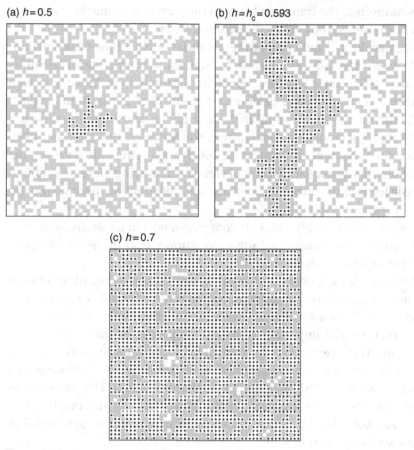

**Figure 20.2** Isotropic percolation. Results from simulations using the rules depicted in Fig. 20.1(a). The initial site was in the middle of the lattice. The sites occupied by the species in equilibrium are denoted by dots. The density of good sites $h$ varies to show an example from (a) the subcritical region, (b) the critical threshold, and (c) the supercritical region.

most quantities in this chapter, unless mentioned otherwise, are defined in the limit $L \to \infty$. To use unequivocal terminology, the lattice cells will be called "sites", and the emergent structures will be called "patches". For example, a set of contagious good sites, surrounded by bad sites, is a "good patch".

Consider a species spreading from an initial good site (like $*$ in Fig. 20.1a). How far can the species reach, provided that it can live in good sites only, and bad sites are forbidden to enter? When the density of good sites $h$ is low, then the area for spreading is confined: any initial good site is part of a finite-sized good patch (Fig. 20.2a). Therefore, the reachable distance is finite even if the lattice size is infinite: the habitat is fragmented. Conversely, when $h$ is high (Fig. 20.2c), then it becomes likely to find a good patch which spans across the lattice: the habitat is connected. The transition between the fragmented and the connected state has been studied thoroughly in *percolation theory*.

Landscape ecology is only one of the potential applications of percolation theory. It was originally established in statistical physics (Broadabent & Hammersley, 1957). Later it gained several applications in technology as well (ferromagnets, semiconductors, gelation, etc.; Deutscher, Zallen & Adler, 1983; Stauffer & Aharony, 1992 ). Its applicability in studying landscape structures has been suggested by a number of papers (Gustafson & Parker, 1992; Andrén, 1994; With *et al.*, 1997; chapter 6 in Turner *et al.*, 2001), but a systematic review of the phenomenon from an ecological point of view is still missing. Here we summarize the basic features of percolation systems, and call attention to some straightforward consequences in ecology.

To establish a common ground, a random map model in landscape ecology is analogous with a two-dimensional site percolation model in physics. A "good patch" is the same as a "cluster".

One of the basic messages of the physical theory is that the transition between the fragmented (disordered) and the connected (ordered) state is a *critical transition*. Increasing the density of good sites $h$ continuously, we reach a particular value at which several important statistical properties of the patch pattern change abruptly. (Nevertheless, the transition is continuous; therefore, it is a second order phase transition.) Numerical simulations have estimated the critical threshold $h_c = 0.592\,746$ (Stauffer & Aharony, 1992). The value of the threshold depends on the geometry of the lattice and on the definition of neighborhood, but other important statistical properties (the values of scaling exponents; see later) are invariant.

Consider first the *probability of percolation* ($P$). This is the probability that a randomly chosen site belongs to a good patch that spans across the landscape. Put differently, we ask whether a colonizer species (e.g. an invasive weed) that lands in a random place could spread to arbitrary distance without being confined by the barriers of nonhabitable sites. As Fig. 20.3(a) shows, $P = 0$ up to $h_c$, and increases beyond that critical point. (The control parameter is $x \equiv h$, and the order parameter is $R_1 \equiv P$ in Fig. 20.3a.) The increase is sharp, threshold-like ($\frac{dP}{dh} \to \infty$ as $h \to h_c+$). Finally, $P$ converges to 1 as $h \to 1$.

It is interesting to have a closer look at the supercritical region close to the threshold $h_c$ (denoted by a thin, solid line in Fig. 20.3a). The increase of $P$ in this region follows a power law,

$$P \propto (h - h_c)^{\beta}. \tag{20.1}$$

Theoretical considerations suggest that $\beta = 5/36$ (Stauffer & Aharony, 1992). As

$$\log(P) \propto \beta \cdot \log(h - h_c), \tag{20.2}$$

$\beta$ would be the slope of a linear function in a log-log plot.

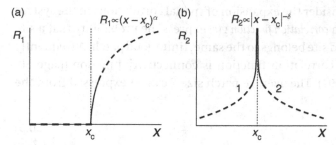

**Figure 20.3** Scaling laws at a critical transition. The horizontal axis shows the value of a control parameter $x$. In our model on habitat fragmentation, $x$ is the proportion of good sites ($x \equiv h$). In the model on population fragmentation, $x$ is the local rate of spreading of the population ($x \equiv \lambda$). Vertical axes ($R_1$ and $R_2$) show macroscopic statistical properties of the system. The figures are general illustrations about the shapes of the curves; the actual statistical properties will be discussed in the text ($R_1 \equiv P$, $R_2 \equiv S$, etc.). Tuning the control parameter $x$, the system undergoes an abrupt transition at the critical point $x_c$. The solid-line parts of the curves follow scaling laws (power laws), shown by the formula. The transition between the solid-line and dashed-line regions away from the threshold is smooth (characterized by a crossover between functions). $\alpha$, $\delta > 0$. (a) $R_1$ declines to zero with the decrease of $x$. (b) $R_2$ diverges (increases to infinity) as $x$ approaches the critical point $x_c$.

This scaling relation can be better understood if we study the sizes of the good patches. In the fragmented region ($h < h_c$), the average size[2] $S$ is increasing monotonously with the increase of $h$, and finally approaches infinity at $h_c$, at the emergence of the infinite good patch (curve 1 in Fig. 20.3b; $x \equiv h$ and $R_2 \equiv S$). The dependence of $S$ on $h$ can also be described by a power law (the solid line in curve 1),

$$S \propto (h_c - h)^{-\gamma}, \tag{20.3}$$

where $\gamma = 43/18$ (Stauffer & Aharony, 1992). In the connected region ($h > h_c$) a certain proportion of the area is occupied by the spanning good patch, but solitary, finite good patches may also be found. The mean size of these patches has been found to follow a power law with the same exponent (solid line in curve 2),

$$S \propto (h - h_c)^{-\gamma}. \tag{20.4}$$

Therefore, the equation in Fig. 20.3(b) is a general expression for the mean size of the finite good patches close to the critical transition. This quantity diverges, and the patch pattern has a fractal structure in the critical point. That is, one can find all sizes of patches, up to infinite size. The fractal dimension is $D = 91/48 = 1.897$ (Stauffer & Aharony, 1992).

---

[2] This is defined as the expected size of a good patch containing a site which was chosen randomly from all good sites which do not belong to a spanning (infinite) patch (page 20 in Stauffer & Aharony, 1992).

It is interesting to consider the expansion of spatial correlations in the system as $h$ approaches $h_c$. Let a *correlation function* $g(r)$ express the probability that a site at distance $r$ from a good site belongs to the same, finite good patch. A frequently used synonym for the correlation function is connectivity function (page 60, Stauffer & Aharony, 1992). The average patch size $S$ can be expressed from the correlation function as

$$S = \sum g(r),$$                                      (20.5)

summing over all lattice sites. The correlation length (or connectivity length) $\xi$ is defined as

$$\xi^2 = \frac{\sum r^2 g(r)}{\sum g(r)}.$$              (20.6)

Therefore, $\xi$ is a cutoff length, beyond which it is not probable to find pairs of good sites belonging to the same (finite) patch. Within $\xi$, the habitat structure can be approximated by a fractal with the above-mentioned dimension $D = 1.897$. Beyond $\xi$, it can be considered as homogeneous: its dimension is equal to the lattice dimension, $d = 2$.

The correlation length $\xi$ also diverges at the critical point (Fig. 20.3b; $x \equiv h$ and $R_2 \equiv \xi$),

$$\xi \propto |h - h_c|^{-\nu}$$                          (20.7)

with a scaling exponent $\nu = 4/3$ (Stauffer & Aharony, 1992). The correlation expands rapidly as the critical transition is getting near. Therefore, the spatial domain within which the habitat has fractal structure dilates rapidly.

The scaling exponents are not independent (Stauffer & Aharony, 1992). For example, knowing the dimension of the lattice ($d = 2$), $\beta$ and $\gamma$, we can calculate

$$\nu = \frac{2\beta + \gamma}{d}.$$                      (20.8)

The fractal dimension can be calculated as

$$D = \frac{(\beta + \gamma)d}{2\beta + \gamma}.$$        (20.9)

The exponents show that the transition from connected to fragmented habitat structure belongs to the *isotropic percolation* universality class of critical phenomena (Box 20.1). The existence of universal features is important from the perspective of ecological modeling: several conclusions are independent of the details of the model, therefore, even simple models can give reliable predictions about complicated real-life situations. For example, the aforementioned scaling laws apply for any landscape structure that can be approximated by random disorder. The elementary scale is arbitrary: one site can represent a square centimeter or several square kilometers as well. An attractive feature of using

## Box 20.1 The scaling hypothesis and universal phenomena

The scaling relations expressed by Eqs. (20.1–20.4) and (20.7–20.9) can be explained by the "scaling hypothesis". Suppose that the density of good sites, $h$, is near to the critical value; therefore the correlation length is much larger than the distance between the adjacent sites. Imagine that we see our system on an aerial photograph conveniently scaled to study the patches. When the patches are large, individual sites and their local patterns cannot be seen on the photo. Scaling hypothesis postulates that these unrecognizable details do not affect the patch structure on the scale of the correlation length. As we do not see the individual sites, we cannot assess how far our scale is from the elementary scale (set by the distance between adjacent sites), i.e. this ratio should not matter. Shift the value of $h$ even closer to $h_c$. This will increase the correlation length $\xi$. Nevertheless, we cannot see any change in the photo after rescaling it appropriately. That is, the patch structure is "scale invariant" under the scaling hypothesis, which mandates the fractal structure and the power-law scaling.

The scaling hypothesis has a further consequence: *universality*. Near to the critical transition, when the correlation length is large, details of the model specifications (e.g. defining the model with 4- or 8-neighborhood) do not matter. By analogy, fine-scale differences would be unrecognizable on the photo on the scale of $\xi$. The lattice can be triangular, hexagonal, etc.; even continuous space can be assumed. The state of a site can also be represented in various ways; discrete (presence versus absence of the species) or continuous (local population density). In general, if $\xi$ is large, then the macroscopic behavior becomes largely independent from the local rules: the microscopic details of cell-to-cell configurations become insignificant.

The scaling hypothesis and universality are well-established concepts in statistical physics to describe critical transitions (Stanley, 1971). They are strongly supported by simulations and theoretical studies. The theory of criticality was originally developed to describe "second-order" phase transitions. Later it was generalized to nonequilibrium phenomena as well as to many other transitions outside the domain of physics (Deutscher et al., 1983; Milne, 1998; Marro & Dickman, 1999; Hinrichsen, 2000a, b; Stanley et al., 2000). Critical transitions are characterized by diverging correlation length at a critical point (Eq. 20.7). If two models are identical on large spatial scales, their behavior becomes similar as the critical point is approached, where large-scale correlations dominate. In particular, the models will have identical scaling exponents. Such models are considered to belong to the same "universality class" (Stanley, 1971). This part of the chapter has discussed one of the universality classes: isotropic percolation. The next section will introduce another class: directed percolation.

> The values of the exponents, and the relations between them (Eqs. 20.8 and 20.9) are ubiquitous within a universality class. But the value of the critical threshold (in our case, $h_c$) depends on the actual definition of the model, as the control parameter ($h$) is defined in the context of the local details (Stauffer, 1979).

a percolation model as a null model is that we do not introduce any arbitrary assumption about the patch sizes, the distances between patches, or any other macroscopic, statistical feature of the landscape pattern. These features change continuously as we tune the control parameter $h$. Fragmentation is also not introduced arbitrarily: it emerges spontaneously with the decrease of $h$.

Let us summarize some direct ecological consequences of the occurrence of a critical transition in the landscape structure.

## Consequences

Figure 20.3(a) suggests that creating *ecological corridors* can increase landscape connectivity significantly in a narrow range of parameters only. If $h$ is far below $h_c$, then adding a few connections (even if added preferentially) cannot increase connectivity significantly ($P$ remains zero). If $h > h_c$ then the landscape is connected anyway. Merging solitary, finite patches into the spanning patch can still be important. However, it should be realized that the number and average size of these connectable patches declines rapidly as $h$ increases. Basically, it is the region around $h_c$ (solid lines on Fig. 20.3) where the addition of corridors can cause significant changes in the statistical properties of the landscape structure. In this critical region, even a small change in the local connections can have far-reaching effects because of the rapid increase of spatial correlation ($\xi$).

Several papers on landscape management have expressed doubts about the efficiency of ecological corridors, referring to case studies in which the creation of corridors could not promote the persistence of a species at the desired extent (Harrison & Bruna, 1999; Fahrig, 2003). Our study supports this view in a large region of the parameter space, but emphasizes the existence of a critical region, in which the corridors can be very efficient. Recognizing this region and targeting the effort to these cases would be vital in landscape management. The scaling relations predicted by percolation models may prove suitable for detecting this region.

Stepping through the percolation threshold makes a sudden change: the network of habitat patches becomes open for spreading. Thus, the range size of a species can expand rapidly. The proportion of good sites $h$ may increase for various reasons. Deliberate human action, such as the creation of corridors or restoration of habitats, is only one of the possibilities. The appearance of new habitat sites may be a by-product of human influence on the landscape; recall, for example, the ever-increasing amount of ruderal habitats for weeds. *Climate change* is another reason why *h* may increase: formerly unsuitable sites may become suitable. An important message of percolation theory is that even a small, continuous change in *h* may cause a sudden change in landscape connectivity in the vicinity of $h_c$. In this region, any trend-like increase in *h* should be seriously considered when predicting the future range of distribution of a species. Random fluctuations in *h* may also be important. For example, a single extreme year, when *h* becomes higher than $h_c$, may let an invasive species spread across large distances in the landscape.

The change in the opposite direction, *habitat loss*, is also interesting. As *h* is decreasing towards $h_c$, the spanning patch is thinning to a filamental structure (Fig. 20.2b; see also chapters 3.4 and 5.2 in Stauffer & Aharony, 1992). The filaments break up, and the system becomes fragmented when *h* decreases below $h_c$. Those species that are sensitive to habitat fragmentation are challenged at $h < h_c$. But even the supercritical region close to $h_c$ can be harmful. A filamental structure is obviously more exposed to edge effects. In addition, living in a filamental structure is typically an "ant in the labyrinth" situation (page 11 in Stauffer & Aharony, 1992). Those species that are bad at *habitat tracking* may suffer from missing the good patch at migration or dispersal, or getting into dead ends of filaments. Typical examples are those plant species which can only move by seed dispersal into random direction. A large proportion of the seeds can be wasted by landing in a bad area.

From an evolutionary perspective, it can be expected that near-to-threshold landscapes impose selection pressure for better habitat tracking; below-threshold landscapes select for longer dispersal distance, i.e. the ability to jump through the percolation barriers.

## Population fragmentation: an analogy with directed percolation

The previous section was dealing with the pattern of the landscape. In this section, we study the pattern of the population. For the sake of simplicity, we assume that the area is homogeneously good ($h = 1$). Only the next section will unite the two approaches to model a population in a heterogeneous landscape.

Merging spatial models on landscapes and populations in a common theoretical framework is not a trivial task, even if the models are relatively simple. While similar phenomena, *critical phase transitions*, can be expected in both spatial processes, they belong to different universality classes. As we have shown above, the model on landscape pattern belonged to the *isotropic* percolation universality class. Now we show that some basic questions concerning population or metapopulation dynamics in space are related to another universality class, *directed* percolation.

A new aspect which enters into consideration now is *time dependence*. To represent this, let us add a third dimension, time, to the two spatial dimensions. Survival of the species in a cell can be considered as advance in time. Sideways colonization complements this with advance in space. Altogether, we have a three-dimensional percolation problem, in which one of the dimensions, *time*, is directed in the sense that turn-back is impossible. (Directed percolation is illustrated in Fig. 20.1b in one spatial and one temporal dimension, in a heterogeneous landscape.)

In this simple model, a site can be in either of two states: empty or occupied by the species. Occupied sites become empty by local extinction with a constant rate *e*. Empty sites become occupied by colonization from neighboring occupied sites with rate *c*. The neighborhood is the same as in the previous model (four cells). This model is called a *contact process* (CP). (The numerical details are specified in the Appendix.)

The CP was originally introduced in physics to investigate the spreading of localized effects through neighborhood contacts (Harris, 1974), and later gained several applications in epidemiology (Harris, 1974; Anderson & May, 1991; Levin & Durrett, 1996; Holmes, 1997) and in population ecology (Crawley & May, 1987; Barkham & Hance, 1982; Franc, 2004; see also Durrett & Levin, 1994 for review). In fact, the CP is the simplest spatial extension of the well-known patch occupancy model in metapopulation dynamics (Levins, 1969),

$$\frac{dn(t)}{dt} = c \cdot n(t) \cdot [1 - n(t)] - e \cdot n(t), \qquad (20.10)$$

where $n(t)$ denotes the density of occupied sites over the whole area at time $t$. The term in square brackets expresses that only empty sites can be colonized. This introduces density regulation into the system: as the density of potential donor sites for colonization, $n(t)$, increases, the density of potential recipient sites, $[1 - n(t)]$, decreases.

Note that Eq. (20.10) is formally equivalent with the classical logistic equation of population growth, only the interpretation differs. In the classical model of logistic population growth, $n(t)$ is interpreted as population density. In the Levins model, $n(t)$ is the density of occupied sites.[3] Although the Levins model and the CP do not take into consideration the local population sizes within sites (only presence versus absence is considered), we will show later that several features of the CP can be generalized for structured metapopulations as well.

Equation (20.10) expresses a spatially implicit (mean field) model: spatial positions are not taken into account. It is assumed that any empty site is reachable for colonization from any occupied site with the same probability (*c*). The CP makes a step further: it considers the exact positions, and assumes that colonization is distance dependent. Only the four neighboring sites can be colonized in the square

---

[3] For a further clarification of terminology, it is worthy of note that a "patch" in the Levins model is the same as a "site" in our chapter. We had to introduce a distinction between "site" and "patch", because some of the models consider heterogeneous landscapes, where a single good/bad cell ("site") can be part of a larger-scale good/bad cluster of cells ("patch").

lattice within one time step. The CP is, therefore, a very basic model for studying spatial population dynamics. Its chief value is the incorporation of spatial limitations: no effect (and no species) can spread arbitrarily fast over the landscape. (See more about the spatially implicit versus explicit approach, and the use of CP as a null model in Durrett & Levin, 1994; Levin & Pacala, 1997; Keymer, Marquet & Johnson, 1998; Hanski, 1999; Snyder & Nisbet, 2000; Ovaskainen et al., 2002.)

The CP has been studied thoroughly in statistical physics, and numerous important scaling laws have been revealed in its behavior (Broadabent & Hammersley, 1957; Marro & Dickman, 1999; Hinrichsen, 2000a).

Let us first investigate the dependence of the equilibrium density of occupied sites, $\hat{n}$, on the values of parameters $c$ and $e$. The rate of colonization $c$ may decrease, for example, due to a climate change whereby the reproductive success decreases, or the probability of establishment of the offspring becomes lower. In those cases where colonization occurs by the migration of adult individuals, increased mortality during migration can also account for a decrease in $c$.

As the time unit is arbitrary, it is convenient to define $1/e$ as a time unit. Thus we have a single control parameter,

$$\lambda = c/e. \tag{20.11}$$

When $\lambda$ is high, local extinctions are rapidly compensated by colonization, and thus the species has a good chance of survival. Starting from a single site, it is likely to spread in space (Fig. 20.4a). By analogy of a diffusion process, the number of occupied sites increases as $N(t) \propto t^2$.

As $\lambda$ is getting lower, the probability of survival decreases, and finally, we reach a threshold value $\lambda_c$ at which the probability of survival becomes zero. The decline of the equilibrium density, $\hat{n}$, follows a power law, as presented in Fig. 20.3(a) (having $x \equiv \lambda$ and $R_1 \equiv \hat{n}$),

$$\hat{n} \propto (\lambda - \lambda_c)^{\eta}. \tag{20.12}$$

Monte Carlo simulations (Broadabent & Hammersley, 1957; Marro & Dickman, 1999; Hinrichsen, 2000a) have estimated $\eta = 0.583$. Extinction is certain below $\lambda_c$ from any initial pattern of occupancy, over infinite time, even in an infinitely large lattice. Numerical simulations have estimated $\lambda_c = 1.6488$. This value is considerably higher than the threshold predicted by the spatially implicit model (Eq. 20.10), where $\lambda_c = 1$. The difference is caused by the spatial limitation of spreading in the CP. Colonization requires an occupied (donor) site and an empty (recipient) site in the neighborhood. Therefore, density regulation is, essentially, a local process. The local densities of occupied sites are statistically higher than the global density, $n(t)$, because neighborhood colonization causes clumping. The discrepancy between the local and the global densities becomes especially serious as $\lambda_c$ is approached. For example, in the equilibrium population in Fig. 20.4(b) (time = 500), the local densities within the population fragments are still rather high, whereas the population inhabits only a small part of

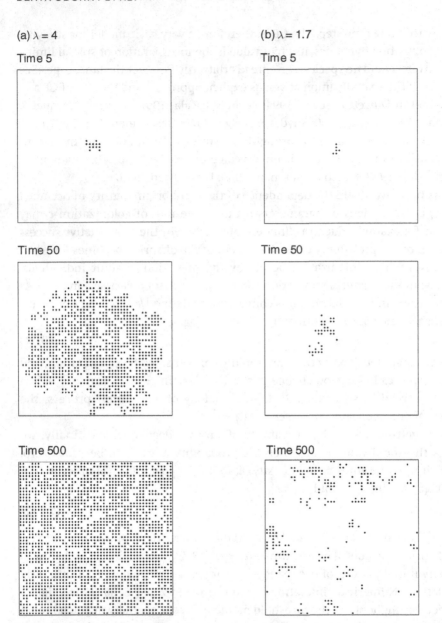

**Figure 20.4** Contact process in a homogeneous landscape. Occupied sites are marked by dots. The initial site of colonization at time 0 was in the middle of the lattice. The pictures show snapshots at three instants of time: (a) high above the threshold, at $\lambda = 4$; (b) slightly above the threshold, at $\lambda = 1.7$.

the area, exploiting only a small proportion of the carrying capacity (Oborny, Meszéna & Szabó, 2005).

Empty areas can only be colonized from the edges of existing population fragments, which become more and more scattered as extinction is getting near. Exactly at the threshold, the spatial structure is a fractal with rather low dimension, 0.7334. The fragments move randomly, and split and merge in a random fashion (branching–annihilating random walk; Hinrichsen, 2000a).

The correlation length in the pattern of empty and occupied sites changes characteristically as the extinction threshold is approached. Since we study a dynamically changing pattern (in contrast with the previous section, where we had a constant pattern), it is worth introducing a notation for correlation length in time $(\xi_t)$, and another for correlation length in space $(\xi_s)$. Analyses (Marro & Dickman, 1999; Hinrichsen, 2000a) revealed the following power laws:

$$\xi_t \propto (\lambda - \lambda_c)^{-\nu_t}, \tag{20.13}$$

where $\nu_t = 1.2956$; and

$$\xi_s \propto (\lambda - \lambda_c)^{-\nu_s}, \tag{20.14}$$

where $\nu_s = 0.733$ is equal to the fractal dimension at the threshold.

As the extinction threshold is approached, correlation extends over the system (curve 2 in Fig. 20.3b; $x \equiv \lambda$, and $R_2 \equiv \xi_s$ or $\xi_t$). At $\lambda_c$, the autocorrelated region becomes comparable to the system size. This result has important implications for stability against perturbations. Consider an infinitesimally small perturbation that happens at this stage, for example, a local extinction event that can naturally occur due to environmental or demographic stochasticity. Equation (20.13) predicts that this small perturbation has long-lasting effects when $\lambda$ is low ("critical slowing down"; Itoh et al., 2004). This is the proximate reason for extinction. The self-regulating ability of the population becomes weak, and fails completely when $\lambda = \lambda_c$.

A well-detectable symptom, showing this failure, is the divergence of fluctuations. Compare, for example, the variance ($V$) in the density of occupied sites to the mean ($M$) within finite samples of fixed size[4] ($A$). In this case,

$$\frac{VA}{M} \propto (\lambda - \lambda_c)^{-\mu}, \tag{20.15}$$

where $\mu = 0.934$ (calculated from data in Broadabent & Hammersley, 1957; Stanley, 1971; Harris, 1974). As the fluctuations increase, stochastic extinction becomes increasingly probable (Itoh et al., 2004). For any actual value of $\lambda > \lambda_c$, we can still find an area $> \xi_s$ which provides a statistically good chance for survival. But this area is increasing rapidly with the decrease of $\lambda$. Finally, even an infinitely large area cannot sustain the population at $\lambda \leq \lambda_c$.

## Consequences

These results have important implications for the protection of species (Oborny et al., 2005). Figure 20.4(b) demonstrates that fragmentation of a population is not necessarily a consequence of fragmented habitat structure. It is an

---

[4] $\sqrt{A}$ should be larger than the correlation length in space $(\xi_s)$, so as to gain a significant sample.

inevitable consequence of low rate and limited distance of spreading even in a homogeneous habitat.

A direct consequence of spontaneous fragmentation is that local fluctuations cannot be damped by local compensatory processes. The regulation of density breaks down as the density decreases. This drives the population into a vortex of extinction.

Consequently, low density is a potential danger in any dispersal-limited population, even if the population size is not particularly small (in the limit $\lambda_c$, it can even be infinite). The dangers of small population size have received serious attention in the literature of conservation biology (Primack, 1998), but the hazards of *low density* have received little emphasis so far (except for the Allee effect: Allee, 1931; Stephens & Sutherland, 1999). The danger of low density presented here is fundamentally different from an Allee effect.

The failure of density regulation is apparent when we compare the CP with the Levins model (Eq. 20.10). The Levins model assumes unlimited spreading, therefore, its density regulation is perfect. The threshold of extinction is $\lambda = 1$, and the decline of equilibrium density can be approximated by a linear function as the threshold is approached. By contrast, the spatially explicit CP predicts a significantly higher threshold, $\lambda_c = 1.6488$, and an accelerating decline. This suggests that nonspatial or spatially implicit models, which do not incorporate the distance dependence of dispersal and migration, can easily be overoptimistic in predicting the future of a population.

In addition to the perils of low density, small-sized populations are exposed to an additional challenge: stochastic extinction. As $\lambda$ decreases, the amplitude of fluctuations becomes comparable to the average (Eq. 20.15). Therefore, extinction may occur well before reaching the theoretical $\lambda_c$.

A practical problem associated with the rapid increase of fluctuations is that it becomes difficult to estimate population size (or the density of occurrences) near to extinction. The endangered species, for which we need reliable estimations, may lack sufficient data. Reaching the extinction threshold, the correlation length becomes infinite; therefore, no finite sample can be statistically representative for the system. Even long-term observations are likely to be weak for the prediction.

It is vital to be able to monitor endangered species before getting near to the critical threshold. Scaling laws help to extrapolate from the off-threshold behavior to the process of extinction at the threshold (by regression in the solid-line region in Fig. 20.3). The universality of the scaling laws is quite encouraging: the exponents are the same for a large variety of population dynamics.

## Unifying the two models

Both habitat fragmentation and population fragmentation are critical transitions. Tuning a control parameter ($h$ or $\lambda$), we can find a critical value ($h_c$ or $\lambda_c$) at which the order parameter ($P$ or $\hat{n}$ ) declines abruptly to zero, and the

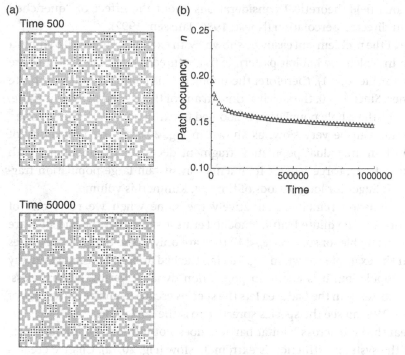

**Figure 20.5** Contact process in a fragmented landscape: $h = 0.5 < h_c$. The pattern of good and bad sites is constant: $f = 0$. The population is viable in the good sites: $\lambda_g = 6.67 > \lambda_c$. The bad (grey) area is totally unsuitable: $\lambda_b = 0$. The simulation started from an all-occupied initial state. (a) Snapshots after long periods of time. Note the persistence of occupancy in large habitat fragments. (b) The total density of occupied sites over the area as a function of time: $n(t)$.

correlations ($\xi$ or $\xi_s$, $\xi_t$) diverge. These processes follow power laws (Figs. 20.3a,b). Nevertheless, habitat fragmentation and population fragmentation belong to different universality classes, because the values of the corresponding critical exponents are different ($\beta \neq \eta$, $\nu \neq \nu_s$).

It would be tempting to unify the two models, and thus be able to study a spatially structured population living in a spatially structured habitat. The need for a common theoretical framework for studying metapopulation processes together with the underlying landscape structure has been emphasized by several authors (e.g. Hanski & Simberloff, 1997; Wiens, 1997; Keymer et al., 2000). But theoretical considerations in statistical physics suggest that the link between the two types of models is not trivial, since we are connecting two different universality classes.

The first step in this direction was made in statistical physics. Dickman and Moreira (1998) studied the CP in a "diluted" lattice, which, in our terminology, consisted of good and bad sites (in densities $h$ and $1 - h$, respectively). They concluded that dilution crucially disturbs the critical transition: the system did not show any universal power-law behavior. This result was in accordance with previous field-theoretical considerations about the effect of "quenched disorder" in directed percolation (Noest, 1986; Janssen, 1997).

The core of the problem can easily be shown by an example. Figure 20.5 shows a simulation in which the habitat pattern is fragmented ($h < h_c$). The bad sites are unsuitable for life ($e_b = 1$), therefore, the population is confined to live in finite good patches. Since $e_g > 0$, the survival time in any of these good patches is finite. Consequently, the whole population is doomed to extinction over infinite time.[5] But extinction can be very slow, as shown in Fig. 20.5(b). The probability of extinction of an individual population fragment decreases exponentially with the increase of size. Large habitat fragments can sustain large population fragments, which linger for long periods of time (cf. Kunin, this volume).

This phenomenon remains qualitatively the same when we relax one of the restrictions of the diluted lattice model. Let us assume that the bad sites are not totally unsuitable for survival ($e_b < 1$); they are only worse than the good sites ($\lambda_b < \lambda_g$). In the example shown in Fig. 20.6(a), the bad area cannot maintain any persistent population; it is a sink in population dynamic terms. Nevertheless, temporary existence in the bad area lets the species escape from the enclosures of bad patches. We can see the species spread across the landscape.

This breakthrough across habitat barriers does not influence a fundamental feature of the system: extinction is extremely slow (Fig. 20.7a). Chance creates regions in which the density of good sites is higher than the average $h$. The population finds these regions during its spreading, and occupies them in higher density than the average, $\hat{n}$ (Fig. 20.6a). This phenomenon is called habitat selection in the plant ecological literature (cf. Salzman, 1985), or localization in physics (Noest, 1986). The population fragment is more localized, of course, when the bad sites are completely forbidden ($e_b = 1$), but some degree of localization occurs even if $e_b < 1$, depending on the contrast between good and bad ($\lambda_g$ versus $\lambda_b$). This localization is the primary reason for the deviation from the power law behavior.

A further step in the study of this system is to relax the assumption that the pattern of good and bad sites is constant. We have made several numerical experiments with randomly changing patterns (Szabó, Gergely & Oborny, 2002; Fig. 20.6b). In each time step, a certain proportion of the sites, $f$, was selected at random. The selected sites gained new qualities randomly (good with probability $h$, and bad with $1 - h$). Therefore, the proportion of good versus bad sites remained stationary over time; $f$ characterized the frequency of change in the environment.

The simulations showed that the CP in a changing environment is a critical system, and belongs to the directed percolation universality class (Fig. 20.8). This is a very advantageous feature. Introducing spatial heterogeneity destroyed the

---

[5] When $h > h_c$, there is some chance for the population to spread across space to infinity, and thus live infinitely long.

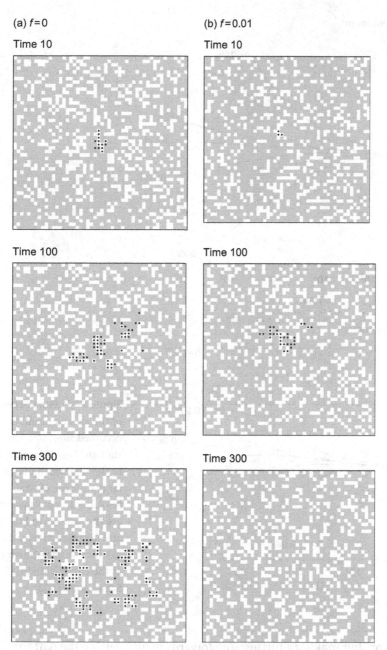

(a) $f=0$

Time 10

Time 100

Time 300

(b) $f=0.01$

Time 10

Time 100

Time 300

**Figure 20.6** Contact process in a fragmented landscape. The notations are the same as in Fig. 20.5, only the parameter values differ: $h = 0.22 < h_c$; $\lambda_g = 4 > \lambda_c$; $\lambda_b = 1 < \lambda_c$. The simulations were started from a single occupied site. The landscape pattern was (a) constant: $f = 0$, or (b) dynamically changing: $f = 0.01$. In the latter case, the population died out.

**(a) Constant environment**

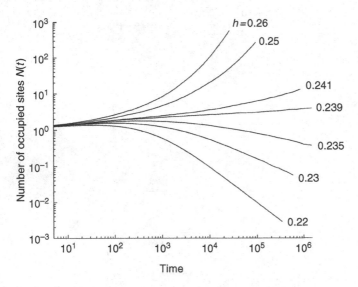

**(b) Changing environment**

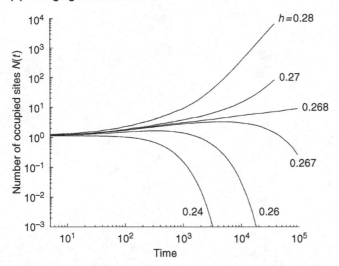

**Figure 20.7** Time dependence of the average number of occupied sites, *N(t)*. The statistical errors are comparable to the line width due to the large number of trials ($10^8$ for $h = 0.22$). The parameter values are the same as in Figs. 20.6(a) and (b), respectively, except for $h$, which varies (shown by labels at the curves). Modified from Szabó *et al.* (2002).

critical transition, but making a further step towards reality, letting the pattern change over time, restored the critical phenomenon. Thus, every universal feature known in directed percolation is applicable again.

Accordingly, we can specify a critical threshold, $h_c$ ($f$, $\lambda_g$, $\lambda_b$) below which the species dies out. Extinction is a fast, exponential process over time (compare $h = 0.22$ in Fig. 20.7a to $h = 0.24$ in Fig. 20.7 b). Figure 20.7(b) suggests that the critical threshold $h_c$ ($f = 0.01$, $\lambda_g = 4$, $\lambda_b = 1$) is about 0.268. Above the threshold, $h > h_c$, the

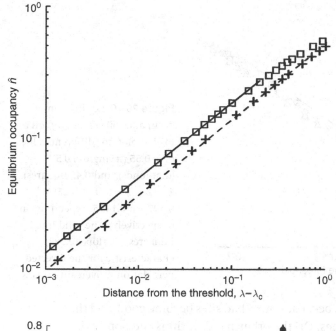

**Figure 20.8** Dependence of the equilibrium patch occupancy ($\hat{n}$) on $\lambda - \lambda_c$ in a homogeneous environment ($f = 0$; squares) and in a heterogeneous, changing environment ($f = 0.02$; crosses). In the latter case, $\lambda$ was defined as the average $\lambda = h \cdot \lambda_g + (1 - h) \cdot \lambda_b$. We manipulated $\lambda$ by fixing $\lambda_g = 4$, $\lambda_b = 1$, and varying $h$. The simulations yielded $\lambda_c = 1.8477$ in the heterogeneous, changing environment. The slopes of both fitted straight lines are consistent with the theoretically predicted scaling exponent of directed percolation, $\eta = 0.583$. Modified from Oborny *et al.* (2005).

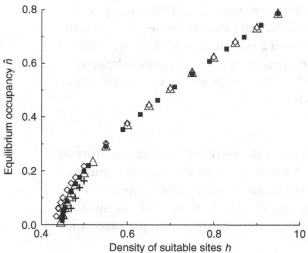

**Figure 20.9** Dependence of the equilibrium patch occupancy ($\hat{n}$) on $h$ in various, changing environments: $f = 0.02$ (black squares), 0.002 (open diamonds), 0.0002 (open triangles), and 0.00002 (crosses). Note that three magnitudes of change in $f$ caused relatively little difference in the curves.

population survives, and spreads by a diffusion process. Note that the function $N(t)$ becomes linear in the log-log plot at high values of $t$. The slope is approximately 2, which indicates diffusive spreading. At the threshold, the slope becomes lower, indicating anomalous diffusion (cf. chapter 1.4 in Stauffer & Aharony, 1992).

Further simulations suggested that the system is not very sensitive for the value of $f$ (when $f > 0$). Three magnitudes of change in $f$ cause only a little modification in the $\hat{n}(h)$ curve (Fig. 20.9). Nevertheless, little is known about the interdependence of $f$, $h$, $\lambda_g$ and $\lambda_b$. An increase in $f$ has a dual effect: on one

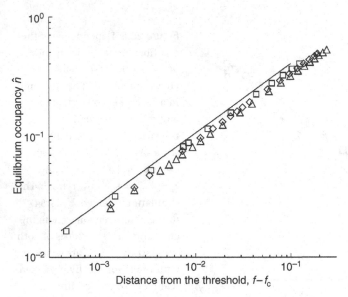

**Figure 20.10** Equilibrium patch occupancy ($\hat{n}$) versus $f - f_c$ on a log-log plot, for different values of $h$: 0.55 (triangles), 0.5 (diamonds), and 0.45 (squares). $\lambda_g = \infty$, $\lambda_b = 0$. $f_c$ is 0.2593, 0.1973 or 0.1435, depending on $h$ (respectively). The solid line indicates the slope (0.583) characteristic for the directed percolation universality class.

hand, it can facilitate spreading, because empty bad sites become good, and thus may serve as new stepping stones. On the other hand, it thins the population, because occupied good sites turn into bad, and become more likely to suffer local extinction. The increase of $f$ beyond a critical threshold, $f_c$, exterminates the population (as $f$ approaches $f_c$, the equilibrium density $\hat{n}$ goes to 0 by a power-law function, shown in Fig. 20.10). The relationship between $h_c$, $\lambda_c$, and $f_c$ is an interesting matter for future research.

**Consequences**

It is obviously important to connect habitat structure with population structure to reflect real biological situations. Many of the spatially explicit population dynamic models do so. This section warns, however, that the connection is not trivial, even in the case of simple, null models. We are likely to meet the challenge of connecting different universality classes: isotropic percolation and directed percolation.

Figure 20.7 suggests that habitat fragmentation is not a great problem per se. Its effect depends on the ability of the population to find and stay in the fragments (localization). When the positions of the fragments are fixed (as in Fig. 20.7a), the population has a good chance for long-term survival, provided that its $\lambda_g$ is sufficiently high. The real danger of extinction emerges when the habitat patches change over time (Fig. 20.7b), and the population is not able to *track* the patches by migration or dispersal. Figure 20.9 warns that even a small fluctuation in the qualities of sites is sufficient for driving the population into extinction.

The strength of selection for better habitat tracking depends on the values of $f$ and $h$, and on the contrast between good and bad patches. When $f$ is very high and $h$ is low, then uniform dispersion over a large area can be more efficient than precise tracking (as we often see in ruderal plants).

## Applicability

These models used serious simplifications. Nevertheless, universalities in a suite of important features suggest that the results are applicable for more complex, and thus more realistic, models of habitats and populations. The scaling laws described above are fairly robust against the particular representation of the habitat and of the population. It is interesting, however, to list some factors that destroy the scaling laws, i.e. fundamentally violate the scaling hypothesis.

First, as we have seen above, localization of the population is one of the factors. This is likely to be more characteristic for habitat specialists than for generalists. Some patch types are fairly immobile on the timescale of population dynamics; therefore, the potential effects of localization are not negligible.

Second, percolation theoretical considerations are based on the assumption that the species can only gradually advance in space. If occasional big jumps are also possible, for example, by far-dispersing seeds, then the dynamics of spreading can change fundamentally (cf. Newman & Watts, 1999; Ovaskainen et al., 2002). "Far" versus "near" depends, of course, on the size of and distance between habitat patches, and on the speed of spreading from neighbor to neighbor ($\lambda_g$ and $\lambda_b$). It may occur that percolation barriers become detectable only when we zoom out to larger distances in the landscape. In addition, even extremely far-dispersing seeds are insufficient for changing some fundamental features. Consider a fragmented landscape ($h < h_c$). A big jump may enable the species to reach a new good patch (percolation cluster), which would be unreachable otherwise. But the new patch is also finite, so the species is still stuck. Only a large number of propagula could inoculate every patch. Recall, however, that the size of patches decreases rapidly as we move away from the threshold (Eq. 20.3; curve 1 in Fig. 20.3b), and the average distance between the patches also increases fast. In spite of the limitations in the usefulness of far-dispersing propagula, it is very important to know whether the particular species for protection has this possibility, and whether it might be subsidized by artificial introductions into distant patches.

Third, theoretical considerations (Henkel & Hinrichsen, 2004) suggest that a specific kind of density dependence can drive the CP out of the directed percolation universality class. When colonization of an empty site requires not one but two occupied sites in the neighborhood, then the transition to extinction falls into another universality class. This assumption may be plausible when a site represents a place (microsite) for a single individual, and two individuals (parents) are needed for the production of a new offspring. In addition, the adults should be sessile, and should only locally interact (which is not applicable, for example, for pollen dispersal). Therefore, the relevance of this modification in the CP is probably very limited, especially when a site represents a place for a whole subpopulation. It is important to remark that only this two-parents assumption has this specific effect; a simple density dependence in colonization or extinction does not divert the system out of the directed percolation universality class (Hinrichsen, 2000a).

It is certain that there are more factors for consideration. The terrane of applicability of percolation theory in ecology is largely unexplored. An example for existing applications is the use of random maps as references ("null models") for the study of real landscapes (Gardner *et al.*, 1987; Gustafson & Parker, 1992; Andrén, 1994; With *et al.*, 1997; chapter 6 in Turner *et al.*, 2001). Plotnick and Gardner (1993) applied percolation models to highlight some ecologically important features of landscapes, for example to explore the edge structure of patches and to identify bottlenecks which may hinder species' migrations. He and Hubell (2003) used percolation theory for studying the relationship between the patterns of distribution and abundance. The CP and its derivatives are also rather widespread in spatial ecology (see the previous two sections). Universal phenomena suggest that these simple models (the random map, the CP, and their combinations) are more than just statistical references: they show interesting behavior, and several features of this behavior are directly applicable for more complex systems.

## Implications for the conservation of biodiversity

The models clearly show that there are several *ways to extinction* according to $h$, $f$, and $\lambda$.

Let us start from a stable population which covers a large, uniformly good area ($h = 1$, $f = 0$, and $\lambda$ is high), and review some ways how human activity can lead to the extinction of this population. The species is limited in spreading: $\lambda$ is finite, and the distance of colonization is also finite.

1.  The first is a general decrease in $\lambda$, as it has been demonstrated in the homogeneous CP. The decrease can have various reasons, for example a climate change due to human activity. Some local disturbances that affect living organisms directly and leave the habitat unaffected can also be modeled by this simple CP. For example, hunting can be regarded as increasing $e$; collecting the flowers of a plant species can be taken into account as increasing $e$ and decreasing $c$. The CP predicts a sudden collapse of the population at $\lambda_c$: the dispersal-limited population cannot exploit the carrying capacity of the area, it gets fragmented into small subpopulations, and loses its capacity for self-regulation. This way of extinction could be called *falling apart*.

2.  The second way is to get *dissected*. Building highways, cutting forests, and making large agricultural fields lead to the fragmentation of habitats for several species. The most worrying case is when the nonhabitat area is not suitable even for temporary survival ($\lambda_b = 0$). When $h$ decreases below the critical $h_c$, the population is confined to live in enclosures. Each finite subpopulation has a finite lifetime; therefore, extinctions from the habitat patches are inevitable. Having $\lambda_b = 0$, the empty good patches are unreachable for the species. Thus, a larger and larger proportion of the carrying capacity remains unexploited. If $h$ is not far from $h_c$, and $\lambda_g \gg \lambda_c$ then the population can linger in the largest habitat fragments for a long time (Fig. 20.5). Although the equilibrium state is $\hat{n} = 0$, i.e. global extinction is certain, it may take a long time to reach the equilibrium.

3.  A similarly smooth way of extinction can be expected when the population gets *subdivided* into partially independent subpopulations, and the metapopulation formed by these subpopulations is below the MVM (minimum viable metapopulation size; Hanski, 1997). This is a milder version of the previous case, dissection, because the habitat patches are not completely isolated. Figure 20.7(a) suggests that the behavior of the population is basically the same as in case 2: it is a slow process to reach $\hat{n} = 0$. This is in agreement with the concept of extinction debt (Tilman *et al.*, 1994; Hanski, 1997). Whenever habitat destruction occurs, and thus $h$ decreases, it takes time for the metapopulation to equilibrate. Local extinctions may proceed for a long while, even if the environment does not change any further. If $h$ is too low relative to the actual $\lambda_g$ and $\lambda_b$, then the whole metapopulation can be regarded as a "living dead".

4.  Fast, abrupt extinction can be expected, however, when the qualities of sites change over time. Even if $h$, $\lambda_g$ and $\lambda_b$ remain the same, an increase in $f$ from zero to a positive value can exterminate the population, because the species may not be able to locate the habitat patches.

Human activities can influence $h$, $f$, $\lambda_g$ and $\lambda_b$ simultaneously, so it is possible that all processes (1–4) contribute to the extinction of a species.

Here we disregarded the trivial reason for extinction, when the carrying capacity becomes zero. The above-listed processes share the feature that the carrying capacity cannot be fully utilized because of spatial limitations. Consequently, extinction may occur well before the carrying capacity decreases to zero.

It is logical to ask whether partial utilization of the carrying capacity might contribute to the *increase* of biodiversity in the parameter region where our target population can securely survive. The nonutilized portion of the good habitat patches can be occupied by other species. Tilman (1994) raised the idea that strong competitors in plant communities may be limited in colonization abilities due to a trade-off. The canopy gaps, left open by superior competitors, can be utilized by inferior competitors. Understanding the spatial matching of coexisting species is a major challenge in ecology (Bell, 1984; Herben, 1996; Zobel *et al.*, 1994; see also reviews about spatial effects: Durrett & Levin, 1994; Tilman & Kareiva, 1997; Dieckmann, Law & Metz, 2000). To translate the problem for the CP model, having a competitor species is a further step from the CP in a heterogeneous, changing environment. When we introduced $f$, we simply assumed that the environment was changing for an external reason (e.g. disturbance). The external factor was not assumed to be influenced by the species. In a further step, we may assume that a site can become unsuitable because it is occupied by another species. That is, the medium in which percolation proceeds is active (as in Li, 2002). "Unsuitable" can mean completely forbidden or just worse in quality. Investigations with the homogeneous CP have shown that when the occupied sites are forbidden, then stable coexistence is not possible. The species with the higher $\lambda$ wins the competition (Yu & Wilson, 2001; Mágori *et al.*, 2005). Coexistence can be promoted by introducing spatial and/or temporal heterogeneity in the environment ($h < 1$ and/or $f > 0$). Interestingly, over-colonization of the occupied sites also promotes coexistence (Yu & Wilson, 2001; Crowley *et al.*, 2005). In these cases, the degree of utilization of the habitat patches can be an important determinant of species assembly. Invasibility of a community can also hinge on the spatial and temporal pattern of gaps (vacant suitable sites).

The *threshold*-like nature of extinctions is an important message from percolation theory. All the control parameters, $h$, $f$, and $\lambda$, have their own critical thresholds. (See the caption of Fig. 20.8 for the definition of $\lambda$ in a heterogeneous landscape.) It would be vital to know more about the interdependence of these parameters. Conservation biology should definitely benefit from this kind of information, because management efforts in nature reserves could be targeted to those control parameters which are close to a threshold. In the vicinity of the threshold, even a small management effort can have great effect on the prospects of survival; further away from the threshold, even large efforts are inefficient (see Fig. 20.3).

It has been asked in conservation biology whether it is worthwhile to allocate money and effort into increasing landscape connectivity when there are other alternatives, for example improving the amount or quality of suitable habitat patches. Some studies definitely vote for the second, referring to the relative inefficiency of ecological corridors (Harrison & Bruna, 1999; Fahrig, 2003). Our study supports the view that there is no general order of preferences. It is always possible to find the best parameter(s) for manipulation, depending on the nearness of $h_c$, $f_c$ and $\lambda_c$. *Habitat restoration* increases $h$. Amelioration of the existing habitats raises the value of $\lambda_g$. *Ecological corridors* increase $c$. Connectivity between the patches (larger-scale structures) can also be increased by improving the quality of the nonhabitat area (raising $\lambda_b$). The control of hunting or collecting individuals can generally increase both $\lambda_g$ and $\lambda_b$. The suppression of disturbance decreases $f$. Frustration about a management technique can well be the consequence of choosing a wrong target parameter, that is, a parameter far from its threshold. It is challenging, of course, to choose the best management when we wish to preserve multiple species simultaneously, having different parameter values.

The possibility for a sudden breakdown of a population underlines the importance of *monitoring*, especially in the vicinity of the threshold(s). By contrast, the divergence of fluctuations (Eq. 20.15, Fig. 20.3b) suggests that monitoring becomes more and more difficult as the threshold is approached. Fortunately, scaling laws offer some diagnostic features, which can be used for prediction. The following symptoms may indicate that a population is endangered (i.e. has entered into the solid-line region in Fig. 20.3a):

1.  Large domains in the spatial structure of the population can be described by a low-dimensional fractal of randomly moving clumps.
2.  There are large, spontaneous fluctuations in the population density.
3.  The equilibrium is reattained slowly after perturbation.

Provided that the time of observation is sufficiently long for measuring multiple points on an extinction curve (Eqs. 20.12–20.15), even the exact distance from the threshold can be determined by linear regression on a log-log plot.

Promotion of the survival of valuable species is only one side of the coin. On the other side, we have the need for preventing invasions by weeds, pathogens, or other unwanted species. Percolation theory warns that the standstill (restricted area of distribution) of a potential invader is not evidence that the species is harmless. The limited availability of suitable sites (low $h$, low $\lambda_b$) may keep the species confined in space for years. But a single extreme year can be sufficient for surpassing the percolation threshold, and spreading across large distances. Then the occupancy of new good patches is permanent; that is, the process of expansion is irreversible.

It would be interesting to look at range expansions in historical records from this aspect, relating the area of distribution of a species to the availability of suitable habitat. Some population outbreaks in recent history are thoroughly documented. Another potential source of data is the consideration of local population dynamics in widespread species, across environmental gradients (as suggested by Holt & Keitt, 2000). Percolation theory predicts that the variance of population density diverges towards the edge of distribution.

## Conclusions

The scale dependence of ecological patterns is a well-established notion in ecology (Addicott *et al.*, 1987; Wiens, 1989; Juhász-Nagy, 1992; chapter 2 in

Turner et al., 2001). Scaling laws warn, however, that not everything is scale dependent: there are patterns that span across multiple spatial scales.

Spatial population dynamics abound in scale-invariant phenomena in the vicinity of extinction. As a population is declining, the correlation length expands in space and time, and thus the behavior of the population becomes dominated by large-scale structures. Since the microscopic details become irrelevant relative to these large-scale structures, various kinds of population dynamics can be expected to converge into a single, robust kind of extinction dynamics.

The CP is a good prototype for studying these general dynamics. Its validity is not limited to simple, homogeneous environments. Whenever the environment is patchy, and the patches are not frozen, then the universal features of the CP can unfold. The information accumulated in statistical physics about this universality class (directed percolation) is also applicable in ecological research.

A population living in a patchy environment faces the challenge to spread across patches (percolate in 2D space) and survive in each site (percolate in 1D time). A population can fail in any of these tasks: fragmentation of the habitat prevents percolation in space; local extinction cuts off percolation in time. Nevertheless, both failures can be compensated from the other dimension(s): fragmentation is a milder problem when local survival is highly probable; local extinction is not troublesome when it can be compensated by colonization from the outside. The real process of survival can only be understood when we put together the spatial and temporal dimensions (Fig. 20.1c). The population percolates through corridors in space–time (cf. Keymer et al., 2000). Extinction becomes a serious danger when these corridors become thin (filamental). Importantly, extinction is a critical transition. Changing the parameters of the environment ($h$ or $f$) or of the population ($\lambda$) continuously, we can expect a sudden breakdown of the population.

We have reviewed the possible reasons and ways which can lead to extinction. It is essential that even an infinite-sized population cannot escape extinction beyond the critical thresholds ($h_c$, $f_c$ or $\lambda_c$). Finite-size effects add to this problem. A population can seriously be endangered in the neighborhood of the threshold already, because the density shows diverging fluctuations, and the capacity of the population for self-regulation is deficient.

It is difficult to monitor a population in this region, because of the divergence of fluctuations. Scaling laws might be utilized for extrapolating from the off-threshold behavior to the dynamics of decline at the threshold. The CP suggests some diagnostic signs to indicate that a population is endangered.

Many external reasons can change the values of $h$, $f$ and $\lambda$: environmental stochasticity, a trend-like climate change, etc. As the population is walking in the parameter space, it is crucial to know the places of precipices ($h_c$, $f_c$ or $\lambda_c$), and to find the proper interventions (habitat restoration, amelioration, connection, etc.) which can keep the population away from the edges.

## Acknowledgments

The research was subsidized by the Hungarian National Research Fund (OTKA T035009, T049689, T047003, K61534). B.O. is grateful for an International Fellowship at the Santa Fe Institute, Széchenyi Scholarship from the Hungarian Ministry of Education (until 2004), and a Bolyai Scholarship from the Hungarian Academy of Sciences (from 2004). We are grateful to Gábor Csányi, Balázs Szendrő, and Ulf Dickmann for discussions about the topic, and to David Storch, Pablo Marquet, and an anonymous reviewer for helpful comments on the manuscript.

## Appendix 20.I   Monte Carlo simulations

We studied the CP by Monte Carlo simulations in stochastic cellular automata. The size of the square lattice was $L^2 \geq 10^6$ cells. We applied periodic boundary conditions to avoid edge effects. The cells of the lattice were updated asynchronously. If a cell was occupied, it became empty with probability $e$. If a cell was empty, it became occupied with probability $c \cdot \frac{k}{4}$, where $k$ was the number of occupied cells out of the four nearest neighbors. One time step (one Monte Carlo step) represented $L^2$ updates. The maximum number of time steps was $10^6$ ($=10^{12}$ updates). The maximum number of independent repetitions (trials) was $10^7$. The parameters of the simulations (lattice size, number of time steps, number of trials) were chosen to have $< 10\%$ relative error in $S(t)$ and $N(t)$ in the final time step. For more technical details about the simulations see Szabó et al. (2002).

## References

Addicott, J. F., Aho, J. M., Antolin, M. F., Padilla, D. L., Richardson, J. S. & Soluk, D. A. (1987). Ecological neighborhoods: scaling environmental patterns. *Oikos*, **49**(3), 340–346.

Allee, W. C. (1931). *Animal Aggregations: a Study in General Sociology*. Chicago: University of Chicago Press.

Anderson, R. M. & May, R. M. (1991). *Infectious Diseases and Control*. Oxford: Oxford University Press.

Andrén, H. (1994). Effect of habitat fragmentation on birds and mammals in landscapes with different proportion of suitable habitat: a review. *Oikos*, **71**, 355–366.

Barkham, J. P. & Hance, C. E. (1982). Population dynamics of the wild daffodil (*Narcissus pseudonarcissus*). *Journal of Ecology*, **70**, 323–344.

Bell, A. D. (1984). Dynamic morphology: a contribution to plant population ecology. In *Perspectives on Plant Population Ecology*, ed. R. Dirzo & J. Sarukan. Sunderland, MA: Sinauer Associates.

Broadabent, S. R. & Hammersley, J. M. (1957). Percolation processes. I. Crystals and mazes. *Proceedings of the Cambridge Philosophical Society*, **53**, 629–645.

Crawley, M. J. & May, R. M. (1987). Population dynamics and plant community structure: competition between annuals and perennials. *Journal of Theoretical Biology*, **125**, 475–489.

Crowley, P. H., Davis, H. M., Ensminger, A., Fuselier, L. C., Jackson, J. K. & McLetchie, D. N. (2005). A linear model of local competition for space. *Ecology Letters*, **8**(2), 176–188.

Deutscher, G., Zallen, R. & Adler, J. (1983). *Percolation Structures and Processes.* Bristol: Adam Hilger.

Dickman, R. & Moreira, A. G. (1998). Violation of scaling in the contact process with quenched disorder. *Physical Reviews, E* **57**, 1263–1268.

Dieckmann, U., Law, R. & Metz, J. A. J. (2000). *The Geometry of Ecological Interactions.* Cambridge: Cambridge University Press.

Durrett, R. & Levin, S. A. (1994). Stochastic spatial models: a user's guide to ecological applications. *Philosophical Transactions of the Royal Society of London, Series B,* **343**, 329–350.

Fahrig, L. (2003). Effects of habitat fragmentation on biodiversity. *Annual Reviews of Ecology, Evolution and Systematics,* **34**, 487–515.

Forman, R. T. T. (1995). *Land Mosaics: The Ecology of Landscapes and Regions.* Cambridge: Cambridge University Press.

Franc, A. (2004). Metapopulation dynamics as a contact process on a graph. *Ecological Complexity,* **1**, 49–63.

Gardner, R. H., Milne, B. T., Turner, M. G. & O'Neill, R. V. (1987). Natural models for the analysis of broad-scale landscape pattern. *Landscape Ecology,* **1**, 19–28.

Gustafson, E. J. & Parker, G. R. (1992). Relationships between landcover proportions and indices of landscape spatial pattern. *Landscape Ecology,* **7**, 101–110.

Hanski, I. (1994). A practical model of metapopulation dynamics. *Journal of Animal Ecology,* **63**, 151–162.

Hanski, I. (1997). Metapopulation dynamics: from concepts and observations to predictive models. In *Metapoplulation Biology: Ecology, Genetics and Evolution,* ed. I. Hanski & M. E. Gilpin, pp. 69–92. London: Academic Press.

Hanski, I. (1999). *Metapopulation Ecology.* Oxford: Oxford University Press.

Hanski, I. & Simberloff, D. (1997). The metapopulation approach, its history, conceptual domain, and application to conservation. In *Metapopulation Biology: Ecology, Genetics and Evolution,* ed. I. Hanski & M. E. Gilpin, pp. 5–26. London: Academic Press.

Harris, T. E. (1974). Contact interactions on a lattice. *Annals of Probability,* **2**, 969–988.

Harrison, S. & Bruna, E. (1999). Habitat fragmentation and large-scale conservation: what do we know for sure? *Ecography,* **22**, 225–232.

He, F. & Hubbell, S. P. (2003). Percolation theory for the distribution and abundance of species. *Physical Review Letters,* **91**(19), 198103 /1–4.

Henkel, M. & Hinrichsen, H. (2004). The non-equilibrium phase transition of the pair-contact process with diffusion. *Journal of Physics A,* **37**, R117–R159.

Herben, T. (1996). Founder and dominance control: neglected concepts in the community dynamics of clonal plants. In *Clonality in Plant Communities,* ed. B. Oborny & J. Podani, pp. 3–11. Grangärde: Opulus Press.

Hinrichsen, H. (2000a). Non-equilibrium critical phenomena and phase transitions into absorbing states. *Advances in Physics,* **49**, 815–958.

Hinrichsen, H. (2000b). On possible experimental realizations of directed percolation. *Brazilian Journal of Physics,* **30**(1), 69–82.

Holmes, E. (1997). Basic epidemiological concepts in a spatial context. In *Spatial Ecology: the Role of Space in Population Dynamics and Interspecific Interactions,* ed. D. Tilman & P. Kareiva, pp. 111–136. Monographs in Population Biology, 30. Princeton: Princeton University Press.

Holt, R. D. & Keitt, T. H. (2000). Alternative causes for range limits: a metapopulation perspective. *Ecology Letters,* **3**, 41–47.

Itoh, Y., Tainaka, K.-I., Sakata, T., Tao, T. & Nakagiri, N. (2004). Spatial enhancement of population uncertainty near the extinction threshold. *Ecological Modeling,* **174**, 191–201.

Janssen, H. K. (1997). On the nonequilibrium phase transition in reaction-diffusion systems with absorbing stationary state. *Zeitschrift für Physik B*, **42**, 151–154.

Juhász-Nagy, P. (1992). Scaling problems almost everywhere: an introduction. *Abstracta Botanica*, **16**, 1–5.

Keymer, J. E., Marquet, P. A. & Johnson, A. R. (1998). Pattern formation in a patch occupancy metapopulation model: a cellular automata approach. *Journal of Theoretical Biology*, **194**, 79–90.

Keymer, J. E., Marquet, P. A., Velasco-Hernandez, J. X. & Levin, S. A. (2000). Extinction thresholds and metapopulation persistence in dynamic landscapes. *American Naturalist*, **156**, 478–494.

Lande, R., Engen, S. & Saether, B.-E. (1998). Extinction times in finite metapopulation models with stochastic local dynamics. *Oikos*, **83**, 383–389.

Levin, S. A. & Durrett, R. (1996). From individuals to epidemics. *Philosophical Transactions of the Royal Society of London, Series B*, **351**(1347), 1615–1621.

Levin, S. A. & Pacala, S. W. (1997). Theories of simplification and scaling in spatially distributed processes. In *Spatial Ecology: the Role of Space in Population Dynamics and Interspecific Interactions*, ed. D. Tilman & P. Kareiva, pp. 271–295. Monographs in Population Biology, 30. Princeton: Princeton University Press.

Levins, R. (1969). Some demographic and genetic consequences of environmental heterogeneity for biological control. *Bulletin of the Entomological Society of America*, **15**, 237–240.

Li, B.-L. (2002). A theoretical framework of ecological phase transitions for characterizing tree-grassland dynamics. *Acta Biotheoretica*, **50**, 141–154.

MacArthur, R. H. & Wilson, E. O. (1967). *The Theory of Island Biogeography*. Princeton: Princeton University Press.

Mágori, K., Szabó, P., Mizera, F. & Meszéna, G. (2005). Adaptive dynamics on a lattice: role of spatiality in competition, co-existence and evolutionary branching. *Evolutionary Ecology Research*, **7**, 1–21.

Marro, J. & Dickman, R. (1999). *Nonequilibrium Phase Transitions in Lattice Models*. Cambridge: Cambridge University Press.

Milne, B. T. (1998). Motivation and benefits of complex systems approaches in ecology. *Ecosystems*, **1**, 449–456.

Milne, B. T., Keitt, T. H., Hatfield, C. A., David, J. & Hraber, P. T. (1996). Detection of critical densities associated with pinion-juniper woodland ecotones. *Ecology*, **77**, 805–821.

Nee, S. & May, R. M. (1992). Dynamics of metapopulations – habitat destruction and competitive coexistence. *Journal of Animal Ecology*, **61**, 37–40.

Newman, M. E. J. & Watts, D. J. (1999). Scaling and percolation in a small-world network model. *Physical Reviews E*, **60**, 7332–7342.

Noest, A. J. (1986). New universality for spatially disordered cellular automata and directed percolation. *Physical Review Letters*, **57**, 90–93.

Oborny, B., Meszéna, G. & Szabó, G. (2005). Dynamics of populations on the verge of extinction. *Oikos*, **109**, 291–296.

Ovaskainen, O., Kazunori, S., Bascompte, J. & Hanski, I. (2002). Metapopulation models for extinction thresholds in spatially correlated landscapes. *Journal of Theoretical Biology*, **215**, 95–108.

Plotnick, R. & Gardner, R. (1993). Lattices and landscapes. *Lectures on Mathematics in the Life Sciences*, **23**, 129–156.

Potter, M. A. (1990). Movement of North Island brown kiwi (*Apteryx australis* Manelli) between forest remnants. *New Zealand Journal of Ecology*, **14**, 17–24.

Primack, R. B. (1998). *Essentials of Conservation Biology*. Sunderland, MA: Sinauer Associates.

Salzman, A. G. (1985). Habitat selection in a clonal plant. *Science*, **228**, 603–604.

Snyder, R. E. & Nisbet, R. M. (2000). Spatial structure and fluctuations in the contact process and related models. *Bulletin of Mathematical Biology*, **62**, 959–975.

Stanley, H. E. (1971). *Introduction to Phase Transitions and Critical Phenomena*. Oxford: Clarendon Press.

Stanley, H. E., Amaral, L. A. N., Gopikrishnan, P., Ivanov, P. C., Keitt, T. H. & Plerou, V. (2000). Scale invariance and universality: organizing principles in complex systems. *Physica A*, **281**, 60–68.

Stauffer, D. (1979). Scaling theory of percolation clusters. *Physical Reports*, **54**, 1–74.

Stauffer, D. & Aharony, A. (1992). *Introduction to Percolation Theory*. London: Taylor & Francis.

Stephens, P. A. & Sutherland, W. J. (1999). Consequences of the Allee effect for behavior, ecology, and conservation. *Trends in Ecology and Evolution*, **14**(10), 401–404.

Szabó, G., Gergely, H. & Oborny, B. (2002). Generalized contact process on random environments. *Physical Reviews E*, **65**, 066111.

Tilman, D. (1994). Competition and biodiversity in spatially structured habitats. *Ecology*, **75**(1), 2–16.

Tilman, D. & Kareiva, P. (eds.) (1997). *Spatial Ecology: the Role of Space in Population Dynamics and Interspecific Interactions*. Princeton: Princeton University Press.

Tilman, D., May, R. M., Lehman, C. L. & Nowak, M. A. (1994). Habitat destruction and the extinction debt. *Nature*, **371**, 65–66.

Turner, M., Gardner, R. H. & O'Neill, R. V. (2001). *Landscape Ecology in Theory and Practice: Pattern and Process*. New York: Springer-Verlag.

Wiens, J. A. (1989). Spatial scaling in ecology. *Functional Ecology*, **3**, 385–397.

Wiens, J. A. (1997). Metapopulation dynamics and landscape ecology. In *Metapopulation Biology: Ecology, Genetics and Evolution*, ed. I. Hanski & M. E. Gilpin, pp. 3–68. London: Academic Press.

With, K. A., Gardner, R. H. & Turner, M. G. (1997). Landscape connectivity and population distribution in heterogeneous environments. *Oikos*, **78**, 151–169.

Yu, D. W. & Wilson, H. B. (2001). The competition-colonization trade-off is dead; long live the competition-colonization trade-off. *American Naturalist*, **158**(1), 49–63.

Zobel, M., Palmer, M. W., Kull, K. & Herben, T. (eds.) (1994). *Vegetation Structure and Species Coexistence*. Uppsala: Opulus Press.

CHAPTER TWENTY-ONE

# Biodiversity power laws

PABLO A. MARQUET
Pontificia Universidad Católica de Chile, CASEB, IEB, The Santa Fe Institute
SEBASTIAN R. ABADES
Pontificia Universidad Católica de Chile
FABIO A. LABRA
Pontificia Universidad Católica de Chile

## Introduction

The last ten years have been marked by important discoveries and scientific advances in our understanding of biodiversity. The emergence of new fields, such as bioinformatics, ecoinformatics, and computational ecology (Helly et al., 1995; Spengler, 2000; Green et al., 2005) has brought about an informational revolution by making available massive data sets on the composition, distribution and abundance of biodiversity from local to global scales and from genes to ecosystems. This has in turn changed biodiversity sciences, expanding the scale of analysis of ecological systems wherein biodiversity resides. While the 1970s and 1980s were marked by studies at local scales, the 1990s were marked by gaining access to regional, continental and global scale analyses. In parallel, and in part as a consequence of the above trend, there has been a shift from approaches that emphasize the highly variable and idiosyncratic nature of ecological systems to a view that emphasizes the action of first principles, natural laws and zeroth order approaches (the macroscopic approach hereafter).

The small-scale approach can be illustrated by a representative quotation from Diamond and Case (1986, p. x): "The answers to general ecological questions are rarely universal laws, like those of physics. Instead, the answers are conditional statements such as: for a community of species with properties $A_1$ and $A_2$ in habitat B and latitude C, limiting factors $X_2$ and $X_5$ are likely to predominate." Macroscopic approaches, in contrast, emphasize the existence of statistical patterns in the structure of communities that are thought to reflect the operation of general principles or natural laws. Prominent among these principles is the identification of scaling and power-law relationships with similar or related exponents, which as pointed out by West and Brown (2005) imply "the existence of powerful constraints at every level of biological organization. The self-similar power law scaling implies the existence of average, idealized biological systems, which represent a "0th order" baseline or

*Scaling Biodiversity*, ed. David Storch, Pablo A. Marquet and James H. Brown. Published by Cambridge University Press. © Cambridge University Press 2007.

point of departure for understanding the variation among real biological systems". These regularities underlie two related research programs in ecology: the first is macroecology (Brown & Maurer, 1989; Brown, 1995; Gaston & Blackburn, 2000; Marquet, 2002a; Storch & Gaston, 2004) and the second is the recently dubbed Metabolic Theory of Ecology (Brown *et al.*, 2004). The change in the conceptualization of ecological systems entailed by these approaches, as opposed to the idiosyncratic view expressed by Diamond and Case (1986), is apparent in the following excerpt (Brown *et al.*, 2004, p. 411): "Our own recent research is based on the premise that the general statistical patterns of macroecology are emergent phenomena of complex ecological systems that do indeed reflect the operation of universal law-like mechanisms." According to this view the law-like mechanisms are intrinsic to life itself and reflect the geometric, physical, chemical, and thermodynamic principles that affect the performance of living entities in different biotic and abiotic settings.

It is not at all unexpected that the macroscopic approach emphasizes the search for power laws and scaling relationships, for it is well known that these are quintessential to complex systems that emerge as statistical regularities not affected by the specific details of the interaction among system components (e.g. Stanley, 1995; Stanley *et al.*, 2000). Despite their potential importance, however, power-law distributions remain little explored in ecology, where most of the attention has been put into the analysis of simple scaling relationships, which although related, are fundamentally different, as we shall see below.

In general, relationships where some quantity can be expressed as some power of another according to the following functional form

$$y = \beta x^{\alpha} \tag{21.1}$$

are called power-law relationships. Power laws are well known to biologists in the form of bivariate relationships of power-law type called scaling relationships (e.g. Peters, 1983; Marquet, Navarrete & Castilla, 1990; Brown & West, 2000; Brown *et al.*, 2002; Chave & Levin, 2003) by which molecular, physiological, ecological, and life history attributes relate to some attribute of organisms raised to a power as in Eq. (21.1). Further, scaling in ecology has been usually associated with relationship where the independent variable is the size of an organism (Peters, 1983; Calder, 1984; Schmidt-Nielsen, 1984). I will call these "allometric scaling relationships" and will differentiate them from power laws that represent probability or frequency distributions, of the form $p(x) = Cx^{\alpha}$.

In this chapter, we will show that power laws are ubiquitous in ecological systems, and although they represent a challenge for understanding, at the same time they provide an interesting interdisciplinary research venue for identifying the general principles underlying biodiversity patterns and dynamics. We will start with a brief description of power laws and scaling relationships and the importance of extreme events (those occurring in the tail of probability distributions) and then provide a couple of selected examples on the existence of power laws in the abundance and population dynamics of species.

## The power is in the tails

Power laws are closely related to fat-tail distributions. A distribution $P(x)$ is said to be a "fat-tailed" distribution if the probability associated with larger values of $x$ contain a larger fraction of the probability mass or density than a Gaussian distribution or any other reference distribution with thin tails, typically a Gaussian or exponential (see Fig. 21.1). The importance of distributions with fat tails is that any distribution with "sufficiently fat tails" is a power-law distribution (J. D. Farmer and J. Geanakoplos, unpublished manuscript), although in a strict sense this is true for a particular class of non-Gaussian Lévy stable distributions only (see Mantegna & Stanley, 2000). In general, we can say that a random variable $X$ follows a power-law distribution if

$$P[X > x] \sim x^{-\alpha} \text{ as } x \to \infty, \tag{21.2}$$

which is equivalent to say that it follows a power law above some threshold $x$. Following Newman (2005), a continuous random variable with power-law distribution will take a value in the interval $x + dx$ with probability $p(x)\, dx$ where

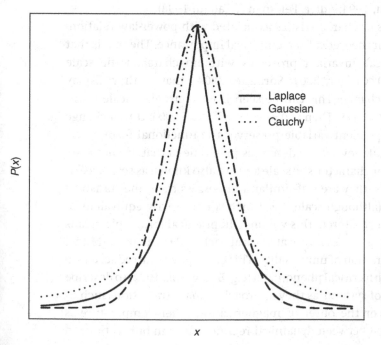

Figure 21.1 Gaussian, Laplace and Cauchy distributions showing the fat tail of the Cauchy, which is well described by a power law.

$$p(x) = Cx^{-(1+\alpha)}, \tag{21.3}$$

which holds for $\alpha > 0$ and above some lowest value $x_{min}$. Interestingly, if $\alpha \leq 1$, the first central moment of the distribution, or its mean, is not finite (i.e. is undefined). Similarly, if $\alpha < 2$, the variance does not converge to any finite value but increases with the sample; a phenomenon commonly observed in ecological time series of abundance and dubbed the "more time more variation effect" (e.g. Pimm & Redfearn, 1988; Inchausti & Halley, 2003). Power laws are ubiquitous in physical and social systems, emerging in phenomena such as the frequency of earthquakes of different magnitudes (the Gutenberg–Richter Law), the distribution of income among individuals (Pareto's law), and the rank–frequency distribution of words in natural languages and city sizes (Zipf's law) (see Mantegna & Stanley, 2000; Sornette, 2004; Newman, 2005, for a discussion of these and other power laws).

Fat-tail distributions are becoming increasingly important in ecological research, especially in the analysis of plant and animal dispersal data (Kot, Lewis & van den Driessche, 1996; Viswanathan *et al.*, 1996, 1999; Clark *et al.*, 1999; Mårell, Ball & Hofgaard, 2002; Gautestad & Mysterud, 2005; Katul *et al.*, 2005; Borda-de-Água *et al.*, this volume). Considering the wild behavior of power-law distributions, their existence represents a challenge to ecologists fascinated with Gaussian distributions with central tendencies and finite variances, and who are therefore used to statistical tools based on them. Fortunately, theory and statistical methods to work with fat-tailed distributions are being developed (Samorodnitsky & Taqqu, 1994; Adler, Feldman & Taqqu, 1998).

There are two notions or characteristics associated with power-law relationships that single out their theoretical and empirical importance. The first is that power laws describe scale-invariant processes with no characteristic scale (e.g. Stanley *et al.*, 2000; Gisiger, 2001; Sornette, 2004), that is, they display invariance under scale change. This can be seen if we consider a scale transformation in $x$ such that $x \to \lambda x$. Then $p(x) = \beta x^{\alpha} \to \beta \lambda^{\alpha} x^{\alpha} = \lambda^{\alpha} p(x)$; thus a change in the scale of the independent variable preserves the functional form of the original relationship. Scale invariance describes phenomena that are not associated with a particular or characteristic scale and are also known as scale-free or true on all scales; that is, they are self-similar and possess the same statistical properties at any scale (although scale invariance is not exactly equivalent to self-similarity; see Šizling & Storch, this volume). In practical terms this means that the same principles or processes are at work at each scale of analysis (Milne, 1998). The second is the notion of universality. This concept was introduced into physics in association with critical phenomena (e.g. Biney *et al.*, 1992) to describe the state and dynamics of systems as they approach a phase transition (such as water turning into ice or the onset of magnetization when temperature is changed or the transition between dynamical regimes through bifurcations in deterministic dynamical systems). Near phase transitions, systems are said to become critical and relevant quantities that describe their state (e.g. magnitude of fluctuations, correlation length) have power-law probability distributions with critical exponents (e.g. Stanley, 1971, 1995, 1999; Maris & Kadanoff, 1978; Solé et al., 1996; Oborný et al., this volume). Interestingly, it has been shown that systems which are completely different away from a critical point, show similar critical exponents and their macroscopic phases become indistinguishable at the critical point (e.g. Biney et al., 1992). These nonarbitrary exponents are said to be universal and define disjoint classes (universality classes) into which different physical systems can be classified. A system can arrive at a critical state through changes in a variable external to it (e.g. temperature), but also as a result of its own internal dynamics, in which case we speak of self-organized criticality, a concept introduced by Bak, Tang and Wiesenfeld (1987). During the last decade or so, several empirical and theoretical investigations have suggested that biological systems in general, and ecological systems in particular, seem to operate near a critical state, which results in the ubiquity of power-law behavior in several descriptors of their dynamics (e.g. Miramontes, 1995; Bak, 1996; Keitt & Marquet, 1996; Rhodes, Jensen & Anderson, 1997; Ferrier & Cazelles, 1999; Solé et al., 1999; Gisiger, 2001; Solé, Alonso & McKane, 2002; Roy, Pascual & Franc, 2003; Pascual & Guichard, 2005), and might even belong to the same universality class as other complex systems such as economic systems (Stanley et al., 2000). Thus the analysis of power laws and scaling relationships can help us to identify general principles that apply across a wide range of scales and levels of organization, revealing the existence of universal principles within the seemingly idiosyncratic nature of ecological systems. However, it should be borne in mind that power laws might emerge as a consequence of several processes not necessarily related to critical points and phase transitions (Brock, 1999; Mitzenmacher, 2001; Allen, Li & Charnov, 2001; Sornette, 2004; Newman, 2005; Perline, 2005; Solow, 2005), so that whether ecological systems are maintained near a critical state or not is still an open question.

## Power laws in ecological quantities

As reviewed by Marquet et al. (2005), power laws are common descriptors of several ecological quantities. They emerge for example in the size and duration of epidemic events (Rhodes & Anderson, 1996; Rhodes et al., 1997), in patterns of abundance, distribution, and richness (e.g. Frontier, 1985; Banavar et al., 1999; Harte, Kinzig & Green, 1999; Harte, Blackburn & Ostling, 2001; Marquet, 2002b; Labra, Abades & Marquet, 2005), in food web attributes (e.g. Garlaschelli, Caldarelli & Pietronero, 2003; Brose et al., 2004), and in disturbances such as landslides and fire (Malamud et al., 2004; Malamud, Millington & Perry, 2005; Moritz et al., 2005). In the following paragraphs we will present and discuss some power laws associated with population abundance and dynamics.

## Abundance

One of the characteristics of the frequency distribution of species abundance is the appearance of heavy tails, such that there is a nonnegligible probability of finding extreme values in abundance. These patterns have been usually modeled more or less accurately by means of lognormal distributions, or by fitting exponential functions in order to describe their tail behavior (Williamson, 1972; May, 1975; Dennis & Patil, 1998; Diserud & Engen, 2000; Halley & Inchausti, 2002; Marquet, Keymer & Cofre, 2003). However, recent theoretical developments have called attention to the possibility that they may also conform to a power-law form (Brown, Mehlman & Stevens, 1995; Ives & Klopper, 1997; Solé & Alonso, 1998; Sornette, 1998; McGill & Collins, 2003; Niwa, 2003; Labra *et al.*, 2005; Marquet *et al.*, 2005), which opens a different scheme of interpretation.

To illustrate the existence of power-law signatures in the distribution of abundances across space at a continental geographical scale we used the North American Breeding Bird Survey (hereafter BBS; Sauer, Hines & Fallon, 2005), which comprises several thousand routes of approximately 24.5 miles long each, sampled once a year during the breeding/nesting season (mainly June) across USA and southern Canada (Sauer *et al.*, 2005). We analyzed three different levels of description representing different ways of analyzing data: intraspecific, interspecific and no-specific. The first level was simply analyzed by constructing probability plots from local abundances measured at different locations in space for a single species. In the second approach, we used the total number of individuals per species measured at the continental level. Finally, we avoided using any taxonomic membership and constructed frequency distributions for the total number of individuals observed in different locations across the continent, irrespective of species identity. For all analyses we used BBS raw counts of individuals, only excluding routes that have remained inactive since 1982. Probability plots were done for every level of description and for years 1982 and 2002. These years were chosen in order to check the robustness of the pattern. In addition to power laws, we also fitted an exponential distribution, since it captures the rapid probability decay in the tails when no scale-free dynamics is present (Newman, 2005). In order to illustrate the intraspecific distribution of local abundances we used as focal species the American coot (*Fulica americana*), a social bird that lives in flocks. This species is a migratory bird found in freshwater lakes and ponds across USA and Canada in summer and in the southern portion of the USA in winter (Terres, 1980; Udvardy, 1994). It is important to keep in mind that the BBS data may suffer from strong biases regarding the effect of habitat complexity upon bird counts, which may affect the effective survey radius (Hurlbert, 2004), and observer quality (Sauer, Peterjohn & Link, 1994). If these were important we would expect significant deviations from a power-law relationship, as scale invariance would be violated. Such deviations may manifest themselves as regime shifts or cutoffs in the observed distributions.

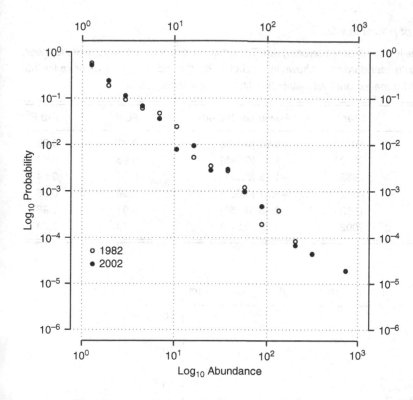

Figure 21.2 Empirical probability distribution for local abundances observed across USA for the American coot (intraspecific level of description).

Interspecific probability patterns were explored for a total of 534 and 595 species (years 1982 and 2002, respectively), summing all individuals counted per species across all routes in the USA. As in the intraspecific case, linear fits in log-log scale and exponential fitting were used to test for the presence of a power-law relationship. Finally we constructed empirical probability distributions for local abundances irrespective of taxonomic identity, by counting the total number of individuals observed in every route sampled across the USA. We fitted the models for years 1982 (1769 routes) and 2002 (2676 routes), but, as is clear in Fig. 21.3, only the right tail was used for the power law fit, given that a small "rollover" is present at low abundances.

The empirical probability distribution for the intraspecific case is shown in Fig. 21.2. Both the exponential and power-law distributions provided significantly good fits, but the power law explained a larger amount of variance than the exponential (Table 21.1). The power-law regime ranged over three orders of magnitude, with a consistent tail exponent of 1.85 for both years compared (Table 21.1). In general, the tail exponent value indicates the number of finite moments of the probability distribution, which in this case implies the existence of a mean but no bounded variance (e.g. Stanley, 1971; Newman, 2005). The lack of finite second and upper moments is indicative of a strong scale-free phenomenon, with a heavy tail towards high abundances. In practical terms,

**Table 21.1** *Summary of power law fits*

Aggregation indicates the level of description analyzed. Tail index corresponds to the slope of the linear regression on log-log scale (standard error shown in brackets). PL $R^2$ is the explained variance for the power law fit and Exp $R^2$ for the exponential distribution fit; $P$-value $< 0.05$.

| Aggregation | Year | Power-law tail index | PL $R^2$ | Exp $R^2$ |
|---|---|---|---|---|
| Intraspecific (Fig. 21.1) | 1982 | −1.85 [0.075] | 0.97 | 0.69 |
| | 2002 | −1.85 [0.045] | 0.98 | 0.53 |
| Interspecific (Fig. 21.2) | 1982 | −1.15 [0.031] | 0.96 | 0.54 |
| | 2002 | −1.11 [0.030] | 0.96 | 0.56 |
| No-specific (Fig. 21.3) | 1982 | −3.43 [0.350] | 0.91 | 0.96 |
| | 2002 | −3.78 [0.216] | 0.96 | 0.73 |

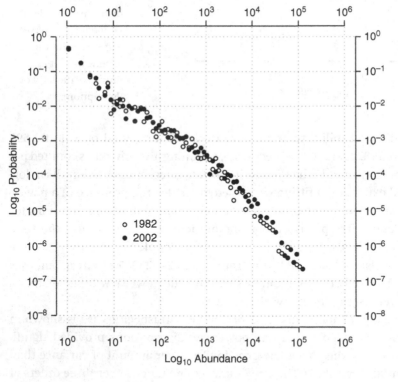

**Figure 21.3** Empirical probability distribution for the total number of individuals per species across the USA (interspecific level of description).

a distribution with an infinite second moment indicates that no matter how much sample size is increased, variance will always keep on increasing (Stanley, 1971; Newman, 2005). A power-law probability distribution in local abundances captures valuable information about the internal structure of a species' geographical range: all abundance levels are present in inverse proportion to its

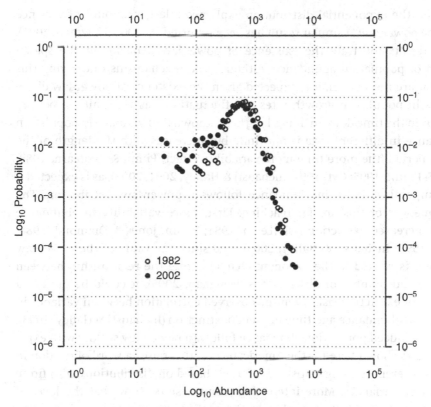

**Figure 21.4** Empirical probability distribution for the total number of individuals observed across the USA irrespective of taxonomic membership (no-specific level of description).

size, similar to the well-known Gutenberg–Richter law for earthquakes (Gutenberg & Richter, 1944; Christensen *et al.*, 2002). Thus, abundances described at a geographical scale would be characterized by a few very abundant local spots and many less abundant sites (see Brown *et al.*, 1995) covering a large spectrum of local realizations and departing from what would be expected under a "normal" fast exponential decay (Newman, 2005; McGill & Collins, 2003).

In the interspecific case (Fig. 21.3), a power law ranging five orders of magnitude also characterized distributions better than exponentials, with tail exponents of 1.11 and 1.15 for years 1982 and 2002, respectively (Table 21.1). Accordingly, finite first but no second moment exists, thus a heavy right skew governs these distributions. For the no-specific case (Fig. 21.4) the probability distributions for the total number of individuals measured across the USA, irrespective of taxonomic identity, show a power-law decay covering almost two orders of magnitude but only for year 2002, after the small "rollover" at approximately 5000 individuals. The exponent is 3.78, indicating a fast decaying tail, but still differing from an exponential one (Table 21.1). For year 1982, however, the exponential distribution explained a larger amount of variance than the power law. A similar result has been reported for 2003 (Newman, 2005).

Our results illustrate the existence of power-law behavior in the spatial pattern of population abundance. Although the mechanisms underlying this behavior are not known, it is expected given the existence of power-law distributions in population growth rates and fluctuations (as we shall see below). Further, in the time domain, it has long been known that variance in population abundance in different taxa is not finite but increases with the length of the census period (the more time more variability effect; Pimm & Redfearn, 1988; Arino & Pimm, 1995; Cyr, 1997; Inchausti & Halley, 2001, 2002), as is expected if the temporal variance in abundance follows a power-law distribution. The consequences of this are far reaching. First, more variability in abundance means increased extinction risk (Leigh, 1981; Pimm, Jones & Diamond, 1988; Lande, 1993; Inchausti & Halley, 2003). And since the value of the power-law exponent is related to the exponent characterizing the relationship between variance and number of observations (Newman, 2005), it could be used as a measure of extinction risk given the observed correlation between variance in population abundance and time to pseudoextinction (Inchausti & Halley, 2003). Second, if indeed population abundance follows a power-law scaling with exponents <2 as shown here for the American coot, this raises a word of caution in making inferences using statistical methods based on distributions with finite means and variances. More interestingly, our results show that the level of description does affect the value of the scaling exponents, which tend to increase from intraspecific to the interspecific and no-specific level of analyses. The observed rollover and the fact that the power-law behavior may disappear at the no-specific level of description are difficult to explain. These might be a consequence of sample biases as pointed out above. This clearly requires further investigation.

## Growth rates

Standard ecological wisdom asserts that population size is expected to follow a lognormal distribution, given that it is the product of a multiplicative renewal processes (e.g. MacArthur, 1960; Lawton, 1989; Blackburn, Lawton & Pimm, 1993; Halley & Inchausti, 2002; but see Williamson & Gaston, 2005). Furthermore, several single species population models give rise to normal or lognormal population abundance distributions (e.g. Keeling, 2000). If population abundances in different time intervals follow a lognormal distribution, it is expected that the ratio of successive abundances $N(t+1)/N(t)$ also has a lognormal distribution, and hence, the logarithm of such a ratio $r = \ln[N(t+1)/N(t)]$, should show a normal or Gaussian distribution. In other words, under an expectation of lognormal population abundances, population growth rates should exhibit a Gaussian probability distribution.

Keitt and collaborators (Keitt & Stanley, 1998; Keitt *et al.*, 2002), however, have shown that population growth rates of North American breeding birds show a power-law probability distribution. As seen in Fig. 21.5(a), this tent-shaped distribution is symmetric about a zero growth rate, with an equal probability of observing increases or decreases for the species studied. While these findings have been criticized, casting doubts on their generality, recent research shows that they are indeed general. Analysis of population growth rates of local ensembles of birds, small mammals and trees has shown that they share the same power law functional form (Labra, 2005), indicating that they do not depend on the geographic scale of analysis. As a further example, when all fish species found in a local community are considered (Magurran & Henderson, 2003), the same tent-shaped power law distribution of growth rates is once again observed (Fig. 21.5b). The fact that species with very different lifestyles, resource requirements, and phylogenetic history show such a consistent pattern is suggestive of a general set of processes giving rise to this power-law distribution.

The presence of scaling and universality in population growth rates has strong implications for understanding population dynamics in general. In physical systems, scaling is often found in the presence of "cooperative" behavior. In inanimate systems such as ferromagnets near a critical temperature point, scaling relationships arise because each particle interacts directly with a few neighboring particles, and as these neighboring particles interact with their neighbors, interactions can "propagate" long distances, thus resulting in power-law distributions (Stanley *et al.*, 2000). Similar results have been observed for the probability distributions of growth rates of companies, universities and countries' gross national product. In physics, such behavior is interpreted as evidence that the particular details of the interaction among the components of the system have no role in setting the system properties, which depends mostly on the dimensionality of the system. This strongly suggests that there may indeed exist universal principles that underlie the growth dynamics of complex adaptive systems involved in the acquisition, transformation and storage of information, materials and/or energy. Recently, Fu *et al.* (2005) have shown that the shape of the distribution of growth rates may be explained by a general stochastic model, which accounts for both the central part as well as the tails of the distributions observed in business and firms' growth rates. Interestingly, the shape of the business growth-rate distribution is due to the proportional growth in number and size of the constituent units of businesses of a given size. More importantly, this result is claimed to hold both in an open economy (with entry of new firms) as well as in a closed economy (with no entry of new firms). Whether similar mechanisms may hold in ecological systems poses a very interesting research question.

In the case of ecological communities, the scaling in population growth or fluctuation can be brought about either by the spatial dimension of spatial

(a)

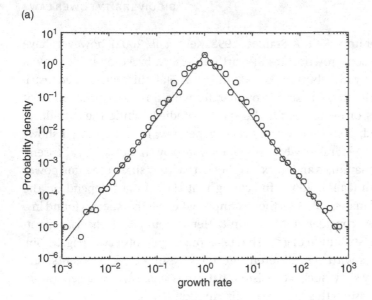

(b)

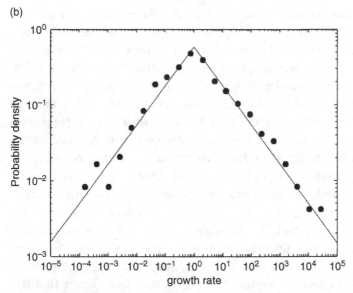

**Figure 21.5** Probability distribution of population growth rates. (a) The distribution of population growth rates across all species in the North American Breeding Bird Survey data set over three decades. The growth rate $r(t)_s$ is calculated by log transforming the ratio of species abundances in successive years, i.e. $r(t)_s \equiv \log[N(t+1)/N(t)]$. Abundances are taken as the total number of individuals of a particular species counted within each survey route. Modified after Keitt and Stanley (1998). (b) The distribution of population growth rates across all fish species in the Hinkley point data set over two decades. The growth rate $r(t)_s$ is calculated by log transforming the ratio of species abundances in successive years, i.e. $r(t)_s \equiv \log[N(t+1)/N(t)]$. Abundances are taken as the monthly average number of individuals of a particular species counted within each year. Data were obtained from the Global Population Dynamics Database. In both cases the distribution of growth rates shows a scale invariant form, symmetric about $r_s = 0$, which indicates a balance in population increases and decreases for the species in the sample over the study period.

population structure, or more importantly, by the physical dimension of energy and material flows. In the first case, it can be argued that interactions in ecological systems may propagate through spatial metapopulation dynamics, with local populations interacting through colonization–extinction dynamics with nearby populations (see Oborny et al., this volume; Kunin, this volume; Borda-de-Água et al., this volume). By contrast, species present in an ecosystem interact directly with some (but not necessarily all) species, which may in turn interact with a second set of species, so that interactions can "propagate" through time and space from the individual to the population, community and ecosystems, and finally to the biosphere scale. The fundamental connectivity of the living makes the existence of power laws plausible.

The relationship between energy and material flows and the emergence of observed power laws in ecological systems can be further highlighted by an important implication, which although remarked by Keitt and Stanley (1998), has not been emphasized by previous authors. In addition to its tent-shaped form and the observed rescaling features, the observed distribution of growth rates is highly symmetrical about $r_s = 0$ in all cases considered (Fig. 21.5). This implies that exactly as many species are increasing in abundance as are decreasing over the 31-year period studied, be it over the whole ensemble, or when grouping by initial abundance bins (although it is not the case at the level of such ecological groups as forest or grassland birds; see Sauer et al., 2005). This result strongly suggests that these species undergo a zero sum dynamics in population size, with demographic gains and losses by all the species balancing over the study period. This is not obvious, nor is it expected from previous theoretical explanations for the emergence of scaling laws in physical systems. The idea of the existence of zero sum dynamics in ecosystems under energy limitation can be dated back to the Red Queen Hypothesis, which predicts that any change in the control of trophic energy by a species is balanced by a net equal and opposite change in the amount of trophic energy controlled by all the other species in the community with which that species interact (Van Valen, 1976, 1977; Stenseth, 1979). In this formulation, trophic energy, defined as an individual's control of a constant amount of the energy available to a group of related species that compete for it, is a proxy for fitness. This implies that, in general, resource (energy) use by the species in a community is a zero-sum game (Hubbell, 1997, 2001; Bell, 2000), with a balance in the energy gained and lost by all the interacting species. In this regard, the Red Queen Hypothesis emphasizes that under a scenario of finite resources zero-sum dynamics must necessarily operate, as an expression of the first law of thermodynamics (Van Valen, 1976, 1977; also see open discussion in Van Valen, 1980).

It is important to note that these results have not been exempt from criticism in the literature, and we close this section by mentioning and discussing the main points made against the existence of power laws in the distribution of population growth rates. It has been argued that the tent-shaped distribution of population growth rates may be the end product of a mixture of lognormal distributions in population size (Allen *et al.*, 2001). This phenomenological explanation, however, does not account for the symmetrical nature of the distribution, nor does it provide a mechanism that accounts for its form and location. Another possible explanation of these results is that the distribution of growth rates in the community arises from a mixture of Gaussian population growth rate distributions for each of the species with different variances (Amaral *et al.*, 1998). This would require, nevertheless, that all the distributions of growth rates be centered with mean zero, so that all species must be, at all times, regulated around an equilibrium point, and hence it does not take into account the fact that in the observed data some species show marked trends in abundance, and thus species increases had to be balanced by decreases in other species.

## Population fluctuations

Power laws in population fluctuations are well known and have been the focus of an increasing number of contributions in recent years, as a consequence of the availability of long time series in population dynamics, such as the Breeding Bird Survey (BBS) and the Global Population Dynamics Database (GPDD). Time series analyses of population fluctuations have shown that the amplitude of fluctuations ($n$) decreases, on average, as the inverse of the frequency ($f$) with which they occur or as "$1/f$ noise" or "pink noise" (e.g. Halley, 1996; Miramontes & Rohani, 1998; Inchausti & Halley, 2001; Storch, Gaston & Cepák, 2002; see review in Halley & Inchausti, 2004) such that the distribution of fluctuation sizes $D(n)$ is described by a power law of the form $D(n) \sim n^{-\alpha}$, with $\alpha$ close to 1, as expected under self-organized criticality (Bak, Tang & Wiesenfeld, 1987).

In addition to $1/f$ noise, one of ecology's most interesting patterns regarding population variablity is Taylor's power law (Taylor, 1961). It has been observed that for many species the variance in population abundance $s^2(N)$ is related to the mean of population abundance $<N>$ by a power law with a fractional exponent: $s^2(N) \propto <N>^g$ (Taylor, 1961; Taylor & Woiwod, 1980; Anderson *et al.*, 1982; Hanski & Tiainen, 1989; Boag, Hackett & Topham, 1992; Keitt & Stanley, 1998). For the vast majority of species, the power-law scaling parameter, $g$, is found to lie between 1 and 2, with many species lying close to the extremes (Anderson *et al.*, 1982). This scaling relationship has been described for a wide range of taxa, in both space and time.

It is interesting to note that, should Taylor's power law hold for temporal variation in abundance, and if the temporal mean abundance follows a negative relationship with body size, the scale invariance in both power-law relationships make it possible to derive the scaling in population variability as a function of body size, and it can be expected that $s^2(N) \propto (<M>^n)^g \propto <M>^{ng}$. Thus, as $n$

is expected to be $-3/4$ and $g$ is usually between 1 and 2, hence population variability should show a negative scaling relationship with body mass, taking values between $-3/4$ and $-3/2$. Although this relationship has not been tested explicitly in the literature, the work by Keitt *et al.* (2002) provides evidence that such a negative scaling may hold for North American birds when studied at the population level. These authors show that the standard deviation $s(r_s)$ of population growth rates in North American birds is strongly related to the average total population size. The relationship follows a power law $s(r_s) \propto <N>^b$, for over four orders of magnitude in $<N>$, the total population abundance averaged across all 31 years studied. Using major axis regression with bootstrap precision estimates, Keitt *et al.* (2002) find $b = 0.36 \pm 0.02$, so that Taylor's exponent (here replicated across species) is found to be $g = 1.28 \pm 0.04$. Again, under the assumption that there exists a negative relationship between average abundance in time and body size: $<N> \propto <M>^n$, with $n = -3/4$, it can be seen that the temporal variance in population abundance should scale approximately as $M^{-1.0}$ ($-0.96 \pm 0.03$). By contrast, the standard deviation in population growth rate should scale as $s(r_s) \propto <M>^{bn}$, which predicts then that fluctuations in growth rates should show a $M^{-1/4}$ scaling (the predicted value is $-0.27 \pm 0.05$), as do other temporal phenomena in ecology and biology (Calder, 1983; West, 1999). It certainly would be interesting to test whether these predictions hold to empirical scrutiny for the species studied by Keitt and collaborators (Keitt & Stanley, 1998; Keitt *et al.*, 2002) as well as for other taxa and at other spatial scales of study.

## Concluding remarks

We have shown that power laws may characterize the statistical behavior of several ecological quantities associated with population abundance, growth and fluctuation. Further, the scale invariance that power-law distributions entail suggests that, despite the idiosyncrasy that might dominate the interaction among system components, there are some general principles underlying the dynamics of the system at different scales. The empirical verification of power-law behavior, however, should not be taken as an end in itself but as the starting point for analyzing the complexity of ecological systems. Power laws are in essence empirical laws that allow for a statistical description of complex systems where the nature of the interaction among system components is unknown. The challenge ahead is to develop theoretical models that on the one hand explain observed patterns and, on the other, make quantitative predictions of new ones. Unless this agenda is carried out, we risk the possibility of being adrift in a sea of empirical relationships and idiosyncratic explanations. This assumes, however, that well-resolved and comprehensive data sets on ecological quantities, which will allow for a good documentation of extreme events that occur in the tail of frequency distributions, are available. Otherwise is the risk of working with truncated distributions that may give rise to false power laws. As recently shown by Perline (2005) truncated lognormal-like distributions can mimic power-law behavior. Unfortunately, the reverse can also be true; that is, a distribution can be a power law but the existence of an exponential cutoff (a fast exponential decay in the tail probabilities) can blur the pattern. Such behavior could emerge as a consequence of the finite nature of the system (but see Laherrère & Sornette, 1998; Fenner, Levene & Loizou, 2005) as is known, for example, in the study of critical phenomena that take place in the thermodynamic limit (infinite system size). Fortunately, information obtained for finite systems can be extrapolated to infinite size by using a phenomenological approximation known as finite size scaling (FSS; Cardy, 1988). In principle, any finite variable showing power-law distribution ought to exhibit finite size scaling and thus the effect of system size dependence can be explicitly modeled, allowing for an assessment of their power-law behavior and the value of its associated scaling exponents. This technique can be of great relevance for the analysis of ecological systems, as demonstrated by recent applications (Banavar *et al.*, 1999; Keitt *et al.*, 2002; Rinaldo *et al.*, 2002; Niwa, 2005). Power laws might provide a new venue for research into biodiversity. It remains to be seen, however, to what extent the challenge of embracing a non-Gaussian world can be met both in theoretical and empirical terms.

## Acknowledgments

We acknowledge support from FONDECYT-FONDAP 1501-0001, Millenium Center Institute Project, Instituto de Ecología y Biodiversidad (IEB) and the Santa Fe Institute. This is contribution #6 to the Ecoinformatics and Biocomplexity Unit. Part of this work was conducted while PM was a Sabbatical Fellow at the National Center for Ecological Analysis and Synthesis, funded by NSF (Grant no. DEB-0072909), the University of California, and the Santa Barbara campus. We thank David Storch for his comments and suggestions on the final version of this manuscript.

## References

Adler, R., Feldman, R. & Taqqu, M. S. (eds.) (1998). *A Practical Guide to Heavytails: Statistical Techniques for Analyzing Heavy-Tailed Distributions*. Boston: Birkhauser.

Allen, A. P., Li, B. & Charnov, E. L. (2001). Population fluctuations, power laws and mixtures of lognormal distributions. *Ecology Letters*, **4**, 1–3.

Amaral, L. A. N., Buldyrev, S. V., Havlin, S., Salinger, M. A. & Stanley, H. E. (1998). Power law scaling for a system of interacting units with complex internal structure. *Physical Review Letters*, **80**, 1385–1388.

Anderson, R. M., Gordon, D. M., Crawley, M. J. & Hassell, M. P. (1982). Variability in the abundance of animal and plant species, *Nature*, **296**, 245–248.

Arino, A. & Pimm, S. L. (1995). On the nature of population extremes. *Evolutionary Ecology*, **9**, 429–443.

Bak, P. (1996). *How Nature Works. The Science of Self-Organized Criticality*. New York: Springer-Verlag.

Bak, P., Tang C. & Wiesenfeld, K. (1987). Self-organized criticality: an explanation of 1/f noise. *Physical Review Letters*, **59**, 381–384.

Banavar, J. R., Green, J. L., Harte, J. & Maritan, A. (1999). Finite size scaling in ecology. *Physical Review Letters*, **83**, 4212–4214.

Bell, G. (2000). The distribution of abundance in neutral communities. *American Naturalist*, **155**, 606–617.

Biney, J. J., Dowrick, N. J., Fisher, A. J. & Newman, M. E. J. (1992). *The Theory of Critical Phenomena*. Oxford: Clarendon Press.

Blackburn T. M., Lawton, J. H. & Pimm, S. L. (1993). Non-metabolic explanations for the relationship between body size and animal abundance. *Journal of Animal Ecology*, **62**, 694–702.

Boag, B., Hackett, C. A. & Topham, P. B. (1992). The use of Taylor power law to describe the aggregated distribution of gastrointestinal nematodes of sheep. *International Journal of Parasitology*, **22**, 267–270.

Brock, W. A. (1999). Scaling in economics: a reader's guide. *Industrial and Corporate Change*, **8**, 409–446.

Brose, U., Ostling, A., Harrison, K. & Martinez, N. D. (2004). Unified spatial scaling of species and their trophic interactions. *Nature*, **428**, 167–171.

Brown, J. H. (1995). *Macroecology*. Chicago: University of Chicago Press.

Brown, J. H. & Maurer, B. A. (1989). Macroecology: the division of food and space among species on continents. *Science*, **243**, 1145–1150.

Brown, J. H. & West, G. B. (2000). *Scaling in Biology*. New York: Oxford University Press.

Brown, J. H., Mehlman, D. W. & Stevens, G. C. (1995). Spatial variation in abundance. *Ecology*, **76**, 2028–2043.

Brown, J. H., Gupta, V. K., Li, B-L, Milne, B. T., Restrepo, C. & West, G. B. (2002). The fractal nature of nature: power laws, ecological complexity and biodiversity. *Philosophical Transactions of the Royal Society of London, Series B*, **357**, 619–626.

Brown, J. H., Gillooly, J. F., Allen, A. P., Savage, V. M. & West, G. B. (2004). Toward a metabolic theory of ecology. *Ecology*, **85**, 1771–1789.

Calder III, W. A. (1983). Ecological scaling: mammals and birds. *Annual Review of Ecology and Systematics*, **14**, 213–230.

Calder III, W. A. (1984). *Size, Function and Life History*. Cambridge, MA: Harvard University Press.

Cardy, J. L. (ed.) (1988). *Finite-size scaling*. New York: North Holland.

Chave, J. & Levin, S. A. (2003). Scale and scaling in ecological and economic systems. *Environmental Resource Economics*, **26**, 527–557.

Christensen, K., Danon, L., Scanlon, T. & Bak, P. (2002). Unified scaling law for earthquakes. *Proceedings of the National Academy of Sciences of the USA*, **99**, 2509–2513.

Clark, J. S., Silman, M., Kern, R., Macklin, E. & HilleRisLambers, J. (1999). Seed dispersal near and far: patterns across temperate and tropical forests. *Ecology*, **80**, 1475–1494.

Cyr, H. (1997). Does inter-annual variability in population density increase with time? *Oikos*, **79**, 549–558.

Dennis, B. & Patil, G. P. (1988). Applications in ecology. In *Lognormal Distributions: Theory and Applications*, ed. E. L. Crow & K. Shimizu, pp. 303–330. New York: Marcel Dekker.

Diamond, J. M. & Case, T. (eds.) (1986). *Community Ecology*. New York: Harper and Row.

Diserud, O. H. & Engen, S. (2000). A general and dynamic species abundance model, embracing the lognormal and the gamma models. *American Naturalist*, **155**, 497–511.

Fenner, T., Levene, M. & Loizou, G. (2005). A stochastic evolutionary model exhibiting power-law behaviour with an exponential cutoff. *Physica A*, **355**, 641–656.

Ferrier, R. & Cazelles, B. (1999). Universal power laws govern intermittent rarity in communities of interacting species. *Ecology*, **80**, 1505–1521.

Frontier, S. (1985). Diversity and structure in aquatic ecosystems. *Oceanography and Marine Biology Annual Review*, **23**, 253–312.

Fu, D., Pammolli, F., Buldyrev, S. V., *et al.* (2005). The growth of business firms: theoretical framework and empirical evidence. *Proceedings of the National Academy of Sciences of the USA*, **102**, 18801–18806.

Garlaschelli, D., Caldarelli, G. & Pietronero, L. (2003). Universal scaling relations in food webs. *Nature*, **423**, 165–168.

Gaston, K. J. & Blackburn, T. M. (2000). *Patterns and Processes in Macroecology*. Oxford: Blackwell Science.

Gautestad, A. O. & Mysterud, I. (2005). Instrinsic scaling complexity in animal dispersion and abundance. *American Naturalist*, **165**, 44–55.

Gisiger, T. (2001). Scale invariance in biology: coincidence or footprint of an universal mechanism? *Biological Reviews*, **76**, 161–209.

Green, J. L., Hastings, A., Arzberger, P., *et al.* (2005). Complexity in ecology and conservation: mathematical, statistical, and computational challenges. *BioScience*, **55**, 501–510.

Gutenberg, B. & Richter, C. F. (1944). Frequency of earthquakes in California. *Bulletin of Seismological Society of America*, **34**, 185–188.

Halley, J. (1996). Ecology, evolution and 1/f noise. *Trends in Ecology and Evolution*, **11**, 33–37.

Halley, J. & Inchausti, P. (2002). Lognormality in ecological time series. *Oikos*, **99**, 518–530.

Halley, J. & Inchausti, P. (2004). The increasing importance of 1/f noises as models of ecological variability. *Fluctuation and Noise Letters*, **4**, R1–R26.

Hanski, I. & Tiainen, J. (1989). Bird ecology and Taylor variance-mean regression. *Annales Zoologici Fennici*, **26**, 213–217.

Harte, J., Kinzig, A. & Green, J. (1999). Self-similarity in the distribution and abundance of species. *Science*, **284**, 334–336.

Harte, J., Blackburn, T. & Ostling, A. (2001). Self-similarity and the relationship between abundance and range size. *American Naturalist*, **157**, 374–386.

Helly, J., Case, T., Davis, F., Levin, S. A. & Michener, W. (eds.) (1995). *The State of Computational Ecology*. San Diego, CA: San Diego Super Computer Center.

Hubbell, S. P. (1997). A unified theory of biogeography and relative species abundance and its application to tropical rain forest and coral reefs. *Coral Reefs*, **16**, 9–21.

Hubbell, S. P. (2001). *A Unified Theory of Biodiversity and Biogeography*. Princeton: Princeton University Press.

Hurlbert, A. H. (2004). Species-energy relationships and habitat complexity in bird communities. *Ecology Letters*, **7**, 714–720.

Inchausti, P. & Halley, J. (2001). Investigating long-term ecological variability using the Global Population Dynamics Database. *Science*, **293**, 655–657.

Inchausti, P. & Halley, J. (2002). The temporal variability and spectral colour of animal populations. *Evolutionary Ecology Research*, **4**, 1033–1048.

Inchausti, P. & Halley, J. (2003). On the relation between temporal variability and persistence time in animal populations. *Journal of Animal Ecology*, **72**, 899–908.

Ives, R. & Klopper, E. D. (1997). Spatial variation in abundance created by stochastic temporal variation. *Ecology*, **78**, 1907–1913.

Katul, G. G., Porporato, A., Nathan, R., *et al.* (2005). Mechanistic analytical models for long-distance seed dispersal by wind. *American Naturalist*, **166**, 368–381.

Keeling, M. J. (2000). Simple stochastic models and their power-law type behaviour. *Theoretical Population Biology*, **58**, 21–31.

Keitt, T. H. & Marquet, P. A. (1996). Extinction cascades in introduced Hawaiian birds suggest self-organized criticality. *Journal of Theoretical Biology*, **182**, 161–167.

Keitt, T. H. & Stanley, H. E. (1998). Dynamics of North American breeding bird populations. *Nature*, **393**, 257–260.

Keitt, T. H., Amaral, L. A. N., Buldyrev, S. V. & Stanley, H. E. (2002). Scaling in the growth of geographically subdivided populations: invariant patterns from a continent-wide biological survey. *Philosophical Transactions of the Royal Society of London, Series B*, **357**, 627–633.

Kot, M., Lewis, M. A. & van den Driessche, P. (1996). Dispersal data and the spread of invading organisms. *Ecology*, **77**, 2027–2042.

Labra, F. A. (2005). Uso de energia desde los individuos a las comunidades: escalamiento y universalidad. Ph.D. dissertation, Pontificia Universidad Católica de Chile, Santiago.

Labra, F. A., Abades, S. R. & Marquet, P. A. (2005). Scaling patterns in exotic species: distribution and abundance. In *Species Invasions. Insights Into Ecology, Evolution, and Biogeography*, ed. D. F. Sax, J. J. Stachowicz & S. Gaines, pp. 421–446. Sunderland, MA: Sinauer Associates.

Laherrère, J. & Sornette, D. (1998). Stretched exponential distributions in nature and economy: "fat tails" with characteristic scales. *European Physical Journal B*, **2**, 525–539.

Lande, R. (1993). Risk of population extinction from demographic and environmental stochasticity and random catastrophes. *American Naturalist*, **142**, 911–927.

Lawton, J. H. (1989). What is the relationship between population density and animal abundance? *Oikos*, **55**, 429–434.

Leigh, E. (1981). The average lifetime of a population in a varying environment. *Journal of Theoretical Biology*, **90**, 213–239.

MacArthur, R. H. (1960). On the relative abundance of species. *American Naturalist*, **94**, 25–36.

Magurran, A. E. & Henderson, P. A. (2003). Explaining the excess of rare species in natural species abundance distributions. *Nature*, **422**, 714–716.

Malamud, B. D., Turcotte, D. L., Guzzetti, F. & Reichenbach, P. (2004). Landslide inventories and their statistical properties. *Earth Surface Processes and Landforms*, **29**, 687–712.

Malamud, B. D., Millington, J. D. A. & Perry, G. L. W. (2005). Characterizing wildfire regimes in the United States. *Proceedings of the National Academy of Sciences of the USA*, **102**, 4694–4699.

Mantegna, R. N. & Stanley, H. E. (2000). *An Introduction to Econophysics: Correlations and Complexity in Finance*. Cambridge: Cambridge University Press.

Mårell, A., Ball, J. P. & Hofgaard, A. (2002). Foraging and movement paths of female reindeer: insights from fractal analysis, correlated random walks, and Levy flights. *Canadian Journal of Zoology*, **80**, 854–865.

Maris, H. J. & Kadanoff, L. P. (1978). Teaching the renormalization group. *American Journal of Physics*, **46**, 652–657.

Marquet, P. A. (2002a). The search for general principles in ecology. *Nature*, **418**, 723.

Marquet, P. A. (2002b). Of predators, prey, and power laws. *Science*, **295**, 2229–2230.

Marquet, P. A., Navarrete, S. A. & Castilla, J. C. (1990). Scaling population density to body size in rocky intertidal communities. *Science*, **250**, 1125–1127.

Marquet, P. A., Keymer, J. E. & Cofre, H. (2003). Breaking the stick in space: of niche models, metacommunities, and patterns in the relative abundance of species. In *Macroecology: Concepts and Consequences*, ed. T. M. Blackburn & K. J. Gaston, pp. 64–84. Cambridge: Cambridge University Press.

Marquet, P. A., Quiñones, R. A., Abades S. R., *et al.* (2005). Scaling and power-laws in ecological systems. *Journal of Experimental Biology*, **208**, 1749–1769.

May, R. M. (1975). Patterns of species abundance and diversity. In *Ecology and Evolution in Communities*, ed. M. Cody & J. Diamond. Princeton: Princeton University Press.

McGill, B. & Collins, C. (2003). A unified theory for macroecology based on spatial patterns of abundance. *Evolutionary Ecology Research*, **5**, 469–492.

Milne, B. T. (1998). Motivation and beliefs of complex systems approaches in ecology. *Ecosystems*, **1**, 449–456.

Miramontes, O. (1995). Order-disorder transitions in the behavior of ant societies. *Complexity*, **1**, 56–60.

Miramontes, O. & Rohani, P. (1998). Intrinsically generated coloured noise in laboratory insect populations. *Proceedings of the Royal Society of London, Series B*, **265**, 785–792.

Mitzenmacher, M. (2001). A brief history of generative models for power law and log normal distributions. In *Proceedings of the 39th Annual Allerton Conference on Communication, Control, and Computing*, pp. 182–191. Urbana-Champagne: University of Illinois.

Moritz, M. A., Morais, M. E., Summerell, L. A., Carlson, J. M. & Doyle, J. (2005). Wildfires, complexity, and highly optimized tolerance. *Proceedings of the National Academy of Sciences of the USA*, **102**, 17912–17917.

Newman, M. E. J. (2005). Power laws, Pareto distributions and Zipf's law. *Contemporary Physics*, **46**, 323–351.

Niwa, H-S. (2003). Power-law versus exponential distributions of animal group sizes. *Journal of Theoretical Biology*, **224**, 451–457.

Niwa, H-S. (2005). Power-law scaling in dimension-to-biomass relationship of fish schools. *Journal of Theoretical Biology*, **235**, 419–430.

Pascual, M. & Guichard, F. (2005). Criticality and disturbance in spatial ecological systems. *Trends in Ecology and Evolution*, **20**, 88–95.

Perline, R. (2005). Strong, weak and false inverse power laws. *Statistical Science*, **20**, 68–88.

Peters, R. H. (1983). *The Ecological Implications of Body Size*. Cambridge: Cambridge University Press.

Pimm, S. L. & Redfearn, A. (1988). The variability of population-densities. *Nature*, **334**, 613–614.

Pimm, S., Jones, H. & Diamond, J. (1988). On the risk of extinction. *American Naturalist*, **132**, 757–785.

Rhodes, C. J. & Anderson, R. M. (1996). Power laws governing epidemics in isolated populations. *Nature*, **381**, 600–602.

Rhodes, C. J., Jensen, H. J. & Anderson, R. M. (1997). On the critical behavior of simple epidemics. *Proceedings of the Royal Society of London, Series B*, **264**, 1639–1646.

Rinaldo, A., Maritan, A., Cavender-Bares, K. K. & Chisholm, S. W. (2002). Cross-scale ecological dynamics and microbial size spectra in marine ecosystems. *Proceedings of the Royal Society of London, Series B*, **269**, 2051–2059.

Roy, M., Pascual, M. & Franc, A. (2003). Broad scaling region in a spatial ecological system. *Complexity*, **8**, 19–27.

Samorodnitsky, G. & Taqqu, M. S. (1994). *Stable Non-Gaussian Random Processes: Stochastic Models with Infinite Variance*. New York: Chapman and Hall.

Sauer, J. R., Peterjohn, B. G. & Link, W. A. (1994). Observer differences in the North American Breeding Bird Survey. *Auk*, **111**, 50–62.

Sauer, J. R., Hines, J. E. & Fallon, J. (2005). *The North American Breeding Bird Survey, Results and Analysis 1966–2004*. Version 2005.2. Laurel, MD: USGS Patuxent Wildlife Research Center.

Schmidt-Nielsen, K. (1984). *Scaling: Why is Animal Size so Important?* Cambridge: Cambridge University Press.

Solé, R. V. & Alonso, D. (1998). Random walks, fractals and the origins of rainforest diversity. *Advances in Complex Systems*, **1**, 203–220.

Solé, R. V., Manrubia, S. C., Luque, B., Delgado, J. & Bascompte, J. (1996). Phase transitions and complex systems. *Complexity*, **1**, 13–26.

Solé, R. V., Manrubia, S. C., Kauffman, S., Benton, M. & Bak, P. (1999) Criticality and scaling in evolutionary ecology. *Trends in Ecology and Evolution*, **14**, 156–160.

Solé, R. V., Alonso, D. & McKane, A. (2002). Self-organized instability in complex eco-systems. *Philosophical Transactions of the Royal Society of London, Series B*, **357**, 667–681.

Solow, A. R. (2005). Power laws without complexity. *Ecology Letters*, **8**, 361–363.

Sornette, D. (1998). Linear stochastic dynamics with nonlinear fractal properties. *Physica A*, **250**, 295–314.

Sornette, D. (2004). *Critical Phenomena in Natural Sciences. Chaos Fractals, Selforganization and Disorder: Concepts and Tools*. Heidelberg: Springer-Verlag.

Spengler, S. J. (2000). Computers and biology: bioinformatics in the information age. *Science*, **287**, 1221–1223.

Stanley, H. E. (1971). *Introduction to Phase Transitions and Critical Phenomena*. Oxford: Oxford University Press.

Stanley, H. E. (1995). Power laws and universality. *Nature*, **378**, 554.

Stanley, H. E. (1999). Scaling, universality, and renormalization: three pillars of modern critical phenomena. *Reviews of Modern Physics*, **71**, 358–366.

Stanley, H. E., Amaral, L. A. N., Gopikrishnan, P., Ivanov, P. Ch., Keitt, T. H. & Plerou, V. (2000). Scale invariance and universality: organizing principles in complex systems. *Physica A*, **281**, 60–68.

Stenseth, N. C. (1979). Where have all the species gone? On the nature of extinction and the Red Queen hypothesis. *Oikos*, **33**, 196–227.

Storch, D. & Gaston, K. J. (2004). Untangling ecological complexity on different scales of space and time. *Basic and Applied Ecology*, **5**, 389–400.

Storch, D., Gaston, K. J. & Cepák, J. (2002). Pink landscapes: 1/f spectra of spatial environmental variability and bird community composition. *Proceedings of the Royal Society of London, Series B*, **269**, 1791–1796.

Taylor, L. R. (1961). Aggregation, variance and the mean. *Nature*, **189**, 732–735.

Taylor, L. R. & Woiwod, I. P. (1980). Temporal stability as a density-dependent species characteristic. *Journal of Animal Ecology*, **49**, 209–224.

Terres, J. (1980). *Audubon Society Encyclopedia of North American Birds*. New York: Alfred A. Knopf.

Udvardy, M. (1994). *National Audubon Society Field Guide to North American Birds: Western Edition*. New York: Alfred A. Knopf.

Van Valen, L. (1976). Energy and evolution. *Evolutionary Theory*, **1**, 179–229.

Van Valen, L. (1977). The Red Queen. *American Naturalist*, **111**, 809–810.

Van Valen, L. (1980). Evolution as a zero-sum game for energy. *Evolutionary Theory*, **4**, 289–300.

Viswanathan, G. M., Afanasyev, V., Buldyrev, S. V., Murphy, E. J., Prince, P. A. & Stanley, H. E. (1996). Levy-flight search patterns of wandering albatrosses. *Nature*, **381**, 413–415.

Viswanathan, G. M., Buldyrev, S. V., Havlin, S., DaLuz, M. G. E., Raposo, E. P. & Stanley, H. E. (1999). Optimizing the success of random searches. *Nature*, **401**, 911–914.

Williamson, M. (1972). *The Analysis of Biological Populations*. London: Arnold.

Williamson, M. & Gaston, K. J. (2005). The log-normal distribution is not an appropriate null hypothesis for the species–abundance distribution. *Journal of Animal Ecology*, **74**, 409–423.

West, G. B. (1999). The origin of universal scaling laws in biology. *Physica A*, **263**, 104–113.

West, G. B. & Brown, J. H. (2005). The origin of allometric scaling laws in biology from genomes to ecosystems: towards a quantitative unifying theory of biological structure and organization. *Journal of Experimental Biology*, **208**, 1575–1592.

# Index